Health Care Ethics

D1468263

Health Care Ethics:
A Theological Analysis

FOURTH EDITION

Benedict M. Ashley OP, PhD, STM
Kevin D. O'Rourke OP, JCD, STM

GEORGETOWN UNIVERSITY PRESS / WASHINGTON, D.C.

Imprimatur:
+ Paul A. Zepfel
Archdiocesan Administrator
September 26, 1996

Georgetown University Press, Washington, D.C.
©1997 by Georgetown University Press. All rights reserved.
Printed in the United States of America

10 9 8 7 6 5 4 3 2 1   1997

THIS VOLUME IS PRINTED ON ACID-FREE OFFSET BOOK PAPER

Library of Congress Cataloging-in-Publication Data
Ashley, Benedict.
    Health care ethics : a theological analysis / Benedict Ashley, Kevin O'Rourke. —
4th ed.
        p. cm.
    Previous ed. has title: Healthcare ethics.
    Includes bibliographical references and index.
        1. Medical ethics. 2. Medicine—Religious aspects—Catholic Church.
    3. Christian ethics—Catholic authors. I. O'Rourke, Kevin D. II. Title.
    R724.A74 1997
    241'.642—dc20
    ISBN 0-87840-644-1 (pbk.)   96-46599

Contents

Preface   ix

Introduction   xiii

Part 1: The Health Seeker   1

1 On Being Human   3
OVERVIEW 3
1.1 WHAT DOES IT MEAN TO BE HUMAN 3
1.2 PERSONAL HEALTH IN COMMUNITY 7
1.3 POLITICS OF HEALTH CARE 10
1.4 PRIORITIES IN HUMAN NEEDS AND VALUES 17
CONCLUSION 21

2 Health and Disease   22
OVERVIEW 22
2.1 CONCEPTS OF HEALTH AND DISEASE 22
2.2 BIOLOGICAL HEALTH AND BIOLOGISM 31
2.3 THE HIGHER LEVELS OF HEALTH 34
CONCLUSION 36

3 Personal Responsibility for Health   38
OVERVIEW 38
3.1 THE PERSON AND HEALING 38
3.2 PREVENTIVE MEDICINE AND LIFESTYLE 42
3.3 STEWARDSHIP AND CREATIVITY 44
3.4 FORMING A PRUDENT CONSCIENCE AND INFORMED CONSENT 47
3.5 PATIENT'S RIGHTS 62
CONCLUSION 65

PART 2: The Healing Profession: Response of the Community to the Health Needs of Persons   67

4 The Health Care Profession   69
OVERVIEW 69
4.1 PROFESSIONS: DEPERSONALIZING TRENDS 69
4.2 TRADITIONAL IDEALS OF THE MEDICAL PROFESSION 77
4.3 MEDICAL EDUCATION AND ITS BIASES 81
CONCLUSION 86

5 Personalizing the Health Care Profession   89
OVERVIEW 89
5.1 THE COUNSELING RELATIONSHIP 89
5.2 PROFESSIONAL COMMUNICATION 97
5.3 PEER RELATIONS AND PROFESSIONAL DISCIPLINE 102
CONCLUSION 106

6 Social Organization of Health Care   107
OVERVIEW 107
6.1 THE POLITICAL SITUATION OF HEALTH CARE TODAY 107
6.2 PRINCIPLES OF PUBLIC HEALTH CARE POLICY 112
6.3 HEALTH CARE ETHICS AND PUBLIC POLICY 120
6.4 THE HOSPITAL AS COMMUNITY 123
6.5 THE HEALTH CARE TEAM 127
6.6 ETHICS COMMITTEES IN CATHOLIC HEALTH CARE FACILITIES 131
6.7 THE IDENTITY OF CATHOLIC HEALTH CARE FACILITIES 134
CONCLUSION 135

PART 3: The Logic of Bioethical Decisions   137

7 The Logic of Bioethical Decisions   139
OVERVIEW 139
7.1 THE LOGIC OF BIOETHICAL DEBATE 139
7.2 DEONTOLOGICAL (DUTY) METHODOLOGIES 149
7.3 TELEOLOGICAL (MEANS-ENDS) METHODOLOGIES 156
7.4 PRUDENTIAL PERSONALISM 166
7.5 EVALUATION OF MORAL METHODOLOGIES 172
CONCLUSION 176

8 Norms of Christian Decision Making in Bioethics   177
OVERVIEW 177
8.1 IS THERE A CHRISTIAN ETHICS? 177
8.2 NORMS OF CHRISTIAN FAITH AND PRUDENCE 181
8.3 NORMS OF CHRISTIAN HOPE 200
8.4 NORMS OF CHRISTIAN LOVE 213
8.5 COORDINATION OF THE PRINCIPLES 221
CONCLUSION 222

PART 4: Difficult Bioethical Decisions   225

9   Artificial Reproduction, Fetal Testing, Abortion   227
OVERVIEW 227
9.1 WHEN DOES HUMAN LIFE BEGIN? 227
9.2 REPRODUCTIVE TECHNOLOGIES 240
9.3 AMNIOCENTESIS AND FETAL TESTING 248
9.4 ABORTION 252
9.5 THE LAW AND ABORTION 264
CONCLUSION 270

10   Conception Control, Contraception, and Natural
Family Planning   271
OVERVIEW 271
10.1 CONTRACEPTION 271
10.2 STERILIZATION AND OTHER METHODS OF CONTRACEPTION 287
10.3 RESPONSIBLE PARENTHOOD THROUGH NATURAL FAMILY PLANNING 297
10.4 CARE OF RAPE VICTIMS 302
10.5 PASTORAL APPROACH TO MEDICAL SEXUAL PROBLEMS 307
CONCLUSION 314

11   Reconstructing and Modifying the Function
of the Human Body   316
OVERVIEW 316
11.1 MODIFYING THE HUMAN BODY 316
11.2 GENETIC INTERVENTION 320
11.3 GENETIC SCREENING AND COUNSELING 323
11.4 ORGAN TRANSPLANTATION 331
11.5 SEXUAL REASSIGNMENT 339
11.6 EXPERIMENTATION AND RESEARCH ON HUMAN SUBJECTS 344
CONCLUSION 354

12   Neurological and Psychological Therapy of Mental Illness   355
OVERVIEW 355
12.1 THE CONCEPT OF MENTAL ILLNESS 355
12.2 PSYCHOSURGERY, ELECTROCONVULSIVE THERAPY, AND PHARMACOTHERAPY 364
12.3 PSYCOTHERAPEUTIC MEANS OF THERAPY 369
12.4 ETHICAL PROBLEMS IN TREATING THE MENTALLY ILL 376
12.5 ADDICTION OR CHEMICAL DEPENDENCY 384
12.6 SEX THERAPY AND RESEARCH 387
CONCLUSION 392

13   Suffering and Death   394
OVERVIEW 394
13.1 MYSTERY OF DEATH 394
13.2 FEAR OF DEATH 397
13.3 DEFINING DEATH 400

13.4 TRUTH TELLING TO THE DYING 405
13.5 CARE FOR THE CORPSE OR CADAVER 407
13.6 ASSISTED SUICIDE AND EUTHANASIA 411
13.7 LETTING DIE 419
CONCLUSION 432

PART 5: Pastoral Ministry in Health Care   433

14 Pastoral Care and Ethical Decisions   435
OVERVIEW 435
14.1 PASTORAL MINISTRY AND THE HEALTH CARE TEAM 435
14.2 MINISTRY TO THE HOSPITAL STAFF 440
14.3 SPIRITUAL COUNSELING IN HEALTH CARE 442
14.4 CELEBRATING THE HEALING PROCESS 447
14.5 ETHICAL COUNSELING AND PASTORAL CARE 456
CONCLUSION 462

Bibliography   463

Name Index   519
Subject Index   523

Preface

Since the last edition of *Health Care Ethics, A Theological Analysis* was published in 1989, many things have happened in the field of health care medicine and theology to necessitate a fourth edition. In the field of theology, the Church has issued several significant documents: the encyclicals "The Splendor of Truth" (*Veritatis Splendor*) and the "Gospel of Life" (*Evangelium Vitae*); the "Instruction on the Vocation of Theologians"; the *Catechism of the Catholic Church*; and the *Revised Ethical and Religious Directives for Catholic Health Services*. These documents have clarified many teachings of the Church in regard to ethical and moral theory and the various modes of authoritative teaching issued by the Church. Moreover, they have made more definite statements concerning some specific actions long prohibited by Church teachings such as abortion, euthanasia, suicide and physician-assisted suicide. Seeking to present the thoughts of these documents which to some extent verify material in previous editions, we have rewritten significant portions of the book. In an effort to simply the treatment of principles, we consider all principles in Chapter 8, rather than considering some of them in other chapters of the book, as we did in earlier editions.

Insofar as health care is concerned, there have also been several changes introduced since 1989. First of all, the federal government sought to renew and restructure the entire health care system. This unsuccessful effort gave rise to efforts to reduce the cost of health care through managed care techniques, which dominate the provision of health care at the present time. Unfortunately, there has been little effort to date to recognize health care as a right for all citizens. These recent and contemporary efforts to reform health care are considered in the light of Catholic social theory in Chapter 6. We believe that problems in the social responsibility to provide adequate access to health care and quality health care are more serious and significant than they have been in the past generations.

Insofar as the theory of medicine is concerned, several changes and developments deserve consideration in this new edition. Physicians and other health care professionals have a new vision insofar as ethical norms for health care professionals are concerned. There is a more open attitude on the part of many health care professionals to accept ethics as an integral element of medical care. Preventive care and involvement of individuals in their own care, are much more significant consideration in the patient-physician relationship than before. Moreover, hospice care is now a recognized phase of quality medical care. The revised and enlarged vision of personal and professional ethical integrity serves as the basis for much of the revision of Chapters 4 and 5.

The practice of medicine has also changed. The changes are no where more evident than in the practice of psychiatry, which has been enhanced by the use of pharmaceuticals in addition to "talk therapy." In addition, the Human Genome Project has identified the source of some genetic diseases and will lead to greater ability to cure or alleviate these genetic anomalies. Overall, the role of genetics in diagnosis and prognosis has increased dramatically. The new role of genetics influences not only the ethics of psychiatry practice, but the somatic aspects of medicine as well. The changes in psychiatry are addressed in Chapter Twelve and the influence of the Genome Project is addressed in Chapter Eleven.

The present literature on medical ethics is so vast that no one can claim mastery of it all. In an effort to be current and somewhat comprehensive, the bibliography has been thoroughly revised; however; significant citations from previous editions have been retained. Thus we hope to present contemporary sources of the development in medical ethics, retaining continuity with the recent past. For most of the topics discussed, we have cited authors having various points of view. Some of them confirm our own arguments, whereas others differ. Consequently, the citation of an author is not intended to mean that the article or book always confirms our own statements, nor that the author's data or analysis has been incorporated into our own text, but rather the desire to enter into dialogue with other authors and to provide the reader with additional resources on the topic.

Our effort in this revision is to provide a contemporary study of health care and the ethics of health care from the perspective of Catholic teaching and theological investigation. What started out to be a timely and manageable revision of our text became as intricate and involved as writing the first edition in 1979 because of the changes already discussed.

Through the fourth edition of this book we have been aided by our colleagues at the Saint Louis University Health Sciences Center, Aquinas Institute of Theology, and the Institute of Religion at the Houston Medical Center. The friends and scholars who helped us with this edition of *Health Care Ethics: A Theological Analysis* are: Erin Bakanas, MD; Mary Lou Bennett, MA; Rodney Coe, PhD; Leon McGahee, MD; Reverend Gerard Magill, STD; Monsignor John Naumann; Dermott Smith, MD; Eleanor Stump, PhD; Vallee Willman, MD; and Reverand Charles Bouchard, OP. The friends who assisted in producing past editions were: Phillip Boyle, PhD; Rodney Coe, PhD; Coy Fitch, MD; Peggy Donovan, RN, BSN; William Stoneman, MD; Alberto Galofre, MD; Manual Comas, MD; Larry Lewis, MD; James Monteleone, MD; Noreen D'Souza, MD; Kenneth Smith, MD; Betty Diehl, MD; Arthur Baue, MD; Alice Kitchen, MD; and Albert Moraczewski, OP, PhD.

During the course of this revision we have been aided by the patient and grace-filled cooperation of Donna Grace Troy and Charlotte Donovan Ruzicka, administrative assistants at the Center for Health Care Ethics and of John Morris, PhD, Rockhurst College, Kansas City, Missouri. In thanking the many people who have helped us through the years, we assume full responsibility for any errors or shortcomings in the book.

INTRODUCTION

PURPOSE OF THE BOOK

Modern medicine has unprecedented power to heal human beings of physical and mental diseases, to keep them healthy, and even to improve the human race. This power can be used to humanize life or to dehumanize and destroy it. It can be used justly to benefit all, or it can be used unjustly to benefit the few at the expense of the many. How to use such power is a question of values and, therefore, of individual and group decisions that are not merely technical but ethical.

Two reasons have induced us to add to the already extensive literature on medical-ethical and bioethical topics. First, too much of this literature focuses on a few controversial but sometimes minor topics, while neglecting the broader and major issues affecting human health and the health care professions. Second, we want to assist Christian, and especially Catholic, health care professionals and health care facilities faced with the difficult and often puzzling responsibility of giving witness to a long tradition of humanistic health care, while working with other professionals and government agencies committed to diverse value systems.

OUTLINE AND METHOD

We believe each person bears primary responsibility for personal health and the right to retain ultimate control over personal health. We also believe each person has the right to the help and care of the community in achieving personal health, as well as the reciprocal obligation to assist other members of the community in the same search. Thus in Part 1 of this book we question: What does it mean to be human? Secondly, we consider the meaning of health and illness, and the personal responsibility to strive for health.

In Part One it becomes clear that persons can not achieve health unless they have the help of others. Thus, Part 2 deals with the responsibilities of the community, of the government, and particularly of the health care profession to assist persons in the search for health.

We use the broad term *health care* profession rather than medical profession because this book addresses not only physicians but all those engaged in serving others in their search for health. If sometimes we devote more attention to physicians than to other members of the health team, it is only because physicians are more visible and their responsibilities more clearly defined by professional traditions. What we say of them the reader should apply to other health team members, the respective differences having been considered.

Because of its emphasis on the individual's primary responsibility for health, this book can also help the general public understand their own rights and responsibilities in relation to the health care profession, which exists only to serve them.

After dealing with the mutual relations between the health seeker and the health care professional, we turn in Part 3 to the process of ethical decision making, which involves both health seeker and professional.

Too often today, bioethical controversies are confused and frustrating because the participants do not define the value systems to which they are committed. Scientifically educated health care professionals know how to deal with facts, but often they are untrained in any method of dealing with values. Consequently, Part 3 deals with the logic of ethical decision making, showing that currently many such logics do not necessarily contradict one another, but are often very one-sided.

Two traditions of medical ethics are used in the United States, the deontological and teleological (Pellegrino and Thomasma, 1988). These traditions were represented by two pioneers of medical ethics, Paul Ramsey (died 1988) and Joseph Fletcher (died 1991). They opposed each other on most issues because Ramsey worked from a *deontological* ethics (duty ethics) of abstract, universal, rational rules of moral obligation, whereas Fletcher worked from a *teleological* (means-ends utilitarian, consequentialist, situationist) ethic, which emphasized pragmatic decisions in unique contexts. To escape this polarization of ethical debate, we propose what we call *prudential personalism*. As with teleological ethics, it is prudential because it makes intelligent practical decisions about the means to meet concrete human needs; but as in deontological ethics, it rejects a merely pragmatic, utilitarian calculation of consequences as an adequate method of moral decision making by human persons. This ethics is not a deontology, however, but a personalism. Rather than basing ethical decisions on axiomatic rules, prudential personalism bases such decisions on principles derived from our experience of the needs of human persons as they share in the historically developing human community.

It is not enough, however to choose a logic or formal procedure for ethical decision making; such decisions must be made in the context of some specific value system. Many assume today that the theological value systems of the various religions— Catholic, Protestant, Jewish, and so forth—will always be pitted against each other on polemics that have no rational solution. Many also assume that if there is to be any public debate and consensus, it must be in terms of a neutral, philosophical, secular, and humanistic value system.

CHRISTIAN VALUES

We take a different view, and in Part 3 we propose a system of values or ethical principles that are frankly Christian and Roman Catholic (not denying room for pluralism even here). We believe that every human being has some type of value system that is either religious or equivalent to a religion. To label one of these as neutral or humanistic is, from the outset, to give it a privileged position, which can only frustrate honest debate and any effort to achieve some measure of sincere cooperation in a pluralistic society. For a long time in the United States, the Protestant value system was taken as self-evident, and all efforts of Jews and Catholics to defend their own value systems were rejected as the intrusion of a private religion on public civil debate. Today the academic community and the media assume that humanism is self-evident (just as Marxism is assumed to be self-evident in some countries), and any effort to speak up in the name of a "religious" value system is decried as an imposition.

Catholics reason ethically in terms of a value system rooted in a view of reality contained in the Christian Gospel, interpreted by the Church in its life of faith and authoritatively formulated by the pope and the bishops (Vatican II, 1964a). Catholics believe this Gospel with the commitment of faith, and they accept its ordinary formulation and application by the pope and bishops with "religious assent" (Vatican II 1964a), even when this lacks the final authority of solemn definition. This commitment to authoritative teaching, as well as respect for a long tradition of Catholic theological reflection, however, cannot exempt educated Catholics from listing honestly to other systems of belief, nor from comparing beliefs with the discoveries of science and history and with the personal experience of life (Vatican II, 1965c). For the Catholics, therefore, faith and reason are complementary, not contradictory, sources of truth and value.

Testing of belief affects the way Catholics understand and apply their fundamental convictions. Catholics who are professionals in any field have a serious responsibility to accept the teaching of the Church but also are responsible to contribute to its development and application. The same must be said of those who adhere to other beliefs and value systems; they also have an obligation to be open to dialogue undertaken in a truth-seeking spirit. None of us has the right to say to another, "You are biased because you are committed to the truth." Each of us seeks the truth through a belief and value system in which we think and, if we are honest, which we seek to deepen, broaden, and make more realistic. Since the Second Vatican Council, Catholics have experienced how fruitful such an ecumenical approach can be, not so much for *conversion* of others as for a *convergence* of insight. In this book we attempt to follow that method, which requires both an openness to the opinions of others and a deepening of our own Christian and Catholic identity.

PARTICULAR ISSUES

Part 4 applies this method of seeking truth to major controversial issues ranging from birth to death. This requires engaging in a type of ecumenism internal to the Catholic community since its introduction by the Second Vatican Council, namely, theological pluralism within a Catholic framework. Today the Catholic ethical system is not viewed as complete and absolutely fixed, but as essentially historical and dynamic in character. At any given historical moment there exists in the Catholic community an authoritative moral teaching that provides a firm basis for any ethical discussion. In medical ethics, remarkably, this teaching developed even before the Second Vatican Council (1963-1965) in the writings of Pope Pius XII (died 1958), who was keenly aware of such issues. The National Conference of Catholic Bishops (NCCB) has applied some of these teachings to health care in the *Ethical and Religious Directives* (1971; 1994). Because we hope that our book will be useful to those working in such facilities, we give due recognition to the pastoral guidance of the Second Vatican Council and to the teaching of the popes and bishops, especially as expressed in the *Directives*.

Nevertheless, at any given moment in the history of the Catholic Church, developing moral understanding is in response to current problems. This development is not always well-balanced or even healthy. Catholics may learn by pragmatic needs from the value system of others, but we may also lose much in the process. A frequently cited example of this is the distortion suffered by Christian sexual ethic from the influence of Stoicism when it was the popular value system of the Roman Empire.

In this process of development there is no easy way to distinguish progress from retrogression; neither conservatives nor liberals have any guarantee that they are automatically in the right. Consequently, along with an exposition of the authoritative position of the pastors of the Roman Catholic Church, we have included various interpretations of such positions and of proposals for their refinement and revision made by committed Catholic theologians. We hope that in doing so we are in line with the intellectual independence, combined with respect for authority and tradition, that seems to us one of the chief features of a Catholic and Christian value system.

Because our ethical discussion of concrete issues is presented within the Catholic value system, we have subtitled this book *A Theological Analysis*. We define *analysis* in this case as an effort to solve concrete ethical problems in terms of principles rooted in Sacred Scripture and tested by the experience of individuals and communities motivated by faith. We believe these principles are discovered most effectively when we employ every form of insight available to us: historical and personal experience, scientific discovery, philosophical reflection, and the Gospel light shining in Scripture and in the living tradition of Christian community.

PASTORAL CARE

Such an analysis leads us to complete the book with a discussion of health care precisely as it is a Christian ministry, this final Part 5 shows that in a health care team that aims at healing the total human person, spiritual ministry must play an integral part. The chaplain in any health care facility or the pastoral care department has the essential function of assisting health care to take on a fully human and Christian vitality. This cannot be achieved if the chaplain and the department monopolize this ministry, but only if they can convince all members of the health care team that as Christian professionals, they are also engaged in a Christian ministry. Physicians, nurses, administrators, and the variety of auxiliaries in a Catholic health care facility are gifted with talents and professional competence through which they truly minister the healing power of Jesus Christ present to our Suffering and hoping world.

PART 1

The Health Seeker

The first concern of health care ethics should be the persons who seek health care rather than the professionals or institutions that provide it. Thus, Part 1 of this book deals with *The Health Seeker*.

Chapter 1 examines the quest to be fully human, because the search for health is only one aspect of that search from complete humanness with which all ethics is concerned. The sum and substance of Chapter 1 is found in the question: What does it mean to be human? As this chapter relates, to be human means to strive to fulfill, in an integral manner, the needs we share with others. Chapter 2 develops the notion of health that is rooted in the natural desire to be fully human. In order to understand health however, we must also understand the concept of illness or sickness. Chapter 3 concludes that each person has the primary responsibility for his or her own health and examines some activities needed in the quest for health insofar as making good ethical decisions is concerned.

1
On Being Human

OVERVIEW

This chapter argues that the basic goal of health care ethics is fulfilling the needs of the human person; to be healthy is to fulfill human needs (1.1). However, the human person can be healthy and whole only in a human community, because to be a person is to be capable of interpersonal relations (1.2). By implication, an ethics of health must also be a politics of health; that is, a community must establish values, norms, and standards to help its members achieve health. There are many competing ethical systems in the United States and in the world. For many this seems to make a workable health care ethics impossible. Even in pluralistic societies, however, progress can be made toward ethical consensus (1.3). The chief obstacle to forming such a consensus is not disagreement about the human values to be sought, but a disagreement about priorities among these values. Thus, to resolve some of the ethical conflicts in the field of health care, a hierarchy of values must be established (1.4).

1.1 WHAT DOES IT MEAN TO BE HUMAN?

Ethics concerns the needs and values of human persons. Health is a vital human need; nothing is more human, more personal. Health is and always has been one of the main concerns of the human community, and health is sustained through health care. To develop an ethics of human health care, we must have an accurate notion of what it means to be human, because health care is directed toward sustaining our human functions (Chapter 1).

Concern about human health goes beyond physical well-being. In 1958 the World Health Organization (WHO) declared: "Health is a state of complete physical, mental, and social well-being and not merely the absence of disease or infirmity." That definition has been widely criticized (Callahan, 1973b, Gillon, 1986c), but at least it has advanced the notion that human health is not limited to physical concerns. Physical health is only one aspect of total human health.

What other aspects are involved in *human* health? Today it is no longer easy to explain what the term *human* means. We live in a technological age in an artificial environment, and we view the world through scientific eyes. To understand the *human* being, we need to recover a sense of our own humanity, our difference from the machine and even from the world of nature, which has become subject to scientific probing and technological manipulation (Moyers 1993). In trying to determine what makes human beings different from animals, plants, and the dust of the earth and stars, we need not isolate or alienate human beings from the natural world of physics or biology. Rather, we must try to locate ourselves in the universe of things to which we are related in countless ways and yet in which we sometimes feel so alone, both as human beings and as an individual being who asks: Who am I?

Perhaps the best way to approximate a working definition of the human person in the ethical context of this book is to begin with the notion of human need. The human being is not definable as a static entity, but as a dynamic system of needs (Maslow, 1970). Human beings have many of the same needs as plants and animals, but we experience these needs in a distinctive way. Animals experience need when they hunger, thirst, gasp for air, or pursue a mate. Human beings not only feel such needs, but we also have at least some understanding of *why* we have them. We also devise alternative ways of satisfying these needs, puzzle over what we need most, and even create needs never experienced by human beings in the past.

To ascertain which human needs and capacities are genetically determined and common to the whole human species and which have been created by human culture is not easy (Gazzaniga, 1992). Sociobiologists such as E. O. Wilson (1978; 1992) argue that the evolution of the human species from its primate ancestors verifies to some degree the biological origin and survival of human behavioral tendencies. Nevertheless, even sociobiologists recognize that the evolution of the remarkable human brain has given humankind the capacity to break through the largely fixed and genetically determined types of behavior characteristics of even our closest primate relatives. Human beings have the need and the capacity to use symbols, invent tools, communicate by speech with its variety of invented languages, and create and modify social and political systems in a manner only faintly foreshadowed in the behavior of other animals (Goldschmidt, 1991).

This need and capacity to develop a diversity of cultural patterns, however, masks the genetically inherent and common needs and capacities that might serve to define human nature. Anthropology and history have found it difficult to verify cross-cultural universals; also, we do not have recourse to the behavior of so-called primitive peoples because their cultural history is as long as ours. Even the study of infant behavior yields only equivocal results, since infants behave only in response to the culture into which they are born (Nugent, 1989).

Nevertheless, the very difficulty we experience in trying to separate human nature from human culture gives us a clue. What defines us as human beings is precisely this limited but real transcendence of rigid biological determinism. We are indeed bodily, biological, animal beings with inherent needs for food, shelter, and reproduction, but we also have the types of brain and intelligence that make it possible and necessary to choose from a vast range of ways to satisfy these needs. Culture is only the expression of our nature, which is to be intelligently free. *This embodied intelligent freedom* defines us as human and gives unity and continuity to the human family across time and space.

To Be a Person

To have this need and capacity for intelligent freedom is to be a *person*. The reason ordinary language does not apply the term *person* to an animal, even a pet, is because human beings do not experience animals as self-conscious autonomous beings. Animals do not talk back. This is why some philosophers today want to broaden the definition of person to include not only "intelligence" and "freedom" but also "ability to communicate," "to care," and "to be called forth." Note, however, that in ordinary usage the terms *person* and *personality* are not identical. A person *has* a personality; that is, persons are the kinds of beings that understand and feel for each other in a human, freely intelligent manner. It is this *expression* of personhood that is personality.

Health care ethics is confronted by the obvious fact that many human beings hardly seem to be persons as we have just defined that term—the infant; the seriously defective, the senile, and the unconscious human being; and even ourselves when we are asleep. Is health care ethics concerned with those who are not fully persons? Certainly such human beings exhibit little that can be called personality, since their behavior seems to be only at the animal or even the plant level. We sometimes say of a comatose, brain-damaged victim of an accident, "He is now in a vegetative state."

Such difficulties highlight the fact that in the human organism, intelligent freedom is intimately linked to the central nervous system and more precisely to the frontal lobes of the cerebral cortex (Cranford, 1988). When the normal functioning of this relatively small but extremely complex part of a human being is inhibited, that person ceases to be actively, intelligently free. He or she sinks back into the deterministic reflexes or physiological reactions of the animal or vegetative level of functioning. As long as the higher brain centers function, however, a human being manifests a personality even when the rest of the body is largely destroyed. Such a person seems to need little from the rest of the body except a supply of oxygenated and nutritive blood to bring energy to the brain and carry away its wastes. But the body is always an integral component of human personality.

Some ethicists recently have proposed a distinction between being *human* and being a *person* (Engelhardt, 1986; Bole, 1992). They define "person" as a self-conscious, free, moral agent; thus infants or victims of senility, although human (i.e., biologically members of the human species), are not, at least in a proper sense, persons. Engelhardt (1977) goes so far as to entitle one essay, "Some Persons Are Humans, Some Humans Are Persons, and the World Is What We Persons Make of It." Does this imply that "moral agents" are free to grant personal status or to deny it to their inferiors—a position that elites have always found very convenient in justifying their neglect or oppression of the powerless?

Such a view is very difficult to reconcile with any scientific account of the unity of human nature and does violence to ordinary language (McHugh, 1992). According to our ordinary use of language, to be a human person does not require that here and now one is functioning as an intelligent, free, moral agent, but to have that *innate power* to develop such capacities and to exercise them more or less effectively under favorable and appropriate conditions. We are actually persons, in the sense of having human rights, even when we are not actually, but only potentially, moral agents.

Indeed the very notion of a living being is that, given the proper environment and matter–energy input, it has the innate capacity to develop itself to maturity long before it is able to function in the adult way characteristic of its species, and many living things have periods of dormancy during which their characteristic activities are not apparent. Nor is it correct to say that the immature or dormant living thing is only "potentially" a member of a given species. Rather, it is *actually* a member of its species because it is already actually capable of developing mature and effective behavior characteristic of that species, though the exercise of that behavior remains only potential. Thus an infant human being is already actually, not potentially, a member of the human species.

The static view that humanhood is separate from personhood fails to recognize that a human person is not a pure intelligence as is an angel—as Plato and philosophical idealism have always contended—but a *bodily being,* evolving out of the natural world yet never separated from it. Consequently, human self-awareness and freedom emerge only at high points of a very complex process, much of which is subconscious and dependent on bodily development and function. When a human organism is conceived, his or her uniqueness is genetically determined by a novel combination of traits. At that moment, a unique human body comes into being and is continuously identifiable. In refutation of idealistic conceptions of the human person as a "self-conscious mind," recent philosophy insists that bodily identity is necessary to the notion of the human person (Howsepian, 1992). Even the medieval scholastics who argued for the survival of the human soul after death did not consider the soul a complete human person. They believed the soul received its identity from its relation to the body it would receive again at the resurrection. The whole life process involves a development of this unique body–mind in constant interaction with its environment.

Personal Biography

Every individual has a *biography* that consists in mature actualization of intelligent freedom and the manifestation of a unique personality. This life story passes through many phases of fetal and infant development before the brain can function at higher levels. Even during adult life, persons function with intelligent freedom only at certain times and in certain relations to their environment. Much of the adult's life is taken up with routine—sleep, eating, relaxation—when intelligence is working at a level below that of creative freedom. Yet this same person carries on the total process of living in all its phases. Getting sick and getting well are both parts of this continuous, struggling process of living development. Thus defining human personhood as "embodied intelligent freedom" presupposes a developing life process that goes on at many levels of activity, but that is more clearly manifest and definable by its maximum, its high point of integration. Health care ethics must always take into account that the person who needs help in a particular crisis of illness is a being who exists not merely here and now, but who also has a history and a future.

The term *personality,* as typically used, also emphasizes the individuality of each member of the human race. Because the essence of human nature is embodied intelligent freedom, each human being transcends the commonalities of this nature and attains a unique biography of personal choices. To be truly human, I must also be truly *myself.* I must live out my life, taking responsibility for its ultimate direction. Individual differences between one human being and another are immense, resulting in a vast range of personalities. Even monozygotic twins, who are genetically very similar, are still able to live personal lives and have distinct biographies. Twins can disagree, can go separate ways. No doubt if someday science produces human clones—a test-tube production of several individuals of the same genetic makeup—these human beings would each still have a life to live and would live it in a unique way.

This account of what it is to be a human person leads to a *preliminary* formulation of human health and of the goal of health care:

Human health enables a person to function as an embodied, intelligent, free person. The goal of health care is to contribute to the full development of human persons in all aspects of their being, that is, *to help human beings become intelligently free.*

1.2 PERSONAL HEALTH IN COMMUNITY

Every ethical problem about health care ultimately may be reduced to the conception of what it is to be human and to actualize personhood. However, this must not lead to the error of individualism (so influential in American culture), which conceives of the person in isolation, continually defending himself or herself against the encroachments of society (Bellah, 1986; 1992). What then is the relation of human person to human community?

The classical definition "man is a rational animal" makes sense only if the terms *animal* and *rational* are understood as tags for a vast, ever-increasing body of information gathered by the behavioral sciences and the humanistic disciplines. *Animal* refers to man's evolutionary origin and complex physiochemico-biological structure. *Rational* describes very complex human behavior at peak moments that rises to a freedom that transcends the instinctive life of animals. To say "man is a rational animal" is to say men and women of every race belong to a single, interacting human community that is not only able to eat, drink, and procreate, but also to think scientifically and creatively, to debate and make political decisions, and to make love personally. Aristotle suggested this by saying "man is a *political* animal" (*Politics* 1, 1253a), giving the word *political* a much broader connotation than it has today.

Thus the notion of person cannot be satisfactorily defined except in relation to its correlative—the notion of society or community. As the Bishops of the United States declared (USCC, 1986):

> Human dignity can be realized and protected only in community. In our teaching, the human person is not only sacred but also social. How we organize our society directly affects human dignity and the capacity of individuals to grow in community. The objective to 'love our neighbor' has an individual dimension but it also requires a broader social commitment to the common good. (n. 14)

No human person can exist apart from a human community. Each of us has parents, and no one of us can develop either physically or psychologically without constant interhuman relationships. The human brain cannot develop fully without language, and language is a cultural, social creation (Leahey and Levin, 1992). Even if in the future persons are produced in a test tube, they will be the product of a technological community and will be able to develop only within it.

The correlation of person and community is not merely superficial. People need a community not merely because it supplies them with certain instrumental needs (food, housing, clothing, and defense), but because their personalities can be fulfilled only in the act of communication and sharing. If personhood is embodied intelligent freedom, it can be fulfilled only in the free act of knowing and loving. In the whole universe the most complex, varied, integrated, and beautiful beings are persons; only in them can the desire to know and love find full play. All science's efforts to understand the universe culminate in exploring the mystery of human persons, who, with their complexity, freedom, and potential for intercommunication, are the highest outcome of the evolutionary process.

Our knowledge of each other, however, cannot be achieved by simple observation in the way we can study a rock, a tree, or a dog. To know *you*, to understand you intimately, I must form a specifically human relation with you, whether as an enemy, a master, a slave—or better—a co-worker, a lover, or a friend. Such knowledge also involves feeling, even love. I must freely reveal myself to you if you are freely to reveal yourself to me. This means that a health care professional cannot understand a patient or diagnose his or her ailment as if the patient were a thing, because he or she is a person whose whole mode of health or sickness is *relational*.

For Christians this correlation of person and community has a still deeper significance for two reasons (Kiesling, 1986):

1. The Christian God is a personal God, a trinity of persons who totally share one single being, life, knowledge, and love. Thus the ultimate

reality is a community of persons that sets the pattern for all other realities, including our human reality.

2. The Christian God has created each unique human person *for* himself or herself, that is, with the intention of drawing each of us to share in our own eternal, trinitarian life. "This fellowship of ours is with the Father and his Son, Jesus Christ" (1 Jn 1:3).

Consequently, the Christian health care professional, in his or her effort to heal another human being, is a minister of God helping that patient to share more fully in the everlasting community of the Father, Son, and Holy Spirit.

This emphasis on the intimate relation of person to community, however, should not lead us into the exaggeration of those who argue that personhood is *conferred* on the individual by the community not through reason of some inherent right, but on the basis of conditions set by the community. Thus the philosopher Ronald M. Green (1974), using a "social contract" theory similar to that of John Rawls (1971), argues, "The issue of abortion . . . comes down to the question of whether rational agents could find it rational in the circumstances of moral choice to confer rights on the fetus and, if so, the nature and extent of these rights" (p. 62). The geneticist Joshua Lederberg (1967) locates the beginning of human personhood around the first year of life, because "at this point only does [a person] enter into a cultural tradition which has been the special attribute of man by which he is set apart from the rest of the species." The philosopher and medical ethicist H. T. Engelhardt, Jr. (1986b) argues:

> Not all humans are persons. Fetuses, infants, the profoundly mentally retarded and the hopelessly comatose provide examples of human non-persons. Such entities are member of the human species. . . . They do not have standing in the moral community. . . . One speaks of persons in order to identify entities one can warrant blame and praise. . . . For this reason it is nonsensical to speak of respecting the autonomy of fetuses, infants, or profoundly retarded adults who have never been rational (pp. 107–08).

This theory of personhood, as an explanation of the relation of person to community, fails to take into account that the human person has a capacity and openness to knowledge and love of other persons. Consequently, human personhood is based on innate capacities, not on acceptance of others. Personhood is never completely actualized in this earthly life but is always in a process of growth, which consists primarily in the deepening of communal relations (Doran, 1989).

Community, in its turn, exists to assist each of its member-persons in this process of growth. Thus, as soon as a unique human organism is conceived, he or she begins this actualizing process and has a right to help from the human community to complete this process. The community, therefore, does not confer on or impute personhood to the sleeping, un-self-conscious infant or fetus, but rather responds to its silent demand to live and grow.

By extension, the hospital or any other health care facility is a human community dedicated to the health care of human persons. The health care facility does not confer the power to get well on the patients; this power is inherent in their capacity for personal life. These patients include not only the self-conscious ones, but also the comatose or senile person, the child, the infant, and the unborn person. Each is a human organism in the process of living out a human life. Each has an ethical claim on the health care community for help (which has limits) in his or her growth and struggle to actualize the inherent capacity for knowledge, love, and human relationship, which depend so intimately on physical health. The very purpose and meaning of the health care community, as of every human community, is to help its members grow in personhood.

Similar to the theories of imputation as a source of personhood is the attempt of Joseph Fletcher and others (1974, 1979; Bole, 1992) to enumerate "indicators of humanhood." Along with the biological criterion of "neocortical function," Fletcher selects "self-awareness," "euphoria" (as found in a retarded but happy child), and "human relationships" as essential criteria for humanness. Such signs certainly indicate stages in the process of the actualization of a person, but they do not necessarily mark the beginning of that process. Also they do not indicate when a person with rights first exists and demands the care of the community nor when a person in decline still lingers in the dying process (Grisez, 1992).

1.3 POLITICS OF HEALTH CARE

Christian Ethical Consensus

The intrinsic relation of persons to community implies that there is a *political* aspect to all human events. Therefore the ethics of the human person in community must also be *political*; that is, it must take into account the ways by which human persons develop value systems socially, sometimes through debate and often through conflict (Emanuel, 1991). To develop the ethics of health care means to discern the politics whereby priorities and policies based on those priorities are developed. If we do not realistically face up to this political aspect of ethics, we will find ourselves each defending his or her own subjective ethical stance in endless and fruitless polemics. Today it has become all too apparent that health is a profoundly political issue—not merely in terms of the argument over "socialized medicine," but in the sense that the problems of poverty, food, population, and pollution are national and international health problems (Aday, 1993).

In light of the many political decisions regarding health care, many Christians are tempted to despair and withdraw from ethical controversy. In the pluralistic world of today, how is ethical debate even possible, let alone practical consensus (Engelhardt, 1992)? Warring value systems appear to be irreconcilable. Only political power will prevail; today, however, Catholics are often bitterly opposed by their fellow Christians and are often accused of politicizing religious differences and imposing their own morality on the public. In the health field, this disagreement among Christians is very sharp in matters such as contraception, sterilization, abortion, *in vitro* fertilization, and euthanasia.

Nevertheless, withdrawal by Catholics from ethical debate was not countenanced by the Second Vatican Council (1965c), which recognized the fact of pluralism, renounced any policy of religious imperialism, and proposed an ecumenical approach to differences in faith and value systems. First, Catholics must be convinced that they form a single faith community with all others who acknowledge Jesus as Lord, ordinarily signified by baptism. Within this community, of course, are great differences of opinion on certain ethical questions as a result of the historical divergence and isolation of one church from another. Such differences should not, however, overshadow the profound agreement among Christians that Jesus Christ, portrayed for them in the Scriptures and the living history of his faithful followers, is the norm of ethical personhood and communal life.

We have subtitled this book *A Theological Analysis* precisely because for us the ultimate ethical norm is not a set of ethical rules but Jesus Christ—God become truly human. Therefore he is our model of what it is to be human, as well as the source of grace that empowers us to overcome our sinful inhumanity and become truly human. Thus, in a search for consensus on issues in health care ethics with all those of goodwill, we can honestly join with humanists to make the world more human; we can also join with fellow Christians in prayer, meditation, fraternal dialogue, and cooperation. To lose hope in the possibility of this union of heart and mind in Christ (1 Co 1:10) is to lose hope in Jesus as Savior of all humanity.

Care for the sick, as well as the sinful, was one of Jesus' first concerns. He healed before he preached, and he went out to the lepers, the most neglected members of the community. If Christians embrace this concern for the bodily needs of the alienated, the experience of charity will sweep away many of the one-sided views that divide us. It was no accident that the source of the recent upsurge in the ecumenical spirit was the common opposition of Christians of every denomination to the tyranny of the totalitarian governments of Hitler, Mussolini, and Stalin.

Efforts at a Wider Consensus

The Second Vatican Council (Vatican Council II, 1965a, 1965c) insisted that this spirit of dialogue must extend beyond the Christian family to other religions. Judaism and Islam believe in the same personal God as do Christians and also have the same fundamental convictions about the dignity of the human person in relation to God (John Paul II, 1995). In the history of health care, Jews and Muslims made fundamental contributions which have become part of the tradition of Christian health care (Galdston, 1981; Ullmann, 1978).

The Eastern religions of India and China are beginning to influence American life. At first sight, however, their outlook might appear incompatible with the Christian emphasis on the dignity of the human person in relation to a personal God, since they teach that the individual, after a series of reincarnations, is absorbed into the unity of the Absolute. Closer study, however, reveals that this Absolute is not subpersonal, nor impersonal, but superpersonal. Thus it becomes possible for monotheists to join with believers in these Eastern religions in a common search for authentic spiritual selfhood. Americans are beginning to appreciate how much these religions, with their meditative disciplines, can contribute to personal integration and total health.

In addition, the *nature religions* of Native Americans and others have taught an appreciation of our relation to nature in its mysterious wisdom and cosmic rhythm. Modern medicine is beginning to learn from the ecological experience of such peoples (L. Moore, 1987). We cannot return to Eden, but woe to us if we forget it.

Thus Christians can learn much from other world religions about ethical dialogue and the pursuit of true health. Today, however, these religious systems of values seem to be receding before the worldwide advance of secularization, both in industrialized countries and in third world countries (John Paul II, 1987a). Moreover, this secularized view of humankind seems more congenial to the science and technology on which modern medicine is based than are the older religious views of man. In response to this situation, however, the Second Vatican Council has indicated that dialogue with nonbelievers should be sought (Vatican Council II, 1965a).

The Christian is inclined to judge the agnostic worldview of humanism that prevails in the industrialized countries and the atheistic worldview of the Marxists as absolutely contradictory to Christianity. Tracing the origin of these new world philosophies, however, reveals that they are sociologically equivalent to the older world religions. The religious wars that resulted from the breakdown of Christian unity in the sixteenth and seventeenth centuries and the shock of discovering other ethically admirable religions of the New World and Asia led to a religious vacuum in Europe. Out of this arose the new philosophy of humanism (the Enlightenment, sometimes called *secular* enlightenment to distinguish it from the older Christian humanism), which enthusiastically accepted the rise of science and technology as a more efficient means to solve human problems than prayer, ritual, and traditional dogmas.

Thus, according to the well-known *Humanist Manifesto* (1933), signed by a group of distinguished American thinkers under the leadership of our most famous American philosopher, John Dewey:

> Religion consists of those actions, purposes, and experiences which are humanly significant. Nothing human is alien to religion. It includes labor, art, science, philosophy, love, friendship, recreation—all that is in its degree expressive of intelligently satisfying human living. . . . Religious humanism considers the complete realization of human personality to be the end of man's life and seeks its fulfillment and development in the here and now. This is the explanation of the humanist's social passion (p. 13).

Thus though humanism rejects the notion of an afterlife for human beings and their dependence on a God or an Absolute, it does so precisely in the interest of human dignity (Kurtz, 1983). Believing that the older religions tend to excuse human beings from full responsibility to create a good society here and now, this humanist position has been reaffirmed by an international group in the *Paris Statement of 1966* and, in the United States, in the *Humanist Manifesto II* (1973).

Marxism, still very much alive in China and a few other countries and still influential in the thinking of the political "left" in many democratic countries, is an even more radical form of humanism, which openly denies the existence of God or a spiritual soul in the human person and believes that poverty and oppression cannot be overcome by peaceful means, but only by class struggle and violent revolution. It has even had an effect on some forms of Catholic "liberation theology" and of radical feminism (CDF, 1984). The Catholic Church has always opposed Marxism, as it did the other totalitarian regimes, the Nazis and Fascists, which were extreme reactions to Marxism, for their atheism or paganism, their advocacy of class and race hatred, their offenses against human rights, their militarism and promotion of violence, and their attacks on the institution of the family.

It would be a mistake, however, to think that the Catholic Church is therefore a supporter of an unregulated capitalism or of the individualism that flourishes in so many democratic countries. Even many Catholics are unacquainted with the fully developed social teaching of recent popes (John Paul II, 1987a, 1991; Paul VI, 1967), which is fundamental to any Catholic approach to today's economics and social issues, including those in the medieval field. This Catholic teaching attempts to transcend the capitalist–communist impasse, based in both camps on a materialistic conception of society. The popes urge us to work for a world community based on spiritual goals and economic cooperation. They link human health and world poverty as the most fundamental problems in health care ethics of our time. These problems are often ignored in the United States, whereas much is made in the public press over secondary problems such as eugenics and organ transplants.

The Second Vatican Council (Vatican Council II, 1965c) has emphasized that Christians have much to learn from the humanist's emphasis on human beings' responsibility to use reason, science, and technology to solve human problems. The otherworldly view of religion rightly deserves the accusation that religion is often an "opiate of the people," when it should be a challenge to use the talents given us by God to overcome poverty, disease, and injustice. For this reason, Catholic health care professionals should strive to heal any schizoid dualism in their own thinking between their religious view of life and an enlightened scientific view of the world. Christians cannot accept agnostic and sometimes mechanistic and materialistic interpretations of scientific findings, but they can and should join enthusiastically in the advance of scientific research and its application to the solution of human problems of health (Polkinghorne, 1991).

Catholic liberation theologians (Boff, 1986, 1991; Gutierrez, 1977, 1990) have taken a further step by arguing that Catholics can learn something from the Marxist criticism of capitalism. They point out that when Jesus announced the coming of the Kingdom of God, he was not talking merely about a temporal reality but was declaring the fulfillment of Old Testament prophetic demands for justice to the poor and oppressed. The Kingdom of God begins here on earth with social justice (John Paul II, 1980a), and no one will gain heaven who has neglected to work for social justice on earth (Viviano, 1988). Jesus declared in the parable of the sheep and the goats (Mt 25:31–46), "I was hungry and you never gave me food . . . . Insofar as you neglected to do this to one of the least of these, you neglected to do it to me"; in the parable of Lazarus and the rich man (Lk 16:19–31), Jesus taught the same lesson. Consequently, a genuine Christian ethics cannot be written from the viewpoint of the *status quo*, which in a sinful world tends to reflect the materialistic spirit of domination and possessiveness. Such ethics must view the world from the side of oppressed persons whose needs have been ignored and neglected. Thus Jesus pointed to his preaching of the Gospel to the poor as the best sign of the authenticity of his own mission (Mt 11:5). Therefore a Christian politics of health care must be based on advocacy for the rights of neglected persons.

Why is the conflict between individualism and collectivism so unresolvable? Christian theology ascribes this conflict to a profound misunderstanding of the relation of person to community. The notion of *personal* is often confused with the notion of *private*. Thus it appears that to favor the community is to *sacrifice* the person to the collective. This is true if the community is based on a sharing of material goods. Such goods can be shared among individuals only by dividing them up and giving to each a private share. What one gets, the other loses, and vice versa. This is the way it works in modern societies based primarily on the sharing of material goods such as economic production and military power. Consequently, those who oppose selfish individualism sometimes turn to pure socialism, wherein the person is sacrificed to the society.

Christian politics, however, aims at the sharing of *spiritual* goods: truth and love. Material goods should be distributed so as to promote spiritual sharing, but they are not the primary basis of community. When spiritual goods are shared, no one loses, but each gains, possessing them more perfectly. Only in such spiritual sharing is profound community between human persons possible. Thus the common good is not opposed to the personal good; rather, it is the deepest heart of the personal good of each person. Private goods are actually *less* personal than this common good (Maritain, 1947).

This theory may sound impractical until we realize that scientific truth is a spiritual good. Is it not true that today scientists across the world are united in the advancement and sharing of scientific research, yet they are deeply divided by the politics of their countries' quests for economic and military power?

Therefore a Christian politics today will aim at overcoming world conflict by witnessing to spiritual values and subordinating material ones as instruments for attaining spiritual community. This is why dialogue in an ecumenical spirit has to be the greatest political strategy of the Christian. Health care is directed to improving physiological and psychological function. However, it is also directed to a spiritual goal, the improvement of persons in their intelligent freedom.

Individualism and Human Rights

Now it should be clear why Catholic theology perceives that extreme form of humanism, sometimes called *radical individualism,* as the greatest danger to the development of an ethical consensus in a pluralistic society (Bellah et al., 1991). Typical humanism has a strong concern for social justice, but radical individualism rejects the belief that community as such is a moral value. This ethic—proposed by Hobbes in the seventeenth century, supported in more moderate form by Locke, and given a new form by Nietzsche in the nineteenth century—has had a profound effect on American society from Emerson to its diverse advocates among psychotherapists (Szasz, 1977, 1987) on the left and libertarians such as Ayn Rand (1967), George Gilder (1982), and Robert Nozick (1981).

The ethic of radical individualism is summed up in the principle, "I have a right to live my own life as long as I don't hurt anybody else"—"hurt" meaning direct harm by bodily injury or damage or theft of private property (Bloom, 1987, 1990). According to this ethic, society exists only as a means to protect one individual from another, so as to leave each to pursue his or her private purposes. Moreover, any claim of one human being on another that is not contractual goes beyond the right to be let alone and is therefore unethical. Ethical behavior becomes the consistent pursuit of self-interest within a minimal code of law and contract enforcement. Proponents of this ethic often argue (1) that people really act this way and therefore other ethics are hypocritical and (2) that this system of *laissez faire* actually produces more economic prosperity and human progress than do collectivist and altruistic ethics.

For *laissez faire* capitalists to argue, however, that they have a right to amass a fortune because it is "good for society" is itself hypocritical, since their real belief is that they have a right to their own lives no matter what the social consequences, as long as they do not provoke those more powerful than themselves to destroy them.

This extreme form of individualism is perhaps best labeled *privatism.* Privatism seems still to be growing in American society in the 1990s (Bellah et al., 1986; Bellah, 1992). It is the most difficult value system to deal with, even for a Christian who has the will to try to find some point of contact. However, even here the individualists deserve their due. A generation ago, when Ayn Rand (1967) attacked altruism and proposed the new selfishness, she obviously supposed that Christians teach an altruistic ethics in which the person is called on to sacrifice his or her self-fulfillment to the community. She rightly sees this as unreal and sentimental. What she does not realize is that to Christians the command "Love thy neighbor as thyself" (Mk 12:31) implies that we must *love ourselves* before we can love anyone else. Selfishness is not repudiated because it seeks the good of the self, but because it denies the self access to those goods that can be achieved only by sharing with other persons. Thus Christians can agree with radical individualists that each person has as his or her first moral duty to seek genuine self-fulfillment. This is not sinful selfishness, but a duty to the God who made human beings so they could make good use of their gifts.

Furthermore, Christians should take up the challenge to show by hard-headed, realistic, and rational arguments that this self-fulfillment demands that people not isolate themselves in sinful selfishness, but become open to community, where this self-fulfillment lies. In this way Christians can learn something from privatism about good health care; namely, that (as Chapter 3 argues in detail) each person has the primary responsibility for the care of his or her own health, a responsibility that cannot be passed on to the health care profession or to society.

The rise of recent "conservative" movements that seek to defend traditional Christian family life and a legitimate patriotism but confuse these values with a privatism and nationalism indifferent or antagonistic to social justice (Krason, 1991; USCC, 1986) presents a difficult ecumenical problem. Unfortunately, "liberal" Christians have sometimes compounded this confusion in their zeal for social justice by seeming to reject domestic virtue and sober patriotism (as these are commended in the Scriptures) and to adopt very different attitudes derived from Humanism or Marxism. To overcome these confusions, Christians must demonstrate how the Gospel inseparably unites the virtues of private and social life, loyalty to one's country, and a still greater loyalty to the whole human family.

One Source of Ethical Consensus

This ecumenical search for ethical consensus has its solid legal and political foundations in the United Nations' *Universal Declaration of Human Rights* (1948), signed by almost all the countries of the world and supported by all the major religions as well as by humanists and Marxists. Catholics have been urged by the Pontifical Commission on Peace and Justice (1973), by Pope Paul VI (1974), and Pope John Paul II (1988) to support the *Declaration* as a sound (although not complete) basis for modern ethics. It begins with a fundamental statement that formulates the very notion of person and community for which we have just argued:

Article 1: All human beings are born free and equal in dignity and rights. They are endowed with reason and conscience and should act towards one another in a spirit of brotherhood.

Here "reason and conscience" are equivalent to "intelligent freedom" and "brotherhood" to "community," in terms of which we have defined the human person. The *Declaration* then effectively concretizes this abstract principle by enumerating 29 basic human rights. Among these are the following, which should serve as a magna charta for a modern health care ethics:

Article 3: Everyone has the right to life, liberty, and security of person.
Article 22: Everyone, as a member of society, has the right to social security and is entitled to realization, through national effort and international cooperation and in accordance with the organiza-

tion and resources of each state, of the economic, social, and cultural rights indispensable for his dignity, and the free development of his personality.

Article 25: (1) Everyone has the right to a standard of living adequate for the health and well-being of himself and of his family, including food, clothing, housing, and medical care and necessary social services, and the right to security in the event of unemployment, sickness, disability, widowhood, old age, or other lack of livelihood in circumstances beyond his control. . . . (3) Motherhood and childhood are entitled to special care and assistance. All children, whether born in or out of wedlock, shall enjoy the same social protection.

According to Article 2, all these rights apply to all human beings "without distinction of any kind, such as race, color, sex, language, religion, political or other opinion, national or social origin, property, birth, or other status." Moreover, Article 29 (1) asserts: "Everyone has duties to the community in which alone the free and full development of his personality is possible."

Of course, Christians in the United States, let alone in the whole world, are far from having fulfilled their obligations under the *Declaration*. Nevertheless, it stands as a proof that in the twentieth century a basic consensus in regard to priorities and policies of health care ethics already exists. The aim of this book is to take that consensus very seriously without, however, glossing over the profound differences that continue to divide the Christian and the secular communities and that challenge us to further research and dialogue.

1.4 PRIORITIES IN HUMAN NEEDS AND VALUES

The fact that the nations of the world are at least nominally agreed on a list of human rights or values is an important step toward increasing ethical consensus, but it is only a first step. This is unfortunate, since the adoption of the *Universal Declaration* has shown the diversity in the interpretations of many of these rights. When carefully examined, this diversity reveals that ethics must not only list agreed-on values, but must also deal with the question of priorities. What is the "hierarchy of values"? Some will reply that this question of emphases and priorities is a wholly subjective matter about which rational discussion is impossible. Whether this is the case can be decided only if the concept of value and its relation to objective facts are examined more closely.

We have already argued that ethics has to do with the satisfaction of the *needs* of human persons in their lives as intelligently free social beings. We have now to ask more precisely: What are these needs? Are some needs more basic than others? The general answer is that human needs are satisfied by human goods or values and the most basic needs by the most basic goods or values. But the term *value* is vague. It was originally used in economics but has been extended in usage to cover a spectrum of analogical meanings (Perry, 1980).

A given human value is always correlative to a human need; that is, it is desired to satisfy a need. On the other hand, a negative value is inimical to human need; if it is desired at all, it is desired only as an apparent value. A neutral value neither satisfies nor obstructs a need. A value, therefore, can be something so trivial as a cup of water to satisfy thirst or so sublime as the truth of Plato's philosophy to satisfy thirst for meaning in the cosmos. A behavioral test for a value is the objective human reaction to it, that is, whether the value is rejected or accepted. Human debate about whether something is desirable or undesirable, acceptable or unacceptable, is clear evidence that what is in question is some value or a conflict of values.

Basic Needs

Together with psychologists, biologists, and other human scientists, we recognize the following basic needs (B. Ashley, 1972; Maslow, 1970).

1. The *biological dimension* (Maslow's physiological needs). Human persons share with all living organisms the need to maintain themselves homeostatically in a dynamic relation with their environment, to grow and mature to full biological development as individuals, and to continue the species through reproduction. This is the level usually dealt with by biologists and physicians.

2. The *psychological dimension* (Maslow's safety needs, as well as belongingness and love needs in their more emotional aspects). Human persons are psychic organisms who sense, imagine, and feel. This is the level of need generally dealt with by experimental psychologists and psychotherapists.

3. The *social dimension* (Maslow's esteem needs, as well as the belongingness and love needs in their more developed aspects). This is the level of human free choice within the limits of an existing culture. Social dimension comprises the need of the individual both for self-control and for social relations beyond those determined by the family. This is the level dealt with by lawyers, political leaders, and clergy acting as moral counselors.

4. The *spiritual or creative dimension* (Maslow's need for self-actualization, including needs to know and understand, to contemplate, and to create). Although many refer to this level of need as the spiritual, we add the word *creative* because many people confine the meaning of *spiritual* to our relationship to God. This is the level of commitment, creativity, and transcendence at which persons not only live within a culture, but criticize it, transcend it, and contribute to it. This dimension includes all activity with a creative element—in art or science or political innovation—in addition to religious activity as it extends to ultimate, cosmic meaning. This is the level dealt with by the inspiring teacher and spiritual guide.

Relationship of Needs

The following diagram makes the rather complicated interrelations of these dimensions somewhat clearer:

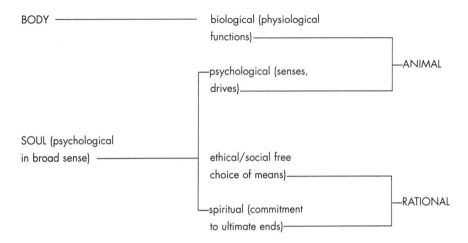

This diagram should not be understood in a dualistic sense, as though the needs and functions more closely related to the soul are independent of the body. They are in fact closely and mutually interdependent, and yet as we shall see in Chapter 12, they cause different problems for human health.

The *biological* dimension focuses on the physiological needs and functions of the body and is especially the field of medicine. The term *psychological* in a broad sense applies to all the psychic (soul) needs and functions and is especially the field of psychiatry and psychotherapy. In the narrower sense in which we use it to name the second dimension of the person, it refers primarily to the needs and functions of our senses, both exterior and interior (imagination, memory, etc.) and to our drives (feelings, emotions, instincts). The biological and the psychological (in this narrower sense) dimensions we human persons share with the other animals. In contrast to these biological and psychological needs and functions, yet by no means independent of them, the ethical and spiritual levels are unique to human beings (hence we are defined as "rational animals"). These levels are either *ethical* (social) and pertain to our knowledge of the various means (functions) to our goals (needs) and our free choices among them, and to the fields of ethical, occupational, and legal counseling; or *spiritual* and pertain to our commitment to our ultimate goals and to the field of pastoral counseling (needs, values) to which these choices are directed.

Each of these levels of human needs contains a complex of natural and cultural needs. The cultural needs are rooted in the natural needs but greatly expand them; e.g., schooling is a cultural development to fulfill the need for knowledge. It cannot be emphasized too strongly that these four levels of needs are not related as stories in a building but rather as *dimensions* in a cube. They can no more be separated from one another than the length, breadth, and height of a cube. Every human act or event has *all* four dimensions. But an act will emphasize one level of need. For example, eating food is primarily directed toward fulfilling our physiological needs, yet the psychological, social, and creative needs of our personality are also fulfilled or not by the manner in which we eat and the manner in which food is prepared. A human spiritual activity, whether the creative activity of a scientist or artist or the graced acts of faith, hope, or love, is at the same time a biological, psychological, and social event. Reciprocally, human biological acts or events, whether eating, sexual activities, or simple physical movement, are not only psychological events but uniquely human social and spiritual events.

Moreover, the reciprocity between these levels of the organization and function of the human personality are hierarchically ordered. Thus spiritual or creative activities are the deepest, most central, and most integrating; biological activities are the least unified and the most peripheral; and psychological and social activities have intermediate positions. At the same time, the higher activities in this hierarchy are rooted in and dependent on the lower ones in a network of interrelations. Studying is very difficult unless one is physiologically healthy. Nevertheless, each level has a certain genuine autonomy and differentiation in its structure and modes of functioning, so it is necessary (as Chapter 2 demonstrates) that persons be served respectively by the different professions of medicine, psychotherapy, ethical counseling, and spiritual direction, which use different healing and helping techniques.

Other Lists of Needs

Others have devised even more elaborate lists of natural needs (Grisez, 1983; John Paul II, 1993). Thomas Aquinas gave a simpler classification of basic needs common to all (*Summa Theologiae*, I–II, q. 94, a. 2): (1) the need to preserve life; (2) the need to procreate; (3) the need to know the truth; and (4) the need to live in society. For the most part in this study, we will correlate the lists of Aquinas and Maslow. Some, however, such as Gordon Allport (1937, 1961), have objected to all such classifications as too heavily based on the notion of instincts. For Allport, the innate tendencies of human beings are so broad, require so elaborate a set of cultural conditions to develop, and develop so much in the context of an individual personality with a personal biography that he wishes to avoid the notion of need or instinct altogether. Allport speaks only of the development, differentiation, and integration of a personality in interaction with natural and social environments. However, Allport cannot avoid discussing different *tendencies* of the human organism in the effort to adjust to or control his or her environment. We consider these *tendencies* to be similar to natural *needs*.

The ethical problem persons face is to plan their lives and engage in political decisions in such a way that *all* these needs are satisfied to some degree in an integrated and consistent manner. This obviously requires the adjustment of priorities in regard to both aims and objectives and adjustment of the practical steps to be taken. This activity also demands the subordination, and even sacrifice, of less important needs to greater ones. The exact mix or proportion will depend on both the culture and the individual.

Thus health as a value cannot be understood ethically in isolation from the whole hierarchy of values of which it is a part.

CONCLUSION

Humans are embodied beings with an innate capacity for intelligent freedom. To be human, it is not required that one is here and now functioning as a free moral agent, but only that one have the innate power to develop these capacities. Thus, the distinction between human being and person is one of reason, not reality. Though the word person may be used to indicate the possession of rights, most of the important rights are due to persons because they are human. Thus, person-hood is not conferred by society. Rather, it is based upon the innate human capacities. Personhood is always in the process of growth, which consists primarily in deepening communal relations. Health aims at the development of all human capacities. Thus, health care is not limited to physiological function alone; rather, it is concerned also with enabling persons to become intellectually free.

In order to understand the quest for health, the concept of person in community must be understood. The concept of person, or human, cannot be understood except in relation to its correlative, society or community. In order to indicate that community is an essential need for persons, Aristotle defined the person as a political animal.

The highest form of community is a spiritual bond, resulting from knowledge and love. Thus, persons have an innate capacity to know and love one another and also to know and love God. Thus, health care may be envisioned as an effort to help patients share in community with God and other persons. Health care seeks to improve the function of the person at all levels of activity, bodily as well as spiritual. Improving human function means fulfilling human needs; when something does fulfill a human need, we call that thing a value or a good. Hence, in order to develop a politics of health care, some consensus is necessary in regard to the needs, goods, or values toward which health care activity must be directed. Developing such a consensus is difficult. Religious and philosophical systems all have theories about the needs, goods, and values which are most prominent in forming healthy individuals and healthy communities. Vatican Council II (1965c) insisted that Catholics join with others of good will in dialogue to search for consensus in regard to human needs, goods, and values. This dialogue should embrace all religions and philosophical theories.

One potential source of consensus in regard to human needs, goods, and values is the *Universal Declaration of Human Rights* (1948), supported by all major religions and countries. In theory, the declaration offers a consensus in regard to the priorities among human needs and values. In practice, it is difficult to encourage consensus in regard to needs, goods, and values in our pluralistic society. But persons of good will must strive for consensus if they aim to live at peace in an ethical and just community.

In our theological analysis of health care ethics, in accord with contemporary psychologists and other human scientists, we recognize four basic human needs: biological, psychological, social, and spiritual or creative.

2
Health and Disease

OVERVIEW

Chapter 1 asserts that the natural and cultural needs of the human person are the basis on which Christian ethics can seek agreement with other ethical systems. Health is the aspect of human need with which this book is concerned. Thus the concept of human health and disease that this chapter develops is grounded in the multidimensional character of the human person in community. Since health is the ultimate goal of all health care, the concept of health and the human right to strive for it serve as the groundwork on which we develop an ethics of health care.

First this chapter deals with the concept of the person as multidimensional (2.1) and then with the various types of health—biological (2.2), psychological, ethical and social, and spiritual (2.3)—and how they are interrelated in total or integral health. The principle of totality and integrity explained in Chapter 8 summarizes the discussion in Chapter 2 and has many applications to concrete medical decisions, such as any type of surgery and transplanting of solid organs.

2.1 CONCEPTS OF HEALTH AND DISEASE

Concepts of Health

The word *health* is related etymologically to the Anglo-Saxon word from which are derived not only *healing* but also *holiness* and *wholeness* (Vaux, 1978; Erde, 1979). The root of that word denotes "completeness," a whole that has all its parts. Such a whole can be considered statically as a *structure* with all its parts— each properly proportioned and all parts in their places. Thus a crippled person lacks wholeness or health because some part of his or her anatomy is missing or deformed. However, health can also be considered dynamically as a *functional* whole, in which all necessary functions are present and acting cooperatively and harmoniously. Thus some sicknesses do not involve any lack of a part or organ or its deformity, but rather a dysfunction; that is, some needed function is suppressed or there is a lack of harmonious balance among functions, as in diabetes or hyperthyroidism.

Since the goal of medicine is fostering and restoring health, the medical profession should certainly be able to explain what health is. One has only to ask the average medical student or student nurse to define health, however, to discover that their medical education is lacking in this area. Medical schools and nursing schools assume that students will glean an adequate notion of health simply from dealing with sick and healthy patients. No doubt this sometimes happens, but such an unexamined presupposition can be dangerous. For a medical professional to be working devotedly toward a goal that is vague and ill-defined is as absurd as for a cancer research team to be looking for a cure without trying first to understand the nature of the disease.

In the actual practice of medicine today, *health* is most frequently defined in terms of standard physiological parameters—the vital signs, various chemicals in the blood, electroneurological readings, and so forth—as well as by gross anatomy and histology (McDowell and Neuell, 1987). Moreover, a complete physical examination and diagnosis of health by means of physiological tests and computerized calculations is anticipated and is partly practical already. Health, therefore, will soon be defined by a model of what is normal.

Such a model will raise some problems, however (Bakken, 1985). First, an exact, universal definition of human health in these terms obviously is impossible, and only a *range* of normal values can be achieved. In the case of some values, such as temperature, this range is not large, but in all cases what is identifiably healthy for one individual does not necessarily indicate a state of health for another person. How can the model of normality be determined? *Normal* is not identical with *average,* since most persons today conceivably are not very healthy. The normal, therefore, is an *ideal* (Lippman, 1992). How can such an ideal be determined in a way that is not arbitrary but that has a sound empirical basis?

This question prompts the notion of health as *optimal functioning.* Clearly, health in the structural sense of absence of anatomical lesion or deformity is the same as optimal functioning because as the axiom states: *structure is for function.* The absence of a functionless part (e.g., the appendix) is not a defect of health but an advantage. Moreover, the deformity of an organ ultimately must be judged in terms of whether it is capable of optimal function. Even appearance can be considered one aspect of function because physical beauty has a social function. Thus a human being is healthy if he or she can function optimally. This implies that each organ and organ system is functioning well and that all are functioning together to form a single life process, of which the diverse functions are harmoniously interrelated yet differentiated phases.

Henrik Blum in a comprehensive study of the concept of health (1983) concluded: "Health is the state of being in which an individual does the best with the capacities he has, and acts in ways that maximize his capacities" (p. 93). Blum contends that this can be measured in terms of eight parameters: (1) prematurity of death, (2) departure from physiological norms, (3) discomfort, (4) disability to function, (5) internal satisfaction, (6) external satisfaction, (7) positive health, and (8) capacity to participate in social activities.

This concept of health is a consequence of the basic concept of a human being as an *organism* (etymologically "a complex of instruments" or organs), that is, a *living whole composed of functionally differentiated parts.* A human being is thus a dynamic or *open system*. A system is a "complex of interacting elements" (Bertalanffy, 1968). A living system is dynamic or *open*, that is, capable of maintaining *homeostasis* (dynamic stability) in relation to its environment by regulating the input and output of matter and energy.

As Ludwig von Bertalanffy shows (1968), the characteristics and behavior of the whole complex cannot be reduced to the characteristics and behavior of the parts, since the parts do not exist or act separately but in mutual interrelation and interaction. Moreover, in more complex systems there are several *levels* of organization in *hierarchical order*, so that the higher levels of function include the lower levels but cannot be reduced to them. The fallacy of reductionism is attempting to explain these higher levels of functioning simply in terms of lower levels or to explain the system merely in terms of its parts. To avoid reductionism, the interrelation and interaction of the parts and the levels of organization in the whole must be considered fully (Hoyninger-Huene, 1989). The whole of the organism is not some mystical or extraneous entity added to the parts of the system; it is precisely the structural and functional interrelation and interaction of the parts.

Obviously, a definition of health in terms of optimal functioning of an open system must include the output of that system. A living thing cannot maintain itself in static existence; it must interact with the environment. This is especially obvious because living individuals must also reproduce to maintain the species, but it is also clear that living things modify the environment in their own interests. Thus animals build shelters and nests, fertilize plants on which they feed, and rid their environment of enemies. In fact, the present earth environment is largely the product of living things that have modified both the soil and the atmosphere in ways favorable to life (Birch, 1981; Wilson, 1990).

In the case of human beings, a further step must be taken. Because they are cultural as well as natural beings, human beings' interaction with the environment is highly creative. They modify the environment with conscious purpose, so that civilization is the production of a city, that is, an increasingly manufactured environment. Today people are beginning to think about living in an environment that is almost entirely artificial (for example, on the moon or even on constructed satellites), where nothing will be natural except the basic raw materials from which the total environment will be humanly constructed.

Still more interestingly, human creativity is not limited to interaction with an external environment. People create not only external things, but also mental and emotional symbols; these fulfill certain needs that cannot be fulfilled by what is merely objective, that is, outside conscience (Cassirer, 1953; Gazzaniga, 1992). Ultimately, human beings need to assimilate the whole order of the external environment. Thus scientists are constantly striving to recreate, as it were, the entire external cosmos in the form of symbols. The great importance of this human life process, from a personalistic point of view, is that such symbols provide communication among persons in the form of language. Human society is ultimately this communication by which we all come to live in the same symbol universe.

This internalization of the environment, however, does not nullify interaction with the external environment. Scientific knowledge can be increased only by experimentation, and communication can be accomplished only through languages, which require an external medium. Moreover, scientific advance is also technological advance. To learn more about the world, we often have to change it. Developing a human culture breaks down the barrier between mind and matter, between the internal and the external. Thus the human organism as a system is progressively opening up to include other human persons and the entire cosmos, as scientific visionaries such as Alfred North Whitehead (1929) and Pierre Teilhard de Chardin (1964) have so vividly shown.

In view of this concept of human functioning, human health as optimal functioning means not only an internal harmony and consistency of function within the organism, but also the capacity of the organism to maintain itself in its environment. Optimal human functioning, however, is something more than the ability to cope with one's environment. An individual's capabilities are themselves open to improvement in view of the fundamental human capacity for intelligent freedom and creativity. Thus, to be precise, a definition of health must also be open, that is, be constantly revised in view of a deepening and enriching vision of human capacities for culture. With the human race especially, this means extending itself creatively to produce an ever-expanding culture. This is why the WHO, in the definition given in 1.1, insists, "Health is a state of complete physical, mental, and social well-being and not merely the absence of disease or infirmity."

In 1.4 the levels of human needs—biological, psychological, social, and creative—are placed in a hierarchical order from primary physical needs to higher cultural needs. Health in the *broad sense* then, corresponds to integrated fulfillment of these needs. A holistic concept of health is thus "optimal functioning of the human organism to meet biological, psychological, social, and spiritual needs." The health care professions are usually concerned with health in the *narrower sense* of optimal functioning at the biological and psychological levels. However, although physicians specialize in biological or psychological functions, they must never neglect or ignore the social and spiritual needs of their patients if they wish to be truly concerned about human health (Pellegrino and Thomasma, 1988).

Concepts of Disease

Given this concept of health as structural and functional wholeness of the human organism in relation to the self and to the environment—a wholeness that extends even to the social and spiritual, to holiness—the notion of disease can also be more precisely defined (Riese, 1953; Mershey, 1986; Gerhardt, 1989). The WHO definition maintains that disease and infirmity are not the exact contrary of health. Health, as we have defined it, is optimal functioning. For an organism to fall short of optimal functioning without actually being diseased or infirm is possible, since an organism can be healthy in a narrow sense without actually being used to its full capacity. However, without optimal functioning, the failure to function soon leads to dysfunction. A person can be healthy in this narrow sense and still be lazy and half alive through lack of full use of personal capacities for living. But a person will not stay healthy even in this minimal way for long because the faculties will atrophy.

The terms *disease, illness, sickness, malady, ailment, disorder, complaint,* and many more synonyms have different connotations (Margolis, 1986; Gerhardt, 1989). Some seem to be more subjective; that is, they designate the feelings of the victim (e.g., illness, sickness, or complaint); whereas others are more objective (disease, malady, ailment, or disorder) (Boorse, 1981). This distinction can be questioned, however, since *disease* comes from *dis-ease,* implying a subjective sense. This book uses the term in its broad sense as the opposite of health.

In the history of medicine, as Owsei Temkin has shown (Temkin, 1963; Lain-Entralgo, 1970), the pendulum has constantly swung between *two concepts* of disease: the ontological and the physiological. The *ontological concept* regards diseases as separate entities (devils, contagions, morbific matters, bacteria, genetic defects, neuroses, and psychoses), which can be classified and named as are plants and animals. The organism constantly fights to throw off such diseases as alien invaders that disturb its homeostasis. Those who think in this way tend to diagnose diseases in terms of clearly classified and labeled entities and to treat them by seeking specific remedies (e.g., specific drugs or specific surgical procedures).

The opposite of the ontological concept, the *physiological concept,* views disease as a breakdown of the internal harmony of the organic system because of hyperfunctioning or hypofunctioning of an organ. Thus dysfunction opens the organism to attack by external agents such as bacteria, but the bacteria are not the primary cause of the disease. If the organism were functioning properly, it would resist such bacteria. Classifying or labeling diseases is dangerous, therefore, because disease is essentially the condition of an *individual* who is internally maladjusted. The advocates of this position thus tend to emphasize regimen or lifestyle and to use drugs and surgery secondarily to assist in the adjustment of the individual organism.

As Temkin and Lain-Entralgo show, the central tradition of medicine (usually identified with that of Hippocrates, the Greek "Father of Medicine") has always tried to reconcile these two extreme positions. In view of the account given of the organism as a dynamic system, such a reconciliation should not be too difficult. The physiologists are correct in thinking of health first as an internal homeostasis or harmony within the organism and disease as an imbalance. The organism as a system is constantly adjusting by means of feedback to changes in the environment. These minor fluctuations are not diseases; rather, they are health itself.

If the system fluctuates beyond a certain range, however, it cannot recover homeostasis without a major readjustment. This may be possible through the internal vital powers, but only at the cost of a period of sickness in which many normal functions must be minimized while the organism uses all its energies to readjust. Such a disease is acute illness. Also, the organism may readjust but at the cost of permanent diminishing of function or suppression of some functions. Then the disease becomes chronic, or permanent crippling or handicap results.

Finally, the adjustment may be greater than the organism can achieve, and death results. Death may be the result of acute disease or aging. Some researchers have hypothesized that aging may result from natural physiological processes that have been genetically programmed as a result of evolutionary selection—the removal of mature organisms after they have had time to reproduce in order to provide more living space for the next generation to mature and reproduce in its turn. As yet this hypothesis has not been confirmed. More probably, aging is the gradual debilitation of a living system exposed to repeated disease and trauma. Thus aging is simply an application of the second law of thermodynamics (the law of increasing entropy) to living systems.

From this point of view, death is always the result of disease. Therefore death cannot be said to be natural if by *natural* is meant, as the Greeks meant, the optimal function or health of the organism. Physiologically speaking, the organism seems to be made to live forever, always recovering from any malfunction. Thus death is caused by injuries inflicted on the organism from the environment, not from any intrinsic tendency. A homeostatic system, by definition, is one that maintains itself perpetually when not disturbed.

Holism and Mechanism

After looking at these various definitions of health and disease, it is important to contrast and relate two points of view which are often seen as irreconcilable: The holistic and the mechanistic. Those who view health holistically emphasize the complex unity of the human organism, its *wholeness*. Their view is also sometimes call "organismic." On the contrary, others view the organism as a combination of *parts* which must be separated from each other and studied in themselves.

Thinking holistically, the human organism is an open system that constantly interacts with the environment. The organism is homeostatic, but limits exist to its power of self-maintenance. Consequently, when the environment is altered beyond a certain normal range, the organism is unable to survive. Thus, when the oxygen content of the air, the temperature, or the number of bacteria in the environment greatly changes, the human organism undergoes stress, then disorganization, and finally death. Therefore diseases can be classified according to various external agents that tax the capacity of the organism to maintain itself. Diseases can be viewed as entities such as plague, pollution, or radiation sickness, that affect all the individual organisms in a given area. From this point of view, disease and death are natural in the sense that the terrestrial environment is a part of the evolutionary process from which no individual, but only the species, is protected. The species itself ultimately yields to the rise of new species. Without disease and death, natural evolution cannot continue.

Organismic vs. Mechanistic

Both the ontological and the physiological concepts conceive of the body as an interactive organism. This organismic concept of the body and the resulting theory of health and disease has been central to Western medicine, but it has had strong competition from the mechanistic theory, which dates back to the Greek Democritus. Even today the thinking of many biologists and medical educators is influenced by the mechanistic theory (Barkow, 1989). This theory of health does not deny that an organism is an open system, but it tends to view it in reductionist terms. *For a mechanist, the parts seem to be more significant and more practically controllable than the whole.* The whole is too complex either to understand or to manage, and its relational character seems tenuous and abstract. One can see and touch the parts, but to mechanists, relations seem to be only mental constructs. Mechanists are more comfortable with anatomy or structure than with function or process. They tend to reduce process to quantitative measurements of results. Their diagnoses tend toward ontologistic views in which disease is the result of alien bacteria, organic lesions, and so forth. In treatment they incline toward a mechanical adjustment of parts by surgery or use of specific drugs. This attitude is encouraged today by three factors: (1) the specialization in medicine, which emphasizes the treatment of particular organs or organ systems rather than the whole patient; (2) the increasing use of a multiplicity of drugs, of complex surgery, and of various measuring devices in diagnosis; and (3) the theoretical success of molecular biology, which promises to give an account of the whole human organism in terms of its ultimate atomic parts.

Maintaining a holistic or organismic view in no way denies the mechanistic view; rather, it includes this view. The notion of dynamic system necessarily includes a detailed analysis of the parts, the interacting elements. To posit vitalistic or holistic forces apart from the interaction of the parts is unscientific (Payer, 1988). An organismic view, however, insists that the relations among the parts are just as real, just as scientifically observable and intelligible, as the parts themselves. Moreover, the parts themselves cannot be observed or understood in isolation but only in the context of the system in which they exist. The eye or the kidney, the cell, and even the macromolecular gene cannot be understood except in the context of the whole organism of which they are parts. Medical specialization, therefore, can never be separated from a medical understanding of the whole person, nor can health or disease be defined except in terms of the whole *and* its parts.

One of the factors that has contributed to mechanistic prejudices in medicine has been the fear of teleology (see 1.4). A homeostatic system necessarily introduces the notion of ends (goals) and means, since such a system tends to constantly achieve a normal state that is the end (goal) or, in Greek, *telos* (optimal functioning). The various vital organs and processes are means tending to an end or goal. They have direction or inherent tendency. This is precisely what the Greeks meant by *nature*. The nature of a thing is its goal-directed tendency. For a living thing, such goal-directedness is its tendency to develop embryologically into a mature, fully differentiated organism—to carry on the various vital functions in an optimal manner, to reproduce itself, to maintain itself in the environment, and to modify the environment and itself in a life-enhancing, or creative, way (Osmond, 1994).

The one-sided mechanist is uncomfortable with these concepts because they seem to introduce purpose into the natural world and to imply some type of psychic dimension even in plants and minerals. Moreover, the mechanist argues that such thinking has been fruitless in scientific research, since science does not deal with purposes but with agents that produce results according to fixed laws. In particular, the theory of evolution, which has been so successful in modern biology, seems to explain all living things purely in terms of agent-causes, that is, the natural selection (without any guiding purpose) of those things most able to reproduce in a given environment.

The fallacy of this mechanistic rejection of teleology is two-fold: (1) the supposition that purpose necessarily implies consciousness in that which tends to a goal and (2) the supposition that the identification of an agent-cause is a sufficient explanation of a process. Teleology simply implies that inherent in agent-causes are tendencies to produce directed or goal-oriented actions and processes. Bertalanffy (1968) and others have shown that homeostatic systems necessarily involve directed and purposeful tendencies controlled by feedback mechanisms. As Bertalanffy states:

> . . . teleological behavior directed towards a characteristic final state or goal is not something off limits for natural science and an anthropomorphic misconception of process which, in themselves, are undirected and accidental. Rather it is a form of behavior which can well be defined in scientific terms and for which the necessary conditions and possible mechanisms can be indicated (p. 46).

In medicine particularly, some have actually wanted to eliminate the term *health* altogether on the grounds that it is normative—a value term rather than a scientific value-free term. Once teleology is admitted, however, then the *goal* becomes the norm or value from which the means to the goal are also evaluated. Having defined human health as optimal functioning and having understood this as the satisfaction of innate and cultural needs or the realization of potentialities, we have defined a norm by which the means to health can be discriminated from what tends toward disease and death, that is, the suppressing or disuse of functions.

Sociologists' View of Health and Illness

A very powerful criticism has been raised against all such definitions of *health* and *disease* by the sociologist Eliot Freidson in his well-known book *Profession of Medicine: A Study of the Sociology of Applied Knowledge* (Freidson, 1971). Beginning with Talcott Parsons (1951), sociologists have been studying the medical profession as the typical profession and have been trying to specify not so much its technical as its *social* function (Aiken, 1986). Eliot Freidson, basing his ideas on the sociology of knowledge of Peter Berger and Thomas Luckmann (1966), develops a theory he calls "the social construction of illness." He grants that some physical disorders such as a broken leg or smallpox, and perhaps some mental ones, are unambiguously and objectively "illness." He emphasizes, however, that these disorders are only a small part of what society considers to be illness and with which the medical profession deals. Freidson maintains that the actual definition of *health* and *disease* in any society is a "social construction" produced by many variable factors and essentially dependent on how society, the medical profession, and the patient behave toward certain phenomena.

Furthermore, Freidson (1971), Conrad and Kern (1981), and other authors emphasize that the tendency in the United States today is to assign the term *illness* to more and more phenomena previously given other labels:

> The medical mode of response to deviance is thus being applied to more and more behavior in our society, much of which has been responded to in quite different ways in the past. In our day, what has been called crime, lunacy, degeneracy, sin, and even poverty in the past is now being called illness, and social policy has been moving toward adopting a perspective appropriate to the imputation of illness. Chains have been struck off and everywhere health professionalism has been raised to legitimate the claim that the proper management of deviance is "treatment" in the hands of responsible and skilled professionals. The labels of sin and crime being removed, what is done to the deviant is likely to be said to be done for his own good, done to help him rather than punish him, even though the treatment itself may constitute a deprivation under ordinary circumstances. His own opinions about his treatment are discounted because he is said to be a layman who lacks the special knowledge and detachment that would qualify him to have his voice heard (Friedson, 1971, pp. 249–50).

If the sociologists are correct, it seems extremely unjust for a society thus arbitrarily to label persons sick because they do not conform to average behavior in that society. Consequently, some people today are demanding that society cease to label any behavior sick or abnormal unless it is obviously dangerous to others. The psychoanalyst Thomas Szasz, whom Freidson quotes with approval, argues that drug addiction and alcoholism should be treated not as diseases but as personal preferences that, if they do any harm, harm only the addict. Similarly, the American Psychiatric Association has removed homosexuality from its list of mental illnesses to avoid stigmatizing the homosexual, whose behavioral tendencies should simply be considered personal preferences (Marmoc, 1980; R. Bayer, 1987).

Some advocates of blind, deaf, crippled, and otherwise handicapped persons even claim that to consider these conditions as less "normal" than able-bodiedness is to stigmatize the disabled and to make their adjustment to their situation more difficult. It is certainly very important to educate the public not to fear persons with such problems, to fully respect their human dignity and rights, and to assist them in living normal lives; nevertheless, denial of disability does not solve the problems they face, but rather amplifies them. Nor does it do much to use euphemistic terms for disabilities, since these euphemisms soon become stigmatizing. Frank acknowledgment of a problem is far healthier, when accompanied by a deep realization that human dignity does not depend on being "just like everybody else."

Thus the approach of Freidson, Szasz, and others, although undoubtedly very useful in uncovering the social processes by which definitions of health and normality are constructed in different cultures, prompts the question of whether all definitions of health are simply cultural artifacts. Obviously, this question raises a broad epistemological issue about *cultural relativism*. Even Freidson, however, admits that some conditions (e.g., broken bones) can be determined as abnormal by objective criteria that are transcultural. His real point is that such definitions are too readily used to cover other conditions that are only *analogously* diseases.

Analogy is a necessary mode of thought and dangerous only when it is not recognized as such. This book deliberately extends the term *health* from its strict medical application at the biological level to the other dimensions of the human personality. This seems necessary to do justice to the wholeness of the human person, who can be sick in many different but closely interrelated ways. At the same time, we have tried to avoid the pitfalls pointed out by Freidson and Szasz by clearly distinguishing the different analogical uses of health and disease in the four dimensions of human personality and to indicate the different criteria of normality appropriate to each. The application of such varied criteria is not always easy or unambiguous or free from arbitrary social construction. With due respect for the cautions of the sociologists of knowledge, however, we hope to improve constantly our transcultural statements of these criteria.

2.2 BIOLOGICAL HEALTH AND BIOLOGISM

This book cannot present even a sketch of the biological criteria of health and human functioning so well known to health care professionals. Biological and medical science are constantly making new discoveries about the tissues, organs, and secretions that constitute the human body—their genetic composition, structure, functional interrelations, and control of their differentiation, development, and modification through the environment and individual biography.

The important question for health care ethics is how this biological level of functioning can be considered truly human and personal, as having profound moral and spiritual significance. Dualistic theories of the human being have been present in all cultures throughout human history (Ashley, 1995). According to these theories, body and soul are in essential conflict with each other (i.e., the biological and psychological levels of human functioning versus the ethical and spiritual levels). Generally, the body is regarded as the negative factor and the soul as the positive factor.

Underestimating the plausibility of this dualistic anthropology would be a mistake (Smythies, 1989). The body is frequently experienced as a burden, as something negative, for two reasons. First, a great part of biological functioning is involuntary and deterministic. People cannot voluntarily control much of what goes on inside them. Even with medical advances, biological life is veiled in mystery. Often uncontrollable, such life becomes deranged and fails human purposes. People find themselves weary and exhausted, unable to do what they would like to do. Suffering from pain and disease, people are painfully conscious that eventually the body becomes subject to age and ultimate failure in death. Thus the body appears as a burden, a liability.

Second, the basic biological drives are urgent, constant, and inescapable—the need for sleep, the fear of insecurity, the demands of hunger and thirst, and the tension of sexual desire. They are so insistent that people feel them as compulsions, limiting their freedom and sometimes overwhelming them against their will.

Since the dignity of human personhood consists essentially in self-understanding and freedom, we find it profoundly humiliating to be the helpless victims of our own bodies, with their limited energies, liability to pain, and their urgent and deterministic demands that arise from unconscious depths and disorganize our self-possession and freedom of action. Our bodies seem to drag us down to the animal level of unfree, instinctive, and blind action. In all religious mythologies this pull is often typified in the fear of sexuality as a regression to the primitive chaos (Highwater, 1990). The sex drive has always seemed especially mysterious; it subordinates the freedom of the individual to the imperious needs of the species. People feel severely disturbed at times by sexual passion, reduced to the level of the animal in heat, and deluded by a promise of pleasure that is very brief and that may be followed by pregnancy, childbirth, and family responsibility. Thus the woman, whose biological functioning is more profoundly determined than the man's by the processes of menstruation, pregnancy, childbirth, and nursing and who in the human species is the more attractive or stimulating partner for sexual activity, is in most cultures mistakenly regarded as somehow negative in contrast to the positive male, who is freer of such biological limitations for other activities.

Thus it is understandable that dualism is so widespread (Foster, 1989). Dualism is essential to certain religious systems (Buddhism, Gnosticism, and Manicheism) and has affected all of them (the Neo-Platonic influences in Jewish, Christian, and Muslim theologies). In the extreme form (Manicheism), the body is thought of as intrinsically evil (Runciman, 1982). In more moderate forms, the body is simply thought of as negative. One might think that such dualistic views are no longer common, since modern society emphasizes the value of sensual pleasure, the dependence of psychic functions on the body, and the equality of male and female.

Today, however, dualism is reappearing under new forms. Thus some sociobiologists (Smythies, 1989) have interpreted the theory of evolution to imply that, in relation to the present environment, the human body is archaic and outmoded. This body was formed by evolution for a primitive environment where human beings had to be highly aggressive and very fertile to survive. Thus the body is badly adapted to modern artificial culture, in which aggressive drives lead to war and antisocial violence, and excessive sexual drives and fertility lead to overpopulation and neurosis. This view has also been supported by Sigmund Freud's belief that a basic antipathy exists between the demands of civilization and the human being's basic drives, and it results in the liability to severe neuroses. To this Freud also added the notion of the death wish, an innate tendency of human beings to regress to the primitive and to ultimate extinction of the individual in the universal rhythm of nature (Freud, 1920).

Armed with these ideas, and especially since overpopulation is an increasing threat, many modern theorists are convinced that the biological level of human life is a threat to human freedom (Hardin, 1993) and must be brought under radical control. Many think of the poor and the people of the Third World as primitives—living an instinctive, almost animal life and reproducing "recklessly" as do rabbits. They also think of the traditional feminine role of the mother and housewife as having this limited, unfree, and subhuman character. They therefore propose that the truly human life for men and women should be similar to what upper-class men have always enjoyed, in which biological activities, especially sexuality, are reduced to simple entertainment to be used or not used at will.

From such discussions one can easily conclude that the facts of human biology as such have no moral significance but derive their moral meaning from the context of culture as a product of human invention and choice. Consequently, many theologians (C. Curran, 1984; Kosnik et al., 1977; J. McNeill, 1976) claim that traditional moral theologians went too far when they attempted to establish moral norms on the basis of a distinction between behavior that is natural and behavior that is unnatural for human beings considered as biological organisms. Such faulty arguments, they say, can be rejected as vitiated by the "fallacy of biologism" or "physicalism." On the other hand, defenders of such traditional positions (e.g., Grisez, 1993; John Paul II, 1993) emphasize the opposite danger of a new dualism in which the animal and the rational aspects of human beings are seen as unrelated or even inimical (Ashley, 1996).

It is fallacious to argue that the moral character of human behavior can be settled simply by asking biologists what is natural or unnatural to animals or even to human beings. The important distinction between the moral and the physical specifications of an act are discussed in 8.1. The morality of any act must be considered in the context of the activity of the human person as a whole, since the biological level of function is only one level of the total system. Conversely, however, this consideration means that the moral or social meaning of a human act cannot be indifferent or neutral to its biological character. Every human act is an act of the whole person, involving spiritual, social, psychological, and biological dimensions. Every human biological function has human (and therefore spiritual and social) significance and, conversely, even the most spiritual activities involve the body and must respect the structure and functioning of the body.

Unity of the Person

A sounder approach to the issue of assessing biological activity as related to free human decision can be found in the Aristotelian tradition, which, in opposition to Platonic dualism, stressed the unity of the human person, of which body and soul are only complementary aspects. Theologians of all the great monotheistic religions (Judaism, Christianity, and Islam) have insisted that this unity is a necessary implication of the doctrine of the creation of the human person by God and of the resurrection of the body. These theologians also have rejected the notion of reincarnation found in polytheistic religions because it seems to imply that the human person is a purely spiritual being and the body only its prison or a garment to be changed. Christianity goes even further by insisting on the Incarnation (through which God becomes truly a human being in bodily existence) and on the Indwelling of the Holy Spirit in the human body as its temple, through which believers become members of the Body of Christ. This same principle leads to the sacramental concept of the human body by which the basic biological functions become signs of spiritual events; birth is reenacted in baptism, eating and drinking in the eucharist, and sexual union in the sacrament of matrimony.

Christian theology, however, recognizes a certain measure of truth in body–soul dualism that can be reconciled with the fundamental unity of the human person. The human person is a complex unity in which conflicts can arise, so that the integration and self-individuation of any man or woman can be achieved only by discipline and a sane asceticism. Such asceticism, however, does not imply that the human body in its biological functions is evil or of little value, but rather that it shares in the spiritual dignity of the total person and therefore needs to be integrated with the other dimensions of human personality (Van Kaam, 1985). Thus the body cannot be suppressed, ruthlessly sacrificed to higher values, or even trivialized as of no moral significance. Instead, Catholic theology has always been concerned to find a middle way between the dualistic extremes of asceticism and antinomianism and to respect the intrinsic teleology of bodily structures and basic biological functions.

2.3 THE HIGHER LEVELS OF HEALTH

The development of modern psychotherapy and of psychosomatic medicine leaves no doubt that, although mental health is intimately connected with physical health, it is not identical with physical health (Moyers, 1993). Chapter 12 states more precisely what this differentiation and interdependence are. It suffices at this point to grant that such a difference exists, since mental disease is not describable in terms of physiological malfunction but in terms of impairment in the characteristic human ability to deal with the environment by *symbolic* activity and communication.

Human beings far surpass animals in the capacity to use symbols (images, feelings, and words) that stand for realities but that can be combined and ordered in many ways that are different from the relatively fixed order of real things. The images and concepts by which a human being represents the world do so only imperfectly, but they can be verified and refined by the use of them as tools to change the world. Physical disease, especially dysfunctions of the central nervous system, can impair this symbolic activity, but it also can be disturbed by social and educational factors within the symbolic realm itself. For example, a physiologically healthy child can acquire prejudiced ways of perceiving reality and neurotic ways of reacting to it emotionally through his or her social environment. This environment cannot be adequately described as just bodies in time and space; it must also be described as a symbolic communication system.

At this level of symbolic or psychic activity, however, there are also differentiated levels of health and disease that are too often lumped together. To reduce human psychic health to emotional adjustment and maturity is a typical fallacy today that can be termed *psychologism*. Psychologism assumes that a physically healthy person who also is free of mental illnesses, which are considered the proper competency of psychotherapy, is totally healthy (Vitz, 1994).

As Chapter 12 shows, psychotherapy has the modest goal of helping patients acquire that degree of self-understanding and emotional integration that will free them from unconscious psychological determinisms that interfere with daily practical life. Psychologically healthy persons are "in touch with their feelings." They perceive the world of ordinary activity as most people do, without manifestly absurd illusions or projections. They are free to choose between practical alternatives and do not have unrealistic expectations. They are responsible for the consequences of their actions.

At this point of freedom from psychological determination, a whole new level of human activity opens up: the level of free, responsible, *moral* activity. Psychotic persons are incapable of moral action (at least within the area of the psychosis), whereas neurotic persons are severely limited in their freedom and responsibility. Only the free man or woman is a person fully capable of either moral good or evil. Don Browning (1983) pointed out that problems of ethical counseling are often confused with those of psychological counseling. Many clergy today seem to have abandoned their traditional role of helping people make ethical decisions and have become amateur psychotherapists.

It is also possible to fall into the fallacy of *moralism*. This error reduces human failure to questions of right and wrong, attributes either mental or physical disease to the victims' sins, and attempts to heal them by moral exhortations. The reaction of many people to the AIDS epidemic follows this pattern of thought. A more subtle form of this same fallacy is the assumption that the highest wholeness in the human personality is achieved at the level of practical ethical life. Some people identify the good person with the responsible, prudent, decent man or woman.

This fallacy ignores the deepest and most central fact of the human personality—the aspect that is spiritual, intuitive, and creative (Ashley, 1995). Some psychotherapists of the Jungian and existentialist schools do concern themselves with this level, but only to free such activity from neurotic and psychotic impediments. To deal with this spiritual level of human existence in its own terms is the task of neither the psychologist nor the moralist, but of the philosopher, theologian, and spiritual guide as Chapter 14 shows. Spiritual health and disease, therefore, cannot be reduced simply to moral or psychological terms.

Even at this spiritual level it is possible to fall into the fallacy of what the philosopher Jacques Maritain (1929) called "angelism"—treating human persons as bodiless angels, or pure souls, as Plato and Descartes conceived the true human self. Human problems cannot be treated in purely spiritual terms, in which the lower levels of functioning, human physiology, human symbolic activity, and human practical responsibility are ignored. Today it seems that this fallacy has influenced those mystical and religious enthusiasts who attempt to heal all bodily, psychological, and moral ills by purely spiritual means.

Thus trying to understand the fullness of human health requires being on guard against those reductionist fallacies that ignore health's many dimensions. For example, to determine whether alcoholism is a sickness without reductionism or arbitrary social construction, first alcoholism must be defined in behavioral terms and then four questions must be asked. First, is it a biological disease in terms of biological criteria, for example, a change in physiology that puts a strain on biological homeostasis? Second, is alcoholism a psychological disease in terms of psychological criteria, for example, a persistent emotional conflict that restricts the victim's capacity for intelligent free choice? Third, is it a moral disease in terms of social criteria, for example, free choice of behavior that is contradictory to the full actualization of the person in community? Fourth, is alcoholism a spiritual disease by spiritual criteria, for example, closure to intuition, creativity, and commitment? Moreover, how are these different levels of functioning interrelated? The terms *disease* and *health* are used at each of these levels in very different but analogous ways.

CONCLUSION

The etymology of the word "health" indicates that health is derived from holiness or wholeness. Today, health is usually used in regard to human function. If human function is measured by physiological tests and computerized calculation, then the average of these functions is presented as normal or healthy function. A more realistic notion of optimal functioning begins with the personal capacities of an individual. In this perspective, health is the state of being in which an individual does the best with the capacities he has and acts in a way to maximize his capacities. In assessing human health, recognition must be given to the various levels of human function. The higher levels of human function, the social and creative levels, depend upon the lower levels, the physiological and psychological, but cannot be reduced or explained by these lower levels. To avoid reductionism when assessing health, the interrelation and interaction of the parts and levels of organization in the whole body–soul entity must be considered.

To be healthy, a living being must interact with its environment and maintain itself in the environment. Humans do this by external activity, for example by creating industries or cities, and by internal activity, for example, by creating language and theoretical explanations of the universe. With this concept of human function in mind, it is clear why the WHO definition of human health extends far beyond mere biological function.

Disease may be considered as an ontological entity which can be classified and named, as are plants and animals, or as an entity which results from the breakdown of the physiological harmony of the organic system because of hyper- or hypofunctioning of an organ. The central traditional medicine reconciles these two extreme concepts.

The mechanistic theory, which tends to reduce human health to the function of unrelated organs, is popular today. Mechanistics are more comfortable with anatomy or structure than with functions or process. Their diagnoses tend toward ontologistic views in which the disease results from alien bacteria or organic lesions. In treatment they tend to reduce purpose, they incline toward a mechanical adjustment of parts by surgery or use of a specific drug. One of the factors that contributes to a mechanistic view of disease is a fear of teleology. Teleology predicates a goal-directed activity leading toward optimal functioning. This is what the Greeks meant by *nature*. Teleology does not deny the separate agent-cause, favored in scientific explanation by mechanistics, but simply implies that agent-causes have purposeful tendencies controlled by feedback mechanisms.

In the latter part of the twentieth century, sociologists have been influential in the study of the medical profession, health, and disease. According to sociological concepts, the actual definition of health and disease in any society is a social construction produced by many variable factors and dependent on how the medical profession and society behave in face of certain phenomena. While sociologists point out the cultural aspects of illness and disease, the concepts do not weaken the objective notion of illness and disease, the experience of dysfunction, and personal conviction that "something is wrong."

The criteria for biological health are many and are beyond the purpose of this study. The important question for health care ethics is how the biological level of function can be considered personal, free, and truly human. Dualism does not answer this question. Rather the Biblical and Aristotelian concept of the unity of the human person, spirit and body, must be invoked. In this concept the body and spirit are complementary powers. In opting for the unity of the human person, however, Christian theology does not deny that conflicts can arise between body and spirit, so that integration of body and soul demands discipline and asceticism.

Mental health is intimately connected with physical health but is not identified with it. Mental illness is described as impairment of the person in dealing with the environment by symbolic activity and communication. In assessing human health, it is clear that persons need more than emotional maturity in order to be truly healthy. When one is free from psychological determination, the level of free responsible moral activity opens up. Only the person who is free from psychotic or neurotic determination is capable of moral good or evil.

The deepest and most central function of the human person, and thus the deepest level of human health, is the spiritual or creative level. Spiritual health and disease cannot be reduced to moralism or psychologism. Thus striving for human health, especially at the most profound levels of human function, requires that we avoid reductionism that ignores the many dimensions of human health.

3
Personal Responsibility for Health

OVERVIEW

Chapter 1 points out that person and community are correlative terms and that community has some responsibility for enabling its members to pursue health at every level of human need or function. Chapter 2 explains further that this responsibility includes biological health, as well as the higher levels of human functioning that depend on it. However, the primary responsibility for a person's health rests on the individual, not upon the community, even though the community has a serious responsibility to support individuals in their quest for health. In this chapter, after considering the need of each person to take responsibility for his or her health (3.1), we explain the implications of this responsibility for daily life (3.2) and the meaning of stewardship (3.3). Having discussed some of the activity pertaining to the pursuit of health, we then consider the elements required to exercise personal responsibility by making prudent decisions in regard to health care. Because Catholics believe that one element in forming a prudent conscience involves "thinking with the Church," we will examine the various ways in which the Church teaches. Another element in forming a prudent conscience is the process of obtaining informed consent, which will also be considered in section 3.4. Finally, we delineate the rights of patients which enable people to exercise personal responsibility for health (3.5).

3.1 THE PERSON AND HEALING

Biological health concerns what is most individual and private to me, namely, my own body. My body, by its very materiality, its space–time limitations, is mine and mine alone. It identifies me as *not* anybody else. Someone can share a room with me, a table, a bed, even my clothes, but that person cannot truly share my body. Sexual partners exchange the right to use each other's bodies sexually (in biblical language, they become "one flesh," Mk 10:8), but even this intimate union has its limits. Ultimately, it is by reason of my body that I am alone in myself, but it is also by reason of my body that I am in the world of things and persons (B. Ashley, 1996; Shalom, 1985).

My body is profoundly subjective not only because I possess it as my own and know it as myself, but because it is incommunicable. Much of what occurs in my body is hidden even from me; even what I know of it, I know for the most part in a thoroughly subjective way such that I cannot express it. When I consult a physician, I experience the difficulty of relating how I feel. Bodily feelings are vivid, yet so vague and so hard to put into words. I am left frustrated and stammering because no one else can really know how I feel. I am the only final judge of whether I really feel well. When no medical test reveals anything wrong with me, but I do not feel well, then I *am* not well.

Even if my sickness is not physiological but imaginary, that imaginary sickness is real at the psychological level and is a psychological illness (Thompson, 1988). At that level, the criterion of health for the psychotherapist is how the client really feels about himself or herself—it is the depth feelings underlying the surface feelings. At the higher ethical and spiritual levels, health also depends on an individual's own conscience or spiritual discernment. Thus no one but the person ultimately can judge his or her own interior well-being.

Furthermore, this subjectivity is true not only of diagnosis, but also of treatment. The psychotherapist constantly has to remind the client: "No one, ultimately, can help you if you refuse to help yourself." Even the ethical and spiritual counselor must say, "God will help you by his grace, but you must open yourself to that grace." Jesus says in Revelations 3:20: "Here I stand, knocking at the door. If anyone hears me calling and opens the door, I will enter his house and have supper with him, and he with me."

Healing is a living process that must occur within the organism. Near the end of life patients may be unconscious and purely passive to the surgery, medication, and injections thrust on them, but these treatments seldom result in healing. Convalescence is an active process on the part of patients, and staying well is clearly something that they alone must do. No physician or nurse can make patients take pills, stick to a diet, or take necessary rest and exercise.

In a profound way the will to life and health is the fundamental element in all healing, and this will to life must be intelligent, that is, a realistic search for the means to health. A noted surgeon once said that he dreaded operating on patients who doubted their chances of recovery because in his experience such patients did *not* recover. Most physicians and nurses seem to believe that the patient's fighting spirit is a critical factor in recovering health (Kaplan, 1991).

Therefore, whether working to prevent sickness, to maintain optimal health, to assist recovery from disease, or to rehabilitate oneself after a crippling trauma, a person must make a personal commitment to life and health. It might seem that no special commitment needs to be made, since everyone has an instinct to live. No doubt the need to live, to grow, and to function well is innate; it is the very teleology of any organism. In the human person, however, whose inmost depth of being is not instinctive but free, this commitment is not a given; rather, it must be freely made by the person. Are there not persons who make the opposite commitment to suicide in open or hidden form?

Karl Menninger, in his classic book *Man Against Himself* (1938), has shown that suicide is only the last step of an intensifying process of self-destruction, of hatred turned away from external objects and toward the self. To assist suicide out of a mistaken notion of compassion is to cooperate in this self-hatred.

Clinically, patients who attempt suicide often have a long previous record of psychosomatic illnesses, such as hypertension or ulcers, and of "accidents." Unconsciously, they have been self-committed to death rather than to life.

This unconscious commitment to death means that everything associated with the medical profession becomes attractive to some neurotic or psychotic persons and symbolizes their own unconscious drives. They often seduce medical professionals into satisfying their morbid needs. They seem to enjoy being sick or at least to enjoy constant complaining, obscure ailments, medication, and even painful procedures. A life otherwise empty is at least filled with the drama of disease and therapy. Physicians and nurses may be tempted to pander to these patients, both because of financial gain and because it is flattering to be needed (codependency). In the home, such a neurotic person may induce the whole family to build its life around "tender loving care." One can only wonder whether the tremendous preoccupation of modern American society with the drama of medicine, as displayed on television and in novels, is not evidence that this neurosis has become social as well as individual.

The same neuroses appear in the social and spiritual arenas of politics and religion. Jesus attacked the legalism of some of the Pharisees of his time because these people, who were both political and religious guides, had imposed a moralistic scrupulosity that expressed self-destructive guilt. Puritan and Victorian morality exhibited similar tendencies. In the spiritual sphere, such seductions are reflected in extreme dualistic asceticism with its hatred of the body, the self, and the world. Psychotherapists often are antireligious because they have been so shocked by the way in which moralistic religion seems to have maimed some of their patients.

Neurosis, however, is a counterfeit normality, and it is absurd to blame either medicine or religion as such for these aberrations, however widespread. Surgeons are not usually sadists, although sadism is unconsciously present in a few surgeons and leads to needless surgery. The clergy are not moral sadists, although unconscious sadism may be found in moralistic sermons, unsound ascetical practices, and aberrant rituals.

Affirmation of Life

The commitment to life, which overcomes such commitments to death, is an affirmation of the value not only of pleasure, but also of freedom, intelligence, creativity, and love (John Paul II, 1995). As Yahweh says through Moses:

> I call heaven and earth today to witness against you: I have set before you life and death, the blessing and the curse. Choose life, then, that you and your descendants may live, by loving the Lord, your God, heeding his voice, and holding fast to him. For that will mean life for you, a long life for you to live on the land which the Lord swore he would give to your fathers Abraham, Isaac, and Jacob (Dt 30:19–20).

Such a commitment to life has to proceed from the spiritual level, although it is ordinarily manifest at lower levels as well. This deep commitment can be so blocked that persons profoundly dedicated to life in their spiritual center can yet suffer from an unconscious will to death at the psychological level (Marmer, 1988).

The Old Testament presents the Jewish view as profoundly life-affirming. It constantly emphasizes the idea that God gives his friends health, security, children, and long life and that God has created men and women for life and wishes to prolong it for them. Faced by the fact that just persons often suffer persecution and martyrdom, the last books of the Old Testament affirm that God will raise his friends from the dead to everlasting life (see 2 Mc 7:27–29). Jesus approved by saying, "God is God of the living, not of the dead" (Mk 12:27). St. Paul also teaches (Rm 5:12 ff.) that death (and by implication disease and aging) is somehow a consequence of sin (see Ws 1:13–15). Thus disease, aging, and death are not willed by God but only permitted by him as a punishment, the inevitable consequence of the sin of the human race, which has committed itself to death rather than to life. St. Paul joyfully affirms that in Christ all may be born again to everlasting life.

When Jesus prayed in the garden, "O, Father, you have the power to do all things. Take this cup away from me. But let it be as you would have it, not as I" (Mk 14:36), he was affirming his own commitment to life. He was also expressing his willingness, however, to endure death if the Father in his transcendent wisdom knew that only through death could doubting men and women be convinced that God and his Son truly love them for their own sake and not for the sake of honor or power.

Thus a sound theology teaches that the Father and Christ desire only life, a desire that is fulfilled in the Resurrection. Following Jesus, who as St. Paul says, was "never anything but 'Yes' " (2 Co 1:20), Christians must always affirm life while being willing to endure the evil of death: (1) as witnesses to others that faith, hope, and love cannot be overcome by the fear and despair of death and (2) as sharers in Jesus' experience of death, by which we learn to be as unselfish, trustful, and hopeful as he was. The Christian, however, endures death serenely not because death is good, but because resurrection and eternal life are good and destroy death forever.

Also, when Christians feel as St. Paul did in prison, when he longed "to be dissolved and to be with Christ" (Ph 1:23), they are not rejecting life but longing to be freed of the barriers that constrict the fullness of life. A Christian can long for death as an inevitable crisis that has to be lived through to achieve full health and life, not as a Freudian regression to the peace of the womb.

Thus it is essential to realize that Christian health care should never be directed to the passive acceptance of disease or death, as if these in themselves were somehow spiritual goods (OSSI, 1994). Even a distinguished medical historian such as Henry Sigerist (1951) errs in thinking that Christianity thought of sickness as sacred. In authentic Christian belief, every individual has a responsibility to choose life and to fight for it. Christians must fight for a full and abundant life and must accept disease and death only as inevitable incidents in the battle, but not as its final outcome (John Paul II, 1995). Christian acceptance or resignation is not acquiescence, but rather a strategy by which good can be brought out of evil. Sometimes the enemy can be defeated only by patience, turning these evils into opportunities for growth and learning; however, sickness and death should always be perceived as enemies. Christians should stand with St. Paul in condemning death as the ultimate evil: "and the last enemy to be destroyed is death" (1 Co 15:26), especially if *death* is understood as the destruction of the human whole, that is, physical, psychological, moral, and above all, spiritual death.

Spiritual death is nothing more than the commitment to this total death. Deliberately turning from the love of God and neighbor toward a false self-sufficiency is spiritual suicide. This self-sufficiency is so contradictory to the very nature of all persons, to their expansion into community, that this refusal to ask for any help can only end in prideful despair. Physical suicide probably seldom has this character of total death, since usually it seems to be an attempt to escape to some better life or at least to peace and sleep. Spiritual suicide is possible, however, if a person shuts off all others and considers himself or herself entirely self-sufficient.

The person who has made a spiritual commitment to life will strive to achieve wholeness in every dimension of personality. Some are so deceived by dualism that they do not realize that spiritual wholeness requires the care of lower human functions. Thus mystics have neglected social development, moral people have neglected psychological and physical health, and those concerned about psychological health have not perceived its intimate connection with both social and biological health. A true understanding of the commitment to life, however, leads to a balanced concern for the whole person.

3.2 PREVENTIVE MEDICINE AND LIFESTYLE

Personal responsibility for health is often thought of as just going to a physician, but this is only a part of it (Sider and Clements, 1984; Manning et al., 1991). The famous ancient dictum attributed to Hippocrates was that the physician should prescribe "regimen, medicine, and surgery" in that order, meaning by *regimen* the person's lifestyle of diet, rest, and exercise (Edelstein, 1967). Today medical science is largely in the curative stage rather than the preventive stage. In the future perhaps the emphasis will shift from the hospital to a center for teaching persons how to improve their lifestyles (Sanders, 1994). Advances in preventive medicine have mainly taken the form of ridding the environment of infectious diseases and disease carriers. Very few advances have been made to remove environmental pollutants. Civilized human beings, especially those in the twentieth century, seem to be subjecting themselves to more and more unknowns while relying on medicine and surgery to remedy the harm done (Grimes, 1993). A look at current lifestyles in terms of physiological and psychological norms is appalling in view of the extremely unhealthy kinds of lives many people lead.

First, modern life often leaves insufficient time for *rest*, not merely in the sense of lack of sleep, but also in the sense of too much stress. People might seem to have more leisure because machines have relieved them of much hard, servile labor. However, this relief is more than offset by the strange routine of urban life that forces us, for example, to spend hours a day driving to and from work in the hazards of traffic. Clearly, as individuals, people are powerless to escape this system, but within it they do have some freedom to make choices that will gradually give their lives greater simplicity and more natural rhythm, free of excessive competition and the drive for success.

Reduced stress also will contribute to moral and spiritual health by making room for a contemplative atmosphere, for service rather than for ambition for power, for solitude and silence, as well as for more time to give to persons and less to things. In the past men and women suffered from the burden of manual work, from fear of enemies, from disease and hunger, but there remained something of the natural rhythm of effort and rest. Today these natural rhythms are often broken up by artificial pressures and hectic overstimulation. As Rordorf (1982) and Kiesling (1970) note, Jewish and Christian cultural traditions were profoundly shaped by the divine command to keep holy the day of rest and reflection (Ex 20:3–12; Mk 2:27).

A stressful life can lead to addiction, the enslavement of human beings to the pursuit of intense pleasure, or anesthesia as an escape from the pain of life. Not only is this addiction to be found in hard drugs, but also in smoking, alcohol, and tranquilizers (Stroebe and Stroebe, 1995). It is found in milder form in the common addiction to overeating and in a particularly corrosive way in the anxious twentieth-century pursuit of sexual pleasure. In moderation, none of these things is unhealthy, but in addictive form they become obsessive and destructive (Van Kaam, 1983). The U.S. population suffers from many physical and psychological illnesses as a result of these addictions. AIDS and venereal disease are not a negligible problem; however, sexual addiction may have more serious consequences at the psychological and social levels because it promotes behavior that stands in the way of true interpersonal love or loyalty and subverts the human social order traditionally based on the family (Carnes, 1983). Finally, many persons today lack proper physical exercise. Although sports are highly cultivated, they are more watched than played by the average man and woman. The average person does little manual work and seldom walks or jogs.

To assume personal responsibility for health, therefore, requires a scientifically based knowledge of hygiene, good diet, rest, exercise, and moderation. These cannot be imposed from without. People need to design their lives to meet personal requirements, which differ greatly. To be healthy, one's lifestyle must express one's true personality, not a false one or a resignation to being half alive (Aday, 1993).

The problems of mental health are similar. Today people are overstimulated by sensation and passive imagination but impoverished in active imagination, reflection, and meditation. They receive much input, much information, but often little integration of symbols and feelings. They live at the top of their heads, out of touch with their feelings.

Concerning spiritual life, many persons today live without clear commitments or goals and suffer from the emptiness, meaninglessness, and absurdity of life in loneliness, never seeking deep-level communication with others (R. May, 1983). A deceptive kind of pseudohealth is sometimes observed in the comfortable, modern personality whose life is filled with satisfactions when whole anxieties have been alleviated by psychotherapy (Rieff, 1968).

Although each person has a fundamental responsibility for his or her health, some factors detrimental to health are often beyond personal control (Goodman and Goodman, 1986). Some of these factors arise from social situations. For example, workers in an asbestos factory cannot protect themselves from asbestos. But more frequently, the factors that cause illness arise from personal characteristics beyond our control. For example, the results of the Genome Project to date indicate that we may be disposed to certain illnesses by reason of our genetic makeup (Kevles and Hood, 1992). Hence, when we posit a responsibility to maintain and pursue health, we add the qualification "insofar as it is in our human power."

3.3 STEWARDSHIP AND CREATIVITY

"Be fruitful and multiply; fill the earth and subdue it. Have dominion over the fish of the sea, the birds of the air, and all living things on earth" (Gn 1:28). Some ecological enthusiasts have placed on this one verse the blame for the technological ravagement of the natural environment. In the next chapter of Genesis, however, another tradition reports, "The Lord God took the man and settled him into the Garden of Eden to cultivate and care for it" (2:15). Thus, although humankind is lord of lesser creatures, nevertheless its dominion over them and over itself is only a *stewardship* for which human beings remain responsible to the One Lord (John Paul II, 1995).

Classical theology based Christian ethics on the conviction that God endowed all human beings with one common nature, which remains essentially the same throughout all history, from Adam and Eve to the Last Judgment. Human beings are stewards of this nature, as they are of the world in which God has placed them. By studying the God-given structure and dynamics of this nature, it is possible, so theologians in the past thought, to formulate unchanging moral norms binding for every time and culture. Stewardship demanded that human beings abide by these norms lest they destroy the garden of the world and the temple of their own bodies, which were given them to "cultivate and care for."

Today this traditional concept of stewardship is often criticized as follows:

First, since theologians generally accept the view that the Creator produced the human race by an evolutionary process, they have to take into account the fact that human beings are not finished masterpieces but rather a work in progress. Thus it is no insult to God's creative wisdom for people to suppose that they can further perfect the world and even their own bodies. Indeed, it is to God's praise that he has generously called them to be co-workers with him in his creative task.

Second, human behavior is the result of natural instinct and of culture and social determinism. Human nature exists not in the abstract but in the flux of human history and of individual biographies, where it seems subject to endless variations. How, then, can a universal definition of human nature that is more than an empty commonplace be formulated?

Third, with the rise of modern technology, for the first time in history human beings have achieved a real dominion over nature. In principle, at least, the discovery of the deoxyribonucleic acid (DNA) molecule opens the way for producing life and controlling evolution. Moreover, scientists are acquiring mastery of the building blocks out of which all material things are made and may soon tap the sources of energy that will make it possible to reconstruct the world.

The ethical implication of these discoveries seems to be that ethical norms can no longer be based on human nature because that nature itself becomes a matter of people's choosing (Francoeur, 1972). People may be able to select from among various models of human nature the ones they prefer to construct, just as they do between various models of houses. The prophecy of Karl Marx and Frederick Engel in 1848 that humankind will become its own creator seems to be coming true (Hook 1953). Perhaps human beings can even learn to reverse the aging process and make themselves immortal. Then they will no longer be stewards but creators.

Scientific Doubts

Of course the biblical story of the Tower of Babel (Gn 11:1–9) and the Greek myth of Prometheus stealing fire from the gods are evidence that this dream is not new. Before people totally succumb to it, they should take into account certain doubts expressed by scientists themselves. First, it must be noted that these predictions of unlimited human dominion over nature are less convincing now than they were a few years ago when atomic fission and the genetic code were discovered. The ecological crisis has revealed that modern technology in its present form has its limits (Hare, 1987). Every technological advance exacts its price in environmental pollution and depletion of energy resources. Moreover, since evolution has adapted human nature very nicely to its primitive environment, neither that nature nor that environment can be altered without serious risks. Humankind always has to proceed strategically, trying to gain a little more than is lost (Rescher, 1980).

Again, the proposals for genetic engineering, which Chapter 11 discusses from an ethical viewpoint, have yielded some results (Culver, 1993), but to date there is little evidence of extensive therapeutic effect (Leiden, 1995). Therapy for genetic shortcomings lies in the future; beyond the discovery of these anomalies (BMA, 1992). Science has grasped certain basic principles of life, but these principles operate in life systems that are bafflingly complex. The details will be unraveled painfully by long and often frustrating research, as the slow progress in understanding cancer exemplifies.

Furthermore, one ultimate limiting factor is still very little understood. Since human creative intelligence depends on the human brain, any alterations of body structure that might injure the brain will be disastrously self-defeating. Can the human brain be significantly improved? So far as is known, the human brain is the most complex system in the universe. To build it would require far more information than to construct any other system, even the most complex computers so far invented. The brain is relatively very small, however, and unlike a computer, it is capable of self-development and some self-repair. As human beings think, they constantly restructure brain circuitry at the synaptic level (G. Edelman, 1987; Rosenfield, 1987; Blackeslee, 1995).

Perhaps, although some speculate about its future, the human brain is already near the limit of evolution. Thus any kind of improvement that can be made in the rest of the human body must be limited by the requirements of the brain. No doubt people could be turned into brain-persons by replacing most of the other body systems with artificial organs to support the life of the brain. The brain could be fed with information and be allowed to transmit its orders electronically. However, this would eliminate much of the imaginative and affective life that plays so important a part in motivation and interpersonal relations. Would people want, for example, to eliminate sexual reproduction and reduce sex to orgasms produced by direct stimulation of pleasure centers in the brain? This would indeed make one-dimensional men or women (Marcuse, 1964). Thus the principle of totality and integrity discussed in Chapter 8 warns of the ethical limits to human self-creation.

Although such warnings are in order, it would be wrong to conclude, as do such modern critics of technology as Jacques Ellul (1980), that modern technology is the temptation of the Serpent, a sin of pride and rebellion against the Creator. God would not have endowed human beings with creative intelligence and freedom if he did not want them to share in his creative action. They are divinely called not merely to preserve the old, but to produce the new. In the *Pastoral Constitution on the Church in the Modern World* (Vatican Council II, 1965c), the Second Vatican Council teaches that technology is a gift of God that requires stewardship, as do any other of his gifts.

In creative activity, however, people have to respect their own limits and the limits of the materials with which they must work. These limits are not set by God out of any concern for his own authority. God himself is "limited" by his own wisdom and love, which forbid him to do what is contradictory to his own nature. Human beings are far more limited by the fact that their share in God's knowledge and love is finite. No matter how they may progress in science, freedom, and power, they dare not contradict their own human nature without destroying themselves (Davis, 1991).

At any given moment in history, people's limits are set by their knowledge. Once they understand some aspect of nature well, they can freely choose to improve nature and surpass it. When they lack that understanding, however, their efforts to improve on nature may prove disastrous. The evils of modern technology are not the result of creative use of knowledge, but of rash exploitation of a nature little understood. Above all, people have failed to understand themselves, their authentic needs and potentialities. To acquire the knowledge they need, research and experimentation, with all the risks involved, are necessary, but even here they must proceed with reverence for the persons and the environment that are at risk. Thus, the Christian attitude toward the right use of nature and the human person is one of *stewardship*, as indicated in Jesus' parable of the talents (Mt 25:14–30), in which the master (God) requires of his servants a return on his investments in proportion to how much he entrusted to each. We are required to conserve God's gifts, but also to use them creatively.

3.4 FORMING A PRUDENT CONSCIENCE AND INFORMED CONSENT

Moral Objectivity

To make a good medical decision, physicians must (1) carefully inform them-selves of the facts of the case; (2) recall or research the medical principles that may apply to the case; (3) make the best judgment they can in applying this medical knowledge to the facts of the case; and (4) act on their best judgment. In this process they must be motivated to arrive at a decision which is *objectively* true, i.e., which will correctly diagnose the problem and recommend a truly beneficial treatment. Yet they are acutely aware that although they sincerely desire to do what is objectively right, there is always in human judgments a *subjective* factor that cannot be entirely eliminated. They never know enough, nor are sufficiently free from biases, self-interest, emotional "hang-ups," etc., to arrive at the full truth. Good physicians attempt to overcome this subjectivity in judgment by study, research, consultation with others, criticism of their own mistakes, and a mature knowledge of their own biases. When they have taken these precautions to be objective, then they cannot be blamed if sometimes they make mistakes in medical judgment. At least they did the best they knew how to make an objectively true judgment. On the contrary, physicians who do not make this kind of an effort to be objective have no excuse for their errors.

While ethical judgments are not the same as technical judgments, such as a medical diagnosis and prescription, they are analogous to them. To make a good moral decision, persons must: (1) carefully inform themselves of the facts of the situation; (2) recall or research the ethical principles that may apply to this situation; (3) make the best judgment they can in applying this ethical knowl-edge to the facts of the situation; (4) act on their conscience, i.e., their best judgment of what is helpful or harmful for themselves and others in the com-mon search for true human happiness. Persons must also be motivated by the desire to find the *objective* truth about what is really helpful or harmful, and thus to free themselves as far as possible from the *subjective* factors that might blind them to the truth. If they sincerely attempt to do this, then even if they make a mistake in judgment, they commit no sin, since they did the best they knew how after first doing the best they knew how to find out the objective truth.

Ethical judgments, however, differ from medical judgments or any other kind of technical judgment in a profound way, although both are types of practical knowledge leading to action. Technological knowledge tells us how to act so as produce a certain effect (in the case of medicine, a state of health), but it does not tell us whether we ought to act or not act to produce such an effect in a given situation (Pellegrino and Thomasma, 1981). Physicians know techni-cally how to perform an abortion, but their medical knowledge is not sufficient to tell them whether or not they should actually do so. Thus medical norms (and technological norms in general) are *conditional*; they tell how to act *if* one should act. Ethical norms, on the contrary, are *absolute*; they tell persons that they ought to act or not act when faced with a certain situation. Thus when physicians decide to perform an abortion, they make not only a medical judgment about the probable results of their employment of a medical technique, but also an ethical judgment about whether in fact such an action is morally good or bad.

Therefore, modern medical practice must ask not only, "Can it be done?" but also, "Ought we to do what can be done?" The sociologist Freidson, in his book *Profession of Medicine* (1971), and several ethicists and physicians (Lappe 1987; Pellegrino and Thomasma, 1988) have shown from different points of view that the claim of health care professionals to make absolutely autonomous professional decisions about medical matters is invalid. Their professional knowledge makes them experts about the techniques of medicine, but this does not imply that they are experts in the *use* of these techniques, since this use involves social, political, and moral issues about which they are not necessarily well-informed.

Thus individuals who seek the services of a medical professional cannot simply delegate concrete decisions about their health to that professional on the grounds that the physician knows best. For a woman to consent to an abortion because the physician advises it is to take the advice of someone who has special competence in medicine but not in ethics. On the other hand, neither is the individual competent to decide such a question on her own unless she has adequate information about the medical aspects of the decision. There is thus a certain dilemma in medical decisions: Who has the knowledge of both the ethical norms and the medical facts to make a wise decision? And how are these norms and facts to be related to each other (John Fletcher, 1983)?

Rational and Revealed Moral Norms

In Chapters 7 and 8 we will discuss the different theories about how ethical norms can be formulated in ways that are motivated by a desire for objective truth, rather than simply by emotion, custom, public opinion, or self-interest. Here it is sufficient to point out that today there are two main types of ethics: (1) value systems based on human reason, that is on history, philosophy, and the modern sciences; and (2) value systems based on a religious tradition that claims enlightenment from some supernatural source. We will speak of these respectively as *rational* norms and *revealed* norms, although we must emphasize that there are wide divergences among philosophers and theologians as to what is meant by "reason" and by "revelation."

Secularists accept only rational norms, and either reject revealed norms altogether as irrational or relegate them to the realm of private opinion and object to any insertion of them into debates about public policy (Charlesworth, 1993). For example, they accuse opponents of abortion of "imposing" their religious beliefs on the public.

Religious people, however, while generally they do not reject rational norms totally, do subordinate them to revealed norms. Traditional Protestantism, based on a literal interpretation of the Bible, holds that, although the "order of creation" is knowable by human reason, reason has been so corrupted by sin that it is more likely to lead us astray than to guide us to God's truth. Consequently, they attempt to base their ethics entirely on revealed norms found in the Bible. For example, conservative Protestants argue against abortion by citing the biblical commandment, "Thou shall not kill," yet may accept direct sterilization and contraception because it is not explicitly forbidden in the Bible. Liberal Protestants, on the other hand, much impressed by modern critical biblical scholarship, generally hold that because the ethical norms of the Bible are so historically conditioned, they no longer apply in a literal way to modern problems. Hence these liberals claim that the revealed biblical norms are to be taken only as expressing ideal values, while today actual ethical decisions must be based on reason, i.e., modern psychology, sociology, or philosophy.

Recently some important Catholic moral theologians have adopted positions very close to those of liberal Protestantism. In answer to the question, "Is there a specifically Christian ethics?" they deny there are any ethical norms which are specifically Christian. The Gospel, they say, although it accents certain moral values such as compassion, forgiveness, and the "option for the poor," leaves us free to solve modern problems by the purely rational norms we share with nonbelievers (Curran and McCormick, 1980).

The authoritative teaching of the Catholic Church, however, as expressed in the *Catechism of the Catholic Church* (1994, N. 170 ff.) and the encyclical *The Splendor of Truth* (John Paul II, 1993, N. 4 ff.) teaches that Christians ought to live both by rational and by revealed norms, since:

(1) Although sin has obscured human reason, yet human reason remains able to arrive at objective moral truth. Hence, there is a solid ground for ethical discussion based on reason among believers of all faiths as well as nonbelievers. Hence, moral debates belong to the public as well as the private sphere and can legitimately affect public policy. Catholics in public policy should therefore appeal only to rational moral norms, which are common ground for nonbelievers and believers of any faith.

(2) It is true, however, that original sin and historic sin have greatly disturbed objective reasoning about morality by spreading illusions, confusions, prejudices, and lying propaganda. Consequently, God in his mercy has assisted our moral vision by revealing certain moral norms to us in the Bible and the Tradition of the Catholic Church (e.g., the Ten Commandments, and the Great Commandment of love of God and neighbor) which are valid for all people and all time. These revealed norms may sometimes be the same as rational norms, but by revealing them to faith God enables us to understand them correctly, free of the confusion wrought by sin. Thus the norm "Do not kill the innocent" is a rational norm essential to any system of human rights. The fact that this right to life of the unborn is not recognized by everyone today, as many still do not recognize the equal rights of all races and of women, shows why we also need the light of revelation to confirm our faith in the equal dignity of every human person.

(3) Moreover, in creating us God not only gave us the intelligence and freedom to live a good human, earthly life, but has graciously called us to an infinitely higher life with him in eternity. This goal so exceeds our natural goals known to us by reason, that we cannot attain it without God's help and guidance. Consequently, God has not only corrected and clarified the rational goals by which we live but has also modified them in view of a far higher destiny. Christians should witness to those of other faiths or no faith at all to their own faith in

this higher way of life, but should not impose it on them or attempt to make it a part of public policy. Thus faith tells Catholics that abortion is an evil not only because it violates human rights, but also because it deprives the child of the grace of baptism and the child's mother of the great privilege of cooperating with the Creator in bringing forth a new person for the kingdom of heaven.

Thus Catholic moral theology recognizes three types of moral norms: (1) Revealed norms known only by faith; (2) Rational norms known only by reason; and (3) Rational norms known by reason but confirmed by faith.

Recent Revision of Moral Theology

Vatican II, among its other reforms, sought to free moral theology from the too-legalistic approach which had prevailed in moral theology since the late Middle Ages (Vatican Council II, 1965), especially after the Protestant Reformation which had accused the Catholic Church of fostering moral laxity. To answer this charge the Church encouraged Catholics to go frequently to confession and sponsored the publication of manuals or textbooks for confessors which tended to reduce morality to a kind of ethical code of sins and penalties. Vatican II had no intention of changing the moral norms embodied in these manuals, but it wanted to make their purpose and meaning more intelligible to our times by a return to the biblical and traditional sources of Christian morality, just as it wanted to reform the liturgy by returning to these sources. In Chapters 7 and 8 we will explain this renewal of moral theology more fully. When this task of reform was entrusted to theologians, however, they were at first overwhelmed by its magnitude, which required them to catch up with modern biblical and historical studies and with a wealth of new information from psychology and sociology. The catechesis offered by bishops and theologians was often confused. Their confusion has been communicated to the Catholic clergy and laity, often through the work of the public media which has misread what was going on not as a return to the sources of the Christian tradition but as a "catching up with the times," i.e., conforming to the prevalent secularist value system that is often quite alien to that Christian tradition.

This confusion is gradually being clarified. Fundamental to this clarification is the distinction and cooperation between the respective roles of the laity, theologians, and magisterium in the Church, both as regards "faith" ("dogmatic teaching," i.e., God's revelation of himself to us) and "morals" (the response God requires of us to his self-revelation) (CDF, 1990). We will here discuss these three roles as regards the teaching of the Church.

The Role of the Laity in Developing the Teaching

The Second Vatican Council emphasized the biblical teaching that Jesus Christ, risen from death, remains present in the Church he founded. He has given it life and guidance by his Holy Spirit which every Christian receives in baptism and confirmation and which makes the Church a unified community that lives a common life and gives a common witness to the world. The Church, therefore, is not just a collection of individuals who believe in Christ, but a corporate body, "the Body of Christ" (Romans 1:12) who live and act together, "united in one mind and one judgment" (1 Cor 1:10). Because of this presence of the Holy Spirit, Catholics believe Christ's true Church can never be divorced from him (it is *indefectible*) and will continue to witness to the true Gospel he has intrusted to it until he returns, i.e., the whole Church as a unified community is *infallible* in its faith (Mt 28:18–20; Jn 16:4–16; Jn 17:9–26).

Thus the council (Vatican Council II, 1964a) reminded Catholics that Christ's three-fold mission as priest, shepherd, and teacher is shared in appropriate ways by *all* members of the Church. Although not all Christians have a special gift (charism) of teaching (1 Co 12:29; 1 Tm 1:7), by their baptism and confirmation they should all (but in different ways) participate *actively* in teaching and witnessing the faith (Congar, 1977; O'Meara, 1983). For example, Christian parents have an important share in the active teaching mission of the Church when they pass on their faith to their children.

Consequently, the universal judgment of the faithful laity about the Gospel transmitted to them (the *sensus fidelium*) is preserved by the Holy Spirit without error. Note that this judgment is not just public opinion; it is precisely the witness to the revealed Gospel (*sensus fidei*). Hence, to ask, as the media often does, "What percentage of Catholics think contraception is wrong?" does not touch on the *sensus fidelium*. The question would have to be posed first of all to Catholics who strive to live by their faith, and then it would have to be, "What has been transmitted to you through the Christian community of all times as God's word revealed in Jesus Christ about contraception?" Thus, when Catholics say the creed, they are declaring that these truths were transmitted to them as God's revelation, God's Gospel covenant which they freely made with him when they were baptized or confirmed as members of the Church. Similarly, they accept the Ten Commandments and the commandment of love of God and neighbor and all that these imply because these norms are Christ's way of life to which they have committed themselves.

This revelation to the Church was given once and for all in Jesus Christ. As Savior of the whole human race, his teaching on how to live applies to all times and all cultures, and the Church cannot take away anything from it or add anything to it. Yet Jesus' teaching was not given to his Church as a merely static code. It is a word which is "living and effective" (Hebrew 4:12), and through the guidance of the Holy Spirit in the Christian community it develops like a living plant which was already present in the seed but requires time and nature to unfold and mature. For example, even in the New Testament we do not find an explicit condemnation of slavery, a social institution universal in Bible times. Gradually in the course of centuries the Christian people came to see the incompatibility of this institution with the biblical teaching on the dignity of every human being for whom Christ died. Their consciences began to tell them to free their slaves, and finally in our country at last to work for the emancipation of African-Americans. The situation in regard to capitol punishment in the present day is somewhat similar (John Paul II, 1995, N. 27). The laity, therefore, contribute to this "development of doctrine" by their prayer and devotion, their daily living in the changing times, their love of family, friends, and country, their good will and compassion for all human beings, and their heroic witness in the face of a hostile world. A special form of this discernment process is the witness given by those in the community who are especially dedicated to contemplation and intense prayer, which the Bible often refers to as the gift of prophecy (1 Co 14:1–5; Ac 21:9) and which helps the community grow in depth and purity of faith and in the liveliness of hope. Thus Paul VI honored St. Teresa of Avila and St. Catherine of Siena as "Doctors (teachers) of the Church." Also, we should not forget that Christian artists such as Fra Angelico or Michelangelo, scientists such as Teilhard de Chardin or Jerome Lejeune, and philosophers such as Jacques Maritain or Gabriel Marcel help us by their human disciplines to express the faith in its full splendor.

The Role of Theologians in Developing the Church's Teaching

Theologians in the past have generally been bishops or priests, who spoke in the name of the Church as by virtue of their office within the Church. After the secularization of the universities in the eighteenth century, these theologians generally taught in seminaries. Today, they are very often laymen or women teaching in university faculties who often do not think of themselves as speaking in the name of the Church, but as independent scholars. They remain Catholics who hope their scholarship will be of service to the Church, yet often, imitating the value free inquiry of modern academic life. Sometimes in the name of academic freedom and scholarly integrity they claim a "right to dissent" from the teachings of the magisterium (CDF, 1990). When the question is raised by others of the laity how a theologian can honestly dissent from what all members of the Catholic Church have committed themselves to believe and witness, some theologians answer by distinguishing between different levels of the Church's teaching which their scholarship enables them to differentiate, and say that they do not dissent from what has been declared by the magisterium to be revealed and therefore infallible, but only from teachings which are subject to change (Curran and McCormick, 1988). Some moral theologians also argue that in fact as regards morals the magisterium has never made infallible pronouncements such as it has made in matters of faith, and hence the field of moral theology is entirely open to responsible dissent.

The charism of the theologian is to witness to the faith by responsible, scholarly analysis of the Bible and Tradition, relating this perennial teaching to the culture and problems of our time (PBC, 1994). If theologians did not have the freedom to express and exchange honest, well-formed opinions (Theological Commission, 1976), the teaching mission of the Church would be seriously weakened. Although this freedom to express theological opinions is called by some "the right to dissent" (Curran and McCormick, 1988), it is rather "the right of responsible analysis or criticism" (Ratzinger, 1984b, 1987; Grisez, 1983; W. Smith, 1987). As responsible members of the Christian community, theologians have the duty to use their gifts to build up the faith of the community (Ep 4:11–13) by communicating to the public not only their criticisms and difficulties, but also the positive, constructive results of their researches (Theological Commission, 1976; CDF, 1990). This opinion it seems has been strengthened by the recent authoritative statements in the encyclical letter, *Gospel of Life* (John Paul II, 1995, n. 62, 65).

Thus the charism of theologians does *not* extend to the definitive discernment of what is revealed truth from what is human opinion nor to authoritative pastoral instruction, because this is the charism of the bishops and the pope (Vatican Council II, 1964a; CDF, 1990). It is to the college of bishops, as successors of the twelve apostles under the headship of the successor of St. Peter, Bishop of Rome, that Christ entrusted the responsibility to oversee the transmission and development of doctrine in the Church and to pass the ultimate judgment on this process of discernment to which all members of the Church contribute. Theologians in the academic sense play an important but not essential role in this process, and their work must ultimately be submitted to episcopal discernment and judgment.

The so-called "right of dissent" in post-Vatican II times, because it has often been modeled on political dissent and protest, has sometimes distorted the true relation between the magisterium of the bishops and the service of theologians (John Paul II, 1993; CDF, 1990; Dulles, 1991). No doubt with the good intention of assisting in the development of doctrine and in making the Church's teachings on sexuality, reproduction, and euthanasia more acceptable to our individualistic and libertarian culture, some theologians have believed it their duty to "dissent" from Church teaching and to encourage the laity to dissent from Church teaching if it is difficult to follow (cf. Chapter 8, Dissent).

The Role of the Magisterium in Church Teaching

The post-Vatican II debate within the Church on the respective roles of the magisterium and of theologians led to the encyclical letter of John Paul II, *Veritatis Splendor* (1993), which provides a clear direction for the Church in the future in conscience formation. Pastoral ministry makes a very special contribution to the Church's teaching effort (Dulles, 1988). This ministry, taken in a broad sense, is not limited to the ordained but is carried on by many men and women whose experience in applying the faith to actual life is essential if the Gospel is to be effectively preached to the poor and to children (Mt 11:5; 18:5–14). For example, religious sisters and brothers probably have contributed more to the active teaching work of the Church in the United States than have the ordained clergy (John Paul II, 1987b).

Nevertheless, a special leadership responsibility falls on the bishops, together with their priests and deacons in local churches, and on the pope for the whole Church to unify all these different witnessing voices, to express their consensus in clear terms suited to the times, to correct this in the light of the Bible and Sacred Tradition when necessary, and to link it to the tradition of the Christian community throughout the world in its historical development. As St. Paul wrote to Timothy:

> Proclaim the word; be persistent whether it is convenient or inconvenient; convince, reprimand, encourage through all patience and teaching. For the

time will come when people will not tolerate sound doctrine, but following their own desires and insatiable curiosity, will accumulate teachers and will stop listening to the truth and will be diverted to myths (2 Tm 4:2–4).

Without such unifying leadership, the spiritual riches of faith and insight contributed by the members of the Church would be dissipated, and the community would be divided in its faith and life, as history shows. Thus, whereas the role of theologians is primarily critical and analytical, the role of bishops is primarily pastoral and unifying (Theological Commission, 1976).

In particular, bishops have the hard task of reconciling partial and extreme views within the Church that might lead to heresy or schism. If they did not exercise this moderating role, the polarization of opinions would so increase in the Church that it would be torn apart or become so diluted as to lose all meaning and vitality. The bishops rightly prefer to do this not by condemnation but by wise emphasis on those principal truths and values that keep a straggling flock moving toward its goal. In moral matters, prudent bishops do not burden the freedom of individual consciences by insistence on secondary issues (1 Co 10:23–33), since they recognize that the members of the Church are at many different levels of moral development. Rather, such bishops constantly emphasize the primary goals of Christian life.

Levels of Church Teaching

In our individualist culture we are taught that we must "think for ourselves." The dangers of blind faith in charismatic leaders such as Hitler, Stalin, Bob Jones, and David Koresh are too evident. Yet individuals cannot achieve the knowledge they need to live by their own efforts alone. Genuine knowledge is a *social achievement*, requiring us to trust the integrity of experts. What scientist or physician can rely only on his or her own research? The same holds for religion and morals. We are not all prophets or mystics. For adequate religious and moral guidance we have to trust others, not just individual gurus but religious institutions whose records are well-known and time-tested. Thus, faith in any of the great world religions (although not in the countless cults and religious fads) is reasonable, but confronts us with the choice of the best. Faith in Jesus Christ and the Church he founded is not forced on anyone, but Jesus confronts us to decide for him or against him. If his claims are warranted, we ought to follow him and accept the guidance in our lives of the Church in which Christ remains present. The Catholic who fails to accept the guidance of the Church is like the patient who pays the doctor but won't take the prescriptions.

As Jesus Christ was true God and true human, so the Church he founded has a divine and a human element. Because of the guidance of Christ through his Holy Spirit, the Church infallibly teaches and believes the faith given to it for all time. Among these truths, some have to do with facts, such as that there is life after death, others with our response to those facts, such as the command to die for the faith rather than deny it. Nothing can be added to this revelation or taken away from it, but the Church humanly struggles to understand this revelation more clearly and fully in the course of history. In this learning and teaching process there are at any given point in history several levels of teaching in the Church, requiring from believers somewhat different responses. The Congregation for the Doctrine of the Faith (CDF, 1990) has recently distinguished these levels as follows:

1. When the magisterium makes an infallible pronouncement and solemnly declares that a teaching is found in revelation, the assent called for is theological faith. This kind of adherence is to be given even to the teaching of the ordinary and universal magisterium when it proposes for belief a teaching of faith as divinely revealed. (n. 15)

2. When the magisterium proposes "in a definitive way" truths concerning faith and morals, which even if not divinely revealed are nevertheless strictly and intimately connected with revelation, these must be firmly accepted and held. (n. 16)

3. When the magisterium, not intending to act "definitively," teaches a doctrine to aid a better understanding of revelation and make explicit its contents, or to recall how some teaching is in conformity with the truths of faith, or finally to guard against ideas that are incompatible with these truths, the response called for is that of the "religious submission of will and intellect." This kind of response cannot be simply exterior or disciplinary, but must be understood within the logic of faith and under the impulse of obedience to faith. (n. 23)

4. Finally, in order to serve the people of God as well as possible, in particular by warning them of dangerous opinions which could lead to error, the magisterium can intervene in questions under discussion which involve in addition to solid principles certain contingent and conjectural elements. It often only becomes possible with the passage of time to distinguish between what is necessary and what is contingent (n. 24). This level of teaching does not have the authority of the first three. While it must be received with reverence, its authority for the most part is based upon the reasons given for the particular statement.

Why there must be these four levels of teaching if the Christian community is to fulfill its mission of witnessing to the Gospel can be explained as follows.

First, there are truths which are certainly part of God's Word and known to be so because they are (a) clearly stated in the Bible (e.g., the Ten Commandments as stated in *Exodus* and *Deuteronomy* and confirmed by Jesus in the Sermon on the Mount in *Matthew*); (b) in the Sacred Tradition of the Church (e.g., that *Exodus*, *Deuteronomy*, and *Matthew* are the inspired Word of God); or (c) have been solemnly declared by the magisterium to be revealed explicitly or implicitly by God in the Bible and/or Sacred Tradition. This can be either by the Bishop of Rome witnessing for the whole church, or by an ecumenical council of bishops with the pope's consent (then it is said to be "extraordinary" teaching), or by all the bishops with the pope's consent but without a conciliar meeting (this is said to be "ordinary and universal teaching"). Since Christ has promised that the Church is infallible in its faith, teaching of this first level is infallible and must be received by all Catholics by an act of the gift of divine faith.

Second, there is a class of truths whose scope has not yet been precisely defined by the magisterium (Sullivan, 1983), which are not revealed, yet are so intimately connected with revealed truths that to deny them is equivalent to denying what is revealed. For example, Scripture and Tradition do not determine who is pope or what council is ecumenical, yet if such doubts could not be *definitively* settled, the Church could not teach revealed truth with certitude. Hence such definitive declarations are also infallible, not because revealed, but because of their necessary relation to revealed truths. The proper response to such teaching is to hold them to be true with firm conviction not as revealed to faith, but as definitively and authoritatively settled by the Church under the Holy Spirit's guidance.

Third, there are truths which the magisterium presents at a given time in her "ordinary" teaching, *not irreformably,* but with such consistency and universality that it is clear they must somehow involve principles that are true, although the exact consequences to these principles may still be unclear. Hence, to deny them may risk denying the Word of God, but it is not yet certain just what this risk is. Thus, it may not yet be clear how to formulate a certain truth in a way consistent with other truths. For example, the Church could not define the Immaculate Conception as a truth of faith until it was clear how to reconcile it with the truth that all are saved from sin by Christ.

Fourth, the ordinary teaching of the Church contains guidance concerning matters that require a prudential judgment on how revealed principles apply to complex and changing situations. For example, Pius XII at a time of crisis urged the Catholics of Italy to vote against the Communist Party, and the bishops of the United States have expressed strong opinions on certain issues that affect political action. Historically, although the Church applied the revealed, unchangeable biblical teaching against usury to the medieval economy, it had to modify its application when the economic system changed (Noonan, 1993). On such matters Catholics must show respect to the Church's concerns and for the common influence of Catholic action, but may have differing views on what is best to think or do.

It is mistaken, therefore, to claim that a Catholic has the right to dissent from all teaching of the pope or bishops which is not an extraordinary, infallible definition. It is also misleading to assert, as some have done, that the Church has never made any infallible definitions in the area of morals (John Paul II, 1995). Although it is true that it has been the custom of magisterium to define as revealed only matters of faith rather than of morals, without doubt the moral norms of the biblical Ten Commandments, the Sermon on the Mount, and the New Testament Epistles are infallible, and the magisterium has the authority to confirm and interpret these norms by infallible definitions if it chooses to do so.

Certitude in Ethical Decision

Even after we have done what is possible to inform our conscience as to the facts of a situation and the revealed and rational norms that apply to it as the magisterium of the Church interprets them, we can still be mistaken about the *objective* goodness of an action because of ignorance we cannot overcome ("invincible ignorance"). As a result, as many health care professionals today know only too well, ethical decisions may involve anguish of conscience. People may be faced with the realization (1) that although they have tried to get adequate information, they still do not have all the facts or the clear understanding of values that they really need to make a decision that will be objectively correct, and (2) that even when they have acquired the best knowledge available, the best alternative may remain very unclear because every alternative has advantages and disadvantages. Given such uncertainty, many people try to "pass the buck" to someone else. By doing so, however, they do not escape responsibility; instead, they assume responsibility for the decision made by the other person, whose judgment may be even less trustworthy than their own. Such uncertainty also causes many to think that in practical matters, an ethical decision is ultimately nothing but a leap in the dark.

Solving Doubts of Conscience

How can people come to a practical or moral certitude that here and now this is what they ought to do? After they have formed their conscience as well as possible at the time and in the place in which they are situated, it will probably become clear that at least some alternatives are excluded as clearly inappropriate means to ethical goals. Among those possibilities that remain, some may be attractive, but they may still not be sure whether they are right or wrong.

Despite efforts to come to principled moral decisions by which to live in peace of conscience, people may occasionally find themselves with a *perplexed* conscience. This state is not necessarily pathological but rather the result of the human condition in a sinful world wherein finding one's way is not always easy. Some Protestant moralists who stress the total depravity of human nature argue that since persons' actions are distorted by their sinful condition no matter what they do, they should "sin bravely" (to use a paradoxical but often misunderstood expression of Luther's). That is, they trust that God will forgive them no matter what their actions are as long as they have faith in his mercy. Such theologians probably do not intend to deny that Christians still have the obligation to do the best they know how, nor do they intend to excuse sin, but only to underline our total dependence on God's mercy (Thielicke, 1964). But in truth it is never necessary to sin, since there are ways to solve one's perplexity and arrive at moral certitude as to what one ought to do without sinning. Some Catholic theologians have also advocated a "theology of compromise" (Curran, 1977a). But in fact the only kind of moral compromise that is justified is when one is forced to do something less good than one would like, because the situation makes it impossible to do the better. For example, one may compromise by voting for a law that lessens the number of abortions, when one cannot get a law passed that forbids them altogether. In such a case one is not promoting abortion, but seeking the good of fewer abortions (John Paul II, 1995).

It can never be right, however, to compromise by accepting acts that are intrinsically evil (John Paul II, 1993, n. 81), e.g., having an abortion to avoid it becoming known that one has become pregnant out of wedlock. The Christian struggle against the evils of this world cannot be effectively carried out by becoming party to the injustices by which this world often achieves its goals. Consequently, it is never permissible to choose "the lesser evil" as such; a less evil act is still an evil act, which cannot be excused. A physician who finds that a patient is determined to do something wrong may point out that it would be better to do something less evil (for example, to have sex with an antiovulant contraceptive rather than one which is abortifacient), but he must tell the patient that contraception is wrong, although less wrong than abortion. If one is faced with a situation where one seems to have only a choice among evil acts, one should not act at all, unless it seems that not to act is also wrong. In that case, one should not intend to do a lesser evil, but rather whatever seems the better thing to do. Thus it is never necessary to sin, since there are ways to solve one's perplexity and arrive at moral certitude as to what one ought to do without sinning.

Christian Prudence

Thus the Catholic Church recognizes that the moral certitude of a well-formed conscience cannot be achieved simply by knowing ethical norms and blindly obeying them. We have to know how to apply them to changing and often puzzling situations. Veteran health care professionals know very well that knowing the principles of good medicine is not all that it takes to make good medical decisions. One must also have the experience of actual practice to know how to apply these principles in real-life situations in a consistently good way and be skilled in drawing on this experience what is relevant to a given decision. Similarly, knowing the principles of ethics and of moral theology may help one to make a good decision in this or that case and to answer questions correctly on an examination, but it does not by any means guarantee that one will be able to make consistently right moral judgements in new, various, and puzzling situations. We can do that only if we have acquired what is traditionally called "the virtue of prudence" (Cessario, 1991; D. M. Nelson, 1992).

Prudence as a virtue is not simply caution (although it includes that caution), but is facility in taking into consideration all the factors that enter into any particular moral decision, making as objective a judgment of conscience as one can, and then courageously and consistently acting according to that judgment. Persons who have acquired this virtue do not panic in new or difficult decisions, but calmly do all the things necessary to form their conscience well, to arrive at moral certitude, and then to act decisively.

Thus Catholic health care professionals, when they hear that moral theologians disagree, need not think that they are sinking into a theological morass in medical–moral matters. They need only keep in mind that two different levels of moral certitude exist: (1) the level of principles and value priorities and (2) the level of concrete application of these principles to particular problems of moral decision. At the level of principles and values, Jesus Christ has given Christians ample guidance on "the weightier matters of the law, justice, and mercy, and good faith" (Mt 23:23); these are clearly expressed in the ordinary teaching of the Church (Vatican Council II, 1964a; see Chapter 8). If professionals study the official pastoral documents of the popes and bishops in a spirit of faith, prayer, and reflection, they will discover the chief ethical values at which to aim in making practical medical decisions. The clearer their understanding and appreciation of these values, the surer will be their moral judgment. Without such understanding, mere mechanical obedience to laws and rules will not yield prudent decisions.

The second level of moral certitude, concerning the concrete application of ethical principles, is a complex and difficult area where official Church teaching can be of great help, but where perfect clarity or undebatable certitude on all questions would not be expected. Some actions are excluded absolutely, such as those acts contrary to human dignity, that is, abortion, sterilization, and euthanasia. However, in some situations, it may be difficult to distinguish actions which are absolutely prohibited from actions which are acceptable; for example, some people equate the removal of food from persons in a persistent coma with killing, while others believe it is allowable because keeping the person alive in this condition is of no benefit to the person (Grisez, 1996; O'Rourke, 1996). Moreover, in applying some well accepted principles of justice in health care affairs, the application will often be tinged with uncertainty, e.g., assuring a living wage to employees, or assuring the rights of minority employees. Hence, there is no "rule book" which will assure absolutely the correct application of ethical principles, but the heath care professional who makes such judgments prudently can be at peace.

It is essential, however, to understand that a Catholic health care facility has a responsibility quite different from that of individual theologians carrying on scholarly debate and from that of individual Catholic health care professionals forming their personal conscience. As a facility supported and approved officially by the local Church, it has the responsibility of bearing a public witness to Catholic moral teaching as interpreted by the local bishop. It acts in the name of the Catholic Church. It cannot without hypocrisy dissent from the health care aims and norms of the Church. Therefore its policies must be correlated with authoritative pastoral teaching and the *Ethical and Religious Directives for Catholic Health Services* (NCCB, 1994). If it fails to exemplify these Catholic ethical standards, it weakens the Catholic mission in the health care field and is on its way to secularization and loss of Church sponsorship. It must resist economic and social pressures, now greatly increased by the health care crisis in the United States, to compromise its moral standards. If it cannot survive without betraying its Catholic mission, then it has no reason to survive; but it is precisely the need of our times for truly Christian health care that is its best guarantee of survival.

Informed Consent

Closely related to the problem of developing a well-formed conscience is the process of obtaining and giving *informed consent* (Belmont Report, 1978; Faden and Beauchamp, 1986; Pellegrino, 1981). When one person asks another to cooperate or even to allow him or her to act on the other's person—for example, when a physician asks a patient to take a prescription, to undergo surgery, or to act as the subject of an experiment—the other's human dignity must be respected according to the principle of human dignity in community (cf. Chapter 8). By this principle, however, the other person, because of his or her personal responsibility for health, may not consent without an informed conscience. This implies that a health care professional has the duty to supply the patient with the medical information necessary for the patient to make an informed decision. When geriatric patients are concerned, this requires greater sensitivity on the part of the health care professional (O'Rourke, 1988b). The health care professional has no right to ask the patient to cooperate or submit to any medical procedure without first obtaining informed consent from the patient, or if the patient is not competent to give this consent, the informed consent of the patient's proxy (Munetz et al., 1985; PCEMR, 1982a). Chapter 10 discusses in more detail some of the difficulties in making sure this ethical solution is properly satisfied in regard to research programs. More specifically, the ethical and legal requirements for informed consent are:

1. The specific *information* that should be provided for the patient concerns the purpose of the procedure, anticipated risks and benefits, alternative procedures, and hoped-for results. Information should never be withheld for the purpose of eliciting consent, and truthful answers should always be given to direct questions. If a research project is in question, then information may be withheld, provided the subject is informed that some information will not be revealed until the research is completed and that no direct harm results from withholding the information.

2. *Comprehension* of the conveyed knowledge is a requirement more complex than it might seem at first. Because subjects' capability to understand varies so greatly, the material must be adapted to the subjects' capacities. Health care professionals are responsible for ascertaining that the subject has comprehended the information, especially if the risk is serious. If the patient cannot comprehend, then some third party, usually a family member but sometimes a person appointed by the court, should be asked to act in the patient's best interest. Some have maintained that comprehension of difficult medical terms is not possible for the ordinary person, but research has shown that persons unfamiliar with medical terms can understand and retain explanations about medical procedures if the explanations are well-planned and given in plain language.

3. *Freedom* implies that the person understands the situation clearly and that no coercion or undue influence is exercised by the health care professional. However, it is often difficult to determine where justifiable persuasion ends and undue influence begins. The health care professional who believes that some particular treatment is better for

the patient should state his or her conviction but should also explain clearly the reason for this opinion. Voluntariness does not imply that the patient will be free from all pressure or persuasion in a given circumstance. For example, a person with an inflamed appendix is limited insofar as freedom of choice is concerned. But voluntariness does imply that, over and above the limitations arising from the circumstances, no external coercion or moral manipulation is present.

Informed Consent: Testing for AIDS

Recently the presence of the AIDS (acquired immunodeficiency syndrome) virus has resulted in discussion concerning the need for informed consent regarding patients in health care facilities (Dent, 1989). The desire to protect health care professionals leads some to declare that patients may be tested for AIDS without obtaining informed consent. The argument is offered that testing all patients in health care facilities for AIDS would be the same as testing for any other blood disorder. Thus, to alert health care professionals to the presence of a patient with the virus, some physicians and health care administrators allow screening without informed consent. They argue that implicit consent is given to such testing by reason of the fact that one voluntarily enters the health facility (Welsby, 1986).

However, we believe that testing for the AIDS virus without explicit informed consent is unethical for the following reasons:

1. Testing for AIDS is not a routine medical procedure because of the harm that may result from such testing. Many persons infected with the AIDS virus are either homosexuals or intravenous drug users; thus the discrimination and opprobrium that may follow testing for AIDS infection are severe (Cassens, 1985; McCombie, 1986). Many people have lost their housing, jobs, and friends when the presence of the virus in their system has become known (Blendon and Donelan, 1988). Even people who have tested negative have been dropped as clients by insurance companies and suffer other indignities, since people surmise that being tested indicates that the person is in a high-risk group (Kristof, 1985; Oppenheimer and Padgug, 1986). Thus, before testing a person for the AIDS virus, the implications of the testing, whether positive or negative, must be explained clearly and thoroughly. Testing for AIDS is not the same as testing for glucose or iron deficiency.

2. Even if health care professionals do know which patients have AIDS, this knowledge alone does not offer any protection. Health care professionals may best protect against acquiring the virus only by treating all patients as though they had the virus. Such procedures are also necessary to protect against other types of contagion, such as hepatitis B, through body fluids. This advice from the Centers for Disease Control (CDC) must be implemented by health care facilities through provision of protective clothing and equipment (gloves, masks, etc.) (CDC, 1987). Treating everyone as though infected is the only safe course because

even if the patient is tested, the tests could not be positive until antibodies have had a chance to form. Thus there is at least a few weeks' time after infection when a negative result may be inaccurate.

Clearly some testing for AIDS should be done for public health reasons, both to keep an account of the spread of the disease and to prevent its spread insofar as possible (Koop, 1986). To accomplish both goals, however, it seems voluntary and "anonymous" testing, that is, testing accompanied by informed consent and revealed only to the person tested, is more effective. Surveys show that people in high-risk groups are reluctant to submit to mandatory testing. Moreover, since this type of epidemic can be effectively curbed only by changed behavior on the part of those at risk (College of Physicians, 1986), voluntary testing accompanied by counseling is most likely to be effective. The behaviors to be changed are principally sharing infected needles for drug use, having sexual intercourse (anal or vaginal) with infected partners of either sex, or receiving blood transfusions from donors who have not been thoroughly screened (National Academy of Science, 1988). Counselors also should be available to help those who test positive to cope with the shock of knowing they have a fatal disease, and above all to help infected persons realize their grave responsibility not to pass on this deadly virus to others. Although ample justification exists for screening recruits to the armed services (the services depend on their own members for blood transfusions), we believe that mandatory screening of prisoners—except in those facilities where rape cannot be controlled—violates their human rights because no benefit to the public good results from such testing. To date, there is no cure for AIDS, although it seems the fatal effects may be delayed for a time through medication. If a cure is found for the disease, mandatory testing, without consent, would become a necessity because knowledge of the disease's presence then would lead to effective action for its elimination, as with mandatory smallpox vaccination for children.

3.5 PATIENT'S RIGHTS

Choosing a Physician

Since each person has the primary obligation of caring for his or her own health, each also has the obligation to seek and choose professionals to help advise them concerning health care. This does not mean, however, that persons can surrender to others the responsibility of making decisions about their health (King, 1991). Professionals are helpers, not keepers. Frequently health care professionals fail to realize how difficult it is for ordinary persons to select a physician or how uncertain such persons are about their own rights in dealing with health care institutions. Health care professionals have an educational responsibility to help clients know how and where to seek health care and how to protect their own rights in doing so (Rosenberg and Towers, 1986).

Even when people have the humility and courage to seek a physician, they are faced with two very serious ethical problems in choosing a good one. The first arises from their choice possibly being restricted greatly by the complex organization of modern medical care, such as managed care, and the maldistribution of its services (Jecker, 1994). A characteristic of managed care is often the limitation of choice in regard to physicians. At present, choice in regard to selecting a physician is not eliminated, but it is usually circumscribed by making physicians qualify before being eligible to serve a specific group of potential patients. Should this restriction of freedom be allowed, or is there a moral obligation to resist it? This sociopolitical issue is discussed in more detail in Chapter 6.

The second ethical issue in choosing a physician or a health care facility arises from today's widespread doubt about the competence and the character of health care professionals (P. Lee et al., 1988). Some authors, such as Illich (1976), have launched an attack on the whole system of health care in the United States. Others (Katz, 1984) without going as far as Illich, have criticized vigorously the way that American health care professionals live up to their professed standards. Still others seek to outline methods that will improve medical care (Reiser and Rosen, 1984; Pew Commission, 1993, 1995). With due allowance for polemics, however, in the United States, as in most countries, the average citizen experiences difficulty in obtaining satisfactory health care (Aday et al., 1984).

Although Americans are convinced, and with reason, that the billions of dollars spent each year on health care go to support the most advanced medical technology and professional education in the world, this by no means proves that the average citizen is receiving health care of high quality. The life expectancy of citizens in the United States is lower than in a number of European countries and has not improved noticeably in the past twenty years. In some states the death rate is 25 percent higher than in other states.

Available studies of the quality of care (College of Healthcare Executives, 1986; R. Rubin et al., 1988) and of the actual competency of physicians in practice frequently reveal alarming percentages of physicians whose competence is substandard (Bosk, 1986; Strauss, 1984). Again, estimates show that a high percentage of surgery (50 percent in some hospitals) is unnecessary and explainable only by incompetence or greed (Margo, 1986). Finally, the studies also show that among professionals, physicians rate highest in drug addiction, alcoholism, and psychological disorders. When this is added to the growing evidence that a considerable percentage of physicians have an income well in excess of members of other professions, choosing a reliable and competent physician and a high-quality hospital is difficult (Couch et al., 1981; Steel et al., 1981).

The ethical issues raised by such choices are dramatized by the very titles of popular books written in recent years: *Talk Back To Your Doctor* (Levin, 1975); *The Bitter Pill; Doctors, Patients and Failed Expectations* (Lipp, 1980); *Getting Rid of Patients* (Mizratti, 1981); and *Enemies of Patients* (Macklin, 1994). Although we do not endorse these works, they do show the need for a careful, even aggressive, attitude on the part of the patient toward the health care professional and the health care facility. This seems in strong contrast to the attitude of *trust* that has been traditionally regarded as the basis of every profession (a tradition defended in Chapter 4). These authors, however, with evidence to support their position, argue that persons who fail to take this distrustful stance toward the medical profession today are failing in their responsibility to their own health.

Protection of Rights

To escape enslavement to the incompetent or exploitative professional, people need to be conscious of the rights that are correlative to their responsibility to choose professional help prudently. These rights may be summed up as follows (Annas, 1973; Summers, 1985; Gillick, 1992):

1. The right to the whole truth;
2. The right to privacy and personal dignity;
3. The right to refuse any test, procedure, or treatment; and
4. The right to read and copy medical records.

Also, Chapter 12 discusses the right to treatment of persons who are institutionalized, such as prisoners or those involuntarily committed to mental hospitals (Forer, 1982; England and Goff, 1993).

All the rights proposed rest on the fundamental concept of informed consent. If the patient is to give free consent, the patient must also be able to refuse any test, procedure, or treatment. The right to privacy and personal dignity also amounts to the right of patients to refuse to be involved in any professional procedures that make them objects to be examined or discussed for the benefit or convenience of professionals or students rather than for the patient's own therapy.

If this consent is to be not only free but also informed, the patient has the right to the whole truth, including access to read and copy medical records (Adcock et al., 1991; Lee, 1992). Many professionals deny these rights on the grounds that the patient is not able to understand the technical information known to the physician and may be harmed by it. Such difficulties, however, do not disprove patients' right to know but only establish the professional's duty to communicate this information in ways that are helpful, not harmful, to patients so that consent may be truly informed.

Among the facts patients have the right to know is the competency and ethical integrity of the physician or health care facility to which they may entrust themselves. The authors already cited give much good advice on this subject. Generally, they agree that the first consideration is medical competency. In the present state of affairs, they believe such competency is most likely to be found among physicians holding assignments to a medical school-affiliated hospital, since they are most likely to be well-educated and up-to-date in knowledge and skill and subject to some form of peer review. Similarly, these authors generally recommend choosing a larger, accredited, medical school-affiliated hospital, whether a public or a nonprofit private institution, and avoiding small proprietary hospitals.

They also recommend choosing a primary service physician who is concerned with total health and who should be a family practice specialist rather than a general practitioner. Through these primary service physicians, the need for further specialized care can be ascertained and suitable specialists sought. All these authors, however, emphasize that no matter how excellent the physician, people should never hesitate to ask for consultation when doubts arise, especially when surgery is in question (Wertheimer et al., 1985; Horowitz, 1988).

Thus the underlying ethical issue of trust again emerges. Is competency the primary consideration in choosing a physician (Cousins, 1985)? Certainly it is the *specific* qualification most people seek in any professional, including their physicians. If physicians are not also trustworthy, however, in the sense that they are sincerely dedicated to helping the patient get well, then their medical competency is dangerous, as in the case of brilliantly competent surgeons eager for more bodies on which to demonstrate their skill. Thus the careful choice of a primary service physician is highly important, since it is this physician who is most concerned for the patient as a whole person. Also, persons should seek physicians who work in institutions where not only their skill but also their professional dedication to patient welfare is most likely to be tested and evaluated by peers.

People, therefore, should not lightly accept the idea that their personal responsibility for their own health is satisfied merely by assuming a critical attitude toward physicians and demanding their rights from them. Such a responsibility also includes willingness to trust physicians once they have been prudently chosen, to make good use of their advice, and to cooperate with their healing efforts. Although people should never be afraid to protect their rights and to insist that physicians give patients all the information they need to give informed consent to treatment, they should also give physicians a deserved respect. Trustworthy and competent health care professionals perform for people a precious service, for which they deserve profound gratitude, good reputation, and fair and prompt payment.

While retaining primary right and responsibility to give informed consent or refusal to any kind of professional health service, people should also remember the commendatory words of Scripture:

> Hold the physician in honor, for he is essential to you, and God it was who established his profession,
> From God the doctor has his wisdom, and the king provides for his sustenance. His knowledge makes the doctor distinguished, and gives him access to those in authority.
> God makes the earth yield healing herbs, which the prudent man should not neglect;
> Was not the water sweetened by a twig [when Moses sweetened the bitter waters in the desert] that man might learn his power?
> He endows men with the knowledge to glory in his mighty works,
> Though which the doctor eases pain and the druggist prepares his medicines;
> Thus God's creative work continued without ceasing in its efficacy on the surface of the earth (Si 38:1–8).

CONCLUSION

There is a note of subjectivity to health and illness. If optimal functioning at any level of being is a concept of health, whether in working to prevent illness or maintain optimal function, to assist recovery from disease, or to rehabilitate oneself after a crippling trauma, a person must make a personal commitment to life and health. Everyone has an instinct to live and be healthy, but at the innermost depth of our being, we make free choices. In the human person then, a choice to affirm or reject life must be made. God calls us to life, as the Scriptures testify. Jesus gives us the example of commitment to life in his prayers to the Father shortly before His crucifixion.

The person who has made a free spiritual commitment to life will strive to achieve wholeness in every dimension of personality. This involves more than going to the physician. First of all, it requires pursuing a lifestyle which respects our physical and psychological needs. To assume personal responsibility for health requires a scientifically based knowledge of hygiene, good diet, rest, exercise, and moderation. Avoiding stress is also a factor in achieving psychological well-being, but it also contributes to moral and spiritual well-being by making room for a contemplative dimension to daily life. Stress leads to addiction in all phases of life.

Some factors detrimental to health are often beyond personal control. More and more knowledge about genetic factors in maintaining or losing the state of homeostasis, or health, is being discovered. Clearly, judgments about moral guilt or fault in regard to health and illness must be controlled. We simply do not have enough information to make judgments about the behavior of others.

Insofar as the relationship between humans and other living creatures and the universe is concerned, we do not have absolute dominion. Human beings are stewards of nature, not owners. In exercising stewardship and in developing the capabilities of human nature, it is our responsibility to pursue the development of technology and scientific discovery. But there are important limitations to the pursuit. There are values and goods more important than new scientific knowledge and new technology. The present state of ecology in the universe expresses the harm that occurs when limits of technology are not observed.

In order to pursue health and avoid illness, human beings must make both decisions of conscience. The Church provides these norms through ordinary and extraordinary teaching. The power of the Church to make definitive judgments extends to moral teaching, as evidenced in *Evangelium Vitae* (John Paul II, 1995). In respect to norms for health care ethics the bishops in the United States have issued the *Ethical and Religious Directives for Catholic Health Care Services* (NCCB, 1994), which apply the teaching of the Church more concretely.

Finally, in order to make careful ethical judgments concerning health care, one needs the advice and care of a competent, empathetic physician. Choosing a good physician within the limits now imposed by some managed care systems is not without problems. While the moral and legal rights of patients should be recognized, patients must also respect the rights of physicians. Thus the underlying ethical issue of trust always arises in consideration of physician and patient responsibility. Patients therefore should not accept the idea that their contribution to the health care relationship is satisfied on assuming a critical attitude and demanding rights. Rather the responsibility of patients includes a willingness to trust physicians and to cooperate with their healing efforts. Trustworthy and competent physicians perform a precious service.

The Healing Profession; Response of the Community to the Health Needs of Persons

Although individuals have primary responsibility to care for their own physiological health as well as for the psychological, ethical, and spiritual aspects of their personal development, such development can be achieved only with the help of other members of the community. In advanced communities, such help is furnished by persons who have chosen and been educated for the special social roles called the professions. Part 2 considers the chief ethical issues involved in the choice of the health care profession as a vocation and in the educational preparation needed to fulfill the demands of so difficult a vocation.

Because the health care profession is only one among several professions basic to the culture of any advanced community, Chapter 4 considers the nature of the professions in general, and then defines the specific role of the medical profession, and finally identifies its interrelations with other professions. The chief thesis in this section is that medical education must include the development of basic ethical attitudes. Since these attitudes are rooted in the relationship of trust, Chapter 5 considers the changes that must occur in the health care profession to guarantee such trust, with the specific character of this relationship. Finally, since today the profession of medicine, like that of teaching, is exercised largely in institutional settings, Chapter 6 considers the ethical issues raised by the social organization of health care.

4
The Health Care Profession

OVERVIEW

This chapter considers first the concept of a profession in general (4.1) and then the specific task of the health care professional. Traditionally, this profession has been rather narrowly identified as "the medical profession" and with the role of the physician as a medical doctor (MD). The overall emphasis of this book is on the health team, but this chapter deals with the more traditional and narrower concept, considering the historical ideals of the medical profession in 4.2 and the education of physicians as it transmits these ideals today in 4.3. The concern here is not with the scientific knowledge and technical skills so essential to this profession, but rather with its ethical ideals and standards.

4.1 PROFESSIONS: DEPERSONALIZING TRENDS

As stated in the Introduction, the purpose of this book is not to pass moral judgment on the shortcomings of the health care profession in meeting its own standards. Rather, our purpose is to identify some of the ethical issues that are most acute for the progress of this profession today and to suggest some directions in which Catholic health care professionals can give witness and leadership in the resolution of these issues by the profession and by the public.

The medieval professions were divinity (theology), physic (medicine), and law. They were "person professions" centered on a counselor–client relation (Sieghart, 1985). They did not produce goods for sale or works of art for enjoyment, but worked to heal, guide, or protect some person in a life crisis. Industrial society has greatly fostered the professions, but it has also depersonalized them. No longer are they centered on conviviality of persons (Illich, 1972), but on the productivity of an impersonal system. They no longer deal with better interpersonal communication, but with more efficient exchange of energy (Brint, 1994).

This slow depersonalizing transformation of the professions is reaching its completion today, just as industrial society itself seems about to yield to a new postindustrial society (Moline, 1986). Neither progressive capitalism nor revolutionary Marxism has been able to fulfill the promises of scientific technology to produce a society of abundance and freedom. Even this promise begins to seem illusory in view of the ecological doomsday predicted by some authorities (Marco et al., 1987).

In postindustrial society, the source of power will no longer be economic ownership (whether capitalist or socialist), but rather *knowledge and its communication*. Such power means a still greater role for the professions (Callahan, D., 1988). This knowledge can be used to bring about greater social conformism and dependency on professionals, or it can be used to open the system to wider and more genuine social participation by all. In either case, the professions, especially the profession of medicine, must be radically reconstructed (Jones, 1992).

Will professionals become technocrats whose technological mastery must extend itself to behavior control (Brody, H., 1992a)? Or will they become the persons who help others to transcend the depersonalization of technological systems by "putting the good of the weaker party over one's own interests" (Moline, 1986)? If professionals choose the latter alternative, the professions must again be personalized. They must be reconstructed so as to eliminate the three-fold depersonalization that the professions have suffered in the epoch of industrial society.

In medical practice, depersonalization is evident. First, *patients* have been depersonalized by the proliferation of specialization. They are no longer thought of as organisms, but as collections of organs (Charman, 1992). The parts are healed, not the person, such that the very meaning of *healing*—that is, "to make *whole*"—has been lost. Around each profession has grown a host of "para" or "semi" professions. However, the result is not so much integration as competition and confusion. Even the efforts of interdisciplinary healing teams never quite seem to succeed in getting it all together again.

Second, *professionals themselves* have been depersonalized by a loss of clear identity. This loss is notoriously true for the ministry (Hussey, 1988) and is now evident in law, teaching, and medicine (Freidson, 1971; Callahan J., 1988; Brint, 1994). Psychiatrists, psychoanalysts, and psychiatric social workers all perform similar tasks, but are considered members of three different professions (Henry et al., 1971). Even more confusing, many ministers, lawyers, and physicians counsel clients in ways not easily distinguishable from those used by psychotherapists (Freeman, 1967).

Contributing to this confusion of identity today is the tension within the profession between the goals of research and the goals of practice (Katz, 1994; Mathieu, 1993). In addition, many areas of professional practice may soon be handed over to computers. How, then, can a professional make that type of personal commitment always regarded as a mark of a profession if it is not clear to what he or she is professed?

Third, the *validity of the professional–client relation* is being questioned. Professionalism seems to imply an elitism that is ultimately socially destructive. Illich (1972, 1978) masterfully studied the problems of underdeveloped countries and launched an all-out attack on schooling and the concept of the teaching profession, and extends the same criticism to medicine (Illich, 1976). More recently, Beriman and Navarro (1983) and Navarro (1986) offered similar observations. They contend that the industrial model for organizing the professions has progressively restricted access to knowledge and skill, placing them in the hands of elites on whom the public is more and more dependent, but from whom the public receives less and less adequate service (Cahn, 1986). The result is that service institutions have become "production funnels" that proliferate subordinate professions and paraprofessions. Illich wants to free people from such production funnels by giving nonspecialists easier access to the information that is now the prerogative of professional elites. He argues that both capitalist and Marxist politics are based on the same invalid professional ideal, and that the Third World is desperately striving to make the same mistake.

Fourth, the contemporary practice of HMOs or other managed care corporations to contract with physicians in the practice of medicine disposes physicians to be more interested in practicing within economic guidelines than in serving patient well-being (Rodwin, 1995).

These four depersonalizations are most easily illustrated in the case of the medical profession, but they also occur in the most unlikely profession—the religious ministry, which has always claimed to be concerned for the whole person. In recent years many priests, ministers, and rabbis have deserted their calling to serve. The clergy have accepted elitist status and are neither sure of their own role nor competent to give interdisciplinary guidance to other professionals in the service of persons (John Paul II, 1984c).

Personalistic Concept of a Profession

Today the term *profession* is used for almost any prestigious occupation because it has the aura of an ideal (Moline, 1986). It is a symbol rather than a reality. The distinguished sociologist Howard Becker (1960) writes:

> The symbol systematically ignores such facts as the failure of the professions to monopolize their area of knowledge, the lack of homogeneity within professions, the frequent failure of clients to accept professional judgment, the chronic presence of unethical practitioners as an integrated segment of the professional structure, and the organizational constraints on professional autonomy. A symbol which ignores so many features of occupational life cannot provide an adequate guide for professional activity (p. 46).

Nevertheless, the sociologists have devoted much time to developing a good empirical definition of a profession. Merton (1960) explains the social value of a profession very succinctly:

> First, the value placed upon systematic knowledge and intellect: *knowing.* Second, the value placed upon technical skill and trained capacity: *doing.* And third, the value placed upon putting this conjoint knowledge and skill to work in the service of others: *helping* (p. 9).

Barber (1965) proposes the following "relativistic" definition:

> Professional behavior may be defined in terms of four essential attributes: (1) a high degree of generalized and systematic knowledge; (2) primary orientation to the community interest rather than to individual self-interest; (3) a high degree of self-control of behavior through codes of ethics internalized in the process of work socialization and through voluntary associations organized and operated by the work specialists themselves; and (4) a system of rewards (monetary and honorary) that is primarily a set of symbols of work achievement and thus ends in themselves, not means to some end of individual self-interest (p. 18).

Similarly, Underwood (1972) says:

> These four concerns—concern for persons, trained skills, values and basic theory, and public responsibility—are the central themes of professional ideology always mentioned in the sociological literature on the professions and the professions' statement of purpose (p. 422).

Moore and Rosenblum (1970) use a scale to define professionalism. Professionals must rate high on the following six operational attributes:

1. Professionals practice *full-time occupations.*
2. They are committed to a *calling;* that is, they treat their occupation "as an enduring set of normative and behavioral expectations."
3. They are distinguished from the laity by various signs and symbols and identified with their peers—often in formalized *organizations.*
4. They have esoteric but useful knowledge and skills through specialized *education,* which is lengthy and difficult.
5. They are expected to have a *service orientation* so as to perceive the needs of a client relevant to their competency.
6. They have *autonomy* of judgment and authority restrained by responsibility in using their knowledge and skill (pp. 51–65, 174–86).

The problem with these definitions (which fundamentally come down to Merton's "knowing–doing–helping") is that they fail to distinguish clearly the original group of person professions from other highly developed occupations that the term has been extended to, but that do not deal *directly* with persons. Today engineering, accounting, architecture and the other arts, and business are considered professions because they also involve knowing, doing, and helping (Kanigel, 1988). Their immediate objective, however, is not personal but productive. This obliteration of the distinction between the person professions and productive occupations is characteristic of industrial society and its depersonalization of the professions. If they are to be repersonalized, this distinction between personal and productive professions must be drawn once more.

The need for this distinction and the importance of the counselor–client relationship in the professions has been pointed out by the sociologist William Goode (1969), who makes a fundamental suggestion:

> Specifically, I suggest that a category of occupations is set apart (as a profession) by a primary variable, upon which a considerable number of structural consequences hinge: whether the professional must symbolically or literally "get inside the client," become privy to his personal world, in order to solve the problem that is the mandate of the profession (p. 307).

According to this view, research scientists and scholars are not professionals because they are directly concerned with knowing, not doing, and with theory, not practice. The work of laboratory experimentation may appear as a doing, but its purpose is to test a theory, not to apply it practically.

To call the technologies and the arts (engineering, business, and fine arts) professions is confusing and dangerous because this designation disguises the fact that they produce *things* and do not directly help persons. Certainly the technologies should educate their practitioners to be more sensitive to the human uses to which their product will be put. This humanization of technology, however, will be hindered if industrial society continues the previous tendency of lumping the technologies and the person professions together under one name and to judge them all in terms of productivity.

A true profession, therefore, is rooted in theory but aimed at practice—a practice that does not produce things external to persons but a service directly to persons themselves (Shaffer, 1987). Furthermore, this service is not applied to persons who receive it passively but facilitates those persons' own activity. It aims at healing them, at making them whole, at freeing them to act on their own. Counselors should not act on clients, nor dominate them, but enable them to become fully, autonomously themselves. Thus a profession cannot properly be elitist. It communicates power rather than enforces dependency.

Finally, professional help in the full sense is concerned precisely with those problems that are deeply personal, that are matters of life and death. Therefore such help engages both counselor and client in a profound responsibility both to each other and to the community. This personalistic concept of a profession can reconstruct the professions and professional education for the future (Eige, 1986).

Physicians and Patients with AIDS

The practical results of viewing medicine as a profession, as opposed to a trade or a business, are immediately evident when considering the responsibility of physicians and other health care workers to treat patients with acquired immunodeficiency syndrome (AIDS). Treating AIDS patients involves some risk for the health care worker of acquiring the human immunodeficiency virus (HIV) infection if the worker is exposed to body fluids (Marcus and CDC Surveillance Group, 1988). Moreover, if a physician accepts AIDS patients, other patients may determine they do not wish to continue as patients. For these reasons, some physicians refuse to treat AIDS patients (Koop, 1987). If health care were simply another marketplace trade, and if health care workers were engaged merely in business, then there would be no responsibility to treat AIDS patients. Moreover, if medicine were only a business, physicians and other health care workers could refuse to treat AIDS patients either because of personal risk or because profits would be diminished (Angoff, 1991).

Although some answer the question concerning treatment of AIDS patients by opting for a general form of responsibility upon the profession as a whole, most individuals and medical societies have stated that because medicine is a profession in the true sense of the word, AIDS patients must be cared for without discrimination. Thus the Texas Medical Association and the Arizona Board of Medical Examiners were willing to settle for a general responsibility on the profession as a whole, maintaining that the physician fulfilled his or her responsibility if the AIDS patients were referred to another physician who would care for the patient (Arizona Medical Examiners, 1987; Texas Medical Association, 1987).

On the other hand, the American Medical Association (AMA, 1988a, 1994), the American College of Physicians (Scherr, 1987), and several individuals considering the topic (Pellegrino, 1987; Jonsen, 1990; Gerbert et al., 1992) declare that because medicine is a profession, individual physicians and health care workers have ethical and legal responsibilities to care for AIDS patients, even at the risk of personal danger. As Emanuel states (1988): "With the understanding that medicine is a profession committed to the ideal of caring for the sick, physicians can deny emergency care, but not simply because of a person's disease, the inability to pay, or the physician's personal dislike; physicians cannot discriminate against people in accepting nonemergency patients."

If medicine is viewed as a profession, reasonable risks clearly are associated with being a health care worker. One assumes those risks on entering the profession. Such risks are associated with other occupations; for example, being a policeman and fireman exposes one to injury and death. Although the injury resulting from an HIV infection is serious, for most health care workers there is small danger of infection (Zuger and Miles, 1987; Weiss et al., 1988). Thus, health care workers statistically are not being called on to undergo undue risks when proper precautions are used in caring for AIDS patients (CDC, 1987). Many health care facilities have developed policies that state the ethical and legal responsibilities of physicians and other health care workers to care for AIDS patients.

Health Care Counseling

This book is concerned with the way the personalistic concept applies to the health care professions because, although health care counseling has much in common with other types of professional counseling, it is also distinct from them.

Originally, the term *counseling* pertained to rational, moral, and ethical functioning (Pietroferg, 1983) and in particular to the legal profession, as the British use of the term *counselor* indicates. Counseling also found a place in the religious ministry, since the rabbi was a type of religious lawyer, and this role was passed on to Christian priests. As Chapter 1 argues and Chapter 14 develops more fully, however, the specific type of counseling proper to the ministerial profession is deeper than the legal and pertains to the spiritual dimension of the human person. One can argue that the teaching profession, in arousing the creativity of the student, also reaches this level of intuitive life.

The medical professional often performs one or the other of these types of counseling proper to the other professions. A physician may have to discuss with a patient certain ethical and legal issues, such as those involved in an abortion decision. Sometimes a physician is involved in a patient's spiritual struggles about death and the meaning of life. Often physicians must play the role of teacher, helping patients understand their body or psyche. However, all these involvements are incidental and substitutional. A prudent physician is quick to refer the patient to experts in other professions when the issues are ethical and spiritual rather than medical.

The proper task of the medical professional is to deal with problems at the biological and psychological levels of human functioning (Pellegrino and Thomasma, 1981, 1988). At the psychological level, counseling of a certain type plays a major therapeutic role. At the biological level, however, it is not so obvious that the physician's role is still primarily that of a counselor. However, if the thesis argued in Chapter 3 is correct—that all persons have primary responsibility for their own health—then the physician's primary responsibility is to help patients make good health decisions, which requires a counseling process. People cannot make good decisions about how to care for their health unless they have the required information. In more complicated cases, this information can be obtained only by consulting a physician. To some extent the physician is playing the role of a teacher in giving this information. More is involved than this, however, since the information required is not abstract biological truth but a concrete assessment of personal health and the possible ways of dealing with the problems this assessment presents. This form of guidance is required of a physician, and it engages the physician in a special type of counseling.

This basic counseling relation on which the whole medical profession is built is "trusteeship" (Freymann, 1974). William F. May (1983) speaks of a "covenant" between physician and patient, as did Ramsey (1970). Technological progress in medicine has temporarily obscured the importance of trusteeship, making it appear that the physician is a scientist–technician rather than a counselor, but this same technological progress will eventually expose what it covers up (Campbell, 1994). Soon not only the process of treatment, but also diagnosis itself, will become the work of technicians, while physicians will be freed once more to deal personally with patients. Moreover, physicians will be dealing not with patients so sick that they cannot think, but with responsible persons concerned to stay well. In such situations, the physician will play the role of health counselor. As Freymann (1974) states:

> The degree to which a modern patient seeks these two attributes— knower–doer and trustee—in his doctor varies. The victim of an acute

catastrophe may need and want only the knower–doer. But the less clear-cut the clinical picture, the more the patient looks for both. He wants a knower–doer who can solve those problems for which there is an answer. But he wants a trustee who can comprehend *all* his problems and help him to face them, no matter what the outcome. The former calls for a scientist, but much of what the pure scientist can do now will be taken over by the technician–computer teams. The latter calls for a physician or a nurse, for no matter how man-like computers may become, I do not think trusteeship will ever be automated (p. 313).

Nursing is truly a profession because it shares in this counseling task of the physician (White, 1992). Today the role of the nurse has become very ambiguous (Crissman and Betz, 1987; Jecker and Self, 1991). One of the original commentators on the nature of medicine, Freymann (1974), was correct in saying that the medical profession has always had the double dimension of cure and care. Thus medicine always requires a distinction between the curing task of the physician and the caring task of the nurse. What is common to both cure and care is that the patient must consent to both and cooperate actively with both, so that both physician and nurse must enter into the trustee relationship with the patient (Curzer, 1993).

Also, this basic relationship will not be eliminated as patients in managed care plans will relate more and more to a health team rather than one-to-one with a personal physician (Mechanic, 1985; Kassirer, 1995). Chapter 1 shows that personal relationships always have a social character. Group psychotherapy has proved that personalism need not be eliminated just because the one-to-one relationship with a therapist is expanded into a more complex social relationship.

The account of the professions as rooted in the counselor–client relationship, however, is very far from the reality of the professions in society today.

As cited in 2.1, Freidson stated in 1971 that the professions are no longer characterized by service to the client nor by fidelity to a body of expert knowledge, but instead by a drive for autonomy. Thus the medical profession is often unresponsive to the health needs of the public, since the public has no way to make its needs effective in the face of this professional autonomy (AMA, 1986).

Freidson is not alone in this opinion. Berlant (1975) denies that the medical profession in the United States and Great Britain arose to meet a social need, but rather that it developed as a "commercial class" dedicated to achieving monopoly control. He argues that historically the medical profession has gone through all the steps characteristic of any commercial class, such as (1) creation of a commodity, (2) separation of the performance of its service from any necessary satisfaction of the client's interests, (3) creation of scarcity, (4) monopolization of supply, (5) restriction of membership, (6) elimination of external competition, (7) price fixing, (8) unification of suppliers, (9) elimination of internal competition, and (10) development of group solidarity and cooperation. Of course, similar disparaging accounts can be given of the other professions, including teaching and religious ministry, which are supposed to deal with spiritual values. In order to understand what might be done to restore the medical profession to its original identity, the following section considers the sociological nature of the medical profession in more detail.

4.2 TRADITIONAL IDEALS OF THE MEDICAL PROFESSION

Priest or Scientist?

To make sure that the personalistic concept of the medical profession is not a mere ideal requires a brief look at the cross-currents of purpose that have been at work in the historical development of the profession (Reiser and Rosen, 1984; Lyons, 1994).

The standard histories of medicine (Garrison, 1960; Sigerist, 1951) usually divide this history into the prescientific period and the scientific period, which begins only in the seventeenth century after Vesalius and Harvey. Michael Foucault, in his fascinating book *The Birth of the Clinic* (1973), shows that the crucial step was taken as a result of the efforts of the radical wing of the French Revolution to abolish all professions, including the medical profession, as a means to establishing a classless society. The resulting chaos in health care then led to the reestablishment of the medical profession and its hospitals on a new basis under the domination of the scientific ideals of the Enlightenment.

Freymann (1974) has also shown that from 1700 to 1850 health care was fragmented, and the profession was at a low ebb until the Age of Pasteur, with its emphasis on the scientific education of physicians to fight acute diseases. Only now, Freymann believes, is the profession entering the Age of Darwin and Freud, with the emphasis on an ecological, positive health approach. Thus medicine as an effective scientific technology is a very recent development in human history.

On closer examination, however, it becomes evident that this division into prescientific and scientific periods is somewhat misleading because it is only a manifestation of two aspects of medical tradition that have always coexisted and still do. Today, along with orthodox scientific medicine, a vast field of heretical medicine exists, ranging from naturopathy, faith healing, homeopathy, and chiropractic to osteopathy, acupuncture, and "holistic" medicine (Easthope, 1986), not to mention countless forms of pure quackery (S. Callahan, 1993). These therapies evidently complement orthodox medicine because they seem to meet health needs that orthodox medicine does not (Campion, 1993). Also, it is no secret that even within orthodox medicine the field of psychotherapy is a borderline area that many medical physicians consider unscientific.

This duality, on closer examination, reflects the mind–body or psychosomatic duality of the human being who is sick (Moyers, 1993; Hilts, 1995). In early times the learned professions all originated from the one rather confused profession of priest (or perhaps priest-king). Priests were looked on as custodians of sacred wisdom and power over the forces of nature, a gift from the gods, who alone possessed cosmic secrets.

In Greece (whence modern Western medicine is directly descended) the first father of medicine was Asclepius, who was so kind as the "mild god" that he was to prove a great rival of Christ as Christianity spread throughout the pagan world (Edelstein, 1967). Asclepius' priests presided over shrines (the first clinics) where the sick came to worship, sleep, and have their dreams interpreted. The symbol of the medical profession today is still a staff with entwined serpents because the serpent, symbol of wisdom and the healing power of mother earth (i.e., nature) was the cult animal at these shrines. Today in the city of Rome, the Hospital of the Benefratelli of medieval origin is built on an island in the River Tiber over remains of a shrine of Asclepius transferred from Greece in classical times. A great snake is still to be seen carved on the ancient ruins.

This myth manifests a basic truth about the medical profession: the physician to this day retains something of a priestly ministry in the service of the healing forces of nature. Something similar is true of every profession, since all professions deal with the sacred dignity of the human person and rest on the sacred covenant of trust between client and professional. This priestly ministry is especially true of the medical profession because its direct relation to life and death gives it a fundamental, primitive character (Ross, 1994). A person's trust in the physician is almost the same as trust in one's mother; it is a primordial confidence in life support.

No wonder, then, that even today the physician is a charismatic figure, surrounded by a priestly atmosphere (witness the myths of television doctor shows). Although this trust can be abused and exploited, it is valuable when it is authentic. No one can be healed without trust. Thus the most significant distinction in understanding the history of medicine is not between scientific and nonscientific medicine, but between *authentic* medicine and quackery. Authentic medicine has both priestly and scientific dimensions.

Why did it take until the seventeenth and even the nineteenth century for the rapid development of this scientific side of medicine to begin? The empirical rational method was already well understood in the time of Hippocrates, about 400 BC. Hippocrates rejected the designation of epilepsy and other ailments as sacred diseases and attempted to explain them biologically. In the next century Aristotle (himself a son of an Asclepian doctor who was the physician of Alexander the Great), in *De Somniis,* demythologized the notion of dreams, often used to diagnose diseases, by giving such psychic phenomena a physiological explanation. This tradition of scientific medicine was further developed by Hellenistic physicians such as Galen and by medieval Arabian, Jewish, and Christian physicians. Before Harvey (d. 1657) described the circulation of blood, however, the practical fruits of this scientific approach were sparse. Why?

One explanation is that the scientific aspect of medicine was held back by its priestly aspect (White, 1896). It is not inevitable, however, that these two aspects should hinder rather than complement each other. Others have pointed out that scientific medicine could not get far until the development of chemistry and biology. But why were these sciences also so slow to develop? Perhaps the better explanation is given by some Marxist sociologists and other authorities. Greek thinkers clearly recognized the method and value of empirical science, but they were discouraged from engaging in experimentation in science and clinical practice in medicine by a social system based on the sharp division between the liberally educated freemen who despised manual work and the slaves or serfs. This barrier between theory and practice, between the spiritual realm and the realm of matter, was the major obstacle to the development of science and scientific medicine.

Elevation of the physician to the status of a learned professional increasingly separated from the suffering patient was intensified by the university education of the Middle Ages. Nevertheless, the Christian concern for the poor began to break through this Greek contempt. Glaser (1970) has shown that Christianity, particularly in its Roman Catholic form, has been the religion most concerned with organized health care because of its belief in personal charity and the integral relation of the body to the human person. Despite practical efforts to realize this Christian ideal, however, the state of scientific knowledge and the level of social organization were so low that, until the end of the Middle Ages, the chief efforts were directed more to caring for sick and dying persons than to healing them.

Practical and material concerns were clearly seen to have religious and ethical values only with the Renaissance and the development of Christian humanism in Catholic Europe and Calvinist emphasis on work as a vocation in Protestant Europe. Thus the groundwork for the rapid rise of empirical science and modern medical technology was finally laid. Undoubtedly the secular humanism of the Enlightenment built well on this basis, but it did not lay its foundation. The role of the French Revolution was essentially negative. It broke down the old, fixed patterns of the medical profession so that the new model might develop fully (Foucault, 1973; Vogel, 1980).

Does the previous tension between the liberal and the service aspects of medicine exist today? At first glance such a suspicion seems absurd. The modern physician is above all interested in practice, and no class of physicians has greater prestige and remuneration (Hsiao, 1988) than surgeons, who certainly get their hands dirty. A closer look, however, reveals that the emphasis on the specialist, as opposed to the general practitioner, and the building up of a pyramid of paramedical professionals in the service of the physician, who mediate between the physician and patient, is the modern version of this class distinction (Pew Commission, 1993; Institute of Medicine, 1996).

The Christian Physician

On the other hand, the rise of psychiatry and psychosomatic medicine in the twentieth century has strengthened and developed the other, priestly, aspect of medicine in which the physician as counselor becomes less the scientific technologist and more the artist in direct contact with the patient. The current debates about the humanization of medicine reflect the resurgence of this other aspect of the medical tradition, which has never died and will always be part of medicine (Brennan, 1994). Many of the real needs of patients that nineteenth-century medicine tended to abandon to the medical heretics are now being recovered as legitimate concerns of the orthodox medical profession (Moyers, 1993). These debates, however, continue. The problem of the personalization of health care is far from solved (Linzer, 1986), but the emphasis on patient needs speaks well for a repersonalization of medicine (Pew Commission, 1995).

Therefore the charismatic character of the physician, which arises from the priestly side of medicine but is also enhanced by the miraculous power of scientific technology, should be respected. In all professions the charismatic atmosphere is an important element of the professional relation and is essential to the healing process. This atmosphere makes it possible for the patient, often distrustful, to place the necessary trust in professional help. It also gives medical professionals a sense of personal dignity, dedication, and responsibility that immeasurably contributes to their satisfaction and persistence in a difficult vocation.

This charismatic aspect is also a guard of other ethical values, since nothing is so likely to keep medical professionals from abusing their position for financial or other gains as this sense of self-respect. It would be disastrous if the increasing mechanization of medicine or the reduction of the medical professional to an anonymous functionary in a government bureaucracy would destroy the priestly charisma of the profession (Pellegrino, 1987; Crawshaw et al., 1996).

On the negative side, however, as with the clergyman, overemphasis on the special status of the physician is open to great abuses. The physician can become an unquestioned, dogmatic authority in medicine and in all other matters as well (Childress, 1982; Landis, 1993). The medical profession often jealously defends its authority and its prerogatives, refuses to discipline members of the profession, and claims the right to settle ethical and social questions that affect the profession on the grounds that laypersons have no right to opinions in such matters (Axelrod et al., 1988).

Therefore, the physician who wants to develop a sound ethical judgment must have (1) a profound respect for the medical profession as a vocation that has both scientific and priestly aspects, (2) a clear understanding of the limits of this profession (Golub, 1994), and (3) a sense of personal responsibility to develop the attitudes and skills that enable one to personalize the profession (O'Rourke, 1988a).

Christian health care professionals are called by their faith to understand this vocation in a special way, just as professionals of other religions or philosophies of life are called by theirs. Christians think of life as a gift of God and the body as a marvelous work of divine creation to be reverenced as a temple of God (1 Co 6:19, 2 Co 6:16). They also think of the human person not only as a living body, but also as a body living with spiritual life open to a share in the eternal life of God. Consequently, the Christian health care professional thinks of sickness as an evil desecrator of the temple. Even when sickness cannot be overcome, the struggle against it can be lived through as an experience that can further moral and spiritual growth. Thus the Christian physician or nurse is truly a minister of God, cooperating with him in helping human beings overcome their suffering to live more fully.

The Christian medical professional finds a model in Jesus Christ, the Healer. Although physicians do not have supernatural or miraculous powers, they do have medical skill, which is also a gift of God. They can imitate Jesus' compassion for the patient and his reaching out to the most neglected, even the lepers. This Christian attitude cannot be a matter of mere pious words; rather, it is a profound dependence on God, who gives the physician and nurse the inspiration, insight, and courage to carry out their work as professionally and as skillfully as possible.

Moreover, one should not make the mistake of thinking that the ethical aspect of medicine pertains only to its personal, priestly side. It also penetrates its scientific aspect. A scientific approach to disease is built on devotion to objective truth and the courageous, persevering effort to advance this truth through research and criticism. The history of medicine is unfortunately replete with examples not only of outright quackery, but also of superstition and self-delusion. Eminent physicians have sometimes become so enamored of their own theories and personal reputations that they have continued to defend their theories and even to counterfeit evidence concerning them long after their fallaciousness was evident (Engler et al., 1987; Lock and Wells, 1993). Others have stubbornly refused to face new facts and new theories (Schlitz, 1987). On the whole, however, the scientific approach, with its insistence on objective evidence and critical review by peers, has a splendid record. This scientific integrity has been very effective in limiting the excessive charismatic pretensions of some physicians.

Dedication to objective truth and scientific integrity is an ethical value of the highest order. Nothing is gained if the effort to humanize or personalize medicine interjects an unhealthy sentimentalism or occultism into the practice of medicine. Sound ethical judgment can only be based on critical, scientific knowledge.

On the negative side, however, the scientific method, as now understood and practiced, often tends to reductionism, that is, the assertion that the scientific method is the exclusive road to truth. Since the scientific method deals only with the limited aspects of reality that can be measured and experimented on, such a reductionist attitude can compel physicians to ignore and deny facts and experiences outside those rather narrow limits. When reductionism is rigidly applied, the patient is treated as a soulless machine. In the history of medicine, this mechanistic approach has been profitable to the degree that it has used the scientific method intensively, but it has ultimately limited the advance of medicine. Biologists and physicians sensitive to the holistic character of living organisms and the human person have revolted repeatedly against reductionism and opened new, broader, and more fruitful lines of research (Kass, 1985).

Thus sound ethical judgment must completely respect scientifically established medical facts, but it cannot rest on these facts alone. It must be open to all humanistic approaches to understanding and evaluating the human condition.

4.3 MEDICAL EDUCATION AND ITS BIASES

In view of the complex history of the medical tradition, medical education needs to do justice to these person-centered aspects of the profession if it is to prepare medical professionals to make good ethical judgments. Most medical professionals tend to think all their lives in the categories learned in medical or nursing school. This outlook has become so much a part of them through the intensive experiences of their training that they are not likely to reexamine or question it; such an attitude can stifle creativity and growth (Ludmerer, 1985; Fox, 1988).

The medical profession, as well as other professions, recognizes that educational institutions often have glaring biases and defects (Ebert and Ginzberg, 1988). The medical profession in the United States has taken the lead in self-criticism in this regard (Eichna, 1980; Bok, 1984; Petersdorf, 1986; Pew Commission, 1993, 1995). The famous report by Abraham Flexner (1910) led the way for reform in medical education. Flexner emphasized (1) the need for professional self-criticism; (2) the unity of scientific research and medical practice; (3) the advantages of the university-associated medical school; (4) the great importance of a sound liberal education, rich in the basic sciences, as a preparation for medical school; (5) a systematic or logical, but not overburdened, ordering of the curriculum with some limited elective freedom for the student; (6) an emphasis on laboratory and clinical work; (7) the great importance of constant research in special institutes; and (8) the adequate financing and use of a full-time medical staff. On the whole, these recommendations still remain sound. Many authorities today, however, would reject Flexner's emphasis on logical ordering of the curriculum, with theoretical study of the normal body preceding clinical contact with the sick person. They would argue that from the beginning, the program theory should be balanced by clinical experience (Tresolini et al., 1993).

Although Flexner strongly emphasized a sound general education as the basis of scientific medical education, he did not provide equally for the personalistic aspect of the profession. He seemed to presuppose this from other sources. Thus his curriculum has little room for (1) discussion of the nature and limits of the profession itself, (2) study of the counseling skills needed by a physician, (3) study of medical ethics, and (4) sociology and ecology.

A more recent effort at renewing medical education was made under the auspices of the Association of American Medical Colleges (AAMC, 1984). Still more recently, a commission funded by the Pew Foundation has made even more radical proposals for the reform of education and practice of health care professionals (Pew Commission, 1993, 1995). The AAMC Report is too lengthy to summarize here, but the first recommendation of the report is notable. The recommendation, entitled "Shifting Emphasis," states: "In the general professional education of the physician, medical faculties should emphasize the acquisition and development of skills, values, and attitudes by students at least to the same extent that they do their acquisition of knowledge.

Has the AAMC Report had as much practical effect as that of Flexner did? Although there has been an effort to add courses in humanities and ethics to the medical school curriculum in recent years, the success and intensity of this effort has not been uniform (Pellegrino, 1985a; McElhinney, 1993). Even when ethics or other subjects in the humanities are required, they are often on the fringe of the educational effort (Ewan, 1986; Charon and Williams, 1995). The effects of the Pew Commission's reports are not yet available. Judging by past efforts at reform in medical education, however, the proposals of the Pew Commission will be adopted only if the milieu in which medicine is practiced will medical schools change their focus. Hence, if managed care succeeds in the efforts to emphasize primary care and limit the number of specialists, there will be significant changes in medical education. The lack of reflection upon the needs of patients and the inability to introduce progressive changes hamper the efforts of most medical schools in the United States (Enarson et al., 1992). In other words, the focus of medical schools is upon the medical profession, not upon patient care (Pew Commission, 1993; Laine and Davidoff, 1996).

The training of nurses has been forced into the same pattern, with the result that today the nursing profession is undergoing a severe identity crisis (May, 1993; Lumsdon, 1995). In the United States the physician's role has been masculine; the nurse's, feminine. The result is that the nursing profession has had to struggle to achieve the autonomy that characterizes a full-fledged profession. This power struggle has forced many nurses out of an expressive or caring role into an instrumental administrative or technical role. Furthermore, the relation of the registered nurse to the practical nurse and other auxiliaries is far from clear. The AMA, for example, sought to institute a new category of health care worker called "registered care technologist," which would require less training and education than nurses (AMA, 1988c).

The view that the nurse has a role complementary to that of the physician rather than subordinate to it has not yet been generally accepted (J. Ashley, 1976; Fetsch and Minturn, 1994; Bradford, 1989). This role cannot be accepted unless the education of nurses provides them with adequate preparation in the personalistic aspects of health care. Fortunately, in the last fifteen years nursing education has become more and more insistent on (1) good general education, (2) emphasis on the sociological aspects of nursing, and (3) some emphasis on techniques in personal relations (White, 1992; Harbison, 1992).

Medical and nursing schools operated under Catholic auspices have an opportunity and a challenge in our pluralistic society. First, if they are faithful to their Catholic tradition, they have a set of time-tested values on which they can form an ethics of the health care professional. Second, they have a position in the public forum enabling them to witness to the sacredness of human life in word and action. Third, they can commit themselves to a value-centered education that will form health care professionals who are true Christian personalists (Heaney, 1992).

To meet these challenges and opportunities, however, Catholic schools educating health care professionals will need to be sure of their identity (Hesburgh, 1994). If they seek only to imitate other schools or correspond to the popular trends in health care education, they will waste their heritage and never achieve their potential. Unfortunately, Catholic schools training health care professionals have a difficult time effectively stressing the development of a Christian identity because they compete in a society that often sets standards for excellence and proficiency in accord with humanistic standards (Ong, 1990; Barron, 1995).

Biases

In view of medical schools' lack of emphasis in regard to the ethical aspects of medicine, what is the ethical outlook of the medical profession at present? The empirical data of a study by Amasa Ford and associates entitled *The Doctor's Perspective: Physicians View Their Patients and Their Practice* (Ford et al., 1967) led the authors to a series of conclusions. These conclusions have been verified by more recent studies (Colombotos and Kirchner, 1986; Ebert and Ginzberg, 1988; Baldwin et al., 1991). The quotes in the following conclusions are from Ford and associates, but they correspond to the thought expressed in more recent studies.

1. Most physicians have a "strong sense of vocation" rooted in the original priestly character of medicine and reinforced in American culture by the Protestant Calvinist stress on vocation. However, this religious motivation has been covered over: "The vast growth of science and technology in the four hundred years since Luther has obscured the specifically religious conception of most vocations. The physician seldom speaks of God any more when discussing his concern for the patient. Yet he still finds satisfaction in measuring up to personal standards. Vocation, thus, has come to have an ethical rather than a religious basis and to be rewarded by satisfaction rather than by salvation." To be effective, the physicians in this study have said, "they must be motivated and competent and must show concern for the patient" (p. 140).

2. Another important component of this motivation is the physicians' sense of specific competence; that is, they have an important and well-defined service to offer. Much of physicians' personal satisfaction in their work depends on this sense of competence. Competent physicians are happy physicians.

3. Physicians are very convinced of the necessity of a "modern individualism," or a professional one-to-one concern. This conviction has been influenced by American economic attitudes, but it also penetrates even deeper. Most physicians believe they must "care for the whole patient," and a minority of physicians are also highly socially conscious.

4. Physicians tend to think *pragmatically*, so their basic attitude can be characterized thus:

   The physician identifies himself as a professionally competent person who is in a social position to apply scientific knowledge and to exercise impartial control over the situation in order to achieve the rational goal of curing or helping a sick patient. The patient's part of the job is to trust the doctor and cooperate with the treatment (p. 144).

   This element of control implies that the physician retains a detached concern or benevolent, affective neutrality and that the patient should be cooperative and trustful. Physicians are often not very sophisticated about the question of control from a psychological point of view.

Furthermore, studies show that physicians on the whole do not regard themselves as scientists, but rather as *applied* scientists, and that they do not clearly experience a dichotomy between the scientific and the humanistic or affective aspects of medicine. Their satisfactions are not theoretical but pragmatic.

5. Physicians take much satisfaction in their professional position as a mark of achievement. Studies tend to show that this sense of achievement is more important for physicians than monetary rewards, which they do not like to think of as a primary motivation. They resent, however, (a) failure of patients to pay, or failure to receive what they consider just acknowledgment and recompense for the burdens of responsibility, or long education, and of long hours that they have to bear, and (b) limitations on their independence, since these restrictions remove important symbols of their professional position.

Moreover, although physicians gain some satisfaction from scientific interest in their work, they gain more from the therapeutic results. Physicians obtain more satisfaction from giving to the patient (in a parental, nurturing sense) than from a mutual relation. In this way, some physicians perhaps alleviate a sense of guilt over their higher social status. An important element of satisfaction or dissatisfaction is found in the sense of consistency between personal and professional ethics. The modern physician is not inclined to moralize; this factor is associated more with older general practitioners than with younger specialists. This study, however, gives evidence that physicians do have a common sense of ethical purpose.

The studies mentioned indicate some possible biases that medical professionals need to be aware of and that medical education should strive to balance if the medical profession is to make good ethical judgments.

First, on the whole, physicians fortunately continue to exhibit the dualistic balance between the scientific and the humanistic. However, this balance is constantly imperiled by the fact that their scientific training is explicit, detailed, and specialized, whereas their humanistic and moral training is left largely to examples and symbols transmitted to them without explicit reflection or criticism (Scully, 1980; Cassel, 1984; Pellegrino, 1985b). Physicians thus assume that, although science is exact, ethical discourse is vague, subjective, and a matter of opinion (Clouser, 1980). On the one hand this assumption leads to a kind of moral skepticism, and on the other to a dogmatic rigidity, since no method of dialogue or research for critical consensus is available.

Second, physicians tend to take a pragmatic view whereby what is most valued is an immediate, practical solution (Beauchamp and McCullough, 1984). In ethical matters, this pragmatism often causes physicians to act so that (1) they will not be made to feel guilty if an action is taken against their professional or personal standards; (2) they will not seem inhumane toward the patient, yet will not become too involved in the emotional or social problems of the patient; and (3) they will not go beyond the limits of the patient to wider social problems. An example of this simplistic type of pragmatic thinking is found in the statement of the Council on Ethics and Judicial Affairs of the American Medical Association, which declared that vital organs of anencephalic infants may be transplanted to other infants before the anencephalic infants die (AMA, 1994b). The Council later withdrew its opinion but retained the pragmatic assumption that the only value of an anencephalic infant is to be a source of organs for other infants (*N.Y. Times*, 1996)

Third, because the motivation of physicians is so bound up with their sense of vocation, autonomy, and competence, they resent interference in their decisions. They believe that only physicians are in the position to make medical–ethical judgments and that they can be relied on to be decent and humane in these decisions. This belief tends to lead physicians (as in the problem of the dying patient) to follow as their primary rule: *help the patient*, but interpret help as the duty to keep trying by every technique available to improve the patient's physiological condition (SUPPORT Study, 1995). Having done this they can then rest assured and without guilt that they have done all they can do. This attitude leads to deeply felt but simplistic attitudes toward ethical questions.

Fourth, physicians are often resentful that so much is laid on their shoulders. They cannot understand why a wider sociological, religious, psychological, or interrelational view should be their responsibility. Physicians believe that such concerns are someone else's business. Moreover, when medical students select a specialty with its even more well-defined area of competency, their limits of responsibility become even narrower.

None of these attitudes is necessarily wrong. Undoubtedly they are the result of the medical professional's need to live by a clear motivation, with limited responsibilities, and to have sufficient freedom for action and personal judgment. They often result, however, in a closed attitude that renders the physician incapable of learning from others or sharing in a team effort to improve ethical treatment of health problems on a social scale. Thus these attitudes become harmful biases that can lead to gravely mistaken ethical judgments.

The health care profession is noble by reason of its great heritage, its remarkable modern advances, and its great promise for the future. It deserves the type of education that will free it from its own weakness, with which it has been infected by an acquisitive society.

CONCLUSION

Even people who are more or less bystanders realize that health care is changing. The theorists of health care interpret these changes in the terms of paradigms; that is, they maintain that the fundamental model, blueprint, or archetype for health care is changing. For years the paradigm for health care, the basic model for health care, revolved around highly trained physicians and well-equipped acute care facilities. The paradigm could have been phrased in this manner: "Good health depends upon highly trained physicians and acute care hospitals with state-of-the-art technology." Guided by this paradigm, specialists outnumbered primary care physicians, physicians' medical decisions usually were not subject to objective accountability, there was no effort to limit the number of physicians, cost was not a factor in evaluating quality of care, and performing high-tech surgical procedures such as transplant or cardiac angioplasty, which benefit a comparative few, became the standard for excellence when evaluating acute care hospitals. But this paradigm did not respond to the needs of the American public. It resulted in a continual spiral of expenses, and it neglected health needs of several segments of the public such as the poor and elderly.

What is the new paradigm for health care? It seems that two paradigms are vying with each other for acceptance. The first paradigm might be expressed as follows: "Health care is a business, and everything should be structured with a view to making the greatest profit." Those who accept this paradigm bargain with health care professionals, whether physicians or acute care hospital administration, to accept less remuneration for their efforts. In other words, cutting the cost of health care and making a profit receives top priority, even though quality care and patient satisfaction are also mentioned as secondary objectives.

Fortunately, there is another paradigm developing (O'Rourke, 1996b). This new paradigm also features a more cost-conscious offering of health care, but its main perspective is to care for patient needs in a holistic manner. Hopefully, the renewed emphasis upon patient need will lead health care professionals to stimulate society toward a greater effort to make access to health care a reality for all.

The effects of the second paradigm in health care professions will occur in five areas of health care. To wit:

1. *Patient participation:* The emphasis shifts from patient compliance to patient participation. Patients increasingly expect to know not only their diagnosis, but also details of pathophysiology, treatment options, and prognosis.
2. *Medical decision making:* Individual patients differ with respect to the amount of detail regarding their health they wish to know and the degree to which they wish to participate in decision making. Consequently, the art of patient-centered care involves determining the appropriate amount of information and participation from the individual patient's perspective.
3. *Medical law:* The Quinlan and Cruzan cases ignited public interest in advance directives. The mere enactment of state laws recognizing this legal device demonstrates that medical law now bends over backward in order to support patient-centered decision making.
4. *Medical education:* The patient-centered paradigm will demand a change in emphasis and content in the medical school curriculum. Curriculum revision in medical schools has been devoted to utilizing new learning methods. Little attention has been given to preparing young people for a new vision of health care.
5. *Medical Research:* Hard biomedical outcomes have long been the currency of medical research. Over recent years, however, there has been increasing realization that other "softer" outcomes such as functional

states, quality of life, and patient satisfaction may be at least as relevant. The primary difference between traditional outcomes and newer outcomes is that the latter requires patient perspectives.

If health care as a business becomes the dominant paradigm for the provision of health care, then a noble profession will be destroyed. Moreover, the quality of health care for all people in the country will be diminished. One does not need a host of empirical studies to prove these conclusions. When profit becomes the principle goal of any enterprise, all other partial goals, no matter how noble, are sooner or later sacrificed. On the other hand, if the patient-centered paradigm becomes predominant, then we can retain the best qualities from the past, develop a health care system which fulfills our personal and social needs, and hopefully extend access to health care to all in need of it.

5

Personalizing the Health Care Profession

OVERVIEW

Chapter 4 argues that at the center of every profession there is a counseling relation between persons and that this relation takes on a special mode in the health care profession. Chapter 4 also points out that many health care professionals are untrained or not specifically skilled in how to develop and maintain such a relation. However, ethical decisions about health matters depend first of all on a cooperative effort of patients and professionals, without which patients lack the information they need for an informed conscience. Ethical decisions also depend on peer relations among members of the health team, who must pool their information and expertise. Such cooperation between patients and professionals and between professionals and colleagues demands trust and effective communication, which are rooted in sound personal relations. Therefore, unless such relations are established and maintained in the health care facility, there is little hope of ethical, humanistic health care.

This chapter first defines the exact nature of professional–patient relations (5.1) and then deals with the ethical problems of professional communication and confidentiality (5.2). Finally, one basic aspect of peer relations in the health team is discussed—the problem of peer discipline (5.3)—leaving other aspects of this important question to later chapters. Again, what is said of the physician–patient relation must be understood also to apply to nurses and other members of the health team in ways appropriate to the specific role of each.

5.1 THE COUNSELING RELATIONSHIP

Models of Professional–Patient Relationships

In the early studies of the physician–patient relationship, Szasz and Hollender (1956) identified three basic models of this relationship: (1) the model of activity–passivity; for example, the surgeon operating on an anesthetized patient; (2) the model of guidance–cooperation; for example, the physician prescribing medication and the patient taking medication regularly; and (3) the model of mutual participation; for example, the patient engaging in a program of diet and exercise with supervision by the physician. These observations have been confirmed by others (Brennan, 1994, W. F. May, 1983). In all three models the physician as well as the patient achieves certain satisfactions. Thus the physician derives a sense of power from the activity–passivity model and a sense of paternal superiority from the guidance–cooperation model. In a course of treatment for a particular illness, there may be progress from one model to another.

Siegler and Osmond, in a fascinating book entitled *Models of Madness, Models of Medicine* (1974), identified eight potential models of therapeutic relationships in medicine.

1. The *medical model,* whereby the physician diagnoses and treats the disease of a patient, who is relieved of blame, who is free to take time out to be treated, and whose role is to trust and cooperate with the physician.
2. The *impaired model,* whereby the physician must get the patient to accept a permanent and incurable defect and then rehabilitate him or her for a life as normal as possible.
3. The *psychoanalytical model,* whereby the therapist assists the patient to come to a greater self-knowledge, even of unconscious motivation, and to develop a more effective way of living.
4. The *psychedelic model,* whereby the patient undergoes a "trip," an unusual experience, during which he or she needs guidance to achieve personal growth.
5. The *family-interaction model,* whereby the patient is only a part of a family system that is disordered (the patient may be a member) and whereby the therapist tries to improve the quality of the system.
6. The *social model,* whereby the real problem is reform of the social order causing the problem. The therapist is a social reformer and the patient perhaps a corevolutionary.
7. The *conspiratorial model,* whereby the patient is a victim not merely of social disorder but of an actual effort of suppression, and the therapist becomes an advocate to expose the conspiracy.
8. The *moral model,* whereby the patient requires moral reeducation and conversion of behavior under the guidance of a moral director.

In view of the differences in professional roles, the social, conspiratorial, and moral models do not seem directly appropriate to the work of the health care profession. Rather, they appear to pertain to the work of the ethical counselors who deal with the level of conscious, free, responsible behavior, whether it is personal (moral model) or social as well (social and conspiratorial models). The conspiratorial model, although concerned with political behavior, also has a psychoanalytical aspect, since it involves the unmasking of hidden political forces just as psychoanalysis unmasks unconscious personal motivation. On the other hand, the medical, psychedelic, and family-interaction models clearly deal with the psychological level and are the concern of psychotherapy. The psychedelic model also raises questions for the spiritual or pastoral counselor. Similarly, the family-interaction model suggests ethical counseling because the family is the basic unit of social life. Finally, the medical and impaired models deal chiefly with the biological level of human functioning.

Psychoanalytical Model

From an ethical perspective, issues are raised first by the psychoanalytical, psychedelic, and family-interaction models at the psychological level. Psychotherapists are well-trained in the problems of counselor–client relations and are generally well-aware of the ethical issues that arise. Some of the more detailed issues are discussed in Chapter 12.

What are the ethical implications of the remarkable dependence of mentally and emotionally disturbed persons in relation to their therapists? The ethical significance of this relationship can be summarized by a more detailed account of the psychoanalytical model (see 12.3).

In the psychoanalytical model, the client comes to the therapist because of painful anxieties that make normal life difficult or impossible, with the goal of trying to resolve emotional conflicts whose unconscious origin is unknown to the client. The therapist's responsibility is not to diagnose the illness by labeling it, but to help the client come to an understanding of the causes of his or her problems and to cope with them more effectively. To achieve this, the therapist must gradually win the client's trust and help the client step by step to interpret the symbolism of the symptoms. The therapist must grant the client the right to have his or her behavior interpreted as symbolic rather than judged morally and to have his or her sufferings counted worthy of sympathy. The therapist must help the client not to act out symptoms, but to discover their underlying meaning and thus to come to a deep and realistic self-understanding. Finally, the therapist must help the client acquire new skills in coping with the problems of life and terminate dependence on the therapist. To do this, the therapist must personally arrive at self-understanding through the same process.

The client must come to trust the therapist, speaking more and more freely, cooperating by undertaking the task of working through symptoms, and rejecting escape from the process by suicide or even by a flight into health. The client's will to get well and become independent of the therapist must also be reinforced. This process depends on an intense one-to-one relationship in which the client withdraws from the familial and social situation in which he or she has become ill. It also demands toleration by family and society of the client's temporary withdrawal from ordinary relationships and responsibilities.

The client's dependence on the therapist is essentially a recapitulation of the parental relationship, but a healthy one rather than the unhealthy one from which the client has suffered. The therapist is a good mother in taking on the attitude of which Carl Rogers (1951), one of the foremost psychotherapists in America, called "unconditional benign acceptance." The therapist is also a good father in the increasing role of interpretation and confrontation with reality. The libidinal, erotic elements of the transference of the client to the therapist are gradually turned toward the real love objects of the client's independent life. By no means is it easy for clients to come to such total trust in their therapists, since they may have learned to distrust any mother or father. If clients are to get well, however, they have a moral obligation to try to trust, cooperate, and engage in this working-through process. Clients must accept the tasks of (1) trusting the therapist and (2) trying to recover health and normal independence.

Therapists undertake the moral burden of being faithful to this trust reposed in them by their clients. Therapists must listen, not judge, and (to a degree) must sympathize. Therapists must set limits on acting out by clients and must insist on working through. They must approve and reinforce the client's progressive achievement of insight and gradually confront him or her more and more with the demands of reality. Finally, therapists must be willing to let even favorite clients go. For therapists to be ethically true to this trust, they must be personally aware of any tendency toward *countertransference* (i.e., the development of a relationship in which the therapist begins to use the client to meet the therapist's own emotional needs) and must strive to keep this human tendency within limits.

Today these mutual duties, which clearly involve considerable virtue from therapists and a desire for virtue and willingness to grow through suffering from clients, are often formalized in a contract made at the beginning of therapy. In this contract, therapists make sure clients understand and accept the goals and limits of therapy and are aware that they can hold a therapist liable for the therapist's half of the contract. Thus therapists are unethical when they fail to make such a clear contract (which is an aspect of informed consent, as discussed in 3.4) or fail to adhere strictly to it. Therapists should *not* assume moral obligations beyond the limits of this contract. Thus analysts normally should not undertake any responsibility for patients who act out their symptoms outside the therapeutic setting.

Such limitations raise certain difficulties, however, the major ones being: (1) What if the patient is contemplating suicide? (2) What if the patient is contemplating some act injurious to another party, such as physical attack, theft, adultery, or divorce? (3) What if the patient proposes sexual relations with the therapist? (4) What if the patient refuses to work seriously at the therapy or needlessly delays its termination? These problems are discussed at greater length in Chapter 12. Here we need only to point out that these actions constitute a breach (perhaps not culpable) of the contract on the client's part. These actions relieve the therapist from his or her contract, but they leave the therapist obliged (not as a professional, but simply as a citizen) to prevent harm to a third party or to prevent insane persons from harming themselves. Consequently, the therapist can discreetly inform the family or others to guard against suicide or crime. In regard to questions 3 and 4, the therapist can also terminate therapy. If the patient becomes worse or needs commitment, consultants should be called in or the family informed so that the commitment process can be undertaken (Morreim, 1993).

Other forms of psychotherapy do not rest on such a close relationship between therapist and client, but they present essentially the same ethical issues.

Medical Model

In strong contrast to the psychotherapeutic model is the medical model, but it also involves many ethical issues. Today the patient enters both models in much the same type of setting—a private office, clinic, or hospital. Even if patients do not have the same freedom of choice they once had, there are still responsibilities present on the part of physician and patient (AMA, 1995). In the medical model, the professional goal is to treat a physical illness so as to restore normal physical functioning to the degree possible. The physician first seeks to diagnose the disease, then to prescribe a course of treatment (in which the physician is assisted by nurses and others) through medicine, surgery, nursing, or change of regimen. The physician must also make a prognosis and, if possible, offer the patient hope. The patient, on the other hand, is relieved from blame for his or her condition and from ordinary responsibilities to work and family, but is expected to be cooperative with the professional staff. Families and society are expected to support the patient psychologically and to contribute to the expenses (Parsons, 1964; Benjamin, 1985).

The patient is not expected to be as active in the medical model as in the psychotherapeutic models, except in rehabilitative stages of treatment, which pertain more characteristically to the impaired model (Downie, 1994). This patient passivity raises the main ethical issue characteristic of this model. If, as Chapter 3 argues, the health care professional is only a servant to the patient because primary responsibility for the patient's health remains the patient's, then it follows that the professional has no rights over the patient, except those given by the patient's informed consent. Thus, ethically speaking, an implicit or explicit contract must regulate all that occurs in the medical model.

What are the essential features of this medical contract (Pellegrino, 1985b)? First, the contract *limits* the obligations assumed. In the medical model, a physician does not assume the role of a psychotherapist or of an ethical or spiritual counselor. Efforts to repersonalize medicine should not demand that the physician assume all the roles proper to a complete health team. Of course, physicians need to be aware of nonphysical factors that may be affecting the patient's health in order to seek the help of other members of the health team in dealing with such factors. More and more, health care professionals are called upon to be concerned about social and psychic aspects of a patient's life, as well as physiological aspects. The changing nature of health care, which emphasizes a generalist approach as opposed to a specialist approach to the patient, requires physicians to offer therapy at all levels of human need, if at all possible (Pew Commission, 1995).

Nevertheless, the physician who provides primary care has a special relation to the patient. Studies show that 50 percent or more of patients seen by primary-care physicians are not suffering from any physical dysfunction. Some physicians regard such patients as hypochondriacs, are bored with their complaints, and get rid of them as fast as possible or (sorry to say) keep them coming back for an easy fee. Other physicians patiently try to alleviate excessive anxiety by prescribing a placebo or tranquilizer or using a little amateur psychotherapy or a dose of parental advice (Lynoe et al., 1993).

The implied contract between a patient and the primary-care physician, however, obligates the physician to undertake a serious effort to help the patient discover the nature of the problem and the type of help appropriate to it, medical or otherwise. The patient who does not feel well comes to a physician as a first, obvious step in an effort to determine the source of the discomfort. If the possibility of a physical cause can be eliminated, the patient then has the information necessary to take the next step—seeing another type of counselor or taking other action. However, if the physician fails to listen or make an adequate examination, or sends the patient away confused or with a placebo or tranquilizer, the patient still lacks the necessary information for rational decisions (Brahms, 1987). Physicians who deal in an evasive manner with patients are only reinforcing hypochondriacal tendencies.

A well-known study of hospital care (Duff and Hollingshead, 1968) showed that a high percentage of patients were incorrectly diagnosed because of the failure of physicians to listen carefully to patients' complaints and recognize nonmedical factors in their conditions. Moreover, the present system of financing health care has led to problems in sustaining quality of care (Donabedian, 1994; Jecker, 1994).

Second, the medical model, as with other professional relations, is based on trust. The physician, therefore, must establish trustworthiness within the limits of the contract. As it relates to this trust, the contract should have three elements.

1. *Concern.* Fundamental to the contract is the physician's concern for the patient's well-being. Trust will never exist if the patient believes that the physician is concerned only about the fee or is acting out of mere routine as a machine or a bureaucratic functionary. The physician must communicate interest in the patient as a person, not as a kidney or a heart, and a willingness to do for the patient whatever is professionally possible, not limited by mere self-interested motives.

   For this reason, Ramsey (1970) has rightly emphasized that the professional contract is something more than a contract; it is a "covenant" in the theological sense. In the Old Testament, God made a covenant with his chosen people based not on their worthiness but on his generous love for them, and he confirmed this covenant by a promise not to desert them even if they did not meet all their obligations. The professional contract is analogous to such a covenant in the sense that the professional undertakes to help the client not because the client is ethically worthy of help, or even because he or she is able to pay for the service, but primarily because of human need and the essential human rights based on need rather than on merit. The professional contract also implies the promise to continue the patient's care even when the patient is no longer able to insist on its fulfillment.

This concept of covenant, however, should not be exaggerated. God himself insists on the responsibility of his people to respond to their own obligations under the covenant. Thus the physician also has the right to demand cooperation from the patient. Moreover, the physician's contract is not universal but limited by his or her own competence. Therefore the physician is not obligated to do more than inform the patient when a problem exceeds the physician's competence and refer the patient to another specialist or another type of nonmedical counselor.

2. *Knowledge and skill in medicine.* Health care professionals have the fundamental responsibility, within their specialties, to be expert in both the science and the art of health care, up-to-date in knowledge, experienced, of good judgment, and skilled in procedures. Personal warmth does not substitute for medical expertise. Reciprocally, however, one may say that this knowledge and skill cannot be put to their best use if the other humanistic elements are not also present (Pellegrino and Thomasma, 1996). Professionals communicate such expertise to patients by evidence of their education and licensure, by reputation, and also by the care and thoroughness with which they deal with patients.

3. *Communication.* Patients retain fundamental rights over their own bodies and the fundamental knowledge of how they feel not only at this minute, but also throughout the day and in varied situations. Thus physicians cannot hope to make a proper diagnosis, carry on successful treatment, or make an accurate prognosis without adequate patient communications (Katz, 1984). Barnlund (1976) made this observation about communication in medicine:

> When one turns to ask what is currently known about communication between medical personnel and patients, the answer is itself mystification—very little. Here is a profession founded on science, dedicated to truth, committed to inquiry, concerned with the relief of suffering, yet either oblivious or unwilling to examine its own communicative behavior. Is this simply a mote in an otherwise scientific eye? Or is it a defensive assertion of the medical mystique and the preference to do as one pleases (p. 273)?

Finally, in caring for the patient, the physician retains his or her own moral agency. The physician does not become the slave of the patient, especially when ethical issues are concerned (Lyons, 1994).

Health Care Fees

To these basic ethical obligations of the physician, a fourth can be added that applies also to the psychotherapeutic models: to set or refuse an appropriate fee. In a capitalist society, one assumes that a professional should be paid as any other worker is paid, according to the laws of supply and demand. One assumes that a service is just as much a commodity for exchange with a value measured in monetary terms as is any other product. Consequently, some persons argue that nothing is ethically wrong with organizing the medical profession on the basis of profit as in any other industry, and they actually speak of "the health industry." They believe that the stimulus of the profit motive has been the main cause of the rapid technological development of American medicine. Many contend that if the free market were permitted to prevail in health care, the economic efficiency of the American medical system would be greatly enhanced and inflation in medical costs reduced (Ellwood et al., 1992).

Furthermore, some argue that the fee is actually a part of therapy, since it causes the average person to refrain from asking for unnecessary services that might overload the system and deprive others in real need from obtaining proper attention. Moreover, the fee promotes a cooperative attitude from the patient and thus shortens the time of treatment. Freud (Drucker, 1978) scandalized the Jewish physicians of Vienna (for whom the Jewish tradition of caring for charity patients was a cardinal rule) when he insisted on fees from *all* his patients. Freud stated that the subject of psychotherapy who does not have to pay a fee is very likely to waste much time before getting down to the painful task of working through resistances. Freud's practice has become standard in psychoanalysis.

The question can also be raised as to whether this capitalistic assumption is a realistic and practical fact. At no time in the history of medicine has the market system operated fully in the professions, because there have always been people who desperately needed professional help but could not pay for it. Either the professional had to provide free services or payment had to be made by a third party. In fact, since the rise of health insurance and Medicare, most health care *is* paid by a third party, the insurer or the government, who determines standard fees. Chapter 6 discusses the various ways of organizing medical systems to meet the problem of the patient who cannot pay.

If the account given in Chapter 4 of the nature of a profession is correct, it should be clear why profit cannot be the primary basis of any profession but must be considered a secondary and highly variable feature. The medical profession, as with any true profession, must rest not on bargaining but on trust; it provides a service that is concerned with life and death, matters so precious as to be priceless. No monetary value can be set on the spiritual light given by a priest, the defense of human rights provided by a lawyer, the risk of his own life provided by a soldier, or the search for truth shared by a teacher. Similarly, there is no price for the service of a physician in the battle to live.

Just because the health care professional performs so precious a service, it cannot be bargained for. Thus in the past the fundamental principle in all professions was that the professional must be ready to give service free to those who were in need but could not pay. Jesus said with regard to religious ministry, "The laborer is worthy of his hire" (Lk 10:7; see also 1 Tm 5:18); but he meant that his disciples should live from hand to mouth, "freely giving what you have freely received." St. Paul followed this same principle in his own way by supporting himself by manual labor, so that no one might accuse him of preaching for gain

(1 Co 4:12; Acts 18:3). Thus religious professionals deserve to be supported by the public so that they can provide services purely on the basis of the client's need.

The same principle applies to all true professions because they provide services that are life-and-death necessities. Thus professional fees are not payments measured by the value of the service provided (which is truly priceless), but a *stipend* to be measured only by what professionals need to live in a manner that will free them to work without distraction. Therefore medical professionals who set their fees so high as to accumulate wealth in other businesses that distract them from their profession are not faithful to their profession (Eisenberg, L, 1986; Kluge, 1993a).

Official codes of medical ethics used to state that medical fees should be adjusted to the patient's ability to pay. The assumption was that richer patients would be charged enough to compensate physicians for what they would lose in low or no fees charged poorer patients. The inadequacy of this as a principle becomes apparent when the fees are paid by a third party such as an insurance company or the government. Experience shows that in such a situation, physicians are tempted to charge as much as they can get, with a resulting inflation in health costs. The ability-to-pay principle is not unjust as long as it remains within the bounds of the more fundamental principle: professionals are public servants who have no right to expect in return for services anything more than a standard of living that will make it possible for them to perform those services with liberty of mind and health of body and to fulfill family and social obligations adequately. The words of a recent commission studying reform in health care are relevant here: "A health system that is motivated only by competition and quest for profit alone cannot serve the interest of the public. Market forces do not have a proud record of service for the poor" (Pew Commission, 1995).

A Christian physician, lawyer, teacher, or religious minister can only conclude that a professional living is essentially a modest one in which simplicity of lifestyle and freedom to be available to serve others is the only honorable measure of remuneration. Also, one cannot accept the argument so often put forward that since physicians spend long years of difficult study, work long hours, and assume great responsibility, they deserve to make money. The true rewards of any profession are to be found not in some extraneous gain, but in the satisfactions of knowledge and of interesting and absorbing work. For the medical profession, the accomplishments of helping people regain health or prepare for death are the true rewards of the profession. Such an ideal is not easy to realize, nor is it often realized in its purest form. Even when imperfectly realized, however, this ideal is what has given the medical profession its own vitality and health (Roduin, 1993).

5.2 PROFESSIONAL COMMUNICATION

Listening and Truth Telling

In health care, as in all professional relations, adequate communication between professional and client is a fundamental ethical requirement. In the medical model, opportunities for such communication may be rather sharply restricted, but they are still crucial. Within these limits, what are the duties of physicians and nurses?

The first obligation is to listen to the patient. Often in the medical model, however, while professionals concentrate on filtering out medically significant information, patients are attempting to express their malaise in a rhapsody of symptoms, fears, fantasies, evasions, cries for attention, and so forth (Reiser, 1993). The work-pressured professional cannot afford to sit and hear a long and rambling discourse from a self-pitying patient. Requirements issued by HMOs and other managed care firms often restrict the time a physician can spend with patients by requiring that physician see a specified number of patients in each work period (Simmons et al., 1992). Even the psychotherapist, who has a special interest in all sorts of behavioral clues, must insist that patients "get to work" without evading the therapeutic process. Somehow professionals must cut through the noise and get at the real message, but they need to remember that "the medium *is* the message"; that is, the way patients are (or are not) communicating may be the most significant symptom.

Therefore, no matter how busy they may be, ethically, health care professionals may not rush through interviews or simply rely on laboratory tests. They have the responsibility to acquire the art of medical dialogue, by which they can help patients say what needs to be said. The first rule of this art is for the professional to repeat back to the patient what the professional has heard that seems significant and to ask whether it is what the patient meant. This feedback not only reassures the patient but can also gradually train the patient in giving relevant information. A second rule is to obtain the patient's cooperation by explaining the purpose of questions, since unexpected and cryptic questions are threatening and confusing to many patients. If physicians are unable or unwilling to learn this art of dialogue, they must learn to work in a team that includes other professionals with such communication skills.

A professional must not only hear but also *believe* patients, who have the basic right to be believed until they lose that right by clearly proved deception. Thus the temptation of some busy physicians and exasperated nurses to jump to the conclusion that a patient is malingering has to be resisted. Although what a patient reports may not be objectively true, it is subjectively so because it expresses what the patient really *feels* and is therefore medically significant and important.

Professionals also have the right to require honesty and frankness from clients (Nelson, 1994). When professionals suspect deliberate deceit, they should deal with the situation explicitly and directly as a breach of the patient's contract with the professional. In most illnesses, however, psychological factors may cause communication to be distorted by unconscious elements of self-deceit, denial, confusion, or panic. Psychotherapists in particular have to deal with this perplexing inability of some patients to communicate openly, but therapists also experience in themselves something of the same ambiguity. Appleton (1972) states this opinion:

Psychiatrists advocate honest and open communication by physicians with patients but too often do not practice what they preach. Their reasons for silence include uncertainty about the cause, treatment, and prognosis of psychiatric illnesses and unwillingness to depress, demoralize, anger, or alienate their patient (p. 743).

This observation applies to all health care professionals, who cannot expect truth from their patients unless they are equally truthful with them. Lack of frankness by professionals is usually excused as concern to spare the patient, but it is just as often the result of the professional's unconscious fear. Chapter 13 discusses the problem of telling the truth to the incurable or dying patient. Here it suffices to say that the fundamental principle in all such situations is that the patient has the right to the truth, however difficult it may be for the professional to communicate it (Applebaum et al., 1987; Thomasma, 1994).

Confidentiality

Patients have the right to the truth about their health because they have the primary responsibility for their health. They also have the right to privacy about those aspects of life that do not directly affect others. Human community is based on free communication, which is impossible if confidences cannot be shared. Thus health care professionals have a serious obligation to maintain such confidences that protect the patient's right of privacy.

How is a professional to act when questioned by others about a patient's condition? Can confidentiality be protected by lying? All Catholic moralists agree that it is always wrong to "lie," even to protect confidentiality, but not all agree on how to define *lying*. Some (C. Curran, 1975) distinguish between a *falsehood* (i.e., a false statement) and a *lie,* which is not only a false statement but also one made to someone who has the right to a true answer. Consequently, they hold that someone who has a duty to keep a secret can answer falsely to inquirers. It seems better to state, as does Knauer (1967), that the meaning of any human statement must always be determined from the context in which communication occurs. Therefore, when persons ask questions that they have no right to ask, the context renders any answer given essentially *meaningless,* so that it is ethically inconsequential whether that answer in a normal context would be true or false. Thus health care professionals who are questioned about confidential matters may, without lying or even giving a falsehood, reply in any way that protects confidentiality. This fact, however, cannot excuse a physician from frankly answering questions put by a patient or the patient's guardians because these persons have the right to know. Whether one has the obligation to reply to a question with unambiguous and accurate information then depends on the questioner's right to such information (Capron, 1993a).

It is not easy to draw the line between what individuals have the right to keep private and what they may have the duty to make public. Thus the contract between professional and patient should determine this as exactly as possible. If professionals are convinced that, to follow the best course for a patient, they need to discuss the case with consultants or before other members of a team or professional staff, the professionals must obtain the patient's informed consent. Generally, this consent is implicitly contained in the contract. Thus, in most mental hospitals, it is assumed that voluntary (or even involuntary) commitment implies the right to discuss the patient's condition and progress with other members of the therapeutic staff.

Such assumptions, however, are easily open to abuse. Books have been published by physicians and psychiatrists about their famous or notorious patients, living or dead (Chayet, 1966; Carton, 1993). In our opinion, much greater care must be taken to obtain explicit consent from patients with regard to matters that may be embarrassing to them, especially in the present age of medical teamwork and computerized records (Roach et al., 1994). Most patients (or when they are incompetent, their guardians) readily permit the therapeutic use of information, but they should have the opportunity to restrict the use of this information when entering into contractual relations with the professional. It should not be too difficult for a physician or health care institution to work out a regular procedure by which patients are informed of their rights to privacy and asked for explicit consent for any necessary use of confidential information. One of the most difficult problems is researchers' need to have access to records, especially when doing epidemiological studies; even here, however, it should be possible to guard individuals' privacy from public knowledge (Beauchamp and Walters, 1994).

Preventing Harm

Nevertheless, the right of privacy, sacred as it is, is limited by other persons' rights and by the individual's own limited rights of self-disposal. Patients may behave in ways that directly injure themselves and indirectly or directly injure others. For example, patients may commit suicide, seek ways to continue their chemical dependency, spread contagious diseases, or commit acts of theft or aggression against other patients or the staff (Waller, 1993). Some may become so seriously incompetent as to become a public danger on release from an institution, such as the epileptic bus driver who refuses to change his job. In the case *of Tarasoff v. Regents of University of California,* the court held a therapist responsible for not warning third parties that his client might be dangerous (Perlin, 1992, Goldstein, 1993).

In all these cases, the family or society has an obligation to prevent harm both to the patient and to the public because all are members of a community that exists for the good of each of its members in relation to all others. Thus, in general, even when information is given in confidence, professionals have not only the right but also the duty to communicate information to those who may be able to prevent serious harm to the patient or to others.

Thus professional secrecy is not as absolute as the secrecy demanded of a Catholic priest, who may not reveal what he has learned in confession regarding a penitent's sins or defects, even to prevent harm to a third party. Professional secrecy also is not as absolute as that given by law to the confidences between accused criminals and their lawyers. With the priest, the penitent is revealing personal moral responsibility before God, which is beyond human judgment. With the lawyer, the accused is protected in his or her rights by the adversary process. In medical matters, however, patients seldom need to reveal to the professional anything that is essentially incriminating; usually the fact, at worst, might be an embarrassment. Moral fault, however, may incidentally be revealed, as when the patient voluntarily admits an intention to commit a crime or when the medical condition has implications for the health of others (addiction, venereal disease, illegitimate pregnancy, infection with HIV) (Goodwin, 1993).

When what is revealed is an intention to commit a crime (including suicide), the professional has the obligation to reveal to appropriate persons whatever information is necessary to prevent such a crime. When no crime is contemplated, but there is probable danger of harm that can be prevented, the professional should discreetly do what is likely to be helpful in preventing such harm. Ordinarily this should not be done without first warning the patient of exposure if the patient refuses to desist. For example, the professional should keep the fact of addiction confidential if the patient is willing to cooperate with treatment, but the professional may be forced to make it known to the family if cooperation is refused. A professional should protect the confidence of someone illegitimately pregnant unless the intention to secure an abortion is evident. In this case, despite recent court decisions declaring the "right" of minors to free choice of abortion, professionals in some states may be forced to inform the parents of a minor or the father of the child (Minow, 1991). This will at least permit parents to discuss the decision with their child and attempt to protect the rights of their grandchild. In the case of venereal disease of a minor, confidentiality should be maintained unless the minor refuses treatment. In other situations, professionals should first seek to obtain the patient's cooperation and only proceed to inform the third party when this cooperation is refused and the damage feared is both serious and probable. The benefit of the doubt is in favor of confidentiality, which influences the dependence of the patient on the professional.

Certain very serious problems about confidentiality have been raised recently by the computerization of health records and also by the requirement of private and government health insurance plans that physicians report the nature of a patient's illness as a condition of receiving payment (Holleman et al., 1994; Kluge, 1993b). A physician clearly does not have the right to give information of this sort without the patient's permission. This, however, leaves the larger question of how patients are to obtain the benefits to which they are entitled without giving such permission. The insurance or public agency has the right to ask proof from patients that they have used funds for a legitimate medical purpose, but the agency also has the duty to design adequate controls that do not require detailed information possibly embarrassing or injurious to the patient. Computerization of health records should always require the patient's permission, and even when permission is given, care must be taken to limit the availability of these records to a few definitely authorized persons

(Stevens, 1994). Similar problems are raised in the case of peer review, a process that is becoming more and more widespread.

Some professionals (Szasz, 1974, 1977, 1987) argue for an extreme individualistic and libertarian position in regard to patients' rights. For example, they contend that addicts should be permitted free access to alcohol and drugs, and some even believe that suicidal persons should be permitted to take their own lives if they wish. This opinion is based on such notions as: "Freedom is doing what you want with your own life," and "Immorality is only doing harm to another, nonconsenting adult." As shown in 1.2, the very nature of personhood implies involvement in a community. Self-destructive behavior is not merely of concern to the person in question, but to all with whom his or her life is intertwined. In fact, psychology seems to show that such behavior is an often unconscious cry for help (Beck et al., 1986; Gula, 1994). To let such persons destroy themselves because they claim that is what they want is actually to ignore this cry that comes from the true self. The real answer must be a social concern for persons in their real liberty, which consists in becoming more open to others, not more closed. To achieve openness, the trust of the alienated must be gained.

In recent times, the spread of acquired immunodeficiency syndrome (AIDS) (see Chapter 3) has reminded health care workers of the serious responsibility of confidentiality (Creighton Group, 1992). Mainly because of the manner in which AIDS is acquired (people infected with the HIV virus often are homosexual, bisexual, or intravenous drug users), severe discrimination is exercised against AIDS patients (President's Commission on AIDS, 1988). Thus their privacy should be protected. People seem to forget that many people with AIDS have acquired the disease through blood transfusions or were born with it. Moreover, Christian compassion demands that respect be shown for those who acquire the disease through aberrant behavior, even though the activity that brings about the disease is not valued. Jesus never asked those he healed how they became ill.

Health care workers therefore have a serious responsibility to maintain confidentiality in regard to AIDS patients (APA, 1993). Those who minister to AIDS patients must be careful about gossip and casual conversation that would reveal the presence of the disease to those who have no right to this information. On the other hand, those who counsel AIDS patients should follow the same norms discussed on p. 100 concerning revealing the presence of the disease to a third party who might be injured. If possible, the AIDS patient should be persuaded to tell third parties, such as a spouse or any person sharing sexual intimacy, about the disease's presence and the danger of contagion (AMA, 1994). In some circumstances, if the patient will not reveal the disease's presence to concerned third parties, the health care professional might be held in charity and justice to reveal this information.

5.3 PEER RELATIONS AND PROFESSIONAL DISCIPLINE

Health care professionals need good personal relations not only with those they serve, but also with their colleagues on the health team. Problems of leadership and accountability, common decision making and cooperation in carrying out decisions, and adequate communication and mutual support have psychological importance, but they also are profoundly ethical.

Some of these issues are discussed in Chapter 6 and in the concluding Part 5 of this book. This section deals only with the especially sensitive issue of peer discipline because the problem of mutual responsibility is crucial in any group. If health care professionals do not care enough about each other and their common enterprise to accept the painful task of maintaining group standards in a fraternal and humane way and with due regard to the public welfare, they cannot hope to personalize health care, and the general public, especially the legislatures, will begin to exact accountability for practice as well as financing (Greenfield et al., 1992).

The recent phenomenal rise in the number of malpractice suits seems proof that the health care profession is currently in need of stricter discipline. Many propose that allegations of malpractice arise from the litigious character of our society. However, surveys indicate that there are reasonable causes for many allegations of malpractice (Taragin, 1992). When the issue of malpractice litigation seemed to be getting out of hand, a federal commission was formed to study the issue. The Commission of Medical Malpractice of the Secretary of the U.S. Department of Health, Education, and Welfare (GAO, 1987; Powsner and Hemmersaith, 1987) concluded (with some dissenting voices on the commission) that the main factor in this increase in litigation has been the growing number of medical injuries, real or apparent. These simply may result in part from the increasingly complex and risky procedures of modern therapy. However, not all agree with this interpretation (Halley et al., 1989). The commission also concluded that malpractice suits frequently result from (1) poor communication between physicians and patients and thus from inadequately informed consent on the patient's part; (2) patients' frustration because physicians seem unresponsive to their complaints; (3) patients' unrealistic expectations about the benefits of treatment; and (4) growing public conviction that consumers need to defend themselves against arrogant, self-serving professionals. It is noteworthy that the first three of these factors (and perhaps in large part the fourth) reduce to a failure in communication in which physicians are often not well-trained. Recent studies show that most malpractice suits are based upon objective complaints about medical effectiveness, as well as subjective dissatisfaction with the physician's attitude on the part of patients (White, 1994).

Two opposite remedies have been proposed for the malpractice problem. One answer is *peer review* (W. Curran, 1987). It is argued, plausibly enough, that in a field so highly technical as medicine, no one is competent to evaluate professional performance except peers in the profession or even in the same medical specialty. Professionals should judge their peers, set penalties and rewards, and, if necessary, expel serious and incorrigible offenders from the profession (Goldberg, 1984).

On the other hand, some authorities (ABA, 1986) argue that peer discipline has never been successful in protecting the patient or even in maintaining high standards of medical competence (Pilote et al., 1995). A profession, they contend, is too concerned with its own autonomy to be very diligent in disciplining its members. A built-in bias works in favor of protecting members of the profession rather than the interests of patients. Consequently, these critics believe that disciplining a profession first must concern those who suffer from malpractice or neglect. Health care consumers must know and defend their own rights by all available economic, legal, and political means (Pew Commission, 1995).

The first of these two positions, peer review, was adopted long ago by the American Medical Association and the American Psychiatric Association for their membership, but it has been implemented rather perfunctorily (AMA, 1987a). As a result, many states have recently extended the authority of state licensing boards to include reevaluation of physicians' performance. Moreover, under the influence of managed care, more attention is being devoted to variations in medical and surgical procedures across the country (Pilote et al., 1995), and efforts to set uniform standards for medical care are also in vogue (Hagland, 1995).

Calling to Account

Since the primary responsibility for health must remain with each person, to whom the professional is only a servant, the ultimate right to call the medical profession to account must be in the hands of those the profession exists to serve. This is why the users of health services have the fundamental right to the final word in regulating the profession through public law.

In this matter it seems that the physician and the lawyer are in a somewhat different position than the minister, teacher, and scientist. These latter professions deal with objective truth as such, and the public has no right to silence the voice of truth. However, the lawyer is an officer of the court; that is, he or she is subordinated to the government's legislative and judicial officers, who represent the people in determining the law. The medical professional also does not stand for truth as such, as a scientist must, but is providing a service to human physical or mental health, a service that must ultimately be judged in terms of its practical enhancement of human well-being (Siegler, 1987). Consequently, the medical profession must accept a public, practical evaluation of its services. Health care professionals, in their secondary role as scientists, have a right and obligation to speak out for objective truth about biological and medical matters, but this does not give them complete autonomy in the realm of medical practice.

There are many views on how to remedy the rise in malpractice suits and the great increase in insurance rates that this produces. Certainly the tendency to forget that medicine is a practical science and that unfortunate results are often not the result of incompetency must be communicated to the public (Quill and Suchman, 1993). Some blame the legal profession because the courts have too often extended vague legal rules, such as those that relate to the time allowed plaintiffs to report injuries, the application of the *res ipsa loquitur* ("the injury is sufficient evidence of fault") doctrine to medical injuries, the doctrine of informed consent, and liability based on oral guarantees of good results. Some blame the legal system also because lawyers find malpractice suits very profitable, since they receive a high percentage (usually 30 to 40 percent) of the damages awarded, according to what is called the *contingent fee system* (Halley et al., 1989).

Besides the poor communication just mentioned, others blame the medical profession for the unwillingness of many physicians to testify against peers. All admit, including the AMA, that physicians and other medical professionals have the duty to testify in such cases out of justice not only to the claimant, but also to the physician and the profession itself. Compassionate concern for a colleague does not excuse the professional from frank and honest testimony as to the colleague's competence or responsibility when they are in serious question as long as due process is being observed.

The medical profession and every learned profession must have a genuine but limited autonomy. As health care users become more knowledgeable about what is and what is not good medical care, they will become increasingly able to detect serious incompetence or negligence in the service they receive. This awareness will only raise questions, however; it will not be sufficient in most cases to pass judgment. *Res ipsa loquitur* will apply in some cases of medical malpractice, but not in most. People may doubt that a procedure recommended by their surgeon is really necessary, but all they can do is either to ask the surgeon for more convincing answers to their questions or to consult another professional.

Apparently, therefore, a satisfactory system of discipline for the medical profession must be a combination of both *peer* discipline and *consumer* discipline. A medical review board must include both professional peers with requisite technical knowledge and experience and also health care users (along with legal advisers) to ensure that the medical professionals are more concerned for the served than for their own self-interest as the servants. At the same time, it is essential that medical information be made more easily available to all users so that each can know and defend his or her own rights and interests (Katz, 1992).

Since medical professionals now have this information, they have the responsibility to undertake the educational task of informing the public so that it can defend itself against the professionals themselves. Since professionals are inevitably biased in favor of defending their own autonomy, and since any work of public education is difficult in the face of inevitable public apathy, the prospects of such an educational program are not bright. It seems that the public does not want to assume personal responsibility for its own health, but prefers to take pills or have surgery rather than to exercise or stop eating, drinking, and smoking too much.

In the face of this dreary reality, many otherwise compassionate and humanistic health care professionals are inclined to lapse into paternalism. They argue that the profession will have to do what it can for the public on the basis of its own expert judgment while defending itself against annoying or even dangerous lay intrusion into health affairs.

Christian professionals cannot accept this paternalistic and defensive position. The real remedy for malpractice and unjustified malpractice litigation is a more personalized practice of medicine that will reduce misunderstanding between professional and patient and will correct human failure by professionals through mutual cooperation and discipline within the health team itself. The notion of fraternal correction is part of the Christian ethos (Mt 18:15–18). Applied to a profession, it means that the members do not simply ignore or hide the defects of colleagues out of indifference or self-interest, but are seriously concerned to help them overcome these defects and repair the consequences. Fraternal correction also implies that even those workers in subordinate positions have a right and an obligation to correct superiors and that the superiors, when there is objective reason for such action, have an obligation to listen to such corrections.

CONCLUSION

The concern for ensuring ethical behavior on the part of health care professionals continues to mount. To create an ethical atmosphere in the corporate culture of health care, a renewed emphasis upon self-fulfillment through service to patients is needed. In a word, a sense of professionalism must be fostered in order to ensure that ethics leaves the realm of theory and becomes characteristic of everyday activities of health care professionals.

While knowledge and skill are important elements in any profession, for caregivers the distinguishing characteristic is empathy, or the ability "to get inside" the patient or client. Empathy is defined in *Webster* as "the capacity for participation in another's feelings and ideas." Professions are directed toward helping people achieve goods that are fundamental and at the same time esteemed because they are goods that bespeak our humanity. Health, for example, is one of the basic goods of human life. Without health, we have a difficult time performing actions that are an expression of the fullness of our humanity. Pursuing truth or building community are two endeavors by which one measures one's humanity. Cannot one pursue these goods more effectively if one is healthy? Norms indicating the ethical manner to conduct oneself as a health care professional are useful. But they will not be observed unless individuals have a personal commitment to being professionals in the full sense of the term. Being a professional means more than earning a degree or possessing knowledge and skills. It also requires an ability "to get inside another person."

6

Social Organization of Health Care

OVERVIEW

Up to this point, we have developed the notions of the human person and of personal responsibility for health care. The notion of person, however, cannot be understood properly unless persons are related to the community. People belong to many different communities: the family; various social organizations, churches, business organizations; and to the various civic entities, city, state, and national governments. Many of these communities have a direct or indirect relationship to a person's health and health care. Hence these communities have a responsibility to promote the health care of their members. Although the family has a major interest in promoting health and health care, it will not be treated here. Rather in this chapter, we shall consider the ethical obligations of (1) society as a whole expressed through government policies and (2) health care facilities as they are at present the chief locus of health care. First, therefore, in regard to government responsibilities, we will deal with the present situation of health care as a principal social institution in the United States (6.1). Then in 6.2 we shall analyze this situation in light of the social principles of the Catholic tradition. Finally, in 6.3 we will analyze the efforts of the federal government to influence health care through ethical guidelines. Second, in regard to health care facilities as the social institutions which directly deliver health care, in 6.4 we will consider these as human communities, in 6.5 as functioning through professional teams, and in 6.6 as guided in ethical matters by ethics committees. Finally, in view of the increasing pressures on Catholic facilities resulting from the political situation described at the beginning of the chapter, we will then conclude in 6.7 with a discussion of how a Catholic health care facility can maintain its own Catholic identity.

6.1 THE POLITICAL SITUATION OF HEALTH CARE TODAY

Individualism and Resistance to Reform

The emphasis on individual initiative and responsibility has been a strong element in American culture of which we are rightly proud, but it often makes the United States public schizophrenic in its attitude to our community responsibilities and to the necessary role of government in uniting us for common action for the common good. This self-contradiction has been glaringly evident in the recent debate about a national program of health care. While surveys indicate that people in the United States are in favor of providing access to health care for all citizens, when it comes down to framing practical measures, there is a reluctance to put the public's generous attitudes into meaningful legislation. Long ago the principle was accepted that government should promote and regulate universal free education for all children, at least through high school. Good education, it is thought, is beneficial not only for individuals but also for the community. Both the private sector and the public sector are involved in providing education. If persons in families are not able to finance education through private means, then several programs, such as public schools or long-term low-interest loans, are available to support the efforts of individuals to obtain an education. Not many people in the United States would quibble with the statement, "Every child has a right to an education." If this right cannot be fulfilled through private means, it is the responsibility of the public domain, city, state, or federal government, to provide the opportunity to fulfill this right. In regard to health care, however, there is no such unanimity of attitude or program (deBlois, 1995).

Our citizenry tends to think of medicine as the business of the private sector (Reinhardt, 1994). Thus the specter of "socialized medicine" is used as a threat by those who wish to prolong the present system of health care. In reality, of course, much of health care in the United States is already "socialized medicine." For example, all citizens over sixty-five years of age are eligible for the Medicare program administered by the federal government. This program pays for some of the cost of hospitalization and visits to physicians. Medicaid programs funded by the federal and state governments provide health care for the very poor and for mothers and their children. There are also health care programs for Native Americans funded by the federal government. In another mode, the federal government also sponsors socialized medicine through the billions of dollars it distributes every year through the National Institutes of Health (NIH) to fund medical research. Granted, much of health care is funded by the private sector in the form of employer sponsored insurance plans. But even these plans require many people to be enrolled in the programs in order for them to be financially feasible. In a sense, then, employer-sponsored insurance plans are a form of socialized medicine. Only a few people in the United States pay for health care as they do for other goods in the private sector through their own savings or current funds (HCFA, 1993).

Yet in spite of this widespread socialization of health care, the U.S. public, in contrast to that of most advanced countries, has oddly not been convinced that health care, like education, is a fundamental human right, and therefore must be provided for all through public funds when private funding does not suffice. Of course, to say that health care is a right also implies that personal responsibility for health which we have argued in Chapter 3. Thus, preventive medicine and primary care medicine must receive major emphasis in any program providing health care for all. Moreover, people need to qualify for health care in public entitlement programs by being conscientious in fulfilling personal responsibilities. But public reluctance to recognize access to health care as a right for all has produced a situation in the United States in which forty million citizens lack adequate access to health care (Berk et al., 1995). Many of these people are employed, but more and more employers do not provide health insurance, mainly because it is so expensive and costs escalate each year.

Why Efforts at Health Care Reform Have Failed

During the past few years, many people and organizations have sought to reform the provision of health care in the United States. For a more comprehensive view of these activities, one may consult the journal *Health Affairs,* which offers the most complete report and analysis available of government financing and provision of health care. We present only a sketch of the situation. At the level of public policy, the federal government in 1993–1994 sought to design and implement a plan which took health care almost completely out of the private sector. The goals of the health care reform plan were to overcome the continual escalation of health care costs and to provide universal access to health care. But this federal plan was designed by theorists who did not consult the people actually involved in the many aspects of day-to-day medicine (Blendon et al., 1995). The planning team did not adequately represent physicians, nurses, or administrators, or representatives of insurance companies or pharmaceutical firms. Even though several professional groups consisting of health care professionals and health care institutions at first expressed general approval of the new plan, it failed to get congressional support and was never actually debated on the floor of the House of Representatives or the Senate (Yankelovich, 1995). While many reasons have been put forward for the failure of this abandoned plan, the following observations certainly need to be considered in any future effort to reform health care.

1. The funding for the proposed program depended mainly upon employers rather than upon general taxes on corporations and individuals. Hence, the business community rejected the plan because they did not wish to assume the burden of funding health care for the entire population. In most of the health care plans of other countries, Canada and England, for example, the plans are funded by general taxes, known as the "single party payer" system. This system clearly realizes that health care cannot be funded through private sources, whether personal or corporate, because a system covering all citizens will require support by more than private business.

2. The provision of health care was based upon a managed care model. While the managed care model has much to recommend it as far as controlling cost is concerned, it was thought greatly to reduce the personal aspects of medical care. Thus the members of Congress became greatly concerned that managed care would not allow people to choose their own physician, and they considered this freedom of

choice to be the basis of the American health care system. Yet it was by no means clear that these managed care proposals, especially after some revision, would have drastically limited choice of physicians. In fact, as a result of innovations in the private sector, managed care, often without unlimited choice of physician, is rapidly coming to dominate health care. Thus, all efforts to improve public health care policy can be frustrated by a failure to inform the public of the facts.

3. Powerful forces in the private sector were either ignored in the planning phase or relegated to minor roles in the provision of health care. While several of these organizations from the private sector, such as the American Medical Association (AMA) and the Health Insurance Association of America, initially applauded the stated goals of health care reform, cost control, and universal access, they soon realized that the proposed plan would relegate physicians and insurance companies to lesser roles in the overall provision of health care. Thus, they appealed through advertisements and video vignettes for some vague "better way."

4. The health care reform plan never did define "basic health care," claiming only that the basic plan would have to be "rich" enough to attract enrollment by most of the people in the country. On the other hand, the Catholic bishops of the United States, always strong advocates of health care as a right for all, criticized the plan because it included abortion as part of the basic package (USCC, 1993a).

5. Finally, some declared there was "no real crisis" in the access to or provision of health care. The many people without health care insurance of any kind were not heard, proving once again that there are segments of our society, because they have little power or money, who are never prominent in public debate.

Since the failure of efforts by the federal government to initiate health care reform have failed, there have been efforts in the private sector and to some extent at the level of state governments to correct the situation by reducing health care costs. Surprisingly, even though managed care was denounced by many during the health reform debates of 1994, the efforts at the level of the private sector to reform health care have followed a system of managed care.

The Growth of Managed Care

This turn to managed care seems to be taking place in the United States in two phases. Phase one demands efforts on the part of businesses and insurance companies to force the principal providers of health care, namely physicians and acute care hospitals, to charge less. Health care providers have responded to this effort not only by reducing fees, but by forming cooperative ventures, either of hospitals alone, of physicians alone, or of hospitals and physicians entering into single-provider organizations. For example, physicians formed independent physicians' associations (IPA), and accepted discounted fees from insurance companies, businesses, and health maintenance organizations. In phase one of managed care, the method of financing usually remains "fee-for-service"; that is, a fee is charged for every visit, test, procedure, or hospitalization. Hence, health care costs increase as the number of procedures increase.

Phase two of managed care does away with fee-for-service payments. Instead, managed care provides funding based upon a system known as *capitation*. In a capitation plan, people are enrolled to receive care for a specific fee for a set period. In exchange for the fee, the sponsors or managers of the health care plan promise to provide all necessary health care for each person in the plan. Because the health care providers cannot charge for each procedure, this form of funding encourages physicians and hospital administrations to avoid unnecessary medical procedures and over-extended stays in the hospital. If a health care provider utilizes the capitation system for payment, it is usually known as a health management organization (HMO). The HMO form of managed care has for some years been growing in the United States, and government insurance plans such as Medicare and Medicaid are encouraging their constituency to enroll in HMOs in order to reduce health care costs.

One of the more controversial aspects of phase two managed care is that the health care insurers and managers set standards for medical practice to make sure that unnecessary and experimental procedures are avoided. Sometimes physicians are consulted when these standards are set, sometimes they are not. Individual patients are able to select physicians from a panel associated with the health care plan, but physicians must agree to follow practice norms before being admitted to the panel. Hence, physician autonomy, the ability of physicians to make therapeutic decisions with little or no surveillance, is severely limited in managed care plans (AMA, 1995). In addition, managed care plans stress outpatient care rather than hospital care; preventive medicine; primary care; and other care by specialists. Access to specialists is usually allowed only through primary care "gatekeepers" and may be delayed by this process.

The concept and actual experience of managed care have provoked many negative reactions. Some point out its possible dangers: lack of adequate care in order to increase profits, lack of complete freedom to choose one's own physician, and lack of physician autonomy in treating patient illness. Another negative aspect of managed care is the small amount of income spent on medical services, only 58 to 70 cents per dollar, as opposed to the money spent on administration, advertising, and employee compensation. According to a 1995 survey, salaries paid to executives of for-profit managed care corporations, were extravagant. CEOs of the ten leading for-profit HMOs earned an average of 7.3 million dollars in salary and stock options per year (Krieger, 1995). In mitigation of these criticisms, some recall the shortcomings of the health care system of the recent past: the proliferation of unnecessary procedures encouraged by fee-for-service payment; the lack of clear standards for treatment for rather common ailments; the dependence upon specialists for primary care; and the negligence in stressing good health habits as part of the total effort to maintain health and declare that managed care is not all bad. Finally, proponents of managed care maintain that quality of care and patient satisfaction are more carefully moni-tored in managed care systems than under the fee-for-service system.

A final step in phase two of managed care will be the development of integrated delivery systems or community health systems (CHA, 1993b; Robin-son, 1994). These systems call for patient-centered programs designed to meet patient needs, not to keep physicians employed or acute care hospitals open, and they will demand more intimate cooperation among health care profession-als and facilities (Boyle and Callahan, 1995). For example, nurse practitioners and midwives will supplant physicians when possible, and dying patients will be cared for in hospice programs rather than in an intensive care unit in an acute care hospital.

The ethical issues arising from managed care and the capitation system of payment are rather obvious. If a managed care system is a for-profit corporation, it has as its purpose making money for investors rather than the promotion of patient well-being. For-profit health care is essentially unethical because the goal which ultimately determines its decision is not the right of the patient to good health care (O'Rourke, 1987). This right ought not to be subordinated to the financial goals of the corporation, however sincere its claims to meet its obligations to patients. Health is not something which can be bartered or sold, as shoes or popcorn; thus, health care is not a business nor an industry (Ber-nardin, 1995). Even not-for-profit managed care systems are in danger of con-centrating too much on profit and not enough on quality patient care.

One prominent ethical need which will not be served by managed care is the provision of access to health care for those not enrolled in public or private insurance plans. In other words, even if managed care plans are successful in providing quality health care while controlling costs, the problem of adequate access must also be considered. What principles can be derived from Catholic social teaching to guide us to better health care planning?

6.2 PRINCIPLES OF PUBLIC HEALTH CARE POLICY

The American way of life has moved toward a high degree of centralization and monopoly in industry as well as in government. Such centralization has not changed the class structure of American society in any radical way. It would be perfectly possible to set up a centralized model of health care so as to leave considerable choice to both the consumer and the provider. This model could even include voluntary health insurance and fee-for-service features. What is essential to such a system is that it be centralized on a regional basis and involve planning in acquisition and allocation of resources. Given the difficulties with the present system in regard to planning for health care and arranging for financing that would afford adequate access for all, a new model should be considered. Such a model would be based on the view that there must be centralization and planning, but also extensive participation in the planning process. In a planned society, whether governed by a democratic or a socialistic bureaucratic elite, individuals receive health care but lose any real control over how this is done. In a market system, individuals scarcely have any more control because they lack the information or alternatives from which to choose. What is needed, therefore, according to those who seek a third model, is a system in which well-informed consumers play a real role in the planning process (Navarro, 1986).

One great problem in adopting the participatory model is the resistance of health care professionals. They have been educated to believe that the maintenance of high-quality health care demands professional autonomy and forbids interference by lay-persons (AMA, 1995a). Such barriers to a participatory model can be overcome only by a change in medical education to move the physician's ideal away from the exclusively scientific model toward a more humanistic model (Pew Commission, 1995). A humanistic model is superior even scientifically because it relates the individual ecologically to the environment (Annas, 1995). Other researchers believe that a participatory model can come about only by educating consumers to know and aggressively defend their rights. Our line of argument would lead to the conclusion that the essential steps to developing a participatory model are (1) assumption of responsibility by each person for his or her own health, (2) restoration of a sound professional–client relationship, and (3) education of medical professionals to be able to work in this relationship (Pellegrino and Thomasma, 1988).

Common Good

The first step in seeking a better organization of health care in the United States and in the world must be to free ourselves from the ideology that leads Americans to analyze every social issue in terms of the American free-enterprise system and the tyranny of socialism. Many Americans, for example, have received a kind of education that identifies Christian social teaching with the American way of life. Such identification of any human culture with the Gospel is certain to be misleading, since the Gospel stands as a prophetic criticism of every culture, approving some of its features but correcting others.

The authentic social teaching of the Catholic Church has been formulated since Leo XIII's great encyclical *Rights and Duties of Capital and Labor* (1891), in many papal encyclicals and documents, by the Second Vatican Council in *The Church in the Modern World* (Vatican Council II, 1965c), and most recently in the encyclicals of Pope John Paul II, *On Social Development* (1987a) and *Centesimus Annus* (1991). This teaching contains some strong criticisms of socialism, chiefly on three grounds: (1) its materialism, (2) its denial of the right of private property, and (3) its tendency to promote totalitarian government. However, this teaching also contains a vigorous criticism of capitalism on three grounds: (1) its deterministic reliance on economic laws, (2) its advocacy of unregulated competition and the profit motive, and (3) its neglect of the Christian advocacy of the poor. Recent papal documents (e.g., John XXIII's *Christianity and Social Progress* [1961], Paul VI's *The Development of Peoples* [1967], and John Paul II's *On Social Development* [1987a]) have pointed out that capitalism and socialism alike have become colonializing powers either politically or economically and are thus largely responsible for the wars and poverty that oppress the great majority of humankind (Curran and McCormick, 1986). Christian health care professionals, therefore, should base their thinking about the social organization of health care on the principles of the Gospel, not on the principles of the free-enterprise system any more than on those of socialism (NCCB, 1983).

Apart from ideological bias, no one economic system any more than one political system is simply natural, right, or Christian. Such systems are human inventions, each with some advantages and some disadvantages, to be selected according to particular historical circumstances. These merits need to be evaluated both from a theoretical point of view and from a practical, experiential point of view. In judging them ethically, both their congruity with fundamental moral and Gospel principles and their pragmatic results in a given situation must be considered. A theoretically correct system in some circumstances may result in ethical disaster, whereas it is sometimes necessary to tolerate theoretically wrong institutions because they are the best that can be hoped for at the moment. In the long run, however, bad principles will have bad consequences. Christians must constantly strive to test their understanding of principles by experience and to bring the real situation into line with these principles once they are refined.

Catholic health care professionals thus have the responsibility at present to study all proposals for a plan for health care and attempt to judge them in terms of theoretical principles and practical experience. Such a study is beyond the scope of this book, but it may be useful to indicate the first steps in such an ethical inquiry seeking a solution to the problem of providing access to health care for all. To face this fundamental dilemma requires radical thinking, and it is here that Catholic social thought can make an important contribution to finding a new solution. This solution must rest on three propositions that have been previously expounded in this book: (1) every human being does have a fundamental right to health, as acknowledged in the *Universal Declaration of Human Rights* (United Nations, 1948), Article 25, because human rights are based on essential human needs; (2) individual persons have the primary responsibility to promote their own health; and (3) as social beings, however, people also have the right to seek the help of others when necessary to fulfill this responsibility and reciprocally have the duty to give the same help to others as much as they are able.

Subsidiarity

The papal encyclicals and the Second Vatican Council have repeatedly proposed a universal social principle (of which this second proposition is only an application to health care) that is called the *principle of subsidiarity* or, more comprehensively, the *principle of participation* (cf p. 222). This principle follows from the need of the person in community which is to be realized in communal sharing, or in the common good. Each individual, therefore, in order to fulfill human need, has a moral obligation to contribute to the common good and a right to share in it.

Most social evils and injustices are the result of exclusion of some persons from the common good in which they have a right to share (Williams and

Houck, 1987). The ancient evil of slavery was precisely such an unjust institution. The slaves contributed to the common good but were not permitted to share fully in it, not only in regard to economic goods, but also in regard to spiritual goods such as education, freedom, political participation, respect, and even the right to worship the "gods of the city." Thus the distribution of the common good is a fundamental demand of social justice.

Jesus, moreover, taught an ethics that clearly went beyond even this demand for distributive justice based on merit. Jesus proclaimed the coming of the Kingdom of God (Mk 1:15), which was not merely a heavenly kingdom but also the fulfillment of the Old Testament prophecies of the reign of God on earth (Viviano, 1988). When Jesus said to Pilate, "My kingship is not of this world" (Jn 18:36), he did not mean by "world" the earth, but the present sinful order of power struggle. He was saying to Pilate, "I am not competing with you power brokers. I am building a kingdom built on a different principle; on service, not on dominion." He taught his followers to pray, "Your Kingdom come, your will be done, on earth as it is in heaven" (Mt 6:10). The Beatitudes (Lk 6:20–22; Mt 5:3–11), in their original form, were the joyful announcement to the poor (i.e., those excluded from the common good) that at last they were to be included in that common good, not only economically, but spiritually ("The poor have the good news preached to them") (Lk 7:22). Consequently, the principle of the early Church was "from each according to his ability, to each according to his needs," a principle that Marx borrowed from the Acts of the Apostles (4:32–35). Thus the principle of the common good requires love and mercy and the distribution of the common good not according to merit, but according to need. Thus the mark of all Jesus' work was his concern for the neglected, the outcast, the leper, the prostitute, the Samaritan heretic, and the pagan unbeliever.

A Christian ethics of health care distribution must be based not on merit, and certainly not on the ability to pay, *but on need*, because the needy are the most neglected. Those who can care for themselves do not need social help. Moreover, social oppression of the needy is the major cause of their illness, an oppression from which the more affluent members of society profit. Thus those who are helpless by reason of poverty, disease, defect, or age (the unborn or the senile) should be the first consideration of any health plan.

However, all persons should contribute to the plan according to their *ability*. Thus the social responsibility for health care falls first on those who have the ability to heal, the health care professionals, and second on those who have the ability to pay, that is, those who have financially profited the most from society. For such affluent individuals to claim that they have made their wealth simply by their own efforts is an absurdity. They may have worked hard, but their wealth would not have been possible exclusive of the society of which they are a part. Consequently, their debt to the common good is in proportion to the wealth they have received from it.

From this notion of the common good, the idea of subsidiarity follows logically. *Subsidiarity* implies that the first responsibility in meeting human needs rests with the free and competent individual, then with the local group. Higher and higher levels of the community must assume this responsibility (1) when the lower unit cannot assume it and (2) when the lower unit refuses to assume it.

Although all persons are primarily responsible for their own health (cf. Chapter 3), when, because they are too young, too old, too poor, too uneducated, or possessed of any other handicap, they cannot assume this responsibility, the community at higher levels must come to their aid. If a lower level neglects to fulfill the responsibility, a higher level must correct the oversight by punishment or other remedies. The higher level should never be content merely to take over responsibility, however; it must work to return responsibility to a lower level. Thus people should be educated about personal health care, helped to pay for such care, and held responsible for neglecting it. *The main objection to many social reforms has been that they have not provided for this progressive decentralization.* For example, the welfare system in the Untied States has perpetuated poverty rather than helped the dependent to become independent.

The growing criticism of liberalism and the excesses of government bureaucracy, however, should not lead to identifying Catholic social thought with the conservative movement, which has grown more and more powerful in the United States since the Second World War. As Nash (1976) has shown in *The Conservative Intellectual Movement in America Since 1945*, American conservatism is of three varieties: (1) libertarianism, which advocates a *laissez faire* government; (2) traditionalism, which deplores the loss of Western cultural heritage through overrapid social change; and (3) nationalistic anticommunism. Catholic social doctrine has always opposed *laissez faire* capitalism, which the papal encyclicals label "liberalism" in the original sense the term had in the economic thought of Adam Smith and the political thought of the French Revolution. Although Catholicism has conserved the Western cultural heritage, the Gospel message, as Vatican II made very clear, is to build the Kingdom of God on earth by a radical reform of society according to the demands of peace and justice. Likewise, Catholicism opposes communism, not by a program of nationalism but of disarmament and international cooperation. Thus Catholic thinking in social matters must remain independent of both the liberal and the conservative tendencies, both of which arise from the basic assumption of humanism (USCC, 1995a).

Therefore the type of health care program that Catholics can consistently support must aim at preventive medicine, at achieving a healthier people who can care for themselves, rather than an ever-increasing dependence on technical medical care and professional help. As Plato observed, "A society that is always going to the doctor is a sick society" (*Republic* III, 405A).

Functionalism

The popes have also stressed that one of the evils of historical capitalism and socialism alike has been the tendency of both systems to concentrate all the power of decision making in the state. Before secular humanism became the dominant philosophy of modern society, Christian thinking was able to advance the notion that a society is not simply a two-level structure of government and citizenry, but an organic community containing many *functions* that are mutually interdependent.

This concept of the mutual interdependence or solidarity of a community was enunciated by St. Paul in 1 Corinthians 12–13 and linked by him with Jesus' teaching that the greatest should become the servants of the least in the Kingdom of God. Thus the power to make social decisions ought to be kept as close as possible to those who experience those problems and are most strongly affected by the decisions concerning them. Only in this way can the dignity of the least members of a community be acknowledged and their interests effectively served by the greater. A paternalism that decides everything for those it claims to serve is really nothing but a form of domination and tends to become self-serving. Thus St. Paul, without directly attacking slavery, admonished the master that he should treat his slave not as a child, but as a "most dear brother" (Philemon v. 16), that is, as equals by reason of their mutual interdependence in Christ.

The principle of subsidiarity therefore requires us to share decision-making power not only at various vertical levels of local, state, and federal government, but also among horizontal sectors representing various functional bodies. Thus education, as a basic function of society, forms a body of persons, some with expertise (the educators) and others (the students) who are trying to educate themselves through the services of the experts. Decisions about education pertain first not to government but to bodies of cooperating teachers and students mutually dependent on each other. The same holds true for other basic social functions—especially for the economy, with its interdependence of management, workers, and consumers—as well as for the social organization of health care, with its mutual interdependence of professional healers and health seekers. Each person in a society is related to as many such functional bodies as he or she has basic needs. The role of government is to coordinate and encourage the full development of these different organs of society, not to deprive them of their decision-making capacity.

This application of subsidiarity to the organization of society on the basis of social functions, rather than on the basis of a struggle between isolated individuals defending their rights and a centralized government having all the powers of social decision, is usually referred to as *corporatism* in Catholic documents. This term somewhat misleads Americans, who usually view corporations as purely economic organizations. The term has also been discredited because it has been used by fascist political parties in Europe to win Catholic support for its exact opposite, namely, totalitarianism or total state power. The following discussion will use the term *functionalism* instead.

Functionalism is opposed on the one hand to communism and national socialism because they are totalitarian, concentrating all decision-making power in the hands of the state and the military. On the other hand, it is opposed to the competitive individualism of unregulated capitalism or free enterprise, with its hidden tendency toward monopolism, resulting in concentration of decision-making power in the hands of an interlocking power elite (Califano, 1985) or the industrial–military complex. Functionalism is not a mere theory, since it has a powerful influence, through Catholic statesmen, on the formation of the European Common Market and of codetermination by management and labor in West Germany, Japan, and other countries. Some of its implications are also evident in Latin America in the efforts of Catholic theologians and political leaders to develop a theology of liberation that is not capitalist, fascist, or Marxist (Boff, 1986, 1992).

Politically, it might seem that functionalism would have little chance in the United States. Certain features of some institutions, however, are in fact functionalist. For example, higher education in the United States, in contrast to the statism of the lower school system, remains largely functionalist. Decisions about educational policies in our colleges and universities are made independently of government by faculties and accrediting agencies and by the right of students to choose their own schools. The student revolt of the 1960s, however, seemed to show that schools needed to allow students greater participation in policy making, and to a certain extent this has taken place, rendering the system still more functionalist (Dickstein, 1988). On the other hand, the increasing control of the government over schools by reason of their economic dependency is working strongly to destroy their functionalist character.

Similarly, after the Great Depression the growth of labor unions in the United States, to a considerable degree under the influence of Catholic social thought (Cronin, 1950), portended the eventual development of functionalism in the economic sphere. Unfortunately, the unions have largely neglected the social aspects of their original purpose and have been co-opted by the capitalist market system, in which they tended to become just another monopoly. Renewed Catholic leadership in unions, including hospital unions, could remedy this neglect. Fortunately, this trend toward monopoly shows some signs of a reversal in the growth of consumer activism, participatory democracy, and social ecology, as well as in the increasing dissatisfaction with resulting liberal reforms, so many of which have served only to enlarge the power of government bureaucracy. Catholics need to take advantage of this growing criticism of the so-called American way of life to propose a more personalistic and functionalist conception of society.

In health care, these general ethical principles of subsidiarity and functionalism have to be applied to the concrete historical situation of American medical institutions. The medical profession, as it has operated in the United States, has been influenced by three somewhat inconsistent principles: (1) the ancient ideal of a profession as service, which was formulated in the Hippocratic oath and reinforced by Christian ethics; (2) the philosophy of secular humanism, with its strong emphasis on human rights and the duty of man to use scientific knowledge to solve human problems; and (3) the ideology of capitalism, which has been fostered by humanism. Many liberal secularists recognize that this capitalist ideology is at odds with their concern for human rights and the full application of the social sciences to the planning of economic and political life. Conservative humanists, however, have defended this capitalist ideology out of fear of Marxism.

In view of Christian goals, a Catholic should be particularly aware of the lessons learned by the United States. The first of these is that our existing health care system has not adequately cared for the poor nor emphasized preventive medicine (AHA, 1986a; Aday, 1993). Rather, it has tended to foster an exaggerated professional elitism, to place strong emphasis on monopolization and the profit motive, and has produced a system of medical education lacking in humanistic breadth and depth. On the other hand, the existing system should be credited with promoting very rapid technological and scientific progress and with developing many health care facilities equipped to give acute care. It must be noted, however, that this progress has led to greater expenditure of resources on the sophisticated treatment of relatively rare ailments rather than to better care for the health of the majority (Fox and Swazey, 1992).

A centralized system is aimed at correcting some of these defects, but not in a very radical manner. Such a system will probably greatly increase the bureaucratization, which, as evidenced by the welfare system, can cost a great deal and accomplish very little. A centralized system will provide more health care, but there is no certainty it will promote better health. A bureaucracy also is not likely to personalize the health care it gives. Even if this system makes a sincere effort to humanize medicine, such effort will not be guided by a Christian concept of the person but by a secular humanist concept that may express itself not in concern for neglected persons, but in their extermination by abortion or euthanasia (Hardin, 1993).

Therefore, although Christians should favor a national health care program as the only practical way available to extend care to the neglected of society, they should not have any illusions about the adequacy of such programs. Instead, Christians should critically support the new schemes for comprehensive health care, stressing the need to incorporate into these plans as many functionalist features as possible. For example:

1. Comprehensive health care should aim primarily at the promotion of positive health, not merely at the cure of acute disease or the prolongation of life through sophisticated techniques. Therefore, it should work for (a) removal of the environmental and social causes of ill health, including the commercial encouragement of unhealthy patterns of living, and (b) provision of preventive health education that will give persons control over their own health.

2. Priority should be given to the problems of the most powerless, poorly informed, and least able to pay. These persons should not be cared for paternalistically, but should be admitted to participate in the power of decision about their own health needs.

3. Decision-making power should not be confined to a government bureaucracy, nor to autonomous professionals, but should be shared by all concerned in mutual interdependence.

4. Planning should proceed in such a way as to avoid tendencies to increase dependence on higher levels and to promote a gradually increasing decentralization in both control and funding. This decentralization, however, should not be used as an excuse for the govern-

ment to neglect the monitoring of health care and the supplementation and correction of defects at lower levels of organization.

5. Planning must be a continuous process of decision making that adapts to experience and new needs, rather than a fixed plan based on projections that may be mistaken.

Christians may find support for various items of a functionalist program from different and opposed ideological camps. For example, ecology-minded people are convinced that environmental and social factors are the major cause of poor health conditions, but others cite this fact to defend the medical profession against the charge that it is responsible for these conditions. Again, the rights of health consumers are defended not only by civil rights and consumer advocates, but also by individuals who believe that the free market is the best method of controlling health costs. Consequently, Christians should attempt to transcend ideological biases and use a strategy of coalition to promote particular goals.

Above all, Christians should work together through various church agencies to influence the health education of consumers and the medical education of the professionals. Catholic schools, medical schools, and teaching hospitals especially should teach a personalistic approach to health and to the objectives of the medical profession. Catholic institutions must protest against the many current forces that tend to absorb them into the centralized, bureaucratic structure of society dominated by secular humanism. At the same time, Catholics should approach secular humanists with a genuinely ecumenical spirit, which seeks through dialogue to find grounds of agreement and cooperation.

6.3 HEALTH CARE ETHICS AND PUBLIC POLICY

Government and Ethical Guidelines

In funding health care, government finds itself also promulgating ethical guidelines to regulate medical research and therapy. Thus in the late 1960s and early 1970s, Congress became uneasy about the implications of scientific research in human biology. Revolutionary progress in science and technology were predicted, such as genetic engineering and DNA splicing, and it was feared that these advances might have damaging effects on individuals and society (OTA, 1993). At the same time, public outrage arose over some scientific research projects that had violated human rights. For example, a study was made public in which aborted fetuses were decapitated in order to perform pharmaceutical tests. The Tuskegee Syphilis Study, in which the cure for syphilis was withheld from some poor black men afflicted with this disease, was exposed in the press (Jones, 1982). Government recklessness in studying the effects of radiation from nuclear explosions also began to surface.

Because of general apprehension about revolutionary scientific developments and the sharp public reaction to specific abuses in the area of research, Congress established the Commission for the Protection of Human Subjects of

Biomedical and Behavioral Research (CPHS) in July 1974. As its name indicates, the mandate for this commission was to set ethical guidelines for research projects involving human beings, especially those whose rights might be violated. When the life of this commission expired, the Secretary of the Department of Health, Education, and Welfare appointed an Ethics Advisory Board (EAB) in the spring of 1977 to continue the study of ethical issues and public policy. The advisory board was superseded a few months later (November 1978) by another group created by Congress, called the President's Commission for the Study of Ethical Problems in Medicine and Biomedical and Behavioral Research (PCEMR). The commission, having declared its work complete, disbanded on March 31, 1983.

In 1985 Congress instituted the Congressional Biomedical Ethics Board composed of representatives and senators, who were to be assisted in their work by a 14-member advisory committee of scientists, ethicists, and lawyers. The board was to have remained in existence until further legislative action was taken. Selection of the advisory board was delayed because, like every other dimension of American life, the process had become highly politicized. Though funding was allocated for this board and senators selected to serve on it, a panel of experts was never selected because of intense lobbying of special interest groups and reluctance of Congress to displease constituents, and to date no studies have been undertaken. In 1996, President Clinton appointed a National Bioethics Advisory Commission of 15 members to study two issues: the protection of human research subjects and concerns related to management and use of genetic information (AMA News, 1996).

The productivity of the first three federal commissions has been impressive. The CPHS published more than ten studies in its four-year life on subjects such as research on fetuses, children, prisoners, and mentally infirm patients. It also studied psychosurgery, put forth ethical guidelines for delivery of health care by government agencies, and set standards for institutional review boards. In the Belmont Report (1978), the CPHS sought to synthesize the ethical principles concerning informed consent. The EAB, because of its short existence, studied only one ethical issue in depth; that of *in vitro* fertilization. The PCEMR was commissioned by Congress to consider many ethical issues such as brain death, access to health services, withdrawal of life support systems, and screening in regard to genetic diseases. During its existence, the PCEMR published ten studies on these and other topics.

Evaluation of Ethical Guidance by Government

Although we do not attempt to evaluate the documents emanating from these federal commissions (CPHS < EAB < PCEMR), we offer the following general comments.

1. The very fact that Congress recognizes the need for ethical norms in the field of research and therapy is a step forward. For the most part, the norms set forth by the commissions are useful and protect the rights of scientists and physicians as well as subjects and patients.

2. The norms formulated by the commissions are designed with our pluralistic society in mind. Thus these norms seek to enunciate principles on which most scientists, politicians, and religious thinkers can agree. Although the norms do not state it explicitly, it is clear that they avoid controversy, so some of the more difficult and important ethical issues are not considered, such as when human life begins, the purpose of health care, and the difficult decisions that limited public funds will require in the future.

3. Although some of the more important norms concerning physician-patient relationships are considered, such as informed consent and justice in selection of research subjects, there is insufficient consideration of the pressing ethical questions arising from the society–physician–patient relationship, such as: Is there a right to equal health care for all? Should all feasible care be financed publicly? What are the goals for U.S. national health programs?

4. The basis on which these ethical statements are formulated is not the nature of the human person, the covenant between physician and patient, the just society, or religious teaching. Rather, the basis is what is culturally acceptable, that is, what norms seem acceptable to the American public. As a result, the conclusions are pragmatic and usually balance rights rather than defend them. Deciding ethical responsibilities in this manner is dangerous because it justifies whatever is popular. The ethicist should continually question and evaluate what is culturally acceptable, judging it on more fundamental values.

5. Motivation for observing the norms of the federal commissions is mainly monetary. If a person or institution does not observe these norms, the person or institution will not receive federal funding and might be subject to malpractice litigation. Thus, in a certain sense, these "ethical statements" emanating from the federal commissions are legal norms as far as the motivation for observing them is concerned. Although ethicists may differ in detail as to the proper motivation for ethical activity, no ethicist considers avoiding legal sanctions to be the ultimate justification for ethical action.

6. The change in ethical and political attitudes in the United States may be discerned from the recent efforts of the federal government to establish new committees to formulate norms and guidelines for managing new issues in health care ethics (DHHS, 1995). Whereas the first study group mentioned sought to develop a consensus position in regard to issues of health care ethics, a consensus founded upon a common attitude toward the dignity of persons, founded upon natural law and shared religious beliefs, those sources of consensus are no longer acceptable.

At the private level, there is also an extensive effort to influence public policy. At present, more than 50 private centers are sponsored by universities or corporations that seek to educate people in one way or another concerning ethical issues. Although most of these centers serve a local or regional constituency, some seek to serve a national audience. For example:

1. The Pope John XXIII Medical–Moral Research and Education Center in Braintree, MA, considers the ethical issues in medicine, health care, and research from a Catholic perspective. During recent years, the center has published several books on seminars held to probe contemporary ethical issues, in addition to the monthly *Ethics and Medics*.

2. The Hastings Center Institute of Society, Ethics, and the Life Sciences at Briarcliff Manor, New York, studies ethical issues affecting all facets of society. Although the ethical issues arising from medicine and research have been considered by members of the institute's study commissions, such issues as ethics in business, in government, and in the military have also been the subject of their study. The Hastings Institute proceeds from a humanistic perspective and publishes the *Hastings Center Report*.

3. The Kennedy Institute of Bioethics at Georgetown University, Washington, DC, has published the important *Encyclopedia of Bioethics*, sponsors the National Reference Center for Bioethics Literature, and produces *The Bioethics Line*, a computer-assisted method of searching for literature on questions of ethics and public policy. The Kennedy Institute also publishes the quarterly *Kennedy Institute of Ethics Journal*.

4. The Center for Health Care Ethics at Saint Louis University specializes in health care ethics as related to clinical situations. Working in the Catholic tradition, it seeks to interpret this tradition to the pluralistic society of the United States. The Center has a periodical, *Health Care Ethics USA*, and an interdisciplinary PhD program in health care ethics.

5. The Institute for Public Policy and Ethics of Creighton University in Omaha, Nebraska, considers ethical issues resulting from interaction of government with health care and business.

In addition to the publications and services offered by these institutes, more than a score of centers publish articles concerning ethical issues in health care and human research.

6.4 THE HOSPITAL AS COMMUNITY

Cure and Care

So far this chapter has noted that the social organization of health care in the United States is and probably will remain pluralistic, although more careful planning is needed to meet everyone's needs because resources are limited. Now we consider the structure and function of the basic units from which this system is built (Stephens, 1989). At present these units in which health care is concentrated are hospitals and medical centers dedicated primarily to the treatment of acute diseases. While hospitals are decreasing in importance insofar as frequency and length of patient stay are concerned, they are still a focal point of health care. This is especially true of hospitals affiliated with educational medical centers (Ball and Rubin, 1995). Long-term care centers are growing in number, but their existence has little effect on the manner in which medicine is practiced and health care provided in the United States.

A great modern hospital is a world of its own: a strange community in which most members remain only a few days, and where life begins for some and ends for others. Today the trend to hospitalize patients for medical care is being reversed by developing outpatient surgery centers and other facilities designed to care for ambulatory patients. For the immediate future, however, the hospital will be a prominent locus for health care (Dube, 1996). It is therefore necessary to raise some questions about the ethical goals of the hospital as a human community.

According to Sigerist (1960b; C. Rosenberg, 1987), the hospital evolved historically in three stages. First, the Romans established hospitals for soldiers and for work gangs of slaves for the purpose of maintaining manpower for special tasks. Second, Byzantine Christians instituted *xenodochia* (guest houses) or hospitals (hotels, inns) for the poor, a development paralleled in older religions only by the Buddhists in the second century BC under the emperor Atoka. These hospitals were copied and further developed by the Muslim conquerors of portions of the Byzantine Empire, and the Muslim hospitals at the time of the Crusades in turn inspired Western Christians to new efforts. These medieval institutions usually did not supply medical care in the strict sense, but only nursing and spiritual comfort. By the Renaissance, however, Christian hospitals were regularly visited by physicians and sometimes even became retirement homes for the rich. Third, in the eighteenth and nineteenth centuries the Christian hospitals were gradually replaced by modern public and private hospitals, generally under the inspiration of Enlightenment humanism with its emphasis on scientific technology and the free-enterprise system. Thus, historically, the line of development has been from an emphasis on care to one on cure. A fascinating example of this development can be found in the 600-year history of the work of the Alexian Brothers studied by Kauffmann in *Tamers of Death* (1976) and *The Ministry of Healing* (1978).

The Modern Medical Center

Considerable sociological effort has been devoted to understanding this typical modern institution, into which a good portion of the national income is poured each year (Starr, 1982; Rosenberg, 1987; Stephens, 1989). The hospital seems to be a curious mixture of several types of organization.

1. The hospital retains something of its original character as a hotel or temporary residence, with the primary function of care and custody. This purpose is most pronounced in caring for chronically impaired

patients, wherein the hospital becomes a permanent or long-term residence. As such, it is divided into two groups: *hosts* (the administration and staff), who care for the *guests* (the patients).

2. The hospital is also a place of cure in which the medical staff provides diagnosis and treatment for the patients. Thus it consists not only of hosts and guests, but also of *healers* and *sick*.

3. Finally, the hospital is usually also a school in which there are *teachers* and *researchers* (overlapping roles, as in any modern university) with their *students* and *research staffs*. The students are engaged both in class work and in supervised clinical practice, and some are interns and residents in actual full-time practice.

Especially interesting is the fact that the nurses are at the point of intersection of all these functions (Bishop and Scudder, 1996). They are often themselves students in training, but they also provide care; that is, they are the persons who actually carry out the host function of the hospital. At the same time, nurses are an essential part of the medical staff engaged in cure, since nurses execute many of the treatment procedures and cooperate closely with physicians in observing patients and monitoring therapy.

Today the organizational complexity of the hospital is further intensified by the fact that the hospital has become a quasigovernmental agency for the administration of public funds for health care. As such, it is also staffed with social workers, who help patients return to the wider community. Thus the hospital today becomes one of the principal formative institutions of society, providing a model community that is bound to have a profound effect on the average American's understanding of social and personal interrelationships. This is evidenced by the mythical power that television dramas about hospital life seem to have over the American imagination.

If the modern hospital and nursing home are to perform these varied functions effectively, they must solve several basic ethical questions. In discussing total institutions, Goffman (1962) in his well-known work, *Asylums*, has shown that a prison, a small village, or a monastery can never be really total because it lacks the resources to satisfy all human needs. If it is not to foster regressive behavior in its inmates, the total institution must find ways to be open to wider influences. The medieval monasteries found it necessary to develop a complex internal life enriched by the practice of hospitality, which made them centers of communication rather than mere enclosures from the world.

A Healing Community

Thus hospitals and especially nursing homes, in which some patients remain for long periods, have two special obligations. First, they must constantly seek ways for their patients to retain contact with the life of the outside world and to engage in a variety of stimulating and enriching experiences and occupations. Second, they must find ways to involve patients in some genuine participation in making the decisions that affect their lives. Obviously, senile or mentally disturbed patients may have little capacity for such participation, but too often this incapacity has been fostered by patterns of institutional life that have given them no opportunity to express their preferences or to take at least some responsibility for themselves and others.

Today, largely because of the inflation of health costs, great efforts are being made to reduce the hospital stay for surgical patients and even for acutely ill patients, so that now the average stay is less than a week. This is not only less costly, but also better therapeutically and ethically. The hospital has an ethical responsibility not to disrupt the home life of patients. Although sick persons have the right to be relieved of many ordinary social obligations, they need to be helped to experience sickness as a part of life, not as an interruption in living.

Consequently, despite inconveniences to the staff, better hospitals and nursing homes no longer discourage visitors, not even small children, but find ways to facilitate continued family contact and opportunities for the family to share in the therapeutic process. Similarly, when their condition or convalescence permits, patients should be encouraged to assist their fellow patients. The sense of isolation, abandonment, and helplessness is perhaps the most traumatic aspect of being sick, but sickness can also be an important occasion to draw people together in a shared effort of healing. Whenever possible, patients or residents should be given an opportunity to exercise freedom of choice.

Today, within necessary limits, hospitals and nursing homes provide such freedom, but there must also be a constant, imaginative effort to enlarge the scope of patients' activities. This should be measured not by the convenience of the hospital staff, but by therapeutic and human values. Moreover, the public should also share in making the policies by which health care facilities are governed as public institutions. Most members of the public will have to use a hospital or nursing home at some time, and all have an interest in the type of institution their taxes and gifts support.

Staff Relationships

The communal orientation of a hospital or nursing home as described here is primarily patient-centered. Patients will not be treated as persons, however, if the professionals who care for them are themselves alienated by feelings that their own needs are neglected or their rights infringed. Generally speaking, professional freedom in health care institutions, as with academic freedom in universities, must be vigilantly protected (Loewy, 1986). The trustees and administrators not only have such disciplinary responsibilities, but also a positive duty to unify the institution's multiple functions in a manner that permits both the patients and the staff to form a truly human community and not merely a "health factory." Faulty communications among physicians, nurses, auxiliaries, and administration, and within these subgroups, produce an atmosphere of tension deleterious to the services that can directly affect the psychosomatic health of the patients, especially in mental hospitals. Modern administrative and communications theory affords important resources for improving such situations, provided they are used as tools to achieve ethically acceptable goals and not merely to oil an impersonal machine.

Finally, as the inflation of health care costs continues, many ethical questions arise from the economic policies of hospitals, reflecting the severe pressures from which they suffer (Morreim, 1995). Here two important patient rights come into question: the right to emergency care and the right to treatment once the patient is admitted. Courts have generally upheld the legal obligation of hospitals with emergency wards (and even of those not so equipped to the extent of their resources) to care promptly for all persons who come to them in serious need of medical attention and to continue to care for them until they are ambulatory or can safely be transferred to another hospital willing to receive them. The courts are beginning to develop a doctrine on the rights of patients in so-called custodial institutions to treatment as well as to care (Kindred, 1984). In some states there are laws against "dumping" (sending endangered patients to other hospitals), and all health care commentators have through the years declared dumping to be an unethical practice (Friedman, 1982; Schiff et al., 1986). Christian and humanist ethics both have accepted the teaching of the parable of the good Samaritan (Lk 10:25–37), but this concern for one's neighbor must be legally enforced as well.

All these ethical and legal questions, which arise from the ideal of the hospital as a community of care and cure, faced with the realities of modern depersonalized and competitive society, can be solved only at the price of an unremitting effort to give priority to *persons* over institutions and properties. Every hospital suffers from the proliferation of bureaucratic rules intended to protect the institution from exploitation by the crazy or the crafty. This red tape is destructive to patients and staff. The chief remedy against this ever-present danger is training the staff to deal with borderline situations in a flexible and prudent manner and to provide a variety of methods by which self-criticism can be promoted and outside criticism can be heard. To achieve this interplay, it is necessary to develop the staff not merely as a hierarchical structure of command responsibility, but as an interacting *health team*.

6.5 THE HEALTH CARE TEAM

Physicians and Co-Workers

Because of the highly specialized character of modern medicine, health seekers must entrust themselves not to a single physician but to a *health care team* (Brower, 1985). The medical staff of such a team may include physicians, nurses, psychologists, and perhaps paramedics or medical assistants. The nursing staff will include registered nurses, practical nurses, aides, and perhaps nursing unit managers and nursing clerks. The medical departments will include physicians who are pathologists, along with many medical technologists (e.g., specialists in hematology, chemistry, microbiology, serology, histology, and cytology), other physicians who are radiologists and radiation therapists with their assistants, technicians in encephalography and electrocardiography, and finally therapists skilled in occupational and physical therapy. They will be supplemented also by a social services department (staffed by medical social work professionals), a pharmacy, a dietary department, and a health science library.

It is noteworthy that because of the ever-increasing number of drugs, physicians are beginning to give pharmacists a greater role in determining the precise pharmaceuticals to use and the mode of administration according to the physician's diagnosis and general plan of treatment. In addition, in hospitals and nursing homes or rehabilitation facilities, persons will be in charge of patient services such as admissions, hospital records, environmental services (housekeeping), laundry, and purchasing. The business services department involves admissions, accounting, budgeting, and credit and collection, and the buildings are cared for by a plant department. Personnel and public relations departments are essential to secure and care for this complex body of skilled people, and the whole institution requires an elaborate administration, with its governing board and administrative staff. Finally, a health care facility makes use of the services of such outside professionals as architects, accountants, attorneys, special consultants, and sales representatives.

This (incomplete) list of the various diversified professional and subprofessional roles required in a modern health care facility emphasizes that any patient entering a hospital, nursing home, or hospice is confronted with a small army of persons. These people are supposed to serve the patient, but the patient must deal with them and perhaps must protect himself or herself from them. This section discusses only the health care team in the somewhat narrower sense of those members the patient must deal with very directly—the physician, the nurse, and the social worker—in order to determine what reciprocal ethical obligations exist between the patient and these three types of professionals.

Physicians

Traditionally, the chief decision maker in any health team is the licensed physician, the medical doctor (MD). Supposedly, licensure guarantees that physicians have the basic, integral knowledge of the human body and its essential life processes to be reasonably certain about a patient's condition and therefore able to decide (1) what emergency care is necessary and (2) what should *not* be done to the patient without further examination. Consequently, no serious step toward treating the patient can be taken without a physician's permission. Of course, much emergency care is provided by first-aid persons who may have very limited training, but it is generally conceded that any patient has the right to be seen by a physician as quickly as possible (Sanders, 1984).

Today the concept of the licensed medical doctor as a general practitioner has been vastly altered by the growth of medical specialization. In 1950, only about 36 percent of physicians in private practice were specialists (Ginsberg et al., 1984); as of 1996, about 65 percent are specialists (AMA, 1996). This growth of specialization is not clearly related to patient needs. This imbalance is largely the result of decisions by the physicians themselves, who prefer a particular type of work because it is interesting, convenient, prestigious, or profitable. The possibility of a free choice of specialties is one of the features of free-enterprise medicine most valued by the profession. This freedom is not as unlimited as it once was due to the economic standards of managed care. In an effort to control costs, managed care programs do not provide access to specialists unless a need is verified by a primary care physician. Moreover, more physicians are again being encouraged, often due to economic limitations, to go into the primary care specialties of medicine.

In the recent past, the decline of the general practitioner as the primary care professional has deprived patients of the advantages of having their health problems evaluated by someone who knows the patient in his or her family context over a long period and who thinks of the patient as a whole person with a continuous biography. Recently, there was a trend among medical students to specialize in family medicine as a way to reconcile specialization with an interest in primary care. Again, managed care seeks to depend more upon primary care physicians as gatekeepers in order to reduce costs.

None of these developments seems as yet to provide a completely satisfactory answer to the problem of how to provide the kind of primary health care that will keep the total person in clear focus while making use of all the advantages of specialized knowledge and skill.

Nurses, Social Workers, and Patient Advocates

Perhaps the key to this difficulty is to be found in a better understanding of the nurse's proper role, which today has become ambiguous (Bishop and Scudder, 1996). Originally, the nurse was the person most concerned with caring for and having continuous contact with the patient. Therefore, the patient-centered type of health care this book is advocating would dictate that the nurse is the *central* professional figure in the care of the patient, not the physician. Primary care is the nurse's task, not that of a general practitioner, family specialist, or others.

Nurses, however, have been burdened with other tasks. For too long they spent much of their energy in housekeeping chores—making beds, carrying trays, and so forth (Pew Commission, 1995). Today they have been largely relieved of these tasks by auxiliaries, but they are still much occupied with such technical tasks as temperature taking, injections, medications, and intravenous feeding. Moreover, they are oppressed by the sexism implicit in the notion that caring is a maternal role suitable only for women (J. Ashley, 1976). This sexism is reflected in the fact that until recently female physicians were a small minority, whereas in many other countries their number more than equals male physicians. Fortunately, this trend is now reversing, and within the next generation as many as 30 percent of physicians in the United States will be women (NIH, 1996). This freeing of medicine from sexism would also be furthered if men were encouraged to enter the nursing profession in larger numbers.

Under present circumstances, however, as nursing education has advanced, able female nurses have sought administrative and teaching posts as the only way of advancement open to them. They would find nursing itself much more interesting, however, if it became the real focus of health care, so that the role of the nurse, female or male, in direct contact with the patient is seen as primary care and the real source of unity in the health care team. Then the nurse assigned to a given patient would become the authority having responsibility for the patient as a person and assisting the patient in making use of all the resources furnished by the health care team.

This personalistic, mediating function today is often performed by the social worker. Sociological study of the medical profession has led to acknowledging the great importance of the social dimension in treating disease. Thus persons trained in social process have been added to healing teams. The social worker interviews patients to discover possible social factors of ethnic culture, economic status, and family structure that may have caused the disease, may hinder treatment, or may prevent rehabilitation. Such workers typically help patients regarding their legal rights, their opportunities for public financial assistance, and other matters connected with illness. They also act as liaison with the patient's family and help find ways to ensure family stability in the absence of the patient from the home. Finally, social workers undertake the patient's reentry into society. In the case of psychiatric patients, this involvement is of major importance, since reentry into normal life is difficult for mental patients and may lead to recommittal.

If we compare the role of the social worker with that of the nurse, we find that the social worker is chiefly concerned with patients in their normal life patterns, and the nurse with patients undergoing the actual experience of sickness and healing. Consequently, these two roles are very closely connected and together constitute primary care in the strict sense of direct concern with the patient as a person. The physician's role, on the other hand, is more specialized because it is focused precisely on the diagnosis and treatment of a pathological condition or its future prevention. If this analysis is correct, the physician cannot be the sole decision maker on the health team. Rather, the patient has the ultimate decision and is helped in this decision first by the nurse and social worker, who are acquainted with patients in their total personalities and life situation; second by the primary care physician; and third by various specialist physicians.

Recently, more hospitals have begun to recognize the need for pastoral care, not as an occasional intervention of religious ministry from outside the institution by a visiting member of the clergy, nor as a convenience for patients who wish religious ministration by a resident chaplain. Rather, pastoral care is being seen as a regular part of patient care, since all patients, religious or secular, have problems of ultimate concern that affect the success of the healing process. This issue is discussed at length in Chapter 14. Here we only say that pastoral care has to be closely linked to the role of the nurse and the social worker, since it adds depth to their firsthand concern for the patient as a person.

Autonomy and Teamwork

Physicians do not find it easy to reconcile their proper professional autonomy with the requirements of teamwork or to relinquish the idea that they have sole decision-making power in health care and all others are merely their executive assistants (cf. Chapters 4 and 5). The readjustment necessary in their education and self-identity might be compared to what Catholic priests are being forced to undergo since the Second Vatican Council. If the health care team concept is to have real significance, physicians, along with priests, must come to acknowledge that they need the help of others not only in carrying out decisions, but also in making them, if the people entrusted to their care are to be well-served. This is especially true as length of stay in hospital is reduced and patients have less contact with the health care team.

One element fostering team effectiveness is common ethical norms. Often, when continuing education programs on ethical policies are offered to a hospital's professional staff, the nurses take advantage of these, but the physicians are notable by their absence. The most propitious method for introducing ethics into the medical school and specialty training programs seems to be by discussing ethical dimensions of medical problems at conferences and grand rounds. Yet after their specialty training is over, many physicians no longer have the opportunity to attend conferences and grand rounds. Because physicians occupy a leadership role on a health care team, they must be as well-acquainted with the ethical policies of the institution as are other members of the staff; yet they often excuse themselves because of their heavy workload, as if the nurses had it easy.

Therefore, it is entirely reasonable for Catholic institutions to specify as a condition of granting hospital privileges to physicians, or for medical staff and residents, attendance at a certain number of hours of continuing education on the institution's ethical policies. A hospital administration that puts this issue on a professional, rather than an informal, level will find that physicians will accept this responsibility as they do so many others. Further, physicians will soon come to view it as a reasonable and necessary part of the continuing education demanded of all health care professionals today.

6.6 ETHICS COMMITTEES IN CATHOLIC HEALTH CARE FACILITIES

The Need for Ethics Committees

Ethics committees in hospitals received their greatest impetus from the Supreme Court of New Jersey when deciding the Karen Ann Quinlan case. The court, assuming erroneously that most hospitals had ethics committees, declared that such committees, rather than courts, should be involved in decisions concerning the withdrawal of life support. The President's Commission on Ethics in Health Care and Research (PCEMR), writing shortly after the Quinlan decision, recommended the establishment of ethics committees in hospitals of any size. Thus, by 1980 the trend to appoint ethics committees, especially in large hospitals, was well established.

In the 1980s two other influential organizations supported the founding of ethics committees: the American Hospital Association (AHA) and the Joint Commission for Accreditation of Health Care Organizations (JCAHO). The JCAHO required that if the health care facility did not have a committee, "The organization should have in place a mechanism for the consideration of ethical issues and to provide education to caregivers and patients on ethical issues in health care" (JCAHO, 1993). Over the past twenty years this new type of committee has become a fixture in health care facilities of any size. Even large long-term care facilities have ethics committees.

The purpose of an ethics committee is educational, not jurisdictional (Dougherty, 1995). It accomplishes its purpose in three ways:

1. Through education programs for the committee itself and for the various members of the health care facility. For example, a few years ago the federal government set forth certain regulations in regard to advance directives (McClosky, 1991). It was the responsibility of ethics committees to organize lectures and discussions to explain these regulations and to strategize for their application.
2. Through framing ethical policies concerning various aspects of the facilities' activities. Usually, these policies are promulgated by higher authorities, for example, the board of trustees or the medical staff. For the most part, these policies are concerned with issues in clinical medicine, such as informed consent or removal of life support. On the other hand, often issues concerning social justice will require policies, for example, how to settle grievances within the work force.
3. Through consultations which are usually requested by health care professionals and sometimes by families. The committee will usually respond to these requests through subcommittees in order not to overwhelm the people who have requested the consultation. These consultations are not decision-making endeavors on the part of the committee. Rather, the committee members help the decision makers, whether patients, family, or health care professionals, to discern the ethical issues, the options for action, and the course of action which seems to be better in the present situation, all circumstances being considered (Minogue, 1996).

Ethics Committees as Educational

Thus primary purpose of an ethics committee is educational. Education may be fulfilled in many different ways. But a significant function of the committee is to educate its own members. Usually, many of the people called to serve on an ethics committee have little formal formation in the discipline of ethics. Developing a common method of considering ethical issues, whether in regard to lectures, policies, or consultations, is most important. A common method cannot be developed unless there is some effort on the part of the committee to understand the purpose of ethics and the various methods used in considering issues or proposing solutions.

Ethics committees in Catholic health care facilities do not start at the beginning in their deliberations. Rather, each ethics committee has a set of general norms, the *Ethical and Religious Directives for Catholic Health Services*

(ERD) (NCCB, 1994, revised edition). Study of the ERD is a high priority for members of ethics committees in Catholic health care facilities. In fact, all people associated with Catholic health care facilities should be familiar with the ERD, because it lays out a breadth of ethical responsibility which is wider than issues usually associated with medical ethics. For example, the new ERD considers the ethical norms for social justice and cooperation among health care facilities, as well as the norms for using or removing life support.

Moreover, a method of decision making that is directed toward enhancing the dignity of the human person is also traditional in Catholic teaching. This characteristic Christian method of decision making rejects proportionalism and pragmatism, and grounds moral decision making on an analysis of the moral object of a human act (John Paul II, *Veritatis Splendor*, 1993, esp. 70–82). Thus certain kinds of actions such as adultery, lying, and theft must be judged to be morally wrong, no matter what the circumstances or the purposes for which they are performed, as we will explain in Chapter 7. Hence there are some universal, concrete, negative norms which any ethics committee ought to insist can never be ethically violated. The traditional Hippocratic Oath was based on such absolute norms, and its recent abandonment by many medical schools is a sign of the corruption of sound professional attitudes by pragmatism and moral relativism.

Yet even though there are norms and methods consistent with the Catholic tradition, there will often be discussion and difference in how to apply them. For example, it is a well-accepted norm of Catholic ethics that workers should receive a just wage (NCCB, ERD, n. 7). But how does one determine a just wage? Another norm concerns the use of extraordinary and ordinary means in sustaining life. But when does intubation become an extraordinary means? The intelligent, sensitive, and honest application of the ERD to such problems is not easy and requires serious and respectful discussion and debate.

Proposing that ethics committees in Catholic health care facilities have norms and a method to guide them may seem doctrinaire in a pluralistic society (Siegel and Orr, 1995). However, "the purpose of the committee is to serve the institution and patients within the framework of the Catholic tradition" (Brodeur, 1984). Logically then, ethics committees in Catholic health care facilities are to work within the ERD and help people make ethical decisions in accord with its norms. This conclusion is implied in the ERD in the following statements:

> . . . Within a pluralistic society, Catholic health care services will encounter requests for medical procedures contrary to the moral teachings of the Church. Catholic health care does not offend the rights of individual conscience by refusing to provide or permit medical procedures that are judged morally wrong by the teaching authority of the Church (Part I, Introduction).
> . . . Catholic health care services must adopt these Directives as policy, require adherence to them within the institution as a condition for medical privileges and employment, and provide appropriate instruction regarding the Directives for administration, medical and nursing staff, and other personnel . . . (n. 5).

Hence, in the Catholic tradition, there is an assumption that moral reasoning can reach definite conclusions regarding good and bad actions aside from emotional influences. Moreover, in Catholic tradition some actions, such as killing the innocent, are always wrong. The morality of these actions does not change due to circumstances or changing attitudes in society. Because of the relativism and consequentialism in our society, discussions in health care ethics are becoming abstract exercises in linguistic analysis, rather than discussions about patient benefit in light of norms for preserving and promoting human dignity. Maintaining the identity of Catholic health care services will require that the ethics committee accepts and applies the traditions of its Catholic heritage.

There should be a wide perspective represented in the committee. Members of the various health care professions should be represented, as well as persons for administration and other support services. The ethics committee is not concerned with risk management nor with avoiding malpractice litigation. For this reason, if lawyers are members of the committee, their presence will be helpful only if they concentrate upon patient benefit, not upon keeping physicians or the institution out of court. Ordinarily, the ethics committee should not be considered a function of the medical staff, because the medical staff does not have exclusive responsibility for the ethical dimension of the health care facility. Rather, the ethics committee should be responsible to the board of trustees in order to show its concern for all ethical aspects of the corporation's activities. The ethics committee should have a budget which enables it to perform its functions successfully. Too often, its chair is supposed to fund the various needs out of some other budget. But if an ethics committee is to perform its tasks adequately, it needs secretarial help, stipends for speakers, and adequate funding for books and videos to help educate the committee members.

6.7 THE IDENTITY OF CATHOLIC HEALTH CARE FACILITIES

Catholic hospitals and long-term care facilities were founded principally by religious orders of sisters and brothers to give health care to the neglected and, especially in areas where Catholicism was not the chief religion, as a means to witness to the ethical and spiritual aspects of health care in accordance with Catholic values and to carry on the healing mission of Christ (John Paul II, 1995). Health care has always been considered an apostolate of the Church, whether offered in the home or in a more formal institution. Today in the United States, the dominance of secular humanism as a philosophy of life has so influenced and pressured the operation of such Catholic institutions that many wonder whether these institutions are any longer Catholic and are able to be conducted as an apostolic endeavor (CCHCM, 1988; McCormick, 1995a)

What characterizes a Catholic hospital or nursing home? In the United States such a facility has several obvious characteristics.

1. This institution has a Christian and Catholic ministry and therefore receives apostolic direction from the bishop of the diocese. Under his guidance and interpretation, it follows the *Ethical and Religious Direc-*

tives for Catholic Health approved by the United States Catholic Conference (NCCB, 1994).

2. A Catholic hospital or nursing home is usually sponsored by a religious community or a diocese; that is, the community or diocese usually owns the facility and has responsibility for determining policy. A few Catholic hospitals and nursing homes in the United States are sponsored by laypeople, and this will be a growing tendency. At present, many executives of health care corporations are laymen and laywomen (CHA, 1995).

3. The facility offers spiritual and pastoral care to patients, health care professionals, and other employees (cf. Chapter 14), if possible a priest chaplain (resident or nonresident) regularly conducts Mass and is responsible for sacramental administration to the patients and staff.

4. Such institutions usually are marked by various Catholic symbols, statues, pictures, crucifixes in the rooms, evidence of some sisters or brothers and the chaplain in religious clothing, and so forth.

All these characteristics (even the last) are more than superficial. They express the character of the facility as a ministry of the Catholic Church, based on the interrelations of the whole person in all the biological, psychological, social, and spiritual dimensions dealt with in this book.

There is something deeper, however. Catholics essentially conceive of the healing ministry as an extension of the ministry of Christ (USCC, 1981; John Paul II, 1995). Jesus was prophet or teacher, king or shepherd, priest or sanctifier. The Second Vatican Council has taught that this three-fold ministry should be reflected in all the works of the Church and in every member. Healing is part of the shepherding function of the Christian community, since building this community entails concern for each weak member who needs restoration to vital life and participation.

Jesus healed people *radically* by penetrating to the spiritual core of the human personality and liberating the person from original or social sin and also from individual, personal sin, with the more superficial but real effect of healing them also psychologically and physically. A Christian health care facility, therefore, is also concerned with the radical healing of those for whom it cares. The experience of sickness and healing in such a hospital should also be an experience of personal spiritual growth through suffering and redemption.

One of the main methods of ensuring that the Catholic organization, whether a facility or corporate entity, seeks to foster and protect its Catholic identity is the ethics committee.

CONCLUSION

The social organization of health care determines the manner in which health care is provided as well as the overall health of people. While we have sought to consider the principles in the social provision of health care and their ethical responsibilities, there is no doubt that the methods of providing health care are changing and that ethical responsibilities will change as well. A firm foundation for ethical analysis in regard to new developments may be derived from the church's emphasis upon the dignity of the human person, "the manifestation of God in the world, a sign of his presence, a trace of his glory," (John Paul, 1995, n. 34). Social organizations and agencies will be no more ethical than the individual people responsible for their existence and services. Hence, the social aspects of health care depend upon individuals dedicated to preserving the dignity of the people they serve. This truly is the bedrock principle for formulating social policy and organizations involved in health care.

PART 3

The Logic of Bioethical Decisions

In a certain sense, Part 3 is the heart of our study. In the United States today, and indeed throughout the world, there are contradictory answers given to problems occurring in the field of health care. Opinions in regard to the morality of abortion or *in vitro* fertilization are good examples of the differences and controversy. Reasonable people seek some agreement in regard to ethical solutions. At present in our society the solutions to ethical questions are defended by public opinion polls, rather than by rigorous logic. In order to reach some consensus in regard to the several ethical issues besetting the practice of medicine and the delivery of health care, two things are needed: 1) a method or logic of decision making and; 2) a set of values which are used to measure the ability to achieve the goals of human fulfillment discussed in Chapter 1.

Hence in Chapter 7, we consider the various methods used in our time and throughout history to achieve some degree of certainty on ethical issues. We opt for a system which we call prudential personalism. We speak of a personalistic system to indicate that the goal of our logical formula of ethical decision making is fulfillment of the human person. We speak of a prudential system to indicate that even if definite value statements or principles can be formulated, there these principles must be applied by the acting person or the responsible community to particular cases.

In Chapter 8 we describe the need for principles, or values statements, and present the more important principles generated over the years in Christian tradition. Finally, we seek to compare these principles with those offered in the humanistic method of ethical decision making most favored in the United States.

What does Chapter 7 and 8 have to do with Christian decision making? The model for prudential personalism is the person of Jesus. We learn more about concrete decision making from people than we do by studying methods. In Chapter 8, many of the principles we name are developed from the words and examples of Jesus through the mediation of the Church. Thus, while the reader of these chapters may find them at first theoretical, they are extremely practical when applied through the prism of the teaching of Jesus.

The Logic of Bioethical Decisions

OVERVIEW

Chapter 7 discusses the logical *form* of ethical reasoning, and Chapter 8 its *content*. Although it may take us into the deep waters of philosophy, an understanding of the different logical forms of ethical reasoning is important, since sometimes groups with very similar values (the content of ethical reasoning) can still violently disagree on how to solve concrete problems because the forms or methods of their reasoning differ. In order to understand the Christian approach to ethics, special attention should be devoted to the scriptural basis for the various principles, and the manner in which a principle differs from a rule.

7.1 THE LOGIC OF BIOETHICAL DEBATE

Need for Critical Thinking in Ethics

Piaget (1929) and Kohlberg (1973, 1981) have tried to show that almost any group of adults includes persons at different levels of ethical development, corresponding to the three main phases a child must pass through to full ethical maturity.

1. In the *preconventional* phase, decisions are made on the basis of the immediate consequence of an action, its rewards and punishments.
2. In the *conventional* phase, decisions are made on the basis of social approval. Conformity to group norms becomes paramount, and satisfactions can be delayed and suffering incurred to achieve the praise of others.
3. In the *postconventional* phase, maturity increases through the internalization of moral judgments. Decisions are made on personal standards, whereas the standards of society become subject to criticism.

Although the details of this analysis have been widely criticized through the years (Duska and Whaelen, 1975; Philibert, 1975; Gilligan, 1993, 1995), it illustrates the fact that most public ethical controversies seem to be carried on at the "conventional" level of moral thinking. Only when people begin to think critically for themselves do they begin to question society's assumptions about what values are important. To do this, however, I must ask myself, "What method am I following or should I follow in trying to solve my ethical problems?" In seeking a good method for ethics, we must keep in mind that no method of *practical* reasoning can be expected to give the same clarity or even the same certainty that sometimes is achieved in purely theoretical reasoning such as mathematics.

Moreover, not only is ethical reasoning practical rather than theoretical, but it deals with ultimate problems of life and death, of self-fulfillment and self-destruction. Consequently, ethical reasoning is often obscured by our conflicting emotions, our own sinfulness, and the sinfulness of our milieu. Therefore, to think about ethical problems with such clarity and certainty as is possible in so difficult a field, we need a good method, and today bioethicists struggle to find one (Engelhardt, 1986b; Pellegrino and Thomasma, 1988; R. Veatch, 1981; Beauchamp and Childress, 1994). In this chapter we will use examples taken from the abortion question, so hotly debated in today's culture, not to take a stand on that question itself—we will do that later—but to illustrate the different ways people reason ethically.

Religious versus Natural Law Ethics

Ethical theories can first be divided into those based on unaided human *reason* and those based on a *revelation* from some superhuman source. These two types are by no means exclusive. We have to use human reason to understand revelation, and in using human reason we can still remain open to superhuman light. Some Christian theologians, especially those in the Protestant tradition (Tillich, 1957; Bourgeois and Schalow, 1987) who emphasize the corruption of human nature by sin, are suspicious of reason as a basis for moral decision. But Catholic theology, while it admits sin has clouded human reason, emphasizes the essential harmony between faith and reason. God's revelation not only heals and supports human reason, but enables it to gain a deeper insight into God's creation, the Creator himself, and his plan to save humanity from its sinful condition.

In contrast to such theological views, philosophical theories of morality—whether closed to faith or open to it—are constructed on a purely rational basis. Most such rational theories also make reference to what we know by reason about "human nature" and consider it one factor at least in determing whether actions are good or bad. Thus they hold that to act so as to satisfy innate human needs in an integrated way is to act reasonably. At least in a broad sense, therefore, they are "natural law" theories. Yet today there is a good deal of skepticism about this notion of "human nature" because so often certain traits or ways of behaving have been claimed to be "natural," only to be exposed by history, anthropology, and the modern life sciences as highly variable in time and place. Sociobiolgists attempt to trace most items of human behavior to a genetic basis, while anthropologists and sociologists trace the very same behaviors to variations in culture.

Thus many researchers conclude that "nature" and "culture" so interact and condition each other that it is futile to talk about "human nature" or "natural moral law." Hence, they resign themselves to "cultural relativism" in moral evaluation. But to accept such moral relativism seems to surrender any rational grounds for protesting against unjust laws and traditional prejudices. Moreover, how can we reasonably believe that the human race, which forms one recognizable species with one common gene pool, does not have a human nature in common? While we certainly are far from knowing all about this common human nature, it is a reality recognized long before the genome was discovered. Our common humanity has always been identified by our physiology, psychology, and capacity to interbreed. Moreover, these features common to the whole human species are not just a random bundle of traits, but define integrated human organisms which, in spite of all individual differences, have the same essential structures and interdependent life functions.

As Mortimer Adler (1970) has well argued, a sound natural law ethics can be based on a commonsense notion of what it is to be human. Yet such a commonsense understanding of human nature also can and has been improved by scientific study. Although the complexity of our human nature is amazing, and we are constantly learning surprising things about it, we already know a great deal with certitude or high probability. From what we do know now about ourselves we can derive a natural law morality in a strict sense of the term, i.e., a purely rational theory rooted in what is essentially common to all human beings. We can improve and refine this present understanding of natural moral law by coming to a more profound and complete knowledge of human nature.

Some philosophers (Ayer, 1936), however, have argued that it is a logical fallacy to infer statements of what "ought" to be from statements about what human nature "is." It is true that we cannot say that women ought to have abortions from that fact that many do, or that they ought not to have abortions because even more refuse to have one. Nevertheless, there is no logical fallacy in a physician telling an anorexic that she ought to eat because it is a fact that the human body needs food. The logical link between "is" and "ought," fact and value, is the notion of *need*. Since reason tells us that as free and responsible beings we ought to act so as to meet our human needs as individuals and as a human community, and our basic needs are determined by our human nature, a natural law ethics can and must be based on the facts of human nature as now known or perhaps in the future better known.

A simple example of a natural moral law (relevant to the abortion debate but not of itself conclusive) is the norm that parents have the primary responsibility for the care of their own children. This does not refer simply to a "parental instinct" although, no doubt, like higher animals, human parents do have some instinctive feelings about their children. Rather, it refers to the fact that human beings in all times and places have reasoned on the basis of experience that (a) children need a great deal of care to survive and grow up as good members of the human community; (b) a community cannot survive unless it gives its children proper care; and (c) those members of the community who have produced a child cannot expect the community to help them in other matters if they do not assume the primary care of their own children.

The fact that in different cultures at different times there have been different ways of caring for children reflects the creativity of human reason, but it does not contradict this basic norm of parental responsibility. When we see today in our society that not a few parents, especially biological fathers, fail to carry out this duty, we do not conclude that this is all right just because it is seems to be in the process of getting accepted into the "common morality" of modern culture. Instead, we see it to be a great injustice, a sign of moral decadence. Is this merely because there are human laws requiring parental care? Or because public opinion still frowns on the deliquent parent, while it more and more accepts single parenthood as normal? Even if there were no laws, or if public opinion becomes indifferent to the rights and duties of fatherhood, our reason would still tell us that our human nature gives us a need to care for our children.

Human Historicity

Yet, if we are to base a natural law ethics on the truth about human nature, we must be on our guard against confusing what is really natural for us from what is merely a product of our culture. Human beings never exist simply as human, but as members of a particular community with its particular culture, in a given place, at a given time in history. Moreover, we are individuals unique in our temperaments and experiences. Consequently, what it is to be human is variously manifested and can be either developed and enriched or distorted and trivialized by culture. Again, human nature itself is not absolutely unified, as is evidenced by genetic differences among members of the human race; nor is it absolutely stable, since it is subject at least to some extent to the continuing evolutionary process of natural selection, although our species is now many thousand years old. Some of these changes result not from natural causes but from cultural ones, and with increasing knowledge may fall under human control. This means that at any given moment of history for any given group of people, their moral understanding will be profoundly conditioned by their history. One needs only to read the Old Testament to become aware of how differently the ancient Hebrews interpreted the Ten Commandments than Jews and Christians do today.

Nevertheless, historicity itself implies continuity, identity, and community. There would be no biographies if people were mere streams of consciousness. It is only because I remain really myself from cradle to grave that I have personal identity and history. Unless the human race shared a common nature that was at least relatively stable for vast periods of time, there would be no human history nor today a global, interbreeding, intercommunicating human community. Therefore human persons all have some basic common needs that characterize them as human and make possible cooperation as a human family. Yet an adequate moral theory must also take into account the historic context of moral decisions and their probable effect on future generations.

In our example of abortion, history shows us (Noonan, 1970a) that though the pagan Hippocratic Oath (probably of Pythagorean origin, [Edelstein, 1967]) forbids it, it has been the Christian Church which has from as early as the *Didache* of the first century A.D. consistently opposed abortion. The recent legalization of abortion in countries where the majority of citizens are Christians raises a serious question as to what we mean when we declare that all human persons have certain basic rights—first of all a right to life—if in fact others have the right to choose whether we live or not.

Pluralism and Humanism

Keeping in mind this delicate balance between the universality and permanence of human nature on the one hand and its historicity and cultural variation on the other, Christians seek moral standards that are transcultural yet sensitive to existential realities. In the historical postmodern context of today, they find that their value system based on the Bible and Christian tradition no longer controls Western culture, although it is still a major player in the pluralistic dialogue and confidently hopes to achieve a final victory.

At the end of the seventeenth century, the religious wars between Catholics and Protestants and among the reformed churches caused great scandal among the European intellectual elites. From this loss of faith arose the so-called Enlightenment, which sought to replace Christian revelation with a "religion of reason" which it was hoped would transcend religious quarrels. Thus the Founding Fathers of our republic, who were largely products of the Enlightenment, justified their revolution from England in their Declaration of Independence by asserting it to be a "self-evident" truth "that all men are created equal" and have been "endowed by their Creator with certain unalienable rights," including "life, liberty, and the pursuit of happiness."

Christians, both Catholic and Protestant, surprised by this rebellion of the elites against revealed religion, made the tragic mistake of allowing the Enlightenment to co-opt modern science, although this scientific advance had originally been inspired by the Christian vision of God's orderly creation (Ashley, 1985). Thus the Enlightenment has used science as a weapon against the Christian worldview, making it the basis of its own faith that by reason alone, without God's revelation, we can master our world. In our twentieth century the Enlightenment worldview has indeed taken control of the economic system, the universities, public schools, and the public media in the form of "secular humanism."

Thus in our pluralistic world the two value systems that most often clash in the United States are those of Christianity, 2,000 years old, and of the philosophies of the Enlightenment, now 300 years old and culturally dominant in our country and most "developed" countries. Christianity is, of course, now much divided, but in this book we present it in its Roman Catholic form, both because we are Catholics and because it is admitted even by our Protestant colleagues (Gustafson, 1978) that Catholics have produced the most systematically developed and officially formulated version of Christian ethics. On the other hand, it is characteristic of the value systems descended from the Enlightenment that they reject any unified, official formulation as inimical to freedom of speech and conscience. It leaves this coherent formulation of the Enlightenment "faith" up to various formulations by various philosophers.

Historically, most of these "enlightened" ethical philosophies independent of revelation seem to have had their origin in the questions raised by David Hume (d. 1776), of the Scottish school of philosophy that greatly influenced the founders of the United States. John Locke (d. 1784) had attacked the Platonic doctrine of innate ideas as the source of reliable human knowledge, revived by Rene Descartes (d. 1650), generally called the "Father of Modern Philosophy." Locke adopted the more Aristotelian view that all our knowledge begins in sense experience, yet contrary to both Plato and Aristotle, had reduced human intelligence to a kind of sense knowledge. Hence Hume grew skeptical about the ability of our intelligences to know a universal human nature and thus doubted, as we have already mentioned many philosophers still do, that the "ought" of moral norms concerned with values can be deduced from the "is" derived from the facts of human nature. From Humes' doubts have arisen, as we shall see, the major ethical systems that today attmept to replace a natural law ethics: (1) Emotivism, which was Hume's own solution; (2) Formalism, proposed by Immanuel Kant (d. 1804); and (3) Utilitarianism, proposed by Jeremy Bentham (d. 1832). That our American culture is the heir of these Enlightenment philosophers is evident from the fact that our public media take for granted certain values largely derived from their thought, which the media use to interpret our world and its current history. For example, "science says," "human rights," "democracy," "compassion," "economic prosperity," etc., stand for generally recognized values that are used daily to evaluate right and wrong in our society. We may debate whether the pro-life or pro-choice stance on abortion is correct, but no one would dare deny the conception of "free speech" on which both sides base their right to demonstrate against the other party.

We will not attempt here to formulate systematically this Enlightenment value system, but will assume that our readers can recognize it when referred to. The problem is what name to give it, since it refuses to be named. It might well be called "modernity," except that we are now "postmodern." The "religious right" call it "secular humanism," but often with connotations we do not wish to make, since our purpose here is not to attack the very real achievements of the Enlightenment, but to redeem them for Christianity. Therefore, while we believe there is also an authentic Christian humanism, we will surrender the term "humanism" itself to our partners in dialogue. The two worldviews and value systems are both humanisms in that both believe in human dignity, human rights, and the power and freedom of humanity to control its world. Christian humanists, however, believe that this control must be a stewardship in cooperation with the Creator, while humanists, in the sense we will use the term henceforth, believe that we are entirely on our own in the world, whether there be a God or not.

As a new millenium approaches, the awareness grows that while this humanist religion of reason has encouraged the magnificent achievements of science and technology, the advance of democracy, and the defense of human rights, it has also spawned two great world wars, the Holocaust, the threat of nuclear destruction, the rape of the natural environment, the breakdown of the family, and a widespread moral confusion and cynicism. The question raised by this "postmodern" breakdown of values is not whether reason and science are false, but whether they are adequate guides for an understanding of the world and human life. In the discussion of moral systems that follows, we will first deal with those based purely on human reason, which Christians and humanists ought to be able to share, and then with those favored by the Catholic Church, which has always striven to reconcile faith with reason. To present the main ethical methodologies developed in our civilization, a single example will be used: the highly controversial issue of the morality of abortion. The purpose here is not to debate that issue, as we will do in Chapter 9, but to show how different modes of thinking can be applied to an especially difficult problem.

Deontological versus Teleological Ethical Methodologies

Current bioethical writers usually divide ethical methodologies into those that are *deontological* (from the Greek for "reasoning about duty") and those that are *teleological* (from the Greek for "reasoning about a goal"; i.e., the means to be taken to achieve some end) (H. Brody, 1981; B. Brody, 1983; T. Shannon, 1987; Beauchamp and Childress, 1994).

For deontologists, questions of moral right and wrong always reduce to obedience or disobedience to some code of laws, customs, or agreed norms which obliges us because of the authority of some legislative power which can enforce its *will* by appropriate sanctions. Thus deontologists are *voluntarists* who believe that ultimately something is right or wrong because the lawgiver says it is (Bourke, 1970). This does not necessarily mean that the lawgiver is somebody else, since people can set their own laws by willing to commit themselves to certain self-imposed rules.

Teleologists, on the other hand, think of ethics according to the model of the reasoning technologist, who begins with an idea of something to create and then tries to figure out how to achieve that goal. Therefore teleologists trace back the norms of right and wrong not to the will of any authority, but to some *intelligence* (their own or that of a wiser person whom they can trust) that is able to see the alternative means to the end and to select the most effective. They are *intellectualists* rather than voluntarists.

Nevertheless, teleological reasoning about morals differs greatly from teleological reasoning about technological problems, although both are about ends and means. Technological reasoning is always conditional: "If I want to get to the moon, what means should I take to get there?" But teleological ethical reasoning is absolute: "Since I want to be happy, what ought I to do to get there?"

Unfortunately, this clear-cut distinction between teleological ethics and deontological ethics, as these two logical types were historically understood, has become confused in modern ethical literature, as is evident in Kohlberg's theory of three phases of moral development. Both his "conventional" and "postconventional" phases seem to be forms of deontological, legalistic thinking, since the morally conventional person lives by the laws imposed by society; and for Kohlberg postconventional persons also live by laws, though these are self-imposed. As his critics have pointed out, Kohlberg's theory neglects the teleological types of moral reasoning, probably because he was overly influenced by the deontological "formalistic" ethics of Immanuel Kant, which we will soon describe.

This same neglect of teleological thinking in ethics has long had its influence on Catholic moral theology. The theologians of the patristic and medieval periods favored a teleological ethics with an emphasis on the development of the virtues that make consistent actions toward the goal possible. However, after the sixteenth-century Council of Trent, the manuals used in seminaries came to emphasize a deontological ethics based on the commandments and the will of God (Häring, 1966). Protestant theologians during this period also generally taught a duty ethics, to which Immanuel Kant finally gave a philosophical systematization. This widespread theological trend reflected the attitudes of secular society which, in the Age of Reason, stressed the need for centralized sovereign authority acting through codified laws and clear lines of command. Since, as we have already shown, natural law theory bases the "is" and the "ought" on the *needs* fixed in human nature, while deontology replaces *needs* with *authority*, this trend in Catholic thinking weakened the natural law foundation of moral theology.

After the Thomistic revival in Catholic theology and the antirationalistic reaction in Protestant theology at the end of the nineteenth century, a trend back to a means–ends ethics grounded in natural law began, as became evident in the Second Vatican Council (Vatican Council II, 1965c). The Council taught that the "objective criteria" of moral right and wrong are based on "the nature of the human person and human action," not simply on obedience to law (*The Church in the Modern World*, 1965c, n. 51), and this teaching is even more explicitly formulated in John Paul II's major encyclical *The Splendor of Truth* (1993). Although the *Catechism of the Catholic Church* (1994) Part III is structured on the Ten Commandments, it grounds this teaching in a thorough presentation of a teleological, natural law, virtue-centered ethics.

Hence, in reading current bioethical literature, it is important to steer clear of certain mistakes about the difference between deontological and teleological moral reasoning. The first error is to identify all teleological reasoning with *consequentialism* and to say that all teleologists determine whether an action is right or wrong only by its consequences, whereas deontologists maintain it can be right or wrong no matter what its consequences. These two methods of ethical reasoning are not necessarily exclusive. Deontologists need not hold that the authority they obey is *arbitrary*. They may be convinced that the legislator has good reasons for his or her rules, although it is not necessary to know those reasons, just to obey the rules. Teleologists, on the other hand, can admit that laws, customs, and norms are important and sometimes necessary guides to good decisions about which means to use to achieve an end, provided that the authority who made these rules was an expert who should be obeyed because trustworthy.

A second error is to identify deontological reasoning with the acceptance of *exceptionless norms,* that is, rules whose violation no circumstances can justify, while supposing that all teleological reasoning denies that concrete moral norms can be absolute. On the contrary, *The Splendor of Truth* (John Paul II, 1993) distinguishes between "teleology" in general and the "teleologism," a special type of teleological ethics which wrongly rejects absolute concrete moral norms.

A third mistake is to suppose that because these two methodologies are not necessarily exclusive, there can be "mixed" systems. This error results from the failure to see that one really cannot avoid deciding whether deontological obedience to law or teleological choice of means to an end is primary or secondary and merely instrumental (McCullough, 1986). Those who advocate a "mixed form" of ethics (Curran, 1977a) believe they can agree with deontologists that the objective criteria of morality cannot be reduced exclusively to the consequences of an action, while also agreeing with teleologists that these criteria must include such consequences. They propose this mixed model as "an ethics of relationality and responsibility" (Niebuhr, 1963; Jonsen, 1968; Curran, 1988) and argue that we cannot claim complete control over our lives (as means–ends ethics seems to assume), nor can we reduce our responsiblities to obedience to general norms (as duty ethics assumes). Rather, our decisions have to respond to the persons and events that confront us in life in ways that maximize human values, making creative use of the resources available. Such an ethics of response, they say, is more in keeping with a Christian understanding of dependence on the grace of God and encounters with other persons than is a duty ethics, with its danger of legalism, or than a means–ends ethics, with its danger of illusions about our rational control over our lives.

We would argue that such an "ethics of relationality and responsibility" should be classified not as a mixed form, but rather simply as a teleological form of means–ends ethics, since it clearly subordinates the obligation of duties to teleological considerations. We also would insist that any modern Christian ethics must stress that the "ends" of human action are always *persons* and the community of interrelated persons responding to each other. At the center of this community is a Three-Personed God with whom the initiative always belongs and on whose grace we completely depend to make any fully human response (Kiesling, 1986). However, to respond to persons is to direct action to the good of persons, and this always is a matter of free choice of means to ends, i.e., of acts that relate persons to persons or alienate them from each other. Nor need a teleological ethics require that we have total control over our own lives independently of God or other persons, but only that if we try to make decisions within the limits of our own knowledge and freedom we can make them purposefully and reasonably.

On the other hand, any deontological ethics, unless it is merely arbitrary, must be subordinate to a teleological one, since it only traces the criteria of morality back to the will of some lawmaker, whether that lawmaker be God, the government, or the autonomous individual. But this leaves a question still to be asked: "Why am I ethically obliged to obey the will of the lawmaker?" The ultimate answer to this query can only be given in terms of the practical wisdom or *prudence* by which the legislator makes wise rules for the benefit of those who are to obey (Cessario, 1991; Nelson, 1992). If I cannot trust that the lawmaker has good reasons for his laws, why am morally obliged to obey them? To purpose reasons for laws based on "benefit for someone" is go beyond duty ethics and to construct a means–ends ethics, which measures the rightness or wrongness of human action by its helpful or harmful effects, that is, as a practical means to the goals of human life or the satisfaction of human needs.

The importance of this distinction between a deontological and teleological type of ethical reasoning has been starkly evident in the abortion debate. Some have attempted to resolve this debate deontologically by referring to the law, the courts, or majority opinion. Others appeal against the human law to higher "natural law," that is, to teleological reasons drawn from the relation of the act of abortion to the goals of human life in the community.

Classification of Moral Methodologies

Given the broad division of moral methodologies into deontological and teleological, a further subdivision is required. One of the most thorough recent discussions of ethical methodologies in a bioethical context is that of Beauchamp and Childress (1994), who propose the following classification based on the ethical factor which a system chiefly features. Thus, current ethical methodologies emphasize:

1. consequences (utilitarianism);
2. obligation (Kantianism);
3. virtue (character);
4. human rights (liberal individualism);
5. community (communitarianism);
6. human relationships (ethics of care);
7. cases (casuistry); and
8. common morality based on principles.

After evaluating each of these systems in considerable detail, Beauchamp and Childress give preference to the last ennumerated system of "common morality based on principles," which they describe as (a) grounded in the morality accepted in any given culture at a given time, (b) yet open to improvement; and (c) clarified by the formulation of certain principles which cannot be reduced to any single unifying principle. Although they give preference to this common, principled morality (p. 53), they also concede that the special features of all the other seven systems need to be taken into account in any moral decision.

In what follows in this and the next chapter, we will attempt to show that the various current systems do indeed emphasize features which need to be included in a workable theory. But we will also attempt to provide a synthesis based on a firmer foundation than the "common morality" of today's American culture on which Beauchamp and Childress principally rely, since they too

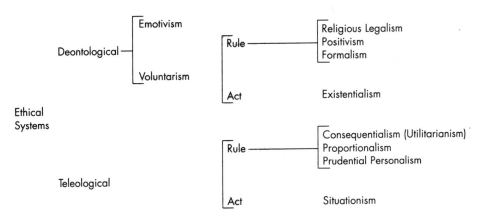

DIAGRAM 1. Types of Teleological and Deontological Ethics

admit that it needs improvement. How is it possible to "improve" our culture, unless we admit that there are ethical standards for improvement superior to this common morality? Diagram 1 assists the reader in following our search for this transcultural moral standard.

7.2 DEONTOLOGICAL (DUTY) METHODOLOGIES

Emotivism

Some ethicists have followed Hume in maintaining that it is a logical fallacy to derive the "ought" from the "is." They insist that while it is possible to decide between conflicting views in the sciences by checking the *facts,* in disputes over ethics it is not facts that are in question but *values.* Hence, they conclude as Hume did that values have no rational basis but are simply based on a *feeling* of preference. Thus the statement, "Abortion is wrong" is not a statement of fact such as "The earth is round," but simply means, "I don't like abortion," or "Abortion is ugly." Hence, they hold that an *emotivist* ethics is the only one possible, since any discussion of values is a discussion about subjective, emotional attitudes (Ayer, 1936). Others have conceded that "ought" statements are not only expressions or descriptions of emotion, but also prescriptions stating what people "feel" ought to be be done, though they still maintain that the grounds for such prescriptions are only subjective feelings, not the knowledge of some special kind of truth (MacIntyre, 1981).

It is certainly the case that at the beginning of most discussions of an ethical issue, people express felt attitudes. For example, I am horrified at the idea of abortion and especially at the way so many people are now ready to approve what they once regarded as a shameful crime. You, on the other hand, may be indignant at the presumption of anyone who would force a woman to bear a child that she does not want, especially when that child will be defective and live a miserable life, or when it was forced on her by incest or rape, or when carrying it to term threatens her life. You may be pleased that more liberal, humane, pro-choice views are beginning to prevail. From the outset it appears that this discussion will get nowhere. How can we discuss the obviously sincere but purely subjective feelings of another person or defend our own?

We cannot rest content, however, with this initial impasse. Feeling cannot be an ethical criterion that is beyond criticism, no matter how sincere it may be. Obviously we are often led by our feelings to do things that turn out to be very destructive not only to others, but even to ourselves. You may "feel" it is all right to destroy a fetus, but what if you, like Hitler, also feel it is all right to kill Jews? I may "feel" it is wrong to permit a woman to have an abortion, but what if I feel it is wrong to permit my child to be given a necessary blood transfusion?

Therefore, this emotivist reduction of moral statements to mere subjective attitudes does not seem very convincing. Yet a more plausible form of emotivism can be defended as follows: Certainly not all feelings can be trusted, but can't we trust our better nature, our humane feelings? Hume himself thought we should follow only those preferences which are felt even when we are not emotionally disturbed. His contemporary, philosopher Jean Jacques Rousseau (1753), argued that if people would free themselves from the prejudices acquired by bad education and the influence of a corrupt civilization and return to their natural human feelings, they would make much better ethical judgments. Such seems the basis of our American confidence in the common sense of the people. We believe that the "common" person is closer to nature and reality than is the sophisticated intellectual. We take opinion polls on many bioethical problems because we assume that what most people "feel" is right probably *is* right. The difficulty with this approach is that it provides no method of public, objective discussion but leaves problems to rhetoric and passion. Whose instincts are sound? After all, some people, even when emotionally calm, feel that all races but their own are subhuman. Consequently, it is important that we try to find an objective and logical method of settling what is right and wrong, even though this method may not be foolproof.

Yet there is much truth in this trust in common decency because natural human feelings of family love, loyalty to one's group, sympathy for the underdog, opposition to arrogance and tyranny, and fairness and compassion are better guides to morality than current fads or the fanatical ideologies of armchair philosophers out of touch with basic human realities (R. Baron, 1981). In discussing abortion, the fact cannot be overlooked or denied that most women are very reluctant to have an abortion, even when they think they have a right to do so. On the other hand, who could be insensitive to the anguish of a woman faced with bringing a deformed child into the world?

If people attempted to live only by natural feelings, however, the progress of civilization would be impossible. Sigmund Freud in his *Civilization and Its Discontents* (1930) agreed with Rousseau that civilized life produces great psychological tensions by its suppression of our primary feelings and impulses, but he also pointed out that this discipline is an absolute necessity if we are not to be destroyed by the contradictions of our own instinctual drives. Without civilization and its discipline, there could be no modern medical science.

Consequently, as Aristotle long ago in *The Nicomachean Ethics* very realistically showed, emotion is to be trusted only when it has been refined, educated, and disciplined by virtue (H. Veatch, 1971). Recently, ethicists have again been insisting that good decisions are not possible merely by following rules. We need *character* if we are consistently to meet the crisis of decision making (Hauerwas, 1981; Palmour, 1988; Cessario, 1991). Decisions made by people who have a respect for persons, reverence for life, and compassion for the suffering are likely to be good decisions, whereas decisions made by persons who are insensitive and lacking in empathy are likely to be morally bad. Jesus said, "Every good tree bears good fruit, and a rotten tree bears bad fruit" (Mt 7:16). Thus what people *do* is the outcome of what they *are* (McCabe, 1969). This is why persons often make the statement, "I would rather trust physicians or nurses of good character to make ethical decisions than all the bioethics experts in the world."

This point is well taken. Ultimately, all ethical decisions do involve a degree of moral sensitivity, fairness, and compassion that is only found in psychologically healthy and mature people, in civilized, decent human beings. Character is all-important. But what is decency? What are the standards or principles by which good characters are formed? The German physicians who carried out Hitler's evil medical experiments thought themselves (and were considered by others) decent, ethical professionals. Probably they were not, however, accustomed to reflecting critically about the ethical standards of their profession (Alexander, 1949; Lifton, 1986).

In view of the foregoing description of emotivism, should it be classified as deontological, teleological, or perhaps some third type of ethics? Since emotivism is essentially *noncognitive* (i.e., it does not rest on what people know rationally but on what they "feel" spontaneously), it cannot be teleological; the teleological method requires us to reason carefully about the relation between means and ends. Neither is emotivism obviously deontological, since deontology implies obedience to the *will* of the lawmaker rather than to one's own feelings. Nevertheless, emotivism is best reduced to a form of deontological ethics because emotions resemble the will; both are noncognitive, affective faculties that differ only in that emotions relate more directly to imagination and will to reason. Thus emotivism is that type of deontologism which teaches that we each have the duty to follow the law of own natural and psychologically healthy instincts or feelings as the surest moral guide.

Religious Legalism

Many theists ground ethics in a direct appeal to the will of God, who is the ultimate authority and who alone determines what is right and wrong. As St. Paul said, "We ought to obey God rather than men" (Ac 5:29). The Jews, Christians, and Muslims believe that God has revealed his will through his prophets as recorded in the Bible or the Qu'ran. This "Divine Command Morality" (Idziak, 1980) is simply defined as "obedience to the commands of God," such as the Ten Commandments (Ex 20:7–17) or the great commandment of love of God and neighbor which Jesus said "sums up the law and the prophets" (Mt 22:40). Thus abortion seems forbidden by the command "Thou shall not kill" (Ex 20:13), although it can be debated whether this law applies to the fetus, since nowhere in Scripture is deliberate abortion explicitly mentioned (Noonan, 1970a).

Among Christians this type of deontologism has been common, and among Protestants it has predominated (Mehl, 1971; Gustafson, 1978, 1983). Paul Ramsey (d. 1988) (1973), a Protestant pioneer in bioethics, used this deontological approach persuasively in opposing abortion, basing his ethics on the commandment to love of God and neighbor. Although there are a great variety of Protestant ethical systems, most of them, as we have already noted, teach that after the fall of Adam into sin we have been blinded to moral truth by our self-righteousness. People can be freed from this blindness only when confronted by the righteousness of God as revealed in the Word of God, especially in Jesus Christ the Incarnate Word. Even with this biblical revelation, the will of God remains essentially mysterious to us, so we ought simply to obey Him in absolute trust.

Although some Catholic theologians have developed similar deontological ethical systems, Catholics generally have not favored this approach because the emphasis on blind submission to God's will does not seem to do justice to the biblical doctrine that humankind is created in the image and likeness of God. True, this image has been profoundly distorted by human sin, so that without God's revelation, we could never arrive at a wholly correct idea of our true nature or divine destiny. Only by the grace given us in Christ are we able to achieve the goal of eternal life with God. But it is also true that in spite of sin, we remain images of God (Gn 1:27). This indelible likeness to God in humanity, constituted by his gifts of intelligence and freedom, opens all human beings to God's call to his friendship (*Catechism of the Catholic Church*, 1994, # 356–57, 705).

After we are reborn through grace, these gifts are again freed to enable us not just to obey God blindly, but to obey him intelligently and freely. God's will does indeed remain in many ways mysterious, but it is not an arbitrary will. It is God's wisdom in which we share so that we can by grace cooperate with the divine plan for our lives. Thus Catholic moral theology strives to go beyond deontologism to an ethics that insists that God wants us to understand his wise purposes and to use our own intelligence and experience in carry them out in our living (Finnis, 1983; Grisez, 1983; John Paul II, 1994). Jesus' parable of the talents (Mt 25:14–23) shows that when God commands us as his servants to carry out a task, he also demands creativity from us in obeying these commands. Legalism does not seem to take this cooperative creativity into account.

Positivism

Those in Kohlberg's "conventional" stage of moral development tend to think of morality in terms of a divine or human code—the Ten Commandments or federal or state laws. The secular form of deontologism identifies morality with what is *legal* by civil legislation. This is what is called *legalism,* or *positivism;* i.e., law laid down (posited) by the will of the sovereign. For many, the Supreme Court decision in *Roe v. Wade* settled the question of whether abortion is right or wrong. Sociologists and anthropologists believe that morality is determined not so much by written laws (which are easily changed) as by unwritten law or custom. For them, morality simply means conformity to the accepted social standards of a particular culture, that is, "common morality" (Varga, 1984, Beauchamp and Childress, 1994). They point out that in some cultures abortion is considered immoral and that in others, at least in some situations, a moral duty. This view—that there is no such concept as a universal, transcultural standard of right and wrong—is *moral relativism* (Sumner, 1986; John Paul II, 1994).

The case for positivism is strong because it is true that people form moral standards only in a social context with the help and guidance of their community. It is unrealistic to suppose that individuals are capable of working out personal systems of values merely on the basis of their own limited experiences and insights. Nor can we live together if each one of us tries to live by a merely personal ethic. Neither a law against abortion nor a law protecting pro-choice can be effectively enforced unless it is supported by public opinion, i.e., by custom.

Human laws or accepted customs, however, are not ultimate criteria of morality for two reasons: (1) Legal morality is always broad, crude, and unrefined, so that in personal life the law must be supplemented by more refined, sensitive standards. (2) Human laws and customs may be destructive, or, even when originally just, in changed circumstances become unjust, so that it becomes necessary to criticize them, refuse to obey them, or work to have them changed. Thus those who believe that abortion is wrong work for laws and stable public opinion to forbid or restrict abortions; those who believe it is a woman's right to choose abortion work for laws and stable opinion favorable to pro-choice.

Formalism

Immanuel Kant, influenced by Hume's skepticism, changed the course of modern philosophy by denying that it is possible for us to know "the thing in itself," including the human self and its nature. We are only conscious of ourselves in a phenomenological way as thinking, willing "subjects" who order and interpret the data of our senses in logical categories that are innate to our minds in order to form a consistent picture of the world. Hence, to escape Hume's arguments for emotivism in ethics, Kant sought to develop a new type of ethics based not on our unknowable human nature but on the logical requirements for reasonable persons of good will to agree on a consistent value system which would make a stable society possible (Shell, 1979; Auxter, 1982). He was a deontologist in ethics in the sense that he accepted the idea, derived from his pietist Protestant background, that morality is a matter of moral law. But he also believed that for human beings to be truly free and truly moral they ought not simply obey some law outside the individual conscience (heteronomy), even though it be revealed from without by God himself (theonomy), but only a purely interior law legislated by the autonomous conscience of each individual (autonomy).

It might seem that this self-legislation could end in the crudest form of emotivism. Kant, however, who was well aware of this danger, insisted that people cannot claim to be moral unless they have the will to legislate for themselves, not merely, as Hume thought, when calm emotionally, but in a completely objective, rational way, free of all self-interest. Thus his system is sometimes called "ethical rationalism," "moral purism," or "altruism." He argued that all truly moral norms (maxims) must take the form of the "categorical imperative:" *Act so that you are willing that your act should be a norm for all other agents.* Thus I must not steal, because I cannot will others to steal from me. Hence, according to Kant, for a woman to choose an abortion morally, she must be convinced, apart from all feelings or personal interests, that her own mother if pregnant in the same circumstances would have had the duty to abort her!

Undoubtedly Kant saw the categorical imperative as a secular form of Jesus' saying, "Do to others whatever you would have them do to you. This is the law and the prophets" (Mt 7:12), but Jesus' "golden rule" is quite different from Kant's, since Jesus clearly indicates that his rule has a definite content, namely, "the law and the prophets," i.e., the Ten Commandments performed, as the prophets had taught, for the right motive of love of God and neighbor. Kant's categorical imperative, on the contrary, is known *a priori* (prior to empirical experience) from the logical categories of human reasoning. Hence it is an abstract mental form that provides no concrete ethical content, but only the *form* of pure disinterestedness or universalizability (Frankena, 1980); thus the name *formalism* for his ethical theory. For Kant, the content for this universal moral form has to be supplied from a consideration of subjective preferences, just as Hume and Rousseau (whom Kant admired) held. Thus Kant argued, "It is our duty never to lie, no matter what the consequences, because I would not want you to lie to me." But this does not tell us why I *ought* or *ought not* want you to lie to me. Thus, after all, formalism, although it aims to be the very opposite of emotivism, does risk degenerating into it, so that rationalism easily turns into sentimentalism, as it did for the Romantic wing of the Enlightenment.

Today Kant's theory in its original form is usually rejected as unrealistic, since psychologists doubt that the total, pure disinterestedness formalism demands for morality is even possible as a healthy human attitude. Nor is it clear how formalism can produce nonarbitrary concrete rules. Hence, numerous modern ethicists have tried to revise Kant's duty ethics in a more acceptable form. A well-known version is that of Rawls (1971), which bases morality on an implied contract by which human persons agree to protect each others' rights. Another version is that of Frankena (1980), who proposes two principles, *fairness* or justice (the duty to respect the autonomy of others), and *beneficence* (the duty to help others even as you expect others to help you). In conflict cases, these principles must be reconciled with each other in *ad hoc* fashion. Robert Veatch (1981) bases medical ethics on a supposed three-way contract between physician, patient, and society.

Beauchamp and Childress (1994) in their system of "common morality" have made explicit a third principle in addition to Frankena's *fairness* and *beneficence,* namely, *autonomy,* the duty to decide responsibly for oneself about one's own interests. They claim for these three principles no other justification than that they help us settle ethical questions in a consistent way, acceptable to our culture at the present time. Such a deontological method, however, still is open to the objections that (1) it does not provide nonarbitrary concrete rules; (2) consistent behavior does not always mean consistently good behavior; and (3) it gives no objective, transcultural criteria for what makes behavior good except universalizability, i.e., common or customary morality.

Existentialism

The foregoing forms of deontology are all characterized by the fact that they are *rule* deontologism (i.e., obedience to general laws). With World War II, when modernity began to crumble into postmodernity, doubts about any general moral rules arose. Hence, existentialist philosophers such as Jean Paul Sartre (d. 1985) developed an *act* deontology which still has considerable appeal to many today. This denies the existence of divine laws, revolts against the injustice of positive laws, and denies the power of human reason to legislate for itself in advance of the unique situations that every individual must confront. For existentialists even the two or three principles of the formalists break down in conflict situations, such as the woman who discovers the unborn child she has long desired is seriously defective. Existentialists believe that it is up to the individual confronted by the absurdity of the world and its injustices to create his or her own values. Morality consists in being *responsible*, that is, in responding to life situations in one's own way and then accepting the consequences without blaming anyone else. Some Christian theologians, notably Bultmann (1958), have given this type of ethics a Christian interpretation. Bultmann argues for the necesssity of a radical obedience to the surprising, unpredictable call of God, going beyond all general moral laws, such as God's command to Abraham to sacrifice his son Isaac in seeming contravention of the moral law (Gn 22).

The strength of existentialism is that it seems to account for the fact that many greatly admired heroes and saints have not been content merely to keep the rules, but rather have been innovative, meeting new problems in new ways. Did not Jesus himself say, "Pour new wine into fresh wineskins" (Mt 9:17)? This existentialist type of thinking is manifest in the abortion debate when someone says, "I think that abortion is tragic, but when a woman is faced with a crisis in her life because of pregnancy, she should have the courage to decide for herself, no matter what others think or what the law or the Church says." If abortion is a tragic choice to which no law can be adequate, who but the mother should make the decision? Hence the notion that "pro-choice" is a woman's right.

The weakness of existentialism, however, is that (1) it gives the puzzled, agonized individual no help in making a decision; and (2) it destroys communal decision making, without which society is impossible. No doubt each of us is responsible for applying general norms to unique situations, and this requires intelligent creativity, not mere conformity. But without general norms people cannot act together for the common good.

All these forms of voluntarism tend to generate unsolvable controversies over whether moral laws are to be applied strictly (*rigorism*) or leniently (*laxism*). Hence in the sixteenth century a great debate among Catholic theologians arose about what were called "moral systems" concerning the relative "probability" that a strict or lenient interpretation of moral laws was obligatory. The effects of this controversy are still felt today: Catholic "conservatives" insist on law enforcement, "liberals" on "ways around the law." But doesn't this mean that *both* sides are thinking *legalistically?*

7.3 TELEOLOGICAL (MEANS–ENDS) METHODOLOGIES

Teleology and Natural Law

Teleologists insist that an ethics of law, whether that be the law of God, the state, or the individual, cannot be the ultimate source of morality because laws, to be reasonable and binding, cannot be arbitrary but must be based on human nature and its needs. If a wise and loving God created us, he must will that we act in accordance with the nature he originally gave us, free of its later distortion by sin. If the state makes laws, these must take into account the inborn needs of its citizens. If I make laws for my own conduct, I must take into account who and what I am in my God-given nature.

Consequently, teleological ethics, more logically than deontological ethics, is a natural law ethics (Finnis, 1983, 1991). At first it seems paradoxical that natural "law" should characterize teleology, which does not make law the ultimate basis of morality, rather than characterize deontology, which does. In fact, the term *natural law* came into common philosophical usage through the Stoics, whose ethics was the most deontological of all the forms of Greek philosophical ethics, but the term probably originated with the great Jewish thinker Philo (Koester, 1968). In a deontological system, the notion of natural law served the purpose of explaining why there is a higher and more universal law that seems to bind all humanity and which therefore is not the positive law of a particular society or the religious law of a particular religion. The natural law, the Stoics believed, is *instinctive* to the whole human race, thus anticipating Rousseau and Kant by an emphasis on intuition rather than ends–means reasoning. The Roman Stoic and jurist Ulpian even believed natural law was common not only to all human beings but also to animals as well (e.g., the laws of self-preservation and procreation).

In the Middle Ages, however, the scholastic theologians, influenced by the strongly teleological ethics of Aristotle, interpreted "natural law" differently. For them it no longer meant some type of instinct for what is right and wrong, but a type of *reasoning* that leads beyond all verbally expressed laws to the nature of the human person. Human beings act morally when they live in such a way as to satisfy in a consistent and harmonious way those needs basic to human life and common to all human beings (Aquinas' *Summa Theologiae*, I-II, q. 94, a. 2). Thus the natural law is our human sharing in God's own wisdom about what kind of living will best fulfill the nature which the Creator has given us by creating us as bodily beings who also in our spiritual intelligence and free will image God (Gn 1:27). Since human culture also is the product of human intelligence, it also tends, for all its creative variety, to conform to the objective requirements of human nature.

Although some influential ethicists such as G. E. Moore (1903) have insisted that the values natural to us as human beings are known directly and intuitively (*intuitionist ethics*), the more nuanced versions of natural law ethics, unlike the political rhetoric of our Declaration of Independence, do not contend that the natural law is "self-evident" (Finnis, 1980; Macquarrie, 1970). It is not self-evident to us whether abortion is always wrong or is sometimes right. This can be decided only by a process of critical reasoning based on what we have learned about human nature and its needs.

Thus a natural law ethics in a strict sense must be grounded in the conviction that from our empirical observation of human persons and their behavior we can gradually come to an understanding of universal *human nature* and its basic needs (teleology). Hence it differs radically from the ethical systems derived from Kant's formalism, which in various ways seek to base ethics on an *a priori* intuition of mental categories or absolute values or our understanding of ourselves as a self-conscious "subject."

Utilitarianism

Hume was the father of emotivism; Kant, influenced by Hume, was the father of formalism; and Jeremy Bentham, also influenced by Hume, was the father of utilitarianism. Since according to Hume the ethical "ought" is founded in a feeling of preference, Bentham drew the conclusion that we decide whether something is good or bad by estimating how much of pleasure or of pain it entails.

In some forms of utilitarianism the needs of a human person are considered to be purely *individual*. This is called egoism, or what Ayn Rand (1964) advocated as "the new selfishness" and others call "libertarianism." This view seems the very opposite of Kant's ethics, which was based on the idea that any self-interested action is immoral by definition, but perhaps it is more realistic. Certainly each person has the responsibility (Section 3.4) to care for his or her own needs and interests. Persons cannot reasonably demand that others do everything for them, nor are they justified in criticizing others because they take care of themselves. Even Jesus Christ, in giving us the great commandment that sounds so altruistic—"Love God and your neighbor"—added "as yourself" to indicate that we must also love ourselves, since God loves us just as he loves our neighbor. The efforts of some theologians who defend duty ethics to explain away that "as yourself" have not been very successful (Frankena, 1985; Outka, 1972).

Section 1.2 shows that self-love is not necessarily selfishness. Genuine self-love not only is consistent with the love of others, but also demands that a person love others, because the deepest human need is for those spiritual goods that can best be enjoyed in community. To seek personal good is not to remain selfishly individualistic, but to learn to share in communal life. Such sharing is what makes persons images of God, since God himself is a communal Trinity of Father, Son, and Holy Spirit who totally share one being and life and who generously share this being and life with us through creation and redemption.

Thus egoism is inadequate not because it approves self-love, but because it proposes an incomplete view of human needs. Hence, the abortion issue cannot be argued merely in terms of the woman's *private* interests. How can she demand her own rights, if she does not respect the rights of the child within her? Both are equally members of the community and share one common good. Yet the Catholic Church has never rejected the notion that self-love is legitimate and does not deny that a pregnant woman with a cancerous uterus may morally choose to have it removed, although she knows the child will die as a *side effect*. What it rejects is the notion that a woman can morally choose to kill her child as a *means* to save her own life. In fact, the Church has condemned as heretical the theory of "pure love" proposed by Quietism, according to which it is holy to be indifferent to one's own salvation (Knox, 1950).

Few ethicists have accepted egoism; rather, they have opposed Kantian duty ethics by a *utilitarianism* based on the notion of "the greatest good for the greatest number" (Singer, 1980), a principle best defended by the philosopher John Stuart Mill (d. 1873). In its current forms, utilitarianism is often called *consequentialism* and is probably the most favored ethics in modern U.S. society, where humanism dominates (Kurtz, 1988). Any teleological ethics is based on evaluating the effects of an action as a means to an end, but there are different ways of estimating these effects. Utilitarian consequentialism uses a calculus of positive and negative satisfactions and dissatisfactions, enumerating these as *quantitatively* comparable items. Its model is that of an economic exchange in which gains and losses can be calculated in terms of a uniform monetary measure. No wonder such an ethics, with its cost-and-benefit analysis, is very understandable and acceptable in American society, accustomed as it is to thinking in this kind of computerizable logic and greatly influenced by the *pragmatism* of the philosopher John Dewey (d. 1952). Some people identify this type of logic with reason itself.

Situationism

One form of utilitarianism is *act utilitarianism,* exemplified by the *situationism* developed by Joseph Fletcher, one of the pioneers of bioethics (1954, 1988). Fletcher's approach is intelligible because he was reacting to the duty ethics prominent in the Protestant tradition, to which many Catholic conservatives also seem to have committed themselves. For Fletcher there is only one absolute moral rule, that of love: "We should always do what is loving and refrain from doing what is not loving." Fletcher settled abortion cases not by saying that abortion is either always wrong or always permissible, but by judging the consequences of an abortion for this particular woman in this particular situation in view of whether her action is "loving."

But what is "loving" action? It has generally been pointed out by Fletcher's critics (Ramsey, 1965; Outka, 1968; Cox, 1968; King, 1970; McCormick, 1981) that in his actual solution of cases, Fletcher was forced gradually to develop various generalizations and rules. Furthermore, he asserted without proving: (1) that the rule of love is a universal rule (egoists do not admit this) and (2) that no other rules are universal. Fletcher's only argument for this second assertion is that, with sufficient ingenuity, a hardship case can always be imagined in which it seems difficult to apply the usual rule. This, however, only proves the obvious that ethical decisions can be difficult. The same objection can be brought against the rule of love, which in many cases is certainly very difficult to apply.

Consequently, most utilitarians, as did Bentham and Mill, reject pure situationism (Engelhardt, 1986b) and advocate some form of *rule utilitarianism* whereby cost/benefit calculations must be made on the basis of experience formulated in normative generalizations; that is, moral rules. Whether any rule admits an exception cannot be decided *a priori*. Even a scientific prediction based on natural physical law is always merely probable because in the concrete instance another law may modify the outcome (e.g., the law of gravitation is offset by the law of electromagnetic attraction when a magnet is used to lift a piece of metal). Why is it surprising, then, that moral natural laws, which have a basis in natural facts, need to be reformulated as knowledge of human needs and situations increases, or that there may appear to be a conflict of laws in concrete cases? Many rule utilitarians make this point by saying that moral rules have only a *prima facie* obligation (Ross, 1930; Beauchamp and Childress, 1994); that is, laws are assumed to be binding unless sufficient reason is found to make an exception. Thus many ethicists today would consider mothers to be bound first by the rule that in general abortion is wrong, but that in some cases special circumstances shift the cost/benefit balance in favor of an abortion.

Ethical debate based on utilitarianism, however, also tends to end in an impasse. To many it seems grounded on a very superficial, overly economic view of the needs of human persons and human communities. It calculates cost/benefit consequences by treating human values as quantitatively comparable items, without taking adequate account of the unified, interdependent structure of the human person or the person's relation to a community sharing higher values, as discussed in Chapter 1. Some utilitarians, such as John Stuart Mill, have tried to introduce a *qualitative* element into their system, but to do so consistently demands an essentially different type of ethics, which is described next.

Proportionalism

David Kelly (1979), in a study of the development of Catholic thinking on medical ethics, contrasts what he calls a "classicist mentality" and a "historical mentality." Kelly sees a post-Vatican II trend among Catholic moralists to abandon an allegedly static worldview based on the concept of an unchanging human nature and to adopt a newer dynamic, evolutionary, historical, and cultural worldview that takes full account of scientific progress, the variety and variability of human culture, the pluralism of value systems, the differences between unique persons, and the novel situations of contemporary life.

To take account of this shift, Kelly thinks, a new system of teleological ethics called by its opponents "proportionalism" has been developed by some German Catholic moralists since Vatican II. Its philosophical roots are to be found in the thought of the German philosopher Max Scheler (d. 1928; cf. Deeken, 1974; O'Connell, 1974), influenced by the founder of phenomenology Edmund Husserl (d. 1938) and the existentialist Martin Heidegger (d. 1976). Scheler accepted Kant's *a priori* ethics with its distinction between the "transcendental" or abstract forms of moral reasoning and the "concrete" norms that actually guide moral decisions. But he rejected Kant's formalism and sought to remedy its abstractness by positing a phenomenological "moral sense" or "feeling" that can intuit certain *absolute* moral values, such as "love," "loyalty," "trust," etc. These transcendental values inform our moral decisions, but they can only be approximated in actual concrete situations by a creative act by which we maximize them, somewhat as a painter maximizes aesthetic values of composition and color in a particular work of art. Thus a woman faced with a decision about abortion in a uniquely difficult situation cannot solve it by some given rule but only by "doing the best she can."

Scheler's moral idealism was influential in Catholic circles even before Vatican II, notably through the writings of Dietrich von Hildebrand (1965). Hildebrand in the *Humanae Vitae* crisis in 1968 vigorously supported the encyclical's ban on contraception. Karl Rahner, SJ (d. 1984), however, starting from the same Schelerian basis, pointed the way to more liberal thinking, notably in his article, "On the Question of a Formal Existential Ethics" (1961), but did not himself develop its implications. This development was the work of another German Jesuit, Peter Knauer (1967); the noted Roman professor at the Gregorian University, Josef Fuchs, SJ (1971, 1980, 1984); Bruno Schuller, SJ (1973); and the Louvain moralist, Louis Janssens (1972).

In the United States Richard A. McCormick has been a tireless promoter of proportionalism (cf. Hoose, 1987; McCormick 1973, 1981, 1984b; McCormick and Ramsey, 1978; Dedek, 1979; cf. Ashley, 1990), but has not stressed its philosophical foundations in German idealism so much as its persuasiveness in pragmatic American culture. Charles E. Curran (Curran and McCormick, 1979, 1988) has arrived at dissenting opinions similar to McCormick's but on the basis of an ethics of "compromise" or a "mixed" deontological-teleological "ethics of responsibility." Curran was a student of Bernard Häring (1973; 1992; reviewed by Ashley, 1992), a Redemptorist Roman professor, schooled in traditional voluntarist legalism, who after Vatican II also promoted dissent from Vatican teachings by liberal use of *epikeia* (the lenient interpretation of moral law in hardship cases).

What then is "proportionalism?" All theologians, including St. Thomas Aquinas, admit that the proportion of good and evil consequences of human acts is morally relevant, but proportionalism goes further. It can be defined as *a moral methodology which guides moral judgments chiefly by the principle of proportionate reason; i.e., Do only those acts for which there is a proportionate reason in their favor; i.e., whose positive premoral values outweigh their negative premoral values.* By a negative "premoral" (or, to use the phenomenological term, "ontic") value is meant "any lack of perfection at which we aim, any lack of fulfillment which frustrates our natural urges and makes us suffer" (Janssens, 1972). Thus proportionalists, following a phenomenological axiology (theory of values), contrast "ontic" premoral values to "ontological" values because they hold that the ontic "facts" of the world are without determinant value in themselves until given "ontological" (human significance) or moral value by the subject. Hence other proportionalists prefer to speak of the premoral calculus of values as a judgment of "right" and "wrong," rather than of "good" and "evil."

Aquinas and Proportionalism

Since Thomistic moral theology has long had such authoritative status in the Church, proportionalists, in spite of the fact that their new system is rooted in a Kantian philosophy quite different than the thought of St. Thomas Aquinas, have tried to present their theory as a legitimate development of his teaching (*Summa Theologiae* I-II, q. 94, a. 2). They agree with St. Thomas that acts are morally specified by their *moral object, circumstances,* and *intention;* but they disagree with his view that an act can be judged intrinsically evil (*malum per se*) and hence always immoral, even before considering its circumstances or other intentions besides the intention of the moral object itself. Rather, they maintain, we should not judge the act to be morally evil until we have considered the moral object *together with* its circumstances and intentions. Thus *before* applying the principle of proportionate reason to specify the act morally, we must first weigh all the foreseen premoral desirable and undesirable values or consequences of the act. Hence, proportionalists argue, it is not fair to accuse them of approving "Doing evil that good may come from it," or "The end justifies the means," since the negative values involved in an act are not moral but premoral, and the moral act, justified by the principle of proportionate reason, although it may entail negative premoral values, is not morally in part good and in part evil, but wholly and simply morally good.

For example, consider the case of a woman who deliberates about acting to terminate her pregnancy (object) because of her age (circumstance) and because she wants better health (intention), and then after weighing these values together reasonably and objectively decides that the premoral positive values of termination are greater than the negative ones of the child's death; and who then applies the principle of proportionate reason, concludes the act is morally justified, and so acts. According to proportionalism, while one might well question whether she has weighed the values of her act correctly, nevertheless one must say that she has done nothing morally evil, but only what is morally good, in spite of the fact that her act involves some premoral negative values (the child's death).

Aquinas insists that if the moral object (i.e., that which is directly intended to be done) is intrinsically evil, it may never be justified by any circumstances or even by some intention better than the intention of the moral object itself. However, proportionalists hold that though the moral object may be *prima facie* evil, it cannot be judged definitively to be evil until the circumstances and additional intentions are also taken into account. We believe that the philosophical grounds for this fundamental difference between the two methodologies is that for Aquinas the moral object is the *essential* specifier, while the circumstances and circumstantial intentions are only *accidental* qualifiers of this essential specification.

Consequently, for St. Thomas, circumstances and circumstantial intentions, while they can accidentally mitigate or aggravate the essential goodness or evil of an act, can never make an essentially evil act essentially good, since a truly good act must not be essentially flawed, but they can make it evil. Thus, according to Church teaching, the direct termination of a pregnancy can be made less evil by circumstances or a good intention, but it can never be anything but a sin. On the other hand, a good act, such as almsgiving, can be made less good by circumstances or circumstantial intention; in the Sermon on the Mount (Mt. 6:2) Jesus rebukes the hypocrite who gives alms (good moral object), but in the wrong circumstances (in public) or with a wrong intention (hoping to be seen and praised). Wrong circumstances or intentions, however, can even make a good act truly evil, as when (Mt 26:48–49) Judas kisses Jesus in friendship (good moral object) when the guards come looking for Jesus (circumstance) to betray him (evil intention).

The reason that the moral object is the essential specifier is that morality consists in the relation of the act as a means to the true goals of human life which are grounded in human nature. But proportionalists, deferring to Kant's claim that the nature of the human self is unknowable, base their ethics not on human nature but on the self-conscious, phenomenological "subject" endowed, according to Scheler, with an intuitive moral sense of absolute moral ideals (values). Since human nature is unknowable, there cannot be any grounds, as Aquinas thought there were, for assigning a priority to the moral object of a human act over its other factors, circumstances and circumstantial intentions.

It also follows that for proportionalists it is impossible to categorically declare that any concrete moral norms, even negative ones, are absolute (i.e., binding without exception in all circumstances and for whatever intention, other than the intention of the moral object itself), since they can only be approximate concretizations of transcendental absolute values. On the contrary, for Aquinas, there certainly are a number of such concrete negative exceptionless moral norms (e.g., the negative norms of the Ten Commandments).

This new proportionalist theory of moral decision became, as McCormick (1995b) puts it, "mainstream" in Europe and the United States, in catechetics, theological schools, and universities, even the ecclesiastical universities in Rome during the 1970s and 1980s. It has been, however, strongly criticized by certain theologians and philosophers, both Catholic and other (Connery, 1981; Grisez, 1988; W. E. May, 1984; Mullady, 1986; Finnis, 1991; Pinckaers, 1995). It has been shown by several scholars to be a radical departure from the Catholic tradition and a sophisticated form of utilitarianism or consequentialism.

The Magisterium and Proportionalism

After the issues had been thoroughly explored by theologians, Pope John Paul II in the *Catechism of the Catholic Church* (1994) and more technically in his encyclical *The Splendor of Truth* (1993) declared that this methodology—at least in any form that implies that concrete negative moral norms, such as those traditionally condemned by the Church as absolute, admit of exceptions—is inconsistent with the Bible, Christian tradition, and natural law. The pope then concretely applied this pronouncement by declaring in very solemn terms in the encyclical *Evangelium Vitae* (1995) that the direct killing of the innocent, the "mercy killing" of sick, and the direct termination of pregnancy are intrinsically evil acts, never morally justifiable by any purpose or circumstance. Although he did not invoke papal infallibility in *Evangelium Vitae*, it seems clear that this type of declaration now has the status of a definitive ordinary teaching of the universal Church and hence is not open to future contradiction (Sullivan, 1994).

Proportionalists, nevertheless, have hastened to criticize these authoritative declarations by claiming that they misrepresent their ethical theory because: (1) Proportionalists do not deny that an act can be called "intrinsically evil" by reason of its moral object "if the object is broadly understood as including all the morally relevant circumstances" (McCormick, 1993, 1994): (2) They do not deny that there are some absolute moral norms, but only that these are either (a) "formal," abstract norms such as "Do good and avoid evil"; (b) "virtually exceptionless" concrete negative norms regarding matters where the negative values so outweigh the positive ones that no exception is imaginable, such as "Do not rape"; (c) absolute norms expressed in terms that do not simply describe the act in premoral terms, but connote a moral judgment, such as "Do not murder."

Thus proportionalists claim they do not disagree with *Veritatis Splendor* that "murder" and "abortion" are intrinsically evil, since it is tautological to say, for example, that "It is always immoral to murder, since 'murder' is defined as to kill immorally." What is really in question, they say, is whether the classical *definitions* of these sins based simply on moral object, abstracting from circumstances and intention, are satisfactory. Thus, in the case cited of the woman who terminates her pregnancy, a proportionalist might claim that in her circumstances and with her intentions the action should not be defined as an "abortion," but as a "decision to terminate pregnancy based on a proportionate reason, namely, my need at this time in my life to save my health."

It seems to us, however, that these criticisms of *Veritatis Splendor* in fact admit that proportionalism *does* teach there can be no concrete negative moral norms that without exception forbid the performance of certain acts essentially specified by their moral objects apart from their accidental circumstances and intentions. This is precisely what John Paul II has rejected (Janet Smith, 1995). Moral theologians, moreover, have also exposed the inherent flaws of proportionalism as a moral theory. Their chief objections—besides questions raised by proportionalism's roots in Kantian idealism and Schelerian intuitism, which we have already indicated—are four-fold.

First, it has been pointed out that proportionalism is impractical and arbitrary as a method of moral decision making that can be subjected to critical public discourse and rational dialogue, because it depends entirely on weighing short- and long-range consequences of an action, and these are infinite and unpredictable (Connery, 1981). Thus, although Fuchs (1971) claims that this is the most "objective" of methods, since it takes all factors into consideration, in fact it is highly subjective and individualistic. When Rahner urged an "existential" ethics, he was opening the way to mere situationism or act utilitarianism. No one questions that foreseen consequences of unique acts in unique conditions have to be taken into account in moral judgment and their proportionate value weighed in some rough manner. That is the task of prudence, rather than the systematic definition of ethical norms (Cessario, 1991; Nelson, 1992). Thus traditionally casuistry has made use of proportionality in applying such principles as those of double effect and material cooperation to hard cases (cf. 8.3); but only to confirm judgments based primarily on essential specification by the moral object intended. Furthermore, some ethicists argue that moral values are in principle "incommensurable" (Grisez, 1983; Finnis, 1983).

A second and more fundamental objection (Pinckaers, 1995) is that the dependence of moral judgments made according to this theory on a premoral calculus of consequences amounts to reducing moral judgment to *technological* rather than ethical judgment. Moral judgment has an absolute character because it judges an act as it is a means to the ultimate, unconditional goal of human life; technological judgment is only conditional since it concerns means to goals that are not fixed in human nature but are a matter of free choice. Thus, the first consideration in moral choice is not the external consequences of an act as in technology, but the relation of that act to the formation of personal character: "Does the act make the actor a better or worse human being?" A woman may foresee some very positive values to be consequent on having an abortion, but the chief moral question is what kind of a person she becomes by that act.

A third objection, closely related to the second, is that proportionalism is self-contradictory because it tries to base moral decisions on a weighing of premoral values, which requires one to evaluate the consequences of the act by relating it as a means to some human end; otherwise it would be a value only in relation to some nonhuman measure and thus utterly irrelevant to moral judgment. But such an evaluation is already a moral evaluation, so the theory claims that such values are at the same time and in the same respect premoral (i.e., not moral) and yet moral! For example, proportionalism requires the woman considering terminating her pregnancy, before she makes a moral judgment, to balance the values involved in being no longer pregnant and the values of bearing a child. Yet the only meaningful way that she can weigh these values is in terms of the dignity of human persons and of truly human living, and this is a moral evaluation. Thus in making the premoral judgment, she has already made a moral judgment.

Moral Dualism

There are two concepts which have become common in current moral theology, especially by advocates of proportionalism, and which are also rejected in *Veri-*

tatis Splendor. We have seen that proportionalism has its roots in Kantian philosophy and reflects the dualism between the *a priori* of absolute transcendental values known intuitively and the categorical level of concrete moral action, as well as the dualism of premoral and moral values. This same dualism appears in the revision of the Thomistic concept of the "ultimate end" of human life by the notion of "fundamental option" presented by Karl Rahner, SJ (Poddimatam, 1986).

Rahner followed Aquinas in holding that for every human acting person there must be a commitment to some supreme good in life, and the search for this supreme good is at least implicit in every free decision one makes; otherwise we would be trying to go in two different directions at once. As Jesus said (Sermon on the Mount, Mt 6:24), "No one can serve two masters. He will either hate one and love the other, or be devoted to one and despise the other. You cannot serve God and money." Mortal sin, therefore, consists in acts by which we choose some creaturely good in preference to union with God as the goal of our lives, whereas conversion to God means again to commit ourselves to him as our supreme goal in life. Thus someone who, by defrauding the poor of their wages, chooses money as the goal of life rather than God who loves the poor commits a mortal sin.

Rahner, however, in accordance with the Kantian transcendental–categorical dualism, sought to revise our understanding of this "fundamental option" of the ultimate end by maintaining that it pertains to the transcendental, not to the categorical level of moral life. Yet he was careful to point out that we can change this transcendental commitment only by some categorical act. Unfortunately, some of his followers drew from this distinction the conclusion that one can perform an act which is seriously immoral at the categorical level, while remaining committed to God at the transcendental level, and sought to use this notion to solve the pastoral problem of dealing with penitents who in spite of seeming good will again and again yield to the same sins. Traditionally, this was explained—and we believe adequately—by saying that these were sins of weakness which are often committed indeliberately or without full freedom because of addiction, and hence were not necessarily mortal. But as John Paul II insists in *Veritatis Splendor,* when these are deliberate and knowing human acts, they are mortal sins that break off our relation with God. Does not the Bible say (1 Jn 4:17), "If someone who has worldly means sees a brother in need and refuses him compassion, how can the love of God remain in him?"

A second type of moral dualism, frequently found in proportionalist writings, is the accusation that the Church in its teachings on sexual morality is guilty of "physicalism" or "biologism" (Curran 1968, 1977b, 1979, 1985, 1988). This charge means that in specifying human acts first by their moral objects and finding some of them (e.g., masturbation) to be intrinsically evil, the Church has given too much weight to the physical aspects of the act and too little to its more truly human, personal meaning of the acts (e.g., to relax nervous tension by sexual pleasure).

Two points must be made in answer to this accusation. First, the body is an essential aspect of the human person, and the way one uses the body, therefore, can have important moral significance. As St. Paul says, "Do you not know that your body is a temple of the Holy Spirit within you, whom you have from God, and that you are not your own? For you have been purchased at a price. Therefore glorify God in your body" (1 Cor 6:19–20). Second, it is simply not true that the Church's documents confuse the physical object of a human act with its moral object. The moral object considers the physical act not as such but as it is a means to achieve the true goals of the human person. This immediate intention of the object (prior to any merely circumstantial, accidental intentions) is what essentially specifies the object and makes it moral. Although the physical act of masturbation is indeed a distortion of the natural sexual act, this distortion as such is not why the Church teaches that it is perverse, but because the act has been distorted as a means to an end not in conformity with the true purpose of human sexuality, expression of married love.

A sound ethics must maintain that the spiritual mind is the depth of the human person and the body its servant. Ethics insists on the unity and mutual dependence of body and soul which both enter into every human act, so that a good human act must be both physically and spiritually in accordance with the truth of human nature.

If moral proportionalism and dualism have failed, as John Paul II has authoritatively declared, what form should the revision of moral theology urged by Vatican II take? The authors of this book favor "prudential personalism," based on the ethics of St. Thomas Aquinas but taking into full account modern "historical consciousness" as urged by Lonergan and Kelly. It is sensitive to the subjective factors in moral judgment urged by proportionalists without succumbing to their Kantian assumptions.

7.4 PRUDENTIAL PERSONALISM

Why Personalism in Ethics?

Prudential personalism is a teleological, natural law ethics based on what we now know of human nature and its integral fulfillment through intelligent and free choices. Thus it accords with the Second Vatican Council, which said (Vatican Council II, *Gaudium et Spes*, n. 51, 1965c) that ethics should be based on "the nature of the human person and human action." Human nature, however, exists only in *persons*, which word (as we showed in Chapter 1) signifies a being endowed with independent existence, which is an end in itself and is endowed with a nature that is at least potentially capable of intelligence and freedom. Human persons, unlike the Divine Persons of the Trinity or the angels, are body-persons that begin as single-celled organisms, develop to maturity, and suffer bodily death, yet survive spiritually and are destined to bodily resurrection.

Therefore, an ethics is a "personalism" when it takes fully into account the reality (a) that our human nature is embodied in each of us in a unique way, has a unique history, and special cultural context; (b) that because we are intelligent and free, we have a role in determining what we become in the course of our lives; and (c) that we live not in isolation, but in a developing network of interpersonal relationships in community where there are always tensions between persons of different temperaments, experiences, worldviews, and value systems.

Because each of us is a unique person and yet we belong to one human species and live in one global—but multicultural—human community, and because our lives are journeys of development, we are constantly striving to attain certain goals which can only be reached by common action. These goals are, on the one hand, determined by the facts that: (1) We all have human nature, all desire happiness, all have certain needs fixed by our human bodily and psychological structure. (2) We all live within some community that has its own culture and traditions, which somewhat limit our own perspectives. (3) Yet to a significant degree we freely determine just how both our innate and encultured needs are to be met by us as unique, free persons acting together with other free persons.

Chapter 1 lists some of these basic needs that must be met if the ultimate goal of living is to be reached. Germain Grisez (1983) has also suggestd seven such "basic goods" of two types:

1. "Reflexive, existential, or moral goods" which are subject to free choice in their use:
   a. self-integration;
   b. practical reasonableness and authenticity;
   c. justice and friendship; and
   d. religion or harmony with God.
2. Substantive goods which we have no choice but to seek:
   e. health, physical integrity, and handing on life to new persons;
   f. knowledge of various forms of truth and appreciation of various forms of beauty and excellence; and
   g. activities of skillful work and play.

Aquinas (Aquinas' *Summa Theologiae* I-II, q. 94, a. 2), however, regarded Grisez's existential goods as objects of prudence and the moral virtues, and hence only means to Grisez's substantive goods. He would have classified the substantive goods of skill and work and play as objects of the arts (technologies) subordinate to ethical goods. Thus he proposed four basic goals of human nature.

1. Life, bodily and spiritual;
2. The propagation of the human race;
3. God-centered community life with other created persons; and
4. Truth about reality, above all about God, ourselves, and other persons.

We need life to be able to strive for the other goals. We need propagation of the race because without it we cannot preserve the human community. We need community because without it we can cannot achieve the other goals nor share our achievements with others. We need truth, because it is necessary to guide our lives and to give them their ultimate meaning in the knowledge and love of God, ourselves, and other persons in the Kingdom of God. Grisez considers the seven basic goods he ennumerates as incommensurable goods and hence does not order them in hierarchy unified by one supreme good. But Aquinas, rightly we believe, though he holds that each of his four basic goods is a good in itself and not a mere means, also believes that they are mutually ordered in the way just indicated, so that the first three are subordinated to the last, supreme good. Thus the ultimate goal of human life to which all other goods are ordered is friendship with God in his Kingdom, which includes all other persons who are God's friends.

Jesus as Model of Personalism

A personalistic ethics, since it must be realistic and historically conscious, cannot be based on mere moral "ideals" or abstract "values" imaginatively or intuitively conceived. To be consistent with the natural law and historic Christian revelation it ought (1) to be based on actual examples of historic people who have achieved integral human fulfillment in their lives, and (2) to be tested by these persons' positive contributions to the just and peaceful life of the human community. Unless we know that this kind of moral life has actually been achieved, it remains a mere dream. Christians believe this historic model of true humanity is first of all Jesus the Christ (Messiah). As the Catholic bishops of the United States have written in their joint pastoral letter *To Live in Christ Jesus* (USCC, 1976):

> All of us seek happiness: life, peace, joy, a wholeness and wholesomeness of being. The happiness we seek and for which we are fashioned is given to us in Jesus, God's supreme gift of love. . . . God reveals to us in Jesus who we are and how we are to live. Yet he has made us free, able, and obliged to decide how we shall respond to our calling. We must make concrete in the particular circumstances of our lives what the call to holiness and the commandment of love require. This is not easy. We know, too, that decisions may not be arbitrary, for "good" and "bad," "right" and "wrong" are not simply what we choose to make them. And so God gives us his guidance in manifold forms (p. 8).

John Paul II, in *The Splendor of Truth* (1993), also writes:

> Jesus' conversation with the rich young man [Mt:16–22] continues, in a sense, *in every period of history, including our own.* The question, "Teacher, what good must I do to have eternal life?" arises in the heart of every individual, and it is Christ alone who is capable of giving the full and definitive answer. The Teacher who expounds God's commandments, who invites others to follow him and gives the grace for a new life, is always present and at work in our midst, as he himself promised: "Lo, I am with you always, to the close of the age" (Mt 28:20).

Even those who do not have Christian faith in Jesus as God often admit that he wonderfully realizes the fulfillment of the human potential, which other faiths, including humanism, also seek to foster. The virtues of the Jewish patriarchs and prophets, of Muhammad, Buddha, Krishna, Confucius, the heroes and sages of folk religion, and the secular benefactors of humankind, women and men, are all strikingly exemplified in Jesus as the Christian community remembers him.

Yet it must also be remembered that Jesus promised to send the Holy Spirit (Jn 16:13–15) in order that we may gradually come to understand fully who Jesus is and what he teaches. We do not merely look to the past for a real model of Christian living; it continues to be realized in Christ's Church. Hence, we do not need to enter into the disputes about the historicity of the Gospel accounts of Jesus to find in the Christian saints throughout the ages many historically verified examples of men and women whose virtues were modeled on Jesus, but each having her or his own unique personal emphasis. Moreover, these Christian saints provide us with the key to identify other Christ-like personalities in other faiths who also are witnesses to the working of the Holy Spirit in the global community, a witness that points to the unity of all humanity in the approaching Kingdom of God.

A Christian ethics, therefore, has a firm foundation in human, historic experience, continues to develop historically, and is open to the ethical truth in other religions and humanism which enables us to more fully understand the Gospel itself.

Why Must a Personalist Ethics also Be Prudential?

In the Bible the realistic, practical effort to understand what the wise God intends us to do with the lives he gave us is simply called "Wisdom." It is personified as a loving, nurturing, strong, and clever woman in contrast to "Folly," a seductive but destructive harlot. Jesus lived in this tradition first of all as a wisdom teacher and then as one who himself lived wisely. This biblical wisdom was first of all *prudence* (a contraction of the Latin *providentia*, foresight) not merely in the sense of "caution" as we often use the word today, but in the much richer sense of an intelligent planning of life in view of the actual situation in which each person finds her or his own self.

We call the teleological methodology of moral decision making which we are about to describe "prudential" to indicate its practical, goal-seeking, situational, contextual character. Therefore, for a prudential ethics, morality ultimately is not simply a matter of obeying rules, but a life-affirming wisdom that intelligently seeks appropriate, concrete behavior by which to achieve human personal and communal goals. Yet it respects the value of laws, rules, or principles (see 8.1); it knows they are to be obligatory only because they help guide our freedom to "integral human fulfillment" (Grisez, 1983). The fact that there are certain basic needs every human has, and therefore certain basic problems of moral decision that everyone must make, justifies the attempt to develop a systematic discipline of ethics which has scientific universality. We need not be content, therefore, with mere casuistry, "creative" exercises of the "moral imagination," or existential crises of decision. A well-worked-out ethics can provide us with a map of life that, although it can never eliminate surprises, some of them very painful, enables us to strive for human fulfillment, happiness and friendship with God through the person of Christ.

A prudential personalism, therefore, proposes that the rightness or wrongness of human actions should be judged by asking, "How does this action in its context contribute to the growth of persons in community?" For the Christian, this community is the Kingdom of God. Thus the effects of any human act must not be evaluated in terms of immediate pains and pleasures, or even in terms of other immediate qualitative values, but referred to the actualization of the human person in relation to other persons. Because consequentialists and utilitarians fail to provide such a conception of full human personhood as the goal of every human action, but content themselves with more superficial, consequential values, they create an ethics of expediency in which the end justifies the means; that is, *any* means. Following consequentialism or utilitarianism risks wasting our lives in the pursuit of unsatisfying and often inconsistent goals, which ultimately leave our deepest human needs frustrated.

As one type of teleological ethics, prudential personalism begins its analysis of a moral act from the ultimate goal of human life—that is, the self-actualization of the person in relation to God, other persons, and the world. People are not free not to want to be happy, but are free to commit themselves to different concrete realizations of happiness (e.g., pleasure, fame, or God). To choose unreasonably as an ultimate goal (or "fundamental option") what cannot satisfy all our basic needs is to "build our house on sand" (Mt 7:26). The Gospel teaches us that by God's help we can attain to life with God and with his friends in the Kingdom of God, a kingdom that is eternal but into which people enter even here on earth. Nothing less will completely satisfy all our human needs.

Hence persons, in making decisions, need to be very clear about the goal of human life set by the Creator for human beings in common and for each of them in their uniqueness. To achieve this self-understanding they need to make use of all the types of information of the conscience described in 3.4. Such an effort at self-understanding does not result in a single principle (e.g., the voluntarists' "Obey the law" or the situationists' "Act lovingly" or the utilitarians' and proportionalists' "Maximize positive values"), but in a number of principles reflecting the complex, multidimensional constitution of the human person (1.4).

Ethics, however, deals not only with the goals of life but with the free choice of appropriate means to these goals. People especially need to reason ethically when they are faced with decisions that demand actions they foresee will have not only good consequences but bad ones as well. Jesus himself said sadly, "I have not come to bring peace, but division" (Lk 12:51), meaning that his very work of peacemaking would also result in quarrels.

The word "consequences," however, is somewhat ambiguous. Most properly, it refers to those effects that follow on the act itself, and a free act, in its very performance, has as its very first effect a modification of the agent. One of the great insights of Christian ethics is that morality originates not in the outward deed but in the inward motive. Jesus said, "The things that come out of the mouth come from the heart, and they defile. For from the heart come evil thoughts, murder, adultery, unchastity, theft, false witness, blasphemy" (Mt 15:18–19). In acting, persons may not actually accomplish the good they intend or suffer the harm anticipated, but the primary effect of the free act is in themselves and follows inevitably by building up or tearing down moral character (McCabe, 1969). The first question must always be, "Will this act make me more truly human as Jesus was, or less so?"

To judge among alternative means, people use their reason (together with the sensitivity of attention that healthy, disciplined feelings promote) to measure each means by the goal toward which it is supposed to lead. To act in this reasonable, sensitive way in view of basic needs, all of which must be met to attain self-actualization, is to act in accordance with our God-given nature, and this is obedience to the natural law. The law of Christ, the Gospel (Ga 6:2) confirms a correct understanding of human nature and, furthermore, calls us to that higher happiness of intimate friendship in the Trinity, which is beyond human powers and attainable only by grace (Kiesling, 1986).

In making an actual moral decision, therefore, three things are necessary:

1. I must first ask myself whether I am acting for the right goal.
2. I must then ask whether the act I am considering is an effective means to that goal. I may discover that the act is intrinsically evil, that is, directly contradictory to one of my basic goals set by human nature. For example, to kill an innocent person by abortion directly contradicts my need for a society in which the right to life of all members, just as my own, is respected.
3. If, however, the act in itself appears to be an appropriate means, I must consider whether in my circumstances and with my circumstantial motivations (intentions), here and now, its normal effectiveness is destroyed, in which case an otherwise morally good act becomes evil.

Thus prudential personalism is "personal" because it grounds moral norms in the dignity and basic goods of the human person, not simply in the will of a lawmaker; and it is "prudential" because as far as practicable it takes into account the circumstances of an action and the proportionality of its consequences. Hence it synthesizes the strong points of the other ethical systems we have discussed, without yielding to their weaknesses. Its first principle can be formulated, *Do those acts, and only those acts, which are appropriate means to the supreme good of true knowledge and love of God, oneself, and the human community in time and eternity.* Note that in this statement "human community" includes the families which are the units out of which the total society is constituted. "In time and eternity" implies the value of the human body in its physical as well as its spiritual life. Therefore, such a moral logic is "prudential" in its practical, intelligent effort to reach goals, and it is "personalist" in that it works not for superficial goals but for the total realization of the inherent needs of the human person in community.

7.5 EVALUATION OF MORAL METHODOLOGIES

Beauchamp and Childress (1994) propose eight criteria for an adequate ethical theory: (1) clarity, (2) coherence, (3) completeness and comprehensiveness, (4) simplicity, (5) explanatory power, (6) justificatory power, (7) ability to generate new insights; and (8) practicability. Does prudential personalism in comparison with proportionalism and other moral methodology meet these criteria? (1) It is *clear*, because Catholic moral theology has developed a very detailed and self-consistent system of precisely stated norms; (2) *coherent*, because it relates all moral questions to the fundamental goals of human life and establishes a hierarchy among these goals; (3) *complete and comprehensive*, because it is based on the Church's centuries-long dealing with moral problems at both public and confessional level; (4) *simple*, in the sense that these norms are closely integrated and exemplified in the historical model of Jesus and the saints; (5) *explanatory*, since it is able to give reasons for its judgments in terms of the relation of means to ends grounded in the basic needs innate to human nature; (6) *justifying*, since it can give definite reasons to support these norms from age-old, universal human experience; (7) *fruitful in new insights*, as is evident from its extensive current literature dealing with new problems, especially in bioethics; and (8) it is *practical*, since it has long guided Catholic institutions, including health care facilities, which have demonstrated their lasting vitality.

Prudential personalism is a strictly natural law ethics, confirmed and perfected by the light of the Christian Gospel. Modern skepticism about whether such a knowledge of human nature transcending culture is really possible has engendered the types of teleological ethics other than prudential personalism. Thus utilitarianism was developed by English philosophers in the skeptical tradition of David Hume, who had denied that we know anything about the human self except our own stream of consciousness. Such philosophers left the study of human nature to the biological and psychological sciences, which *ex professo* refuse to deal with questions of value. Utilitarian ethics was developed as a method of dealing with ethical problems in terms of observable consequences without reference to any human self or any human nature.

Proportionalism originated in the European continental tradition of idealism and phenomenology. It also surrenders to value-free science the study of human nature as an object to be observed and measured. As an ethical method it is grounded not so much in the concept of "human nature" as in the Kantian notion of the self-conscious, free "subject" in confrontation with an objective "world" which must be endowed with meaning and value through the subject's own purposes or intentions.

Prudential personalism, in contrast to these systems that distrust our ability to know the natural law, maintains that we really do know something transsubjective and transcultural about human nature in its biological, psychological, ethical, and spiritual dimensions both from commonsense experience and from our advancing scientific research. We are not, as phenomenologists describe us, just self-conscious, free "subjects" locked into our historical, cultural, and private "worlds," but body-persons who can explore the objective world, our own natures, and the human community of which we are a part in a scientific way so as to break through our culture and discover the underlying natural and social order established by the Creator. We must live in harmony with that order, as stewards of the Creator over our own lives and environment, if we are to satisfy the needs inherent in our nature. Thus an ethics based on human nature can be much more closely integrated with the scientific outlook of modern medicine than can a proportionalist ethics, which regards medical facts as of themselves without inherent moral significance.

By seeing the human person as "embodied intelligent freedom," we retain the classical methodology and stress even more strongly than was traditional the unity of the human person as a body-person. All human acts, however spiritual, are also acts of the body, as the Jewish tradition has always taught (Novak, 1985; Ratner, 1977). Consequently, for an act to be truly human, it must respect the inherent teleology or normal biological functions of the body and its organs, not because these are superior to other dimensions of the person, but because their functions are not merely animal but truly human and absolutely necessary to think, love, and act as human beings (CDF, 1987).

For these reasons, we believe that the classical methodology of moral judgment, which we include in prudential personalism but to which we add more attention to human historicity and subjectivity in our understanding of human needs and the means available to satisfy them, is superior to that of proportionalism. Thus it is understandable why the Church in its official teaching continues to use the classical methodology and deplore the erosion of traditional norms. This erosion has resulted from the ingenuity of some proportionalists in finding exceptions to these norms by weighing supposed values and disvalues without showing how these are related to the universal structure of the human person—the basic needs and innate biological and psychological structure of the human person that classical methodology endeavors to respect.

Abortion: A Practical Example

To complete this evaluation of these moral systems, we now return to the example of abortion to see how these systems work in practice. A deontologist faced with an abortion decision will ask if there are rules requiring or forbidding abortion. If no rule is discovered, the deontologist feels free to do what seems convenient. Thus someone might argue that since the Bible contains no explicit command against abortion, it is permitted. Another might argue that since it is legal in the United States, it is moral. If there is a conflict of rules, the deontologist will seek another rule to resolve the conflict or fall back on the rule to do the lesser evil.

A utilitarian or consequentialist faced with the same situation will consider the probable consequences of having or not having the abortion and will attempt to judge whether it will be of greater or lesser benefit to the persons concerned. The utilitarian will evaluate "benefit" either in terms of subjective satisfaction or in terms of what appears desirable or undesirable, but without seeking to ground such evaluations in any teleology intrinsic to the persons concerned. Abortion will thus be judged in terms of the subjective sufferings or relief of the mother, the possible sufferings of an unwanted or defective child, the various advantages to society, and so forth.

A proportionalist also will look at the proportion of values and disvalues that he or she can foresee as included in the act of abortion and all of its foreseeable consequences. The proportionalist then will judge if, in this case, the values of the abortion outweigh the *prima facie* disvalues that are traditionally attributed to it. Considered premorally, the value of the child's and the mother's lives and the disvalue of their deaths are premoral values which take on moral value only when the agent, if he or she observes the principle of proportion (i.e., if he or she chooses only acts in which the premoral values equal or exceed the disvalues), intends a morally good act.

A prudential personalist will try to take into account all the consequences mentioned but will evaluate them in terms of the self-realization of the persons involved and of the community of persons of which they are a part in their historic context. Thus we must first determine when the individual life of a human person begins, taking into account all available scientific and anthropo-logical data, as well as what theology and philosophy can tell us about the criteria of personhood. Then the various consequences of abortion must be evaluated in terms of the needs inherent in the mother and the child, both as unique individu-als and as part of the total human community. In this search for moral truth we must also be sensitive to the individual, subjective conditions of conscience of the persons involved and the historical development of our moral understanding.

When we speak of inherent needs in the human person, we are brought back to the modern ethicists' puzzlement about how to get from facts to values, from the *is* to the *ought*. As Henry Veatch (1971) has shown, this problem had its origin in the mechanistic view of the world favored by many modern scientists. If a human being is a machine produced by the blind forces of evolution, what is the sense in speaking about inherent goals and purposes in the human person? In such a view, human goals or purposes are simply a matter of indi-vidual choice, or they are imposed on people by the laws and customs of the culture in which they have been raised.

The discoveries of modern science can be accepted, however, including our evolutionary origin, without accepting the mechanistic interpretation of these facts. One also can accept scientific discoveries without denying either the common sense of Christian conviction that human persons have been created for a purpose and that this purpose is manifest in their genetically determined physical and psychological constitution as individuals and as part of the human species. This dynamic structure of human nature with its innate needs is a part of the order of facts that one can determine empirically by the life sciences, if one avoids the sociobiologist's deterministic exaggerations (Barlow and Silverberg, 1980) and interprets philosophically and theologically to provide a unified view of what it is to be human. Such an empirically grounded view furnished the basis for an ethics that goes beyond cultural relativism (Rachels, 1986).

Thus, whenever this book refers to basic human needs or to human nature, it implies a philosophical account of the human person that considers fully the findings of modern biology and psychology and that is in keeping with what health care professionals know about the human body and psyche. It also tries to take into account the fact that we are living in history at the end of the twentieth century in what John Paul II has called a growing "culture of death," where medical practices have important consequences not only for this or that individual but for the social order.

When human needs are viewed not merely as static facts, but as goals to be achieved, they become values, that is, goods to be desired and sought. Thus it is a biological fact that people need to eat in order to live. But when we perceive this necessity and begin to make free choices about how we can best fulfill this need in various circumstances, human intelligence, freedom, and creativity enter into the biological process of nutrition and it takes on a truly human, ethical meaning. Considered in their totality as a system of needs, these genetically inherent requirements of life become genuinely obligatory *oughts* because we need to be ourselves and to use our freedom to achieve self-realization.

This need for self-realization is itself a fact of human biology and psychology. Indeed, self-realization is the central unifying feature of a human person, an embodied intelligent freedom. We act morally when we perceive this fact and freely respond to its practical challenge; we act immorally when we refuse to respond realistically to this challenge and yield to disorganized and inconsistent impulses. As McDonagh (1979) has argued, moral living is an openness to a call and a stewardship of a gift. The gift is our human personhood, and the call is the purpose inherent in that personhood.

Thus, when we discuss such an issue as abortion, an adequate logic of ethics forces us to go beyond mere utilitarianism and to ask such questions as: For what purpose are we gifted with sexuality? Is the unborn child a gift of God, and for what purpose has he created it? For what purpose are we created social beings who are inclined to care for the helpless and also for women in the crisis of pregnancy? For what purpose are we gifted with the intelligence and the skill of medical art, to further life or to destroy it? What effect do our decisions have on our cultural today and on the situation of future generations?

Health care professionals cannot shrug off such questions as philosophical or theological problems outside their field. They have received a predominantly scientific education that may have led them to be suspicious of any philosophical effort to read values into facts. When philosophers speak about the human person, a scientifically educated person may prefer to talk about the human organism, reducing everything directly to observable facts systematized by some mathematical or quasimathematical theory. No matter how foreign to their regular way of thinking it may be for scientists to reflect on the value implications of biological or psychological facts, however, such reflection is inescapable if there is to be harmony between medical–ethical decisions and medical science.

On the other hand, some philosophers and theologians are intensely uncomfortable with any effort to root ethics in biological or psychological structures. They are afraid that this will result in a fixed and static conception of human nature, and they would prefer to relate ethics to history and the humanities rather than to the sciences. To this view we would respond that the evolutionary view of humankind, at both the biological and the anthropological levels, is in no way contrary to the prudential personalism we have outlined here. We do not have in mind some type of timeless human nature, but simply the historically existing human species made up of unique individuals. All have their own biographies or "stories" but nevertheless form a community based on certain common needs that are not the product of culture but its source. For the Christian, this historical community is centered in Jesus of Nazareth, God's Word revealed in perfect humanity and pointing the way to the final realization for us all of the Kingdom of God "on earth as it is in heaven" (Mt 6:10).

CONCLUSION

Ethical decisions are always made within some value system, and American society has a plurality of such systems. Therefore Christians need to be fully conscious of their own value system and to enter into dialogue with others to reduce conflict and to find some area of consensus. Thus bioethical matters require a logic that will help people make decisions consistent with the Christian system of values, but a logic that will also enable them to recognize analogies between their system of values and those of others.

The logic of emotivism solves ethical questions by references to emotional preferences. This can serve as the basis of dialogue if one can distinguish between sincere, humane, decent feelings and the opposite of these. Another logic, deontologism or duty ethics, solves ethical questions by reference to the will of God, to recognized laws or customs, or to personal principles of behavior. This also can serve as a basis of dialogue if the parties can find authorities in common or moral principles with which they can agree, perhaps for their own reasons. The line of reasoning in consequentialism, utilitarianism, or situationism attempts to find a solution that seems to bring the most satisfaction and the least hurt to all in the concrete situation. This type of thinking is pragmatic and must certainly form an important element in every public discussion in a pluralistic society. Utilitarianism may result, however, in proposals that some members of the community will reject as unprincipled, merely expedient, shortsighted, and immoral. Proportionalism attempts sensitively to take all these factors into consideration in its calculus of values and disvalues, but unfortunately seems to have found no practical criteria for weighing these values and is thus liable to become subjective and arbitrary.

To resolve this impasse that arises between those in a community who take their stand on absolute principles or authoritative laws and those who argue for pragmatic solutions, Catholic moral theology has attempted to find a middle course, which we have formulated as a teleological prudential personalism. Such an approach attempts to think in terms of any action's effects for the good of the persons and the community involved. Prudential personalism evaluates these effects, however, according to needs and purposes that have been established not by subjective preference, nor merely by abstract laws, but by the innate constitution of the human person in its individual and communal dynamism.

8

Norms of Christian
Decision Making in Bioethics

OVERVIEW

In this chapter we are concerned with the *content* of Christian ethical reasoning about issues in bioethics. Beginning with a discussion of the relationship between Christian revelation and ethics (8.1), we describe the virtues that form a Christian character and the ethical principles they engender, and relate these to the satisfaction of basic human needs. Our human needs are satisfied through the practice of the theological virtues of faith, hope, and charity, so we discuss the principles of bioethics under these three headings, and with them the four cardinal virtues (prudence, temperance, fortitude, and justice) that support the theological virtues, and the gifts of the Holy Spirit that perfect all these aforementioned virtues. As an expression of faith (8.2) (a form of knowing) and the related cardinal virtue of prudence, we present five principles that pertain to the formation of a sound conscience. Next we consider the three norms directed to the future or concerned with the eschatological aspects of ethics, gathering these norms under the heading of Christian hope with its related cardinal virtues of temperance and fortitude (8.3). Then under the title of Christian love (charity) and its cardinal virtue of justice (8.4), we consider four norms that are concerned with affective needs, whether this affection is for ourselves or others. Finally, we seek to coordinate the principles presented by aligning them with the four basic human needs (8.5).

8.1 IS THERE A CHRISTIAN ETHICS?

Does the Gospel Modify Natural Law Ethics?

Today the question is debated whether there is a distinctly Christian ethics (Curran and McCormick, 1980; Gustafson, 1975; Macquarrie, 1970; MacNamara, 1986; Langan, 1988). Certainly the moral values of the New Testament are also found in other religions and philosophies of life. Section 1.3 illustrates this fact by referring to the list of such values in the *Universal Declaration of Human Rights* (United Nations, 1948), to which all the nations of the world, whatever their ideologies, have subscribed. As 1.3 argues, however, value systems may agree on a list of important values yet differ greatly in their hierarchy of values. Thus

Christian ethics might be specified by the priority it gives to certain values. Christian reflection on the *Universal Declaration of Human Rights* leads not only to agreement but to certain special emphases in the light of the Gospel of Jesus Christ.

The great disciple of Jesus, St. Paul, summarized these Christian priorities as *faith, hope,* and *love* (Rm 13). By "love" (Greek *agape*) he meant specifically the love of God and of one's neighbor in view of eternal life with God. In addition to the theological virtues praised by St. Paul, Christian tradition has recognized the need of four others which are called the *cardinal* or *moral* virtues: *prudence* (intelligent decision making), *justice, fortitude* (courage), and *temperance* (moderation), which relate to self-control and our dealings with other human persons. Their names are derived from Greek philosophy and they are only listed together once in the Bible (Wis 8:7; cf. also 2 Pt 1:5–8), but are often separately commended. They can be also be correlated with the three theological virtues: prudence aids faith, justice aids love, while hope is aided by fortitude and temperance.

For St. Paul these primary values of faith, hope, and love derive from his conviction that the fully human life can be achieved only through a personal union with God in eternal life by incorporation in the risen Christ. Thus for Catholic moral teaching Jesus provides the supreme model of Christian character marked by these seven virtues. A secular humanist, a Marxist, a Muslim, and a Buddhist might all agree that these seven virtues are important human values, but they would not agree on the priority to be given them, nor their Christocentricity. This difference in evaluation often results in striking differences in concrete moral judgment. For example, Jewish and Christian moralists agree that sexual purity is a virtue, but Talmudic Judaism requires males to marry and have children, while Christianity approves celibacy "for the sake of the Kingdom of God." Furthermore, while Buddhism agrees with Christianity and disagrees with Judaism in commending celibacy, it does so for quite different motives.

Hence, although Christians use such terms as "faith," "hope," and "love" with a special meaning that is only analogous to the way non-Christians use them, they need not deny that non-Christians *experience the realities* to which these terms refer just as Christians do. Catholic theology has always admitted that non-Christians may be living by grace as truly as Christians. They may experience the same realities as Christians, yet not name or understand them in the same way (O'Meara, 1973). Moreover, since the Second Vatican Council (Vatican Council II, 1965a), many Catholic theologians admit that grace may act not only on those of other religions, but also *through* these religions in different symbols and language. Christians do not claim a monopoly on the true God or his grace, but only that the gracious God has made himself most fully, explicitly, and intimately known to humanity in Jesus Christ (Vatican Council II, 1964a; DiNoia 1992).

It is important to understand that love and hope, as Christians use these terms, are not mere feelings or sentiments, but are rooted in faith in the Incarnate Word, Jesus Christ, who tells us who God is and what our relation to him and to our neighbor must be. Thus Christian faith moves people from an emotional to a rational level of ethical understanding, since rather than a blind trust, faith is a genuine understanding of God's purpose for us, an imperfect but real share in God's wisdom. Christian faith, therefore, moves beyond a duty ethics of mere obedience to God's will to a means–ends level of intelligent, creative purpose and free choice.

Therefore, in what follows we classify the chief principles which we will use in discussing bioethical problems under three headings derived from the chief Christian virtues of faith, hope, and love, along with the four moral virtues correlated with them, in keeping with the subtitle of this book, "A Theological Analysis." At the same time, we do not address our ethical argumentation only to those who accept the Christian faith, but as we will show, support our positions also by "natural law" arguments accessible to reason and to dialogue with other ethical systems

What Is an Ethical Principle?

Some ethicists contrast three kinds of ethics: (1) an "ethics of principles" which is deductive; (2) a "casuistic (case) ethics" which is inductive; and (3) a "virtue ethics" based on character models. In our opinion, as we indicated in Chapter 7, a sound ethics must be all three. It must be a character or virtue ethics, not merely a decision-making or case ethics, because we cannot consistently make good decisions about individual cases unless we are at least trying to become good persons. "A rotten tree cannot bring forth good fruits," Jesus said (Mt 7:18). But, on the other hand, we cannot arrive at a model of good character except by an inductive examination of good and bad decisions. "A tree is known by its fruit," Jesus also said (Mt 12:33).

Again, we cannot generalize from a virtue model so as to apply that paradigm to particular and often unusual cases unless we formulate universal principles based on the model we have selected, which we can deductively apply to the guidance of our own lives. Thus Jesus, who is our historic model, did not hesitate to express his moral attitudes in laws or norms or principles to guide us, as when in the Sermon on the Mount he laid down the principle, "Judge not, that you be not judged" (Mt 7:1). Therefore, in speaking of principles, we by no means opt for what McCormick (1977) disdains as a "deductive ethics" or what David Kelly (1979) calls a "static classical ethics" in contrast to a historical, existential ethics. In theoretical reasoning, principles are fundamental laws or assumptions which guide our research and which explain our data. For example, the three "laws of motion" discovered by Newton and reinterpreted by Einstein govern the whole of physical science. In practical reasoning, however, the principles are the ends or goals to be achieved which measure the value of any means purposed to achieve them. In practical reasoning in a teleological ethics, as we have shown in Chapter 7, these goals are the integral satisfaction of basic human *needs* as these are determined by human nature. By "human nature" we mean what we now know at this point in history about the traits common to all members of our species, as this has been learned inductively from experience by common sense and scientific research and has been historically exemplified by Jesus Christ and his faithful disciples.

Currently it is common to criticize "foundationalism," by which some mean any attempt to ground knowledge in first principles. Deconstructionists argue that such principles cannot really be "first" because their validity rests on assumptions which in turn rest on other assumptions that form an enclosed and vicious hermeneutical circle. But as others (Martin and Meslin, 1994) have pointed out, this criticism presumes that we accept the idealist notion of Descartes and Kant that we know only our own thought and not the reality of the things we think about. Others criticize what they call "principalism" (Emanuel, 1995), as exemplified by the very influential first edition of Beauchamp and Childress, *Principles of Biomedical Ethics* (1979), on the grounds that what are proposed as a very small number of fundamental principles are neither primary nor complete.

Our position is not Cartesian or Kantian but *realist*, since we deny that ethical thinking is a projection of *a priori* principles on real life. We maintain that by empirical induction one can arrive at a realistic, albeit imperfect, understanding of what it is to be human. This attempt to define the human person, of course, opens us up to the accusation of "essentialism." In our defense of "natural law," however, we have already argued (cf 7.1) that our concept of "human nature" is not merely static or historical but refers to the nexus of characteristics, taken in their organic unity, which are empirically common to all members of the human species as a relatively stable community. This definition of human nature, which is open to progressive refinement by the life and social sciences, specifies the intrinsic teleology of humanness, its basic needs in their hierarchy. From this system of needs we attempt to derive the following moral principles which have proved most relevant to the solution of bioethical problems. Christian revelation supports this concept of humanness and adds to it a view of God's gracious design for our participation in his own eternal Trinitarian life.

Christian Character and the Health Care Professional

The ethical principles which we will explicate can, therefore, be supported by the evidence of human history under God's providence. The Bible, which for the Christian is a privileged interpretation of that history, provides a realistic model for good human character which applies with special force to the health care professional. To be an effective physician or nurse in a truly Christian way, one must be first of all a person of faith who lives by the Gospel as it is taught authoritatively in the tradition of the Christian community. Yet one must also be a person of prudence who knows how to apply faith in the practical situations of life and work. That, of course, means that one keeps thoroughly informed of all that pertains to one's professional competence and its ethical practice. To gain God's aid in such decisions we must pray and receive the sacraments regularly so that the Holy Spirit's gifts of wisdom, understanding, and counsel (Is 11:1–3) will make us sensitive to his guidance.

Christian health care professionals also must be persons of hope and inspire hope in those they serve, since without hope there can be no healing, and when healing is not possible, there must be hope of a future life to make dying a rebirth. Such hope cannot be sustained unless the physician and nurse have achieved self-control over their own bodily urges so that they do not become chemically dependent, sex-driven, self-indulgent, hard-hearted, or negligent, but remain free to serve others. Nor can hope endure unless health care professionals have the courage and patience required to sustain the stress of the suffering and death of others and their own fatigues and risks. Fear of God and fortitude are gifts of the Holy Spirit (Is 11:1–3) that enable each of us to be strengthened and comforted in this spiritual battle.

Finally Christian nurses and physicians, and the Catholic facilities in which they work, must be motivated by a love for those for whom they care that is inspired by the realization that every patient is another Christ. Jesus said, "I was ill and you cared for me. . . . Amen, I say to you, whatever you did for one of these least brothers, you did for me" (Mt 25:36, 40). But this love will not be genuine unless it is also deeply respectful of the dignity and rights of patients and their families, especially the neglected. Again, the gift of piety (religious respect for the rights of God and his creatures, Is 11:1–2)) supports this sense of justice and enables the physician or nurse to be concerned not only for the bodily welfare but also for the spiritual needs of their patients.

We are sure that this model of the Christian in health care is not unrealistic because most of us have known professionals who have exemplified it in remarkable ways. Such a Christian character is not acquired overnight; it is the gradual product of living the Christian life conscientiously. Nothing contributes to this growth in character more than genuine *humility,* an aspect of the virtue of temperance which moderates our self-evaluation, so that although we rightly know our own worth we do not overestimate it and become resistant to guidance, correction, instruction, and help from others, and above all from God. When bioethical debate is shallow and fruitless, it is usually due to arrogance on the part of one or both parties, who make no effort to understand the fundamental human needs, values, and fears which are at least analogically common to the other's value system. By empathy for these common human concerns, many of the impasses into which ethical debates have fallen today can be ecumenically transcended.

8.2 NORMS OF CHRISTIAN FAITH AND PRUDENCE

Ethical principles grounded in human nature can be used to guide intelligent analysis of concrete ethical situations, although moral decisions cannot be mathematically deduced from them. Actual ethical decision (see 3.4) depends not merely on abstract reasoning, but on *prudence,* in which several other factors are also involved. Among these factors, as we noted in 7.2, are our own feelings and what some ethicists (Keane, 1984) call "imagination." Certainly, prudent persons about to make decisions imagine the consequences of their various options, how they and others may feel (empathy) if they make this or that choice, what other people who are their models would do, etc.

Christian prudence (often called "wisdom" in the Bible) is faith in its practical aspect, as it enables us to be open to the guidance of Christ's Spirit, who alone knows the way to God and who alone can overcome those barriers of alienation that divide one person from another. Because of our sinfulness which blinds with prejudices, pride, and gross stupidity our God-given capacity for making realistic, objective judgments, we need to be freed by the Holy Spirit to think with "the mind of Christ" (1 Cor 2:16). Thus the first five principles or norms of a bioethics enlightened by the Gospel pertain to the formation of a prudent conscience.

Principle of Well-Formed Conscience

The distinguished French biologist Jacques Monod, in his book *Chance and Necessity* (1971), argues that there really is only one moral value, namely scientific truth, since any ethics not based on realism and "facing the facts" is an immoral form of self-delusion. Monod's notion of truth is narrow and reductionistic, since the scientific method is only one way of arriving at truth, but he is correct in saying that truth is the deepest need of human nature on which all morality depends. If our real needs are not known to us, we cannot develop a means–ends ethics. This does not mean that the only value of truth is its practical use as a guide to living; truth is also something enjoyable in itself, as even the great pragmatist John Dewey (1920) admitted.

This value of truth, both as practical and as something worthwhile in itself, has been emphasized in the *Universal Declaration of Human Rights* (United Nations, 1948):

> Article 18: Everyone has the right to freedom of thought, science, and religion; this right includes freedom to change his religion or belief, and freedom, either alone or in community with others and in public or private, to manifest his religion or belief in teaching, practice, worship, and observance.

Christian ethics also insists on the fundamental character of truth for all other values (John Paul II, 1995). Critics are inclined to say, "You Catholics talk a lot about reason and natural law in ethical matters, but when it comes right down to it, you really rely only on the dogmas of the Church. Your use of reason is merely a rationalization of what you believe by blind faith." The honest answer Catholics can give to this is to acknowledge responsibility as Christians to be faithful *both* to the light of faith and to the light of reason. They must, therefore, make the intellectual effort necessary to bring these two sources of knowledge into a genuine harmony with each other. To sacrifice one to the other is itself unethical because it betrays a commitment to truth, whatever its source. As scientists struggle to resolve disagreements by looking for better data and better reasoning, so the fact that we often meet disagreements about ethical truth should not make us despair that agreement can be found by research and dialogue.

This commitment to ethical truth can be formulated in the *principle of well-formed conscience*, which simply describes the work of the virtue of prudence enlightened by faith:

To attain the true goals of human life by responsible actions, in every free decision involving an ethical question, people are morally obliged to:

1. Inform themselves as fully as practically possible about both the facts and the relevant ethical norms;
2. Form a morally certain judgment of conscience on the basis of this information;
3. Act according to this well-formed conscience; and
4. Accept responsibility for their actions.

Note that this principle is founded on the basic human need for truth as one of the necessary goals of human life, rooted in human nature as it is intelligent freedom. Jesus said, "If you remain in my word, you will truly be my disciples, and you will know the truth, and the truth will set you free" (Jn 8:31–32). As John Paul II shows in his encyclical, *The Splendor of Truth* (1993), to be intelligent is to seek the truth and to use our freedom in accordance with objective truth, whether that be theoretical truth sought for its own sake or practical truth needed as a guide to action. Practical truth includes the arts and applied sciences, of which medicine is both a science and an art; however, technological truths only guide persons to goals freely chosen, and these goals must be harmonized with ultimate or life goals. The art of medicine may tell a physician how to resuscitate a dying patient, but the ethical question of whether to resuscitate or not remains to be answered by use of the principle of well-formed conscience.

In making a well-informed moral decision, we need much information that is available to us from our own experience and from various kinds of human experts, but above all we need that guidance which only the all-wise God can give, since all truth, even the truth of the wisest human beings, is God's gift. The whole point of Christian faith is that this divine guidance in our lives comes to us through Jesus Christ, who said, "I am the way, the truth, and the life. No one comes to the Father except through me" (Jn 14:6). It is true that in giving us human intelligence God expects us to think hard and creatively about how we are to journey toward him, but he has not left us alone in the dark. "Your word is a lamp for my feet, and light for my path" (Ps 119:105). We have that constant guidance of Jesus through his Church and its authority to teach.

Jesus Christ, is known, both in his historical reality and in his actual presence in the world today, only in the Christian community, its Scriptures, its Sacred Tradition, its official pastors in their teaching role, and its sacraments as they are experienced in the actual life and prayer of individual Christians. Consequently, all these sources of information must be sought and heeded if this principle is to have a full Christian application.

Jesus' Moral Teaching and the Church

The teaching of Jesus, who is the very Word of God himself (Jn 1:1), can never be wrong nor ever change; that is, it is "infallible." Jesus has shared this infallibility in transmitting his teaching to us in the Church, "Whoever listens to you, listens to me. Whoever rejects you rejects me. And whoever rejects me rejects the one who sent me" (Jn 10:16). Thus the Catholic Church can never fail in preserving and transmitting the whole Gospel revelation entrusted to it. Jesus, risen from the dead, said to the Apostles, "Receive the Holy Spirit. Whose sins you forgive are forgiven them, and whose sins you retain are retained" (Jn 20:22), that is, he gave them the power of ultimate decision on moral truth. Undoubtedly, because of the human frailty of Christians this transmission of Jesus' teaching suffers from certain imperfections. Yet under the guidance of the Holy Spirit sent by Jesus to his Church (Jn 14:25), these defects are gradually overcome by a deepening understanding of the Gospel ("development of doctrine").

Although this magisterium (Latin for "teaching authority") of popes and bishops has historically been made up of men just as humanly weak as were St. Peter and the Apostles, Vatican II (1964a, *Lumen Gentium,* n. 25) declared that the magisterium shares in that infallibility which Christ conferred on his whole Church. If its teaching could not be trusted, Christ's Church would have failed. The trustworthiness of magisterial teaching, therefore, is not from human power but from Christ's Holy Spirit working through merely human instruments, just as the Spirit worked through the human writers of the Bible, and as such is a surer guide than any merely human authority.

Dissent from Church Teaching

Catholics generally understand that to be Catholic they must accept those teachings about faith and morals which are taught by the pope or an ecumenical council as "infallible." But they often do not understand that this infallible teaching includes not just one but three types of truths: (a) revealed truths solemnly defined by the "extraordinary" (*ex cathedra*) authority of the pope, such as that polygamy is forbidden to Christians (Council of Trent, 1563); (b) revealed truths taught by the "ordinary and universal" magisterium, i.e., the moral majority of bishops with the pope throughout the world, such as the commandment that forbids adultery, which no pope or council has ever solemnly defined, yet which the whole magisterium has always taught as revealed; and (c) truths which are not revealed, but are so closely connected with revelation that to deny them would be equivalent to denying revealed truth, such as the validity of the sacraments as performed today, since to deny this amounts to denying the revealed truth that God has provided the Church to administer his sacraments. This third class of truth must be accepted by Catholics as infallible, not as truth directly revealed to faith but nevertheless as logically and practically sharing in the infallibility of such truths (CDF, 1990).

What is more common today is that not a few Catholics, misled by faulty theorizing by well-known theologians, suppose that Vatican II justified a "right to dissent" from any teachings of the magisterium not known to be infallible and hence (at least in theory) subject to future change. Since in the history of the Church very little of moral teaching, not even the exact meaning of all the Ten Commandments or the Sermon on the Mount, has ever been infallibly defined, this notion of a "right to dissent" has left Catholics in the dark without any clear moral norms and thus deprived them of Jesus' guidance.

In fact Vatican II (1964a, *Lumen Gentium*, n. 25; *Catechism of the Catholic Church*, 1994, # 888–92; CDF, 1990) rejected this so-called "right of dissent." It is true that the magisterium leaves many details of our Christian living to our own intelligence and to charitable and fruitful debate within the Church, not only among theologians, but among the whole laity, such as the choice of political parties, ethnic customs, and personal vocations and devotions. Nevertheless, according to Vatican II, all Catholics in the formation of their faith and conscience have the obligation not only to believe on divine faith whatever the magisterium teaches by its infallible "extraordinary" pronouncements, but also to accept the guidance of its ordinary teaching. Thus the Congregation for the Doctrine of the Faith (CDF, 1990) in its *The Ecclesial Vocation of the Theologian* (n. 23–24) says:

> When the Magisterium proposes "in a definitive way" truths concerning faith and morals, which, even if not divinely revealed, are nevertheless strictly and intimately connect with Revelation, these must be firmly accepted and held. When the Magisterium, not intending to act "definitively," teaches a doctrine to aid a better understanding of Revelation and make explicit its contents, or to recall how some teaching is in conformity the truths of faith, or finally to guard against ideas that are incompatible with these truths, the response called for is that of the religious submission of will and intellect [Vatican Council II, *Lumen Gentium*, n. 25; Code of Canon Law, can. 752]. This kind of response cannot be simply exterior or disciplinary but must be understood within the logic of faith and under the impulse of obedience to faith. Finally, in order to serve the People of God as well as possible, in particular by warning them of dangerous opinions which could lead to error, the Magisterium can intervene in questions under discussion which involve, in addition to solid principles, certain contingent and conjectural elements. It often only becomes possible with the passage of time to distinguish what is necessary and what is contingent.

Examples of a moral teaching proposed "in a definitive way" are Pope John Paul II's declarations (1995) against abortion and euthanasia in *Evangelium Vitae*. For examples of a doctrine yet not definitive, given "to aid a better understanding" and which nevertheless requires "the religious submission of will and intellect," one might cite some detailed items of the CDF's "Instruction on Respect for Human Life" (1987) such as its rejection of *in vitro* fertilization and embryo transplant as an acceptable form of human generation. As for "intervention in questions under discussion which involve, in addition to solid principles, certain contingent and conjectural elements," an example might be

John Paul II's remarks on capital punishment (*Evangelium Vitae*, n. 56, 1995) in which he says "as a result of steady improvements in the organization of the penal system, such cases [of absolute necessity that require capital punishment to protect the common good] are very rare if not practically nonexistent."

Bioethics has raised new questions to which the Church in the interest of the dignity of the human person and the value of human life has found it necessary to make a response. The ordinary teaching of the magisterium as regards bioethics is to be found in many recent documents, especially in the encyclical *Evangelium Vitae* (John Paul II, 1995) and the instruction *Donum Vitae* of the Congregation for the Doctrine of the Faith (CDF, 1987). They can be found in practical form in the *Ethical and Religious Directives for Catholic Health Services* (1994) of the U.S. National Conference of Catholic Bishops, which have been recently revised, updated, and supplied with fuller theological and pastoral explanations. While Catholic health care professionals may also profitably seek the counsel of theologians in understanding and applying these directives to particular cases, they should be aware that some claiming theological expertise are not in fact in honest conformity with these magisterial directives. Hence, in doubt recourse should be had to the bishop of the diocese, who alone has authority to give a final interpretation to the *Directives*. Of course, the bishops too must conform to the teaching of the Holy See. Their responsibilities are not easy. As the Apostle Paul wrote to Timothy (2 Tm, 4:2):

> Proclaim the word; be persistent whether it is convenient or inconvenient; convince, reprimand, encourage through all patience and teaching. For the time will come when people will not tolerate sound doctrine but, following their own desires and insatiable curiosity, will accumulate teachers and will stop listening to the truth and will be diverted to myths.

Principle of Free and Informed Consent

The *principle of free and informed consent* plays a primary role in bioethical discussions today. It can be formulated as follows:

> To protect the basic need of every human person for health care and the primary responsibility of each person for his or her own health care, no physical or psychological therapy may be administered without the free and informed consent of the patient or, if the patient is incompetent, of a legitimate guardian acting for the patient's benefit and, as far as possible, in accord with her or his known and reasonable wishes.

This principle is really a corollary of the principle of well-formed conscience. If, as a physician or nurse, I must act according to my own informed conscience, it is unethical for me to ask *other* persons to cooperate with me or to permit me to act on them unless I share with them the relevant information required for both of us to decide, each according to his or her own conscience, whether such an act is ethical. Thus I cannot ask for the consent of others unless

I have helped them to have an informed conscience and unless I believe them to be free to act on it. If, however, the person is incompetent, I must decide for this person if I am his or her legitimate guardian or, if I am not, I must obtain the free and informed consent of that guardian before I attempt therapy. The theological basis for this principle, therefore, is the same as for the principle of well-formed conscience.

The principle of free and informed consent is not always easy to apply in cases involving young, senile, or incompetent persons, persons emotionally disturbed, or of a different culture or language, or in emergency situations (Morreim, 1993; Edwards, 1993). What is required is that a serious effort be made to enable the patient to understand what he or she is being asked to consent to and to make a deliberate and free judgment (cf. Chapter 3).

Principle of Moral Discrimination

Granted that we have the responsibility to inform our conscience before acting and to enable others who depend on us for information to do so, how do we go about applying the moral norms we have learned to the facts as we have established them in a particular case? This is the problem of discrimination of what is right from what is wrong in a particular case. The ability to do this well is what we call the virtue of *prudence*.

Moral persons thoughtfully and freely choose what to do or not to do in view of the life goal to which they are committed and its subordinate goals. These goals and their hierarchy are determined by basic human needs. Most people have a rather vague understanding of what the central purpose in their lives may be, and they often act impulsively and inconsistently, obscuring the direction and unity of their lives. Jesus spoke of people as "wandering sheep" (Mk 6:34; Lk 15:4–7) whose lives seem without purpose or plan.

Yet, actually in every person's life, a commitment to some goal that has priority over all others is evident, shaping every important decision. Thus it is often said of a nurse or physician, "She is someone who really cares about people, and it shows in everything she does, in both private and professional life," or "He may be an expert professional, but he is a selfish person who is always acting for personal advancement or money." This fundamental commitment is the foundation of all morality. Jesus said, "Seek first the Kingdom of God" (Mt 6:33). Morality is thus first a matter of fundamental commitment or *intention of the ultimate end*, that is, the general intention that gives unity and pattern to one's whole life.

In classical ethics this supreme goal of human life was called "the ultimate end." Commitment to this goal involves the whole person and may be made implicitly in action rather than by some explicit verbalized decision. Consequently, some authors today, in order to avoid the implication that it is always explicit and coldly rational, prefer to term it the "fundamental option" (Poddimatam, 1986; cf. McInerny, 1987). Unfortunately, this new terminology has given rise to the erroneous opinion of some that it is possible to remain committed to God and neighbor by a subconscious fundamental option while at a conscious level committing objectively serious sins. This theory is supposed to explain why some Christians who seem sincerely committed to God neverthe-less habitually commit what were traditionally called mortal sins, e.g., drunk-enness or masturbation. But classical theology quite adequately accounted for this phenomenon by distinguishing between the *objective* sinfulness of an act and the *subjective* guilt of the agent. Persons struggling to overcome addictive sins of weakness, while remaining committed to God, may repeatedly fall into objectively wrong acts which are not mortally culpable because of lack of free-dom and full deliberation (John Paul II, *Evangelium Vitae,* 1995, n. 18). Hence, John Paul II, in *Veritatis Splendor* (1993) insists that our life commitment, whether it be called our "ultimate end" or our "fundamental option," must be a free and conscious human act which can be changed only by a free and conscious human act.

Some current authors do not clearly explain the difference between what the Catholic tradition has always called "mortal" and "venial" sin. This differ-ence is not just one of degree but of our *relationship* to God and neighbor. When we perform an act which we know is objectively harmful yet not seriously so, or when subjectively we act without full freedom, deliberation, and consent, our action weakens but does not destroy our relation of commitment to God, to neighbor, and to the integral fulfillment of our own human nature. But when we knowingly, freely, and with full consent perform an action that seriously harms our neighbor, ourself, or our relation to God, that is a *mortal* sin which turns us aside from our true goals in life. We then no longer share in the divine life that God gave us in baptism.

It is also a serious mistake to think, as some have done, that we can commit a mortal sin only by sinning seriously against faith, hope, or love of God, because "If anyone says: 'My love is fixed on God,' and hates his brother, he is a liar" (1 Jn 4:20). In biblical language, to "hate" someone is to be willing to do them serious harm. Just as a divorce is usually the result of a long series of lesser quarrels, we ordinarily fall into mortal sin only as the conclusion of a long series of more and more harmful and deliberate sins which have prepared its way. Thus health care professionals who think themselves to be good Catholics or respectable citizens, but who knowingly and deliberately seriously neglect or misuse professional skill or status so that others are harmed or the professional's own development as a person is seriously impaired, commit mortal sins that must be forgiven in the sacrament of reconciliation and, insofar as possible, repaired.

The Determinants of Morality

The relation between an action and its goal, however, is not simple; it is condi-tioned in several ways, as we saw in the discussion of proportionalism and prudential personalism in Chapter 7, but will now illustrate in more detail with regard to bioethical decisions.

First, goals cannot be reached simply by a general intention but only by taking definite steps. As the saying goes, "If you will the end, you must also will the means." It is not enough to intend to love God. As the epistle of St. James says:

> If a brother or sister has nothing to wear and has no food for the day, and one of you says to them, "Go in peace, keep warm, and eat well," but you do not give them the necessities of the body, what good is it? So also faith of itself, if it does not have works, is dead (Jas 2:14–17).

Thus each particular act specifies one's remote and general intention to act for one's ultimate goal by a proximate and specific intention called the act's *moral object* or the *purpose* of that human action. Note that this proximate intention is not different from the general intention, but rather a further, concrete determination of it: I love God by bandaging this patient's wound.

Second, a moral object has both a form and a content. The moral form of the act of bandaging wounds is the intention to help patients regain health through a particular healing procedure; the content of the act, however, is the therapeutic procedure itself, considered as a process of cleansing, medicating, bandaging, and so forth that has an intrinsic teleology, that is, predetermined results. At this point, medical facts and moral values come together to form a single act, which is at the same time a physical, biological, and psychological process and also a moral act invested with human meaning. It is a medical act, but it is also a moral act expressed by the term *care*, which implies not merely technical skill, but also human personal concern for the patient.

How can facts and values meet in this way? It is because the act of health care, taken in its biological and psychological aspects, already has values, or actions that are harmful or beneficial to the human organism. Bandaging is helpful to the human organism because it furthers the natural processes within the organism itself toward health and optimal functioning. There may also be negative values, since the bandage may impede circulation, etc. But if the bandaging is *essentially* helpful to nature, a professional faced with the decision of whether to bandage or not to bandage can ethically decide to do so. When this decision is made in view of the patient's good and the professional's commitment to caring for the patient, then this merely biological and technical act, simple as it is, becomes a moral act with a moral object. Thus, in any moral object, one can distinguish the content of the act and the specific moral purpose that makes the physical act into a moral act (Pellegrino and Thomasma, 1988).

Third, specific moral acts are always performed in a context or situation; for example, the act of bandaging is frequently performed by a nurse in a hospital or clinic during daytime hours. As long as the situation is an ordinary or normal one, the moral character of an action is not modified. Sometimes, however, unusual features of the situation may be morally significant; for example, if the nurse bandages the wound of a fugitive criminal without reporting him, she may find herself an accomplice to his crime.

Thus, in determining the morality of an action, once the specific moral object is known, any special circumstances that might modify the action's moral significance must also be determined. These circumstances can be of place, time, or person (as in the example just cited). They can also be a matter of *intention* when, in addition to the specific intention of the act, the agent has some additional and special motive. For example, the nurse may bandage the patient not only to help the patient, but also to teach an aide how to perform the procedure. Such an intention is a *circumstantial* intention. Note that the term *intention* has now been used in three different senses: (1) the general intention of a person's life goal (fundamental option); (2) a person's specific intention manifested in this particular moral act as a means to that goal; and (3) possible additional motives extrinsic to the action performed. When engaging in ethical discussions, it is essential to specify in which sense the term "intention" is being used.

The special circumstance of an action that is of itself morally wrong can make it worse; for example, it is usually more irresponsible for a nurse to neglect a child patient than to neglect an adult. If the action is good, circumstances can make it better; for example, a nurse deserves more credit for attention to a difficult patient. But can circumstances make a bad act good? As we saw in the last chapter in evaluating the proportionalist methodology, Catholic moral theology has traditionally held that if a moral object in its own specific intention is morally wrong (intrinsically evil), it cannot then be made morally good by any special circumstance or circumstantial intention (John Paul II, 1993). For example, killing a suffering patient, because the act kills an innocent person, can never be morally justified, no matter what the special circumstances of the patient (age, member of one's family, degree of suffering, etc.) or the good intention of the agent (e.g., intention to end the patient's pain).

Thus for prudential personalism the *principle of moral discernment*, which takes the place of principle of maximum utility in utilitarianism or the principle of proportionate reason in consequentialism, can be formulated as follows:

To make a conscientious ethical decision, one must do the following:

1. Proceed on the basis of a fundamental commitment to God and to human persons (including oneself) according to their God-given and graced human nature.
2. Among possible actions that might seem to be means of fulfilling that commitment, exclude any that are contradictory to it (i.e., intrinsically evil).
3. Also consider how one's own motives and other circumstances may contribute to or nullify the effectiveness of these other possible actions as means to fulfill one's fundamental commitment.
4. Among the possible means not excluded or nullified, select one by which one is most likely to fulfill that commitment, and act on it.

The specifically Christian understanding of this principle derives from Jesus' teaching that the goal of human life is to share in the life of the Father, Son, and Holy Spirit (Mt 11:25–30; Lk 10:22; 1 Jn 1:3). Every moral choice must be guided by a longing to reach this goal, which absolutely excludes mortal sin, that is, acts against God or neighbor that would turn a person away from that goal. All intelligent freedom must be used with the virtue of prudence enlightened by faith to facilitate this journey to God for ourselves and others. In this pursuit, we must use our own creativity to the fullest, but we must also respect the creative wisdom of God, which has made us what we are and which guides us providentially in the concrete circumstances of our lives.

Principle of Double Effect

As already noted, a good moral act may involve not only values, but also disvalues. Persons are often puzzled by the undesirable side effects of actions they feel morally obliged to perform. To some it seems that we should never perform any action for which we foresee harmful results, but should insist on performing only those actions that have only good consequences. Otherwise, we would seem to be responsible for the harm and to have done evil as a means to a good end. This position of *moral purism* or *rigorism,* however, makes action almost impossible in a world where even the best actions may have some harmful results. Since refusal to act is itself often a neglect of duty, this kind of purism actually leads to sins of omission or withdrawal from one's responsibilities. Recently the economic pressure on Catholic health care facilities and other facilities having different moral standards to cooperate in joint ventures has provided many unavoidable dilemmas of this sort.

Eventually moralists, relying on the formulation of the principle of moral discrimination already explained, also formulated the *principle of double effect* as a more precise way of applying the former principle to conflict cases (Mangan, 1949; Gillon, 1986a; Connery, 1981). It is usually stated in such terms as follow (Finnis, 1991):

To form a good conscience when an act is foreseen to have both beneficial and harmful consequences, the following conditions should be met:

1. The *directly* intended object of the act must not be intrinsically contradictory to one's fundamental commitment to God and neighbor (including oneself), i.e., it must be a good action judged from its moral object.
2. The intention of the agent must be to achieve the beneficial effects and to avoid the foreseen harmful effects as far as possible (i.e., must only *indirectly* intend the harm).
3. The foreseen beneficial effects must not be achieved by means of the foreseen harmful effects and be not achievable without them.
4. The foreseen beneficial effects must be equal to or greater than the foreseen harmful effects.
5. The beneficial effects must follow from the action at least as immediately as do the harmful effects.

Note with regard to the fourth condition that unless it be met, it would be difficult to conclude that truly one directly intends only the good effect. This condition is sometimes expressed by saying that the good must outweigh the evil effect, but if this statement is considered apart from the other conditions, it can lead to the proportionalist error of thinking that a greater good can excuse doing something intrinsically evil.

Applying the Principle of Double Effect

The first of these conditions follows directly from the principle of moral discrimination as formulated by prudential personalism, but is rejected by consequentialists, situationists, utilitarians, and proportionalists. Proportionalists contend that the third condition, which is their principle of proportionate reason, is the preeminent one. For prudential personalism, however, the first condition is essential and the second condition is also needed to avoid moral purism. Connery (1981) points out that the purpose of both the third and fourth conditions is to guarantee the first two, since unless one refuses to perform an action foreseen as doing more harm than good (third condition) or judged to be the use of an immoral means to a moral end (fourth condition), one cannot honestly claim to be only indirectly intending the harmful side effects. Moreover, Connery shows that the third condition does not require that difficult and perhaps impossible detailed weighing of values and disvalues demanded by proportionalism, but only the assurance that we are not obviously doing more harm than is justified by the good we directly intend.

For example, when physicians decide to remove a cancerous but gravid uterus, they must directly intend to save the mother's life and may only indirectly intend to abort the child. Physicians are not required to weigh the value of one life against another in terms of every possible consequence, but only to decide if they are directly intending a good that is comparable to the harm they know will also result. Unless this rough proportion exists, physicians cannot honestly say that they only indirectly intend the harm to the child; and if they do intend harm directly, they are violating both the first and the second conditions.

The purpose of the fourth condition is to exclude the use of an evil means to achieve a good end, since such action would also violate the first requirement. This final condition is not always easy to verify. Because of these difficulties, there have been several recent attempts to reformulate it. The suggestion that seems the most persuasive is made by Grisez (1970b), who points out:

> . . . The ambiguity of ambiguous actions can be of two kinds. In one type the destructive aspect of the action is the means by which the positive aspect is realized. In the second the two aspects are really inseparably linked in one action; the positive aspect does not produce the destructive, nor does the destructive produce the positive; the act embraces both results directly (p. 140).

Grisez cites as an example of the first condition the Renaissance practice of castrating boy sopranos for the purpose of producing beautiful music. In this case the act of mutilation is one act (a means) intended for the sake of another distinct act (making beautiful music). This is doing evil for a good purpose, because the intention of the first act is to mutilate (an evil), although the intention of the second act is to make music (a good). On the other hand, the second type of ambiguous action is illustrated by castration of a boy to prevent the spread of cancer. In this case only one indivisible act is intended, namely, an act of healing (good) which, however, contains two effects (one good, one bad) inseparably connected. The essential ethical difference between the two cases is that in the second the *evil* need not be intended but only permitted (indirectly intended), whereas in the first case the agent *must* directly intend the evil (otherwise the act would never be performed), although the agent intends it only as a means and not an end.

Sometimes people try to justify actions as "the lesser evil," but it is contradictory to claim it can ever be ethical to do what is evil or unethical in itself, even under duress. In some situations, however, persons find themselves with a "perplexed conscience"; that is, it seems to them that all their options, even the option of doing nothing at all, are unethical—In such a situation they must do what seems to be the least evil, not indeed because it is evil, but because it seems to be a good option. In practice, however, given the needed time to think the matter through and to achieve a well-formed conscience, the principle of double effect may permit an objectively good solution to moral dilemmas by providing an option which is not "the lesser evil" but which is simply good.

We should note also that one may never approve another's doing the lesser evil, since that would be formal cooperation in evil. This is why physicians cannot escape responsibility for abortion or other unethical medical procedure by refusing to perform it themselves but refer patients to other physicians they know will do it. Yet sometimes a counselor who has tried unsuccessfully to prevent another from doing a very serious wrong, may point out that the stubborn sinner still has the obligation to do a lesser rather than a greater wrong. Thus a physician who has failed to persuade a young patient from reckless sexual activity may point out that in his evil activities he still has the obligation to take precautions not to infect others or be infected with AIDS.

Principle of Legitimate Cooperation

From what has been said, it follows that people must be careful not to cooperate in or promote the evil actions of others. However, it sometimes happens that a person may perform an action which is morally good, which will be used by another person to further his evil purpose. What is the moral responsibility of a person performing the good action? Must he or she avoid all cooperation with the person doing evil? Traditional moralists considering this problem offer distinctions which help answer this question (Merklebach, 1949; Prummer, 1958).

First of all they distinguish between formal and material cooperation. Formal cooperation occurs when one assents to the evil intention of the person mainly responsible for performing the evil action. Formal cooperation may occur if one advises, encourages, or counsels the person principally responsible for the evil action, even though one does not take part physically in the action. Of course, if one is in agreement with an evil action and also contributes physically to the action then it is clearly a case of formal cooperation. On the other hand, one may be opposed to the evil action being performed insofar as the intention to do evil is concerned. This would occur if the person who merely cooperates in the evil action does so due to another motive. If one becomes involved in an evil action without having the same intention of the evil doer, then one cooperates not formally, but materially.

In order to understand material cooperation as considered in the more traditional manner, another distinction is needed. The manner in which one is involved in the evil action becomes significant. Does the cooperator participate in the evil act by doing something necessary for the actual performance of the evil act, or does the act of the cooperator precede or follow the evil act (see example below). If one's action contributes to the active performance of to the evil action so much so that the evil action could not be performed without the help of the cooperator, then this is known as immediate material cooperation. This method of cooperation involves the cooperator acting in conjunction with the person primarily responsible for the evil action. If the act in question is intrinsically evil, then immediate material cooperation is always prohibited. If one's cooperation is not needed to perform the evil action, but only assists in the performance of the action, then this is known as mediate material cooperation. This type of material cooperation may be justified if there is a serious reason for it because the action on the part of the cooperator is fundamentally good. A serious reason is required to justify mediate material cooperation because one should avoid cooperation in evil if at all possible. Clearly, allowing mediate material cooperation in the evil act of another is an application of the principle of double effect, though this has recently been denied (Keenan and Kaveney, 1995).

Some theologians use a different nomenclature than that indicated above (Aertnys-Damen, 1947). They identity immediate material cooperation with implicit formal cooperation. Thus, Bernard Häring (1963) distinguishes two kinds of cooperation, formal and material. But instead of describing two different forms of material cooperation, he describes two kinds of formal cooperation. Implicit formal cooperation indicates that a person who cooperates intimately in performing an evil act *should know* the evil he is helping to perform. We do not concur with this nomenclature because it involves an interpretation of another person's subjective state of mind. While we do not concur with the use of this distinction, we recognize it as legitimate. However, we would prefer to keep the analysis in the objective order. For this reason we will continue to use the distinction of immediate and mediate material cooperation, but caution that when applying this principle of cooperation to practical cases, it is important not to confuse the two methods of nomenclature.

An example may clarify the difference between formal and material cooperation and the two kinds of material cooperation. If a person is associated with an abortion clinic, and approves or encourages the practice of abortion, this person cooperates formally in the evil action, whether or not he is physically involved in the abortion procedure. If one does not approve of the procedure, having another intention besides abortion, for example, simply to make a living or to keep one's job, then the degree of involvement in the evil act must be discerned. If one is a nurse physically involved in the abortion process, for example using a suction pump to remove the fetus from the mother's womb, then one is involved in immediate material cooperation even though he may declare vigorously that he is not in favor of abortion but is "only protecting his job." (Häring and others would call this formal cooperation of an implicit nature). On the other hand, the nurse who cares for a woman after an abortion is not intrinsically involved in the evil act of abortion and cooperates in a mediate material manner. She may continue her work in the abortion clinic if there is a justifying reason; for example, if she cannot find other employment as a nurse. In a case of mediate material cooperation one must also consider the element of scandal because it is sinful to lead a third party to sin or think less of the teaching of the Church, even though one may not be committing a sin by reason of one's personal action.

The specifically Christian understanding of this principle of cooperation in evil arises from the Bible's teaching of the origin of evil in the world, which differs greatly from the Buddhist idea that evil is an illusion, or the secular humanist idea that evil is an inevitable part of evolutionary progress (Bowker, 1970). Christians believe that they, as the community of the human race and in some measure as individuals, have rebelled against God's wise and loving will for them and chosen to "know good and evil" (Gn 3:4), that is, to live in an ambiguous world where good and evil are mixed confusedly. To find a straight path through such a world is impossible without the guidance of Christ and the Holy Spirit he has sent. This also requires, however, that people use their intelligence to the fullest in order to separate what is essentially good and accidentally evil from what is essentially evil and accidentally good. Jesus says to his disciples, "Behold, I am sending you like sheep in the midst of wolves, so be shrewd as serpents and simple as doves" (Mt 10:16) and rebuked the witless imprudence of some of his followers (Lk 16:8).

In cases where the cooperation is only mediate, one must still consider whether the cooperation is *proximate* or *remote*. To avoid a common confusion, note that immediate material cooperation is distinguished from mediate material cooperation which in turn is distinguished into proximate and remote. "Proximate versus remote" refers to how closely mediate (i.e.; noninstrumental) cooperation is connected with the evil in some way but not as an instrument of its performance. Thus if we compare the cooperation of a nurse who prepares the operating room in an abortion clinic with that of the janitor who cleans the building, both cooperate only *mediately* because they are not instruments of the physician in his act of performing the abortion, but the nurse's action is more proximate and the janitor's more remote from the evil act of abortion.

Mediate Material Cooperation

Using the distinctions indicated above, we offer the following observations. Mediate material cooperation is ethical if the following conditions are met (McFadden, 1967).

1. The more remotely related the material and mediate cooperative act is to the evil act, the easier it is to justify. For example, the manufacture of morphine is remotely related to drug abuse because morphine also has important and legitimate medical uses. Yet the sale of morphine is closer to actual abuse than is its manufacture and must be carefully regulated to ensure that it is purchased only on prescription for legitimate uses.

2. The good achieved by the material and mediate cooperation must outweigh the degree of evil and also the contribution of the cooperator to that evil. This requirement follows from the fact that the principle of legitimate cooperation is an application of the principle of double effect. Thus persons whose livelihoods depend on a job (because it is impossible or difficult to get another similar job) may be justified in working for certain institutions where some abortions are performed, provided they do not immediately cooperate with an abortion or approve or encourage it. In such institutions there are many different degrees of cooperative proximity, ranging from the nurse who helps prepare a patient for the abortion procedure, to the nurse who cares for a patient after surgery whose involvement is more remote, to the janitor of the building whose cooperation is very remote. Nevertheless, all have the moral responsibility of deciding whether sufficient reason exists to justify their material cooperation with an institution that kills innocent persons, just as the same responsibility rests on participants in a war effort in which obliteration bombing of noncombatants is regularly employed.

3. The evil effects of scandal, that is, the bad example that can be set even by mediate material cooperation, must be weighed. The appearance of cooperation with evil can help this evil to continue. The Christian has a serious duty to take a stand against destructive actions and to share in them as little as possible. Thus Christians should take as active a part as is practicable in protesting against injustices at institutions in which they work or from which they benefit. Catholic hospitals in particular have the duty to consider the example they set in a community by even appearing to condone injustices.

If persons refused even mediate and remote material cooperation in the affairs of a community, they would also sin by *omission*, since doing good also would become impossible. A Christian purist would be unable to act as a citizen or to share in any institution because every government, human institution, and even organized religion commits some evil and unjust acts. By belonging to such an organization, a person cooperates to a degree with such evils. Nevertheless, all of us have a moral obligation to belong to social institutions, ambiguous as they may be, since only through them can legitimate human needs be served.

It has been argued (Curran, 1975) that since Vatican II approved ecumenical worship on the grounds that we should respect the consciences of others even when they seem to us not wholly sound, it seems to follow *a fortiori* that we may cooperate with persons whose consciences differ from ours in matters less grave than the worship of God, such as many of those treated in medical ethics. We would agree with Curran's observation but emphasize that it still does not justify immediate material cooperation in intrinsically wrong acts (e.g., abortion, contraceptive sterilization, and artificial reproduction), especially when they involve the rights of a third party (e.g., abortion). Neither can such cooperation be permitted in religious matters that involve intrinsically wrong acts (John Paul II, 1993) (e.g., ritual murder, idolatry, satanism, and religious polygamy), but only in essentially good acts (e.g., sincere acts of prayer, even if theologically flawed).

As mentioned in Chapter 6, changes in the United States health care system are rapidly forcing Catholic health care facilities into "joint ventures" with institutions which have other ethical standards, especially as regards care of the poor, abortion, contraception and contraceptive sterilization, and artificial reproduction. Moreover, insurance systems, managed health care systems, and federal regulations and funding threaten legal pressure and economic disaster for Catholic institutions unless they compromise Catholic ethical standards.

From what has already been said it should be clear that such pressures ("duress" is the technical term usually used) can never justify formal cooperation, but the question is often asked, "Can duress ever justify immediate material cooperation?" In some of the "manuals of moral theology" immediate cooperation under duress is allowed, but only in cases involving property, not in actions which are intrinsically evil in the objective order. Thus one whose life is threatened could take the property of another without permission because it is thought that the owner of the property would be unreasonable to expect another person to surrender life rather than take the property without permission.

Some moralists have argued for exceptions to the norm against immediate material cooperation in actions which are intrinsically evil when duress exists (National Coalition, 1995; Contra Smith, 1996). For example, could not a Catholic hospital perform contraceptive sterilizations if it feared that it would lose all ob-gyn services because a group of physicians threatens to resign from the staff unless the Catholic hospital performs sterilizations? It is predicted that such a move would endanger the future of the Catholic hospital.

In regard to cooperation, the 1994 revision of the *Ethical and Religious Directives for Catholic Health Services* adds an Appendix, "The Principles Governing Cooperation," which contains the following:

> Material cooperation is immediate when the object of the cooperator is the same as the object of the wrongdoer. Immediate material cooperation is wrong, *except in some instances of duress. The matter of duress distinguishes immediate material cooperation from implicit formal cooperation. But immediate material cooperation without duress is equivalent to implicit formal cooperation and, therefore, is morally wrong.*

The words we have italicized can be seriously misleading if it is understood to say that duress can sometimes justify immediate material cooperation in actions which are intrinsically evil (John Paul II, 1993). In the case of the Catholic hospital just cited, duress threatened by the doctors would not justify the performance of sterilizations. One may never do evil to achieve good.

Therefore, if the arrangement for a joint venture in effect makes Catholics employers of the medical staff which is required or permitted to perform the immoral procedures, or if they profit economically in a significant way from the performance, then even if they disapprove verbally and do have a "good reason" prohibited to allow those surgeries to take place, this remains unethical immediate cooperation (or implicit formal cooperation), because employers are responsible for the actions of their employees and owners for any business from which they profit, since these employees act as their instrumental agents. While it is possible that a large institution might tolerate occasional lesser infractions of moral standards by physicians on the grounds that it is impossible to have total control over its staff, it would be obliged to attempt to enforce its moral standards to the degree feasible. Hence it could not enter into a contractual situation in which such enforcement would become simply impossible.

Short of such formal cooperation, what of arrangements in which the Catholic facility is committed only to management of a joint institution of which some facilities would be obliged to abide by Catholic ethical standards while others would not? It would seem that this in some cases might be permissible if management provided facilities and personnel for care which were in the main licit but did not have to take any direct responsibility for or give approval to the illicit procedures, nor profit significantly from them. This would seem to render the cooperation material, and the duress (i.e., the evil of suffering legal or economic sanctions for not complying) would make evident that this cooperation was mediate, not formal or immediate material, and would also lessen the probability of scandal. However, abortion would not be allowed because of gravity of evil (ERD D. 45).

Arrangements even under duress, however, could not be justified in which the Catholic administration would become subject to control by persons not committed to Catholic moral standards in such a way that the Catholic facility or staff would become agents of the noncommitted persons in performing evil acts, even if this instrumental participation in the evil acts was only material, since this would be immediate material cooperation. "All decisions which may lead to serious consequences for the identity or reputation of Catholic health care services or entail a high risk of scandal, should be made in consultation with the diocesan bishop or his health care liaison" (NCCB, 1994, n. 67).

Thus the *principle of legitimate cooperation* is an application of the principle of double effect to the situation where an act is performed by more than one person with different purposes. It can be formulated as follows:

> To achieve a well-formed conscience, one should always judge it unethical to cooperate formally with an immoral act (i.e., directly to intend the evil act itself), or even to cooperate materially (i.e., to provide means necessary to the act) if this cooperation is immediate (i.e., if one acts as an instrumen-

tal agent of the principal agent of the evil act). One may sometimes, however, judge it to be morally permissible or even obligatory to cooperate materially and mediately (i.e., before or after the evil act, but not as an instrumental agent of the principal agent of the evil act), depending on the degree of the good to be achieved or evil avoided by the cooperation.

Principle of Professional Communication

Truth cannot be arrived at simply by individual effort. No single person has all the information needed for good decisions, nor can one arrive at truth except by a social effort. Every human institution, particularly every modern healthcare institution, is an enormously complex system of *information*. The moment a patient enters a healthcare facility, a process of history taking, testing, chart keeping, record filing, etc. begins. Also an endless amount of research contained in the medical library and in the brains of a network of technologists and specialists begins to be applied to the process of diagnosis and prescription for the patient's treatment. Moreover, because the institution is an administrative network of cooperating personnel, problems of interpersonal relations arise among the staff and the patients themselves.

This whole network essentially depends on good *communication*, which is impossible without (1) trust, (2) contact among the people who have information, (3) clear articulation and expression of information, and (4) continuous feedback by which failures in communication can be corrected. Modern communication theory has shown that this work of communication depends first on good emotional relations among the communicators, since emotional conflict is a powerful barrier to exchange of information and brings into play all sorts of uncontrollable, unconscious factors. It thus becomes a serious moral duty in every institution to promote an emotional openness among both the staff and the patients.

The *principle of professional communication* can be formulated as follows:

To fulfill their obligations to serve patients, health care professionals have the responsibility:

1. To strive to establish and preserve trust at both the emotional and rational levels;
2. To share the information they possess that is legitimately needed by others in order to have an informed conscience;
3. To refrain from lying or giving misinformation; and
4. To keep secret information that is not legitimately needed by others, but that if revealed might harm either the patient or others or destroy trust.

Note that this principle is also founded in the basic human need for truth. If human beings cannot trust one another for the information they must use to guide their lives, this need cannot be satisfied. Since the principle of well-formed conscience requires that persons obtain from others, especially from expert professionals, whatever needed knowledge cannot be achieved by themselves, persons have a right to true and relevant professional advice.

The Christian specification of this principle arises from the Christian understanding of trust and forgiveness. Jesus, in the case of Nicodemus (Jn 3:1–21), the Samaritan woman (Jn 4:1–42), the adulterous woman (Jn 8:1–11), and elsewhere, is represented as dealing with individuals in a way that won their trust and their confidence in his full acceptance of them even in their sinfulness. The Church, in its sacrament of reconciliation, has established the confessional seal of total confidentiality so that people might feel free to unburden themselves not merely of physical and psychological problems but of their real guilt. For the Christian, therefore, professional confidentiality is not only professional; it expresses respect for the dignity of the human person, whom only God has a right to judge (Mt 7:1–5).

This trust is protected also by the obligation to speak the truth. Lying is contrary to the Eighth Commandment, "You shall not bear false witness against your neighbor" (Ex 20:16). Hence lying is intrinsically evil and in no circumstances or for any purpose can be morally good. It is important, therefore, to define "lying" correctly as *asserting as true what one knows not to be true.* We are not, however, required to give others information to which they have no right, and we may be obliged by confidentiality not to do so.

8.3 NORMS OF CHRISTIAN HOPE

The word "Gospel" means "Good News" (Anglo-Saxon for the Greek *evangelion,* "good tidings") and hence the word of faith is also a word of hope. The revelation that God has invited us to share his eternal life in the community of Father, Son, and Holy Spirit, which we hear in faith, inspires us to respond in hope to journey toward that distant goal. Without such hope there would be no use dreaming of such perfect happiness. The virtue of Christian hope manifests what theologians call the *eschatological (eschaton* is Greek for "last things") aspect of the Gospel as it hopes for the final coming of Jesus Christ in the fully realized Kingdom of God. The human person and the human community are not structures of static relations but are dynamic—living, growing, developing, and evolving. This is why we have opted for a teleological, goal-directed, means–ends ethics.

Furthermore, human goals are not always clearly envisioned in advance. As persons progress toward goals, these goals themselves take on a new look. They open out ahead of us as does the horizon of a landscape. John Dewey (1920) made an important contribution to ethics by stressing this dynamic character of human goals, which is vividly experienced in American culture. Sometimes Christian thinkers have not taken this dynamism of life fully into account in their ethical discussions, yet Jesus centered his teaching on the theme of the approach of the Kingdom of God (Mk 1:15), a goal so mysterious that Jesus often expressed it in parables (Mt 13:1–53).

Recently, Christian theologians such as Jürgen Moltmann, Johannes Metz, and Wolfhart Pannenburg (Capps, 1970) have constructed "theologies of hope" to bring out the many ways in which the Gospel is not merely a message about the superiority of heaven to earth, but a call to transform the earth as we journey heavenward. In this way they are finding areas of agreement with humanism and socialism, which also emphasize that to be human is to work for the future. Christian faith sees in every earthly event (even if that event is a crucifixion) a promise, an opportunity to be used, an invitation by a God of the future to share in building the future. In health care this sense of hope is the source of all healing, so that to be a health care professional is constantly to affirm the possibility of turning suffering into a victory over disease and death.

Four ethical norms relate in a special way to Christian hope. First, as intelligent and free beings we seek to achieve control over our world through science and technology. We can do so constructively only if we cultivate the gifts of nature, including our own bodies, with a profound respect for nature and ecology. To do this we are guided by the *principle of stewardship and creativity.* Second, one of the greatest obstacles to this right use of our own bodies is our all-too-common enslavement by compulsive pleasures or destructive fears and inhibitions. These often deprive us of a rational use of our own freedom. Consequently, we need a *principle of inner freedom* which demands that we avoid such snares so we can move forward toward our life's real goals, a principle that has social implications in regard to drug addiction and other addictive behaviors. Third, some of the most dangerous pitfalls on this path of happiness result from the misuse of human sexuality, which through its creation of the basic social unit, the family, is also the source of great hope for the future. Hence the need for a *principle of family-oriented sexuality.* Finally, what if the dangers in life we fear are unavoidable and we actually find ourselves immersed in suffering? It is then that our hope enables us not only to endure the sufferings of life courageously, but to grow stronger as persons through this experience, as shown by the *principle of growth through suffering.*

Principle of Stewardship and Creativity

The hope that leads human beings to endure the inevitable pain of human existence and to overcome the sentence to death by the perpetuation of the human community also leads us to struggle with the environment. The author of Genesis 3 profoundly symbolizes the evil of death by the expulsion from the Garden of Paradise, the burden of sexism by the curse on Eve, and the burden of struggle with the environment by the curse on Adam. These are the fundamental realities of the human situation, but Scripture says they are not what God wanted for humanity. He has given persons the power of intelligence, restored by grace in Christ, the new Adam (I Cor 15:22), by which they deal with these problems. Although persons may meet these evils well or poorly, they cannot escape the struggle and still remain human (Gn 3:16–19).

The concepts of "stewardship" and "creativity" are basic to the ethics of the use of technology to satisfy human needs that would protect the rights of future generations to the earth God gave us. Thus we are ready here to formulate the *principle of stewardship and creativity*, which has become so important today as a guide to the use of modern medical technology:

> The gifts of multidimensional human nature and its natural environment should be used with profound respect for their intrinsic teleology. The gift of human creativity especially should be used to cultivate nature and environment with a care set by the limits of our actual knowledge and the risks of destroying these gifts.

This principle requires us to appreciate the two great gifts that a wise and loving God has given: the earth, with all its natural resources, and our own human nature (embodied intelligent freedom), with its biological, psychological, ethical, and spiritual capacities. Recently, we have come to recognize that our earthly environment is a marvelously balanced ecological system without which human life could never have evolved. Although we certainly have a need and a right to cultivate and perfect our earthly home, to till and irrigate its soil, to build cities, and to use its raw materials for the wonderful devices of modern technology, we should not do this ruthlessly. We must take the utmost care to conserve our ecological system unpolluted and unravished and to recycle its raw materials and its energy supplies. We have already discovered how much damage thoughtless exploitation of natural resources can do to our own lives.

Similarly, our own human nature, our bodies, and our minds are wonderfully constructed. We have the need and right to improve our bodies and to develop medical technologies that prevent and remedy the defects to which they are liable. We must do so, however, with the greatest respect for what we already are as human beings. Our bodily and mental functions have natural teleologies that cannot be eliminated or misdirected without injury to our humanness.

Consequently, a technology based on the false principle, "If it can be done, it should be done," is a misuse of our creative intelligence. Rather, we should ask ourselves, "Should it be done?" and only if the answer is "Yes" develop and use the technology to do it. Thus the God-given gifts of our environment and our humanity are ours in stewardship, but because the greatest of our gifts are intelligence and freedom, the stewardship should be creative. Our creativity should be used as cocreativity with the Creator, not as reckless wasting of his gifts. One very important aspect of ecology is the problem of the "population explosion" related to the Church's stand on the ethical means for responsible parenthood, which will be discussed in Chapter 10.

The specifically Christian character of this principle derives from the risen Christ who is the historic pledge that the Kingdom of God will eventually be fully realized. The coming of his Holy Spirit gives persons the power to share in this construction of the Kingdom, the house built not on the sand of pride but on the rock of faith (Mt 7:24–29). The Gospel does not, as Marxists and humanists have accused it of doing, encourage Christians simply to wait until the Lord returns, indifferent to the world's fate. Christians are called to become involved in God's redemptive action in the world and to play a historical role in the liberation of the human race from poverty, disease, and oppression with the assistance of God's power (Vatican Council II, *Gaudium et Spes*, 1965c). The health care profession is a fundamental part of this mission to heal the world of the effects of sin.

The Principle of Inner Freedom

Health care professionals often confront *addictive* and *compulsive* behavior in their patients—workaholism, eating disorders, hypochondria, etc.—which is far more extensive than chemical dependency. To tell a patient with a habit of smoking that it is bad for health and for the patient to agree about the need to break the habit often has little or no effect on subsequent behavior. The reverse of such addiction to pleasure is *obsessive–compulsion* due to excessive fears or anxieties. When severe, these conditions require psychotherapy, and we will say more about them in Chapter 12. But self-control with regard to pleasure and pain is an element in most human behavior and needs to be formulated in a special ethical principle since it is of great importance for healthy living.

Normally, pleasure, comfort, and peace are the *consequences* and the *signs* of the achievement of authentic human goals and the fulfillment of true human needs, and as such are good and desirable. They are *secondary* signs, however, not the proof or measure of real human well-being. Hence hedonistic ethics is unrealistic. Yet in a consumerist society, health care professionals are sometimes drawn into pandering to patients' bad habits. Moreover, it is notorious that many health care professionals themselves become victims of addictions.

Of course pain typically is a sign of something wrong in the body and comfort a sign of health, but these signs are not conclusive. Pain is often an accompaniment of a healing process, necessary exercise, or the travail of childbirth. Pleasure and comfort may mask a serious disease or a destructive chemical addiction. Psychiatrists also know that clients may claim to be happy and comfortable, but unconsciously may have deep psychological ills. On the other hand, anxiety and crisis may be a part of a healing or growth process or of creative struggle. Thus diagnosticians use pain and comfort as symptoms and clues, but they know that such signs do not prove either optimum or faulty functioning.

A good deal is written today about people learning to enjoy life and free themselves from "puritanical," neurotic guilt about sensual enjoyment. Certainly, we cannot live without some facilitation and recreation of our bodily resources by physical pleasure (C. Williams, 1974). Pleasure is necessary for physical and mental health, for self-understanding (Marmer, 1988; Milhaven, 1977), and for the maintenance of determination and courage for long-run goals. Short-range pleasures and comforts must be present to a moderate degree, and strains and pains cannot be endured too long. Thus leisure recreation (the restoration of human powers through rest and satisfaction) is an essential need of human life, and at an even deeper spiritual level *contemplation*, i.e., the reflective appreciation of the values and meaning of our experiences, ought to become a predominant quality of life (Pieper, 1964). A work ethic by which life is simply striving for a far-off, ever-receding goal is a bad ethic (Adler, 1970).

Addictions and phobias waste human energies. They reduce the freedom of the victims and hence their moral responsibility for their acts, because freedom of choice depends on our capacity to make prudent choices, i.e., by a deliberate, rational, realistic consideration of our options in a given situation. Yet addicts and phobics cannot be wholly absolved from moral responsibility. If, knowing the risk, persons have experimented with addictive chemicals, they remain responsible for their addiction and its consequences. Even if they acquired their addiction or phobias without understanding the risks, when in their freer moments they recognize that these compulsions are leading them to actions objectively harmful to themselves and to others, they cannot simply excuse themselves. Instead, they are ethically obliged to seek help in overcoming their morbid condition so as to cease their irrational behavior. For example, when the chemically dependent begin to recognize their condition, they have a moral responsibility to seek treatment. Likewise, a germ phobic who washes his hands constantly or withdraws from normal contact with others out of fear of contagion has a duty to himself and others to seek therapy.

The ancient Greeks praised the virtues of temperance regulating pleasure and of fortitude regulating fear of pain, and said "Moderation in all things." St. Peter told the early Christians to "rejoice with an indescribable and glorious joy" in the hope of eternal life, but "Live soberly!" (1 Pt 1: 8,13) on this pilgrim journey. In a special way human health depends on this right balance of facilitating pleasure and warning pain, but when these are allowed to take control of our lives we destroy ourselves.

Underlying this enslavement to addiction or obsession is *despair*, sometimes suicidal. The victim has lost hope of recovery. The role of the health care professional, therefore, is above all one of encouragement and inspiration to hope that freedom can be recovered, not just by one's own efforts, but also with the help of others and of a Higher Power. The first step to freedom is the humility to admit that we need such help.

Thus we can formulate the following *principle of inner freedom:*

> In order to be free to follow our conscience, we must avoid actions which may cause addiction to immoderate physical pleasures or obsessive fears that could result in loss of rational control of our behavior; and if such loss occurs, seek therapy and the help of others, who have an obligation to intervene to encourage and support our recovery.

The Principle of Personalized Sexuality

When discussing human sexuality, it is important to realize that "sexuality" is today an ambiguous term. First of all, it is used to denote the capacity of persons to love one another and to be united with them in friendship and community. In this sense of the term, every human being is a social, sexual person. Thus, while sex is one great source of the physical pleasures to which the *principle of inner freedom* applies, it is much more than that.

> [The] human person . . . is so profoundly affected by sexuality that it must be considered one of the principal formative influences in the life of a man or woman. In fact, sex is the source of the biological, physiological, and spiritual characteristics which make a person male or female and which considerably influence each individual's progress toward maturity as members of society. (CDF, 1975a; cf. Lawler et al., 1996; John Paul II, 1981b).

In his instructions on marriage, John Paul II has frequently emphasized that it is in our totality as persons that we are male or female, and this sexuality is the developmental source of our *relationality* as persons. We learn to relate to other persons first of all in our family life based on the sexual commitment of our parents to each other, and by interacting with our mother and father and siblings we learn to love others. Thus we also learn to go beyond the family to form other relationships, culminating for most people in marriage, but for everyone, single or married, in a variety of kinds of friendship and other social relations. In none of these relationships are we neuter persons. Our capacity for affection, communication, and sympathy in all these relationships is rooted in our physical and psychic sexuality (B. Hume, 1995).

Through their sexuality men and women are called by God to either marriage or the single state. John Paul II (1981b) writes:

> God inscribed in the humanity of man and woman the vocation and thus the capacity and responsibility of love and human union. Love (community) is therefore the fundamental and innate vocation of every human being. Christian revelation recognizes two specific ways of realizing the vocation of the human person to love: marriage and virginity or celibacy.

The second way the term "sexuality" is used is to refer to actions which are *genital* and seek orgasmic satisfaction. Here and in subsequent chapters we are principally concerned with ethical questions about genital sexuality within marriage. Therefore, we touch on other extramarital or autoerotic sexual questions only as they help to understand those of married couples.

Human sexuality, in this second sense of the word, is a complex of many values that are generally recognized in every ethical theory, but whose interrelation and ranking are the subject of much disagreement. Because persons have a potential capacity for marriage because of their sexual identity, we often refer to the principle of personalized sexuality and the principle of family-oriented sexuality. These are not two different principles; rather, by using the different terms we seek to signify the different ways in which persons fulfill their "vocation of love." These generally recognized values can be reduced to five major categories:

1. Sex is a search for sensual pleasure and satisfaction, releasing physical and psychic tensions.
2. More profoundly and personally, sex is a search for the completion of the human person through an intimate personal union of love expressed in and through the mutual gift of the lovers' bodies. It is also the mutual complementation of the male and female so that each achieves a more integral humanity.
3. More broadly, sex is a social necessity for the procreation of children and their education in a stable family so as to expand the human community and guarantee its future beyond the death of individual members.
4. Still more broadly, our sexuality opens us, married or single, to all the human relationships of friendship, sympathy, cooperation, compassion, and reconciliation which constitute the network of human society.
5. Symbolically, sex is a sacramental mystery, somehow revealing the cosmic order and our human destiny, since it stands for the creative love of God for creatures and their loving response to God.

The Sexual Revolution and the Crisis of the Family

Because of this cosmic symbolism, these values are celebrated as sacred gifts in all the great religions and philosophies of life and are protected and developed in every viable human culture. In the eighteenth century, however, the Enlightenment abandoned faith in Christian revelation and tried to create a secular religion based exclusively on reason (Ashley, 1985). Hence, many scientific Enlightenment thinkers came to view sex as nothing more than a biological drive for preserving the species, which it was unhealthy to frustrate. Others, more concerned to construct a humanist value system, viewed human sexuality as the mysterious source of romantic love, creativity, and ecstacy. Both types of humanists generally favored permissive attitudes toward sexual behavior. The nineteenth century, however, reacted strongly against the licentiousness of the previous period and committed itself to the "Victorian Compromise." Victorians, although they too had lost faith in Christian revelation, tried to preserve Christian moral standards, especially "family values." They achieved real moral reforms, but also discredited them by much hypocrisy, prudery, and superficial respectability.

After two world wars, the twentieth century has undergone a "sexual revolution" surpassing even eighteenth century license. While Victorian culture tried to cover up sexual misconduct, we have voyeuristically delighted in its total exposure. In the past fifty years, the empirical science of sexology (Kinsey et al., 1948, 1953; Masters and Johnson, 1966; Hite, 1976, 1981; Janus and Janus, 1993) has supplied us with extensive (but not entirely reliable) evidence of how many human beings fall far short of Christian norms of sexual conduct. Before marriage, most Americans seem to masturbate and engage in casual or commercialized sexual encounters or premarital cohabitation. About three percent of the population have sex exclusively with partners of the same sex (Becker and Kavoussi, 1988; Michaels et al., 1994), and this and other sexual options are more and more accepted as normal variations. Serial marriage, divorce, and remarriage has become a common pattern.

In view of these social facts, humanists generally view the traditional morality of the Christian churches as totally unrealistic and even destructive. They ask, "Isn't it reasonable to use our modern medical knowledge to free sexual relationships from all risk of unwanted pregnancy so as to bring human reproduction under the control of free human intelligence rather than chance? Shouldn't we produce children in the laboratory under genetic quality control and then put them in the care of experts to raise, freeing most people from parenthood?" Thus, many humanists believe sexual morality can be reduced to two fundamental norms: (1) All laws or social attitudes that hinder human freedom to achieve sexual values in ways the individual desires are unjust and oppressive; and (2) Sexual behavior, at least among consenting adults, is entirely a private matter to be determined by personal, no-guilt choice (Marcuse, 1972; Kurtz, 1983, 1988).

Historic Tradition of Church Teaching on Sex

The Christian understanding of sexuality is a notable application of the *principle of stewardship and creativity*. Its aim is to guide sexual behavior in cooperation with the purposes of the Creator in designing us as sexual beings. Yet it also seeks to remain open to progressive social and technological ways of improving sexual relationships. The five values of human sexuality which we have identified, not limited to genital activity, but in its full significance for human relationality, are also affirmed by traditional Christian ethics. In his classical work, *On the Good of Marriage*, St. Augustine taught that God intended sex for marriage and that marriage, problematic as it has become in our fallen world, remains a gift of God rich with a three-fold moral goodness, namely, (1) procreation (Gn 1:28); (2) mutual fidelity and help of the spouses (Gn 2: 18); and (3) sacramentality (Eph 5:32). Augustine also acknowledged pleasure as a value, noting that in our fallen state in which we have to struggle to acquire the virtue of chastity, marriage can help the couple learn inner freedom (I Cor 7:9).

Before Augustine, the Eastern Church had acknowledged the New Testament teaching on the holiness of marriage, "Let marriage be honored among all" (Heb 13:4; cf. 1 Cor 7). But the Greek Church Fathers, influenced by Platonic spiritualism and Stoic disdain for the passions, interpreted Genesis 1–3 to mean that if Adam and Eve had not sinned, the human race, like the angels, would have been multiplied by direct creation. In his later works Augustine abandoned this Greek reading of Genesis and taught that a sinless humanity would have multiplied sexually. Yet pessimistically he still believed that in our fallen state sexual intercourse is always flawed by venial sins of selfishness and excess (Hugo, 1968). More positively, Thomas Aquinas taught that if we had not sinned sex would have been even more pleasurable and that, since nature produces the sexes in equal numbers, all humans would have married. Following Aquinas, theologians began to teach more optimistically that not only can marital sex be free of sin but it can promote virtuous, self-giving, sanctifying love.

Thus, down to the twentieth century (Noonan, 1965; Grisez, 1993), theologians generally discussed human sexuality from the perspective of the question, "What is God's purpose in dividing the human race into male and female?" They found the obvious answer in Genesis 1:28, where God's first words to the newly created Adam and Eve are "Be fertile and multiply." Consequently, they ranked procreation and education of children as the primary end of marriage, to which the loving companionship of the couple is secondary, subordinated as a means to that primary end.

They were well aware, of course, that in Genesis 2:18 God also says, "It is not good for man to be alone. I will make a suitable partner [helper] for him." This text, however, does not say why God made Adam male. If God's purpose had simply been to provide Adam companionship, it would have sufficed, some theologians argued, to make humans all of one sex so as to facilitate friendship, since, as Aristotle showed in the *Nicomachean Ethics*, VIII, 3, the best friendships are based on what persons have in common, not on their differences. As for the physical pleasure of sex, an inventive God could have made human companionship sensuously pleasurable without connecting it to the dangerous and inconvenient work of reproduction. Therefore, the only obvious answer to the question, "Why did God make us male and female" is to be found in the advantages of the heterosexual family society for human procreation and education—advantages which, as we have seen, are confirmed today by the life and social sciences. This family school of human love thus becomes the source of all five values previously mentioned, especially sexuality in its broadest sense of human relationality.

In fact the Church never intended to teach that the loving companionship of married couples is simply a *means* to beget children. In its official teaching it never denied and indeed sometimes affirmed (cf. Pius XI, *Casti Connubii*, 1930) that the love of the couple is not only a means to procreation but an end in itself. Yet it is an end in itself that also serves a wider purpose than simply the couple's good. There is no philosophical contradiction in the notion of something being good *in itself*, yet at the same time in some respect subordinated to a higher good. For example, human persons are each ends in themselves, yet their individual good is subordinate to the common good of the community to which they belong. It was in this sense that the loving companionship of married couples was said traditionally to be a "secondary end."

Has Church Teaching on Sex Recently Changed?

In former times (and in some countries even today) marriages were arranged by the families of the couple, and the love relationship was hoped to be a consequence of the marriage, not its cause. Hence the Church, although it always recognized that marriage ought to be a covenant of love, also tended to emphasize the social rather than the romantic, personalistic aspects of this covenant. But in the twentieth century, to respond to our culture's great concern for the subjective factors in human behavior, the Church looks at human sexuality from a new perspective. It no longer simply asks, "Why did God create us male and female," but also, "What do persons as individuals gain from sex?" Sexual difference and mutual desire are assumed, and what implications these have for human fulfillment are queried. Moreover, many look to the health care profession to help them obtain this fulfillment, either by freeing sexual pleasure from unwanted pregnancy or by overcoming infertility or sexual dysfunctions.

Beginning with books by Herbert Doms (1939) and Dietrich and Alice Von Hildebrand (1965, 1984) and culminating in the Second Vatican Council (1965c), Paul VI's encyclical *Humanae Vitae* (1968), and most recently John Paul II's *Familiaris Consortio* (1981b), the Catholic Church has given authoritative status to a new formulation of the purposes of marriage that better balances its social and personal meanings. The former language that spoke of the value of procreation as the "primary end of marriage" has been replaced by the principle of the "inseparability of the unitive and procreative meanings of marriage." Marriage is no longer called only a "contract" but more specifically a "covenant of love" (Code of Canon Law, c. 1983). The characteristics of this covenanted love were listed by Paul VI (1968) as "human, total, faithful, exclusive, and fruitful." John Paul II, in *Familaris Consortio* (quoted in the *Catechism of the Catholic Church*, n. 1643), commented as follows:

> Conjugal love involves a totality, in which all the elements of the person enter—appeal of the body and instinct, power of feeling and affectivity, aspiration of the spirit and of will. It aims at a deeply personal unity, a unity that, beyond union in one flesh, leads to forming one heart and soul; it demands *indissolubility* and *faithfulness* in definitive mutual giving; and it is open to *fertility*. In a word it is a question of the normal characteristics of all natural conjugal love, but with a new significance which not only purifies and strengthens them, but raises them to the extent of making them the expression of specifically Christian values.

Does this very obvious shift in emphasis contradict the older formulation? Vatican Council II (*Gaudium et Spes*, n. 48, 1965c; *Catechism*, # 1652) reaffirmed that, "By their very nature, the institution of matrimony itself and conjugal love are ordained for the procreation and education of children, and find in them their ultimate crown." What it dropped was only the notion that marriage is a means to procreation rather than an end in itself (Grisez, 1993). Thus the new formula does not contradict the former one, though it improves on it by making explicit that married love is no mere means.

Yet the new formula has also caused confusion, because some (Kosnick et al., 1977; Keane, 1977) seem to have understood it to mean that the Church now makes love the primary end and procreation merely an optional consequence. The real aim of this new formula, however, is not to rank the unitive and procreative values of marriage or to subordinate one to the other, but to make clear that they are inseparably connected, so that one value cannot define the marital relationship in isolation from the other. The question to be asked, therefore, "Why are these values inseparable?" is precisely the major point on which humanists and Christians differ about human sexuality.

Of the five values of human sexuality we have enumerated, sexual pleasure cannot be isolated from the unitive or love value of the genital expression of sex because this depersonalizes sex and treats the partner as a mere object or is autoerotic. Also the fourth or symbolic value and the fifth or relational value are achieved only if the genital act is an act of committed love. The question posed by *Humanae Vitae*, therefore, is why the love or unitive meaning is inseparable from procreation and vice versa. This question will be treated at length in Chapter 10.

The Christian Understanding of Marital Sexuality

Taking into account the Church's reformulation of its teaching on marriage, how, in the light of the Christian revelation, are the facts of human sexuality as we know them from long historical experience and from biology, psychology, anthropology, and sociology to be interpreted (Schwartz, et al., 1983; Masters, Johnson, Kolodney, 1986; Ashley, 1995)? Genesis 1–3 teaches that God created us male and female and blessed our sexuality as his great and good gift. Jesus confirmed this teaching and perfected it by demanding men to be as faithful in marriage as the Old Testament required women to be (Mk 10:2–12; Mt 19:3–12; 1 Co 7:10). He also emphasized the dignity and the value of the child as a fully human person (Mt 19:13–15).

What then is the meaning of sexuality for those who have no families because the marriage is infertile or has been deprived of children by death, or for those who for other reasons live a single life? "Spouses to whom God has not granted children can nevertheless have a conjugal life full of meaning, in human and Christian terms. Their marriage can radiate a fruitfulness of charity, of hospitality, and of sacrifice" (Catechism of the Catholic Church, 1994, #1654). The couple who are childless love each other no less, but through no fault of their own cannot enjoy the full generative expression of their love in a family. Yet they can still exercise this generativity by extending their love to the service of others in need. The increasing number of single-parent families in our society should not bear the additional burden of being stigmatized, but ought to be given all remedial support possible. The hard reality, however, is that such households usually suffer serious deprivation.

Modern biology, as we have seen, has remarkably supported, with the addition of rich, concrete detail, this Christian, biblically-based understanding of why we are created sexual. It has done this by showing how necessary in an evolving universe is the differentiation of the human species into men and women, complementarily adapted to each other in body and soul, for the preservation and extension of the human species as it has come to rule its world by scientific understanding and technological control. Hence the bond that holds man and woman together and with their children in the community of the family is not just a bond of self-interest and need, but above all a bond of self-giving love. This love, however, is a special kind of love, specified by human sexuality—its complementarily, bonding, and fruitfulness.

Jesus also taught that while married sexuality is a great gift, its use is only a relative value which can be freely surrendered "for the sake of the kingdom" (Mt 19:12). Thus, for the Christian, the celibate or single life, with its freedom from domestic cares to be of service to others, can be even more personally maturing and fulfilling than marriage. St. Paul (1 Co 7:25–35) praised the holiness of married love as symbolic of Christ's love for his Church (Ep 5:22–23), yet gave preference to the freedom enjoyed by celibates to devote all their energies to the service of God and the human community. We have already shown that human sexuality is something much wider than genital sexuality; it is the source of friendships and other human relationships not directed to genital expression. Like Jesus, St. Paul and countless other Christians have chosen the single life in order in the name of God to devote themselves to the service of others (1 Cor 7). Nor is it true, as some have claimed, that a special charism is required for singles to live a chaste life if they do not marry. The ability to live chastely is made possible for every Christian by baptismal grace, although it may require a long struggle to form the necessary maturity of character.

Hence, the Catholic Church has maintained the institutions of sacramental marriage and of consecrated virginity and celibacy as complementary to each other. In their tension they express the pilgrim nature of the Church as it journeys through this life of birth and death to the kingdom of eternal life. Jesus said, "At the resurrection they neither marry nor are given in marriage" (Mt 22:30). Thus in the ultimate condition of all redeemed humanity the married state related to birth and death will be transcended (Mt 22:30), although the bonds of love which it fostered will endure forever. Through our human sexuality lived as Christians whether married or single, we prepare through our loving human relationships to enter into that everlasting community, God's Kingdom, with Father, Son, and Holy Spirit.

Can the Teaching of the Church on Sexuality Change?

Some theologians, discontent with even the reformulations of the Church's position just explained, call for a "new theology" of marriage more acceptable to the laity. Yet the teaching of Jesus, confirming the meaning of God's creation revealed in Genesis 1–2, is the solid rock on which the Church has rested its doctrine of the God-given purpose of sex and the norms for its use appropriate to this purpose. This revealed truth about God's purpose in creating us sexual is supported by natural law reasoning, but is independent of it and makes its appeal to Christian faith.

This teaching is so firmly grounded in Scripture, so constantly affirmed by the Church's Tradition, so repeatedly reaffirmed by papal and conciliar teaching in the face of vigorous opposition, and recently expounded in the *Catechism of the Catholic Church* after a universal consultation of the bishops, that it seems to bear the marks of an infallible truth which the Church can never change. The unfortunate fact that many Catholics do not understand the authority of this teaching or follow its guidance is not of itself proof that it is not in accord with the whole Church's "sense of the faith" (cf. p. 51). Although it is true that reception by the faithful can be a sign that a particular teaching is a revealed truth (e.g., the reception in the whole Church of the doctrine of the Assumption), its temporary nonreception even by a majority of the faithful or the failure of many to live by it are not conclusive signs to the contrary. Historically, a long time has often elapsed for official Church teaching to be received by the Church as a whole (e.g., the equality of the races and the sexes), and even when received it has not always been put in practice.

Therefore, the gift of human sexuality should be used only in permanent covenant of monogamous, married love as designed to constitute a family and never (1) as a selfish pursuit of pleasure apart from love (masturbation, prostitution, or casual or promiscuous relations; (2) as love which is not true, permanent, and publicly confirmed self-giving (adultery or premarital sex); or (3) as love expressed in ways deprived of its natural relation to the family (contraception, homosexual acts, and other such practices). The reason such actions are ethically wrong is not some repressive rule of the Church or an exclusion from respect of those whose sexual preferences are not those of the majority, but because these actions are contradictory to the intrinsic value and meaning of sexuality as designed and blessed by our Creator. Human culture and customs have undergone many revolutions, but such changes cannot alter the basic structure of human nature without destroying humanity itself.

Thus the principle of the inseparability of the unitive and procreative meanings of marriage which the Church definitively teaches can be formulated as the following *principle of family-oriented sexuality:*

> The gift of human sexuality must be used in marriage in keeping with its intrinsic, indivisible, specifically human teleology. It should be a loving, bodily, pleasurable expression of the complementary, permanent self-giving of a man and woman to each other which is open to fruition in the perpetuation and expansion of this personal communion through the family they responsibly beget and educate.

Principle of Growth through Suffering

On television we witness the extravagant joy of winners in giveaway contests, knowing that such happiness will quickly fade and prove to have been utterly fake. It is also possible for persons to have really achieved goals that are encompassing, profound, and lasting and yet to be in a state of great suffering because circumstances do not yet permit the full satisfaction of achievement. A great writer who has completed a masterpiece, a scientist who has made the discovery of a lifetime, or a statesman who has successfully carried through a great reform may feel exhausted, torn by inner conflict, and depressed. Such persons are to be envied, however, because ultimately they know they have reached the goal of their whole earthly lives.

Therefore the health care profession, although its task is to relieve pain and restore health, should not regard pain and suffering as the greatest of evils. Suffering, whether physical or psychic, is a violation or subversion of a person's bodily integrity or psychic stability. Death is the ultimate and complete violation or subversion of the human person (E. Becker, 1973; Bloom, 1987; Gatch, 1969; A. Mack, 1973). The Christian faith, therefore, looks on suffering and death in two distinct but related ways. On the one hand, suffering is evil because it is ultimately the result of either our own sins or the sins of others of which we are victims. On the other hand, suffering can be a liberating and grace-filled experience if we learn from it to be free of our own sinfulness and grow in love for others. In Chapter 13 we will try to examine this two-fold mystery of suffering more fully. For purposes of ethical discussion, however, the *principle of growth through suffering* can be expressed as follows:

> Just as bodily pleasure should be sought only as the fruit of the satisfaction of some basic need of the total human person, so suffering and even bodily death, when endured with courage, can and should be used to promote personal growth in both private and communal living.

This principle, supremely exemplified in the Cross of Christ, is rooted in the basic human need to preserve life, since people suffer only to achieve a renewed, purified, and enriched life.

8.4 NORMS OF CHRISTIAN LOVE

Motivation

To satisfy fully the human need for truth we must pursue scientific understanding, but even more we must be open to God's revelation of himself and of our road to come to him in his eternal life. Neither scientific research nor growth in faith is easy, and hence we need hope, trust in God's power to help us achieve our goal. Yet we cannot keep up this hope unless we are profoundly motivated. Such motivation has both a structural, or relational, aspect and a dynamic, or processive, aspect. The structural aspect involves the interpersonal relations that bind persons together in community, and the ethical norms that govern these relations can rightly be called norms of *love*, as distinguished from the norms of conscience just discussed. "Love" means not only a feeling, but also the practical *will* that leads one person to be concerned about another person and that person's true needs. Furthermore, love motivates people to help others fulfill these needs by sharing with another the values they themselves enjoy.

In any Christian ethics, the fundamental truth is that there is a Triune God and that "God is love" (1 Jn 4:8). God loves us not because he has first needed our love, but because his love for us has made us lovable:

> In this way God's love was revealed to us: God sent his only Son into the world that we might have life through him. This is love: not that we have loved God, but that he loved us and sent his Son as an expiation for our

sins. . . . If we love one another, God remains in us and his love is brought to perfection in us (1 Jn 4:9–10, 12).

The great theologians have all taught that the essence of the Christian life is the sharing by grace in this love of God, by which we love him and one another through the very same love by which he has created and redeemed us (Gilleman, 1961). God's love is thus a life-giving and healing activity, and the health care ministry is a work of love by which persons cooperate with God in giving life and healing sickness. Love of God can never be merely sentimental because it is built on faith and on all the truths derived from human reason and science. Therefore the health care professional's love must be a love informed by the best available medical knowledge and skill.

Christian professionals know that God loves them and therefore gives them the capacity to love others. This love must be shared, not by a minimal performance of duties, but as a generous concern and competent care for those in need. Yet under the pressures of daily work with its frustrations, this vision and realization of God's personal love as the source and motivation of our work can become very dim and fade into a deadly routine. Jesus, the great physician, found the pressure of the sick so great that he, too, had to retire into a desert place to pray and to regain hope and strength.

The whole town was gathered at the door, and he cured many who were sick with various diseases. . . . Rising very early before dawn, he went off to a deserted place where he prayed (Mk 1:33–35).

In discussing the principle of family-oriented sexuality, it was pointed out that the meaning of human sexuality is not merely genital but extends to all human relationships, yet it has its source in the community of the family as the school in which we best learn to love others. The health care professional who has been privileged to be raised in a truly loving family has learned that fundamental lesson and will not find it difficult to exercise a spiritual motherhood or spiritual fatherhood in tender but realistic care for those she or he serves. Those whose family was deficient need to realize that fact and seek to acquire the qualities of motherhood or fatherhood they may lack, if necessary with the help of psychotherapeutic counseling. The health care profession is the natural ally of the family institution, and it is a tragedy that some trends today have led this profession to connive in undermining family bonds, as we will see in Chapter 10.

Three particular norms help to define the content of Christian love: (1) every person must be valued as a unique, irreplaceable member of the human community (*principle of human dignity in community*); (2) every person must be encouraged to play a role in the common life and fully share its fruits (*principle of participation or subsidiarity*); and (3) all persons must be helped to realize their full potential (*principle of totality and integrity*). These principles are formulated in the following sections, with some reflections on their specifically Christian understanding.

Principle of Human Dignity in Community

Although today the unique value of every human being is affirmed by almost all religions and philosophies of life and the inalienable rights of the person are guaranteed by the constitutions of most governments, these rights are silently contradicted by three trends that seem to characterize contemporary life:

1. Persons are swallowed up in totalitarian, bureaucratic institutions.
2. Persons who are unnecessary for the efficient operation of these institutions—women, the very young, the very old, uneducated and defective persons—are treated as nonpersons.
3. Even successful persons find their happiness not in sharing their lives with others but in private, individualistic satisfactions.

Section 1.5 shows how the right understanding of human personhood and mankind's essentially social nature can help overcome this contradiction. Thus we can formulate the *principle of human dignity in community* as follows:

All ethical decisions, including those in health care, must aim at human dignity; that is, the maximal, integrated satisfaction of the innate and cultural needs, biological, psychological, ethical, and spiritual, of all humans persons, as individuals and as members of both their national communities and the world community.

This principle rests on a basic human need that must be satisfied to attain true happiness, namely, the need of every person for society, since it is only in community that this dignity is recognized and supported. Moreover, this principle not only states one basic need but includes all other basic needs whose satisfaction is required by a person's dignity. In short, human dignity in community sums up the true goal of human life: integral human fulfillment in relation to God and neighbor.

The Christian specification of this principle comes from what Jesus Christ added to our understanding of ourselves as created by God in his own image to share his eternal Triune life in total personhood as bodily and resurrected beings. The community in question, therefore, is not only this temporal human community, but also the Kingdom of God into which even the least and most unworthy human beings are called. Hence, the New Testament warns against "discrimination" against persons, for example, on the basis of whether they are rich or poor.

My brothers, show no partiality as you adhere to the faith in our glorious Lord Jesus Christ. For if a man with gold rings on his fingers and in fine clothes comes into your assembly, and a poor person in shabby clothes also comes in, and you pay attention to the one wearing the fine clothes and say, "Sit here, please," while you say to the poor one, "Stand there," or "Sit at my feet," have you not made distinctions among yourselves and become judges with evil designs? (Jas 2:1–4).

Thus the refusal to respect the rights of others because of their nationality, race, sex, age, or physical or psychological health is contrary to the Gospel and should have no place in the health care profession, whose best traditions have always insisted on helping persons on the basis of need, not of social status. It is a common error in ethical debates today, however, to confuse the equality of persons and their basic human rights with other issues that concern social roles. For example, it is not discrimination to recognize that children have a different social role in the family and society than adults and require special care and protection, nor that mother and father usually play different but complementary roles in raising the children. It is unrealistic to confuse the equal dignity of all human persons with the particular gifts or disabilities which must be taken into account in considering what contribution these differences make to the common good of the community.

This distinction between equal personal dignity and inequalities in abilities applies in an important way to our attitudes toward persons suffering from physical and mental disabilities. In the past such persons were too often treated as cursed by God, touched by the devil, guilty of sin, or more often simply as "inferior" to persons enjoying physical and mental integrity. Today, fortunately, widespread educational and legal efforts are being made to give disabled or "disadvantaged" persons their full human rights and to enable them to live active lives, as normal as possible. Sometimes, however, the approach to these problems is one of denial of abnormality and the use of euphemistic language. To call a cripple a "locomotively disadvantaged person" is mockery rather than justice or compassion.

The root cause of all unjust discrimination is the failure to understand that human dignity is not based on physical or mental health, any more than it is on money or education, but on the single fact that a person is a human being made in God's image. Once this principle is firmly held, no shame or personal inferiority is implied in being blind, deaf, crippled, homosexually oriented, poor, illiterate, black, woman, child, or fetus. All are equally persons, have the same human rights, and have the same claim to justice and dignity. Even persons who are criminal in behavior retain their fundamental dignity as persons and the right to be treated as such, not as "animals" (as they are sometimes called), although as punishment and their rehabilitation and for the common good some of their freedoms must be restricted.

Principle of Participation

The principle of human dignity in community requires that various levels of responsibility be established within the community. Chapter 3 argues that the primary responsibility for health rests with the individual concerned and that the whole work of health care professionals must be conceived as a cooperative service to individuals in their personal search for health. At the same time, individuals are not self-sufficient in this search for health, and they can achieve health only with the help of the community. Consequently, it is also essential to give attention to the *principle of participation*, which can be formulated as follows:

Human communities exist only to promote and share the common good among all their members "from each according to ability, to each according to need" in such a way that:

1. Decision making rests *vertically* first with the person, then with the lower social levels, and *horizontally* with functional social units.
2. The higher social units intervene only to supply the lower units what they cannot achieve by themselves, while at the same time working to make it easier in the future for lower units and individuals to satisfy these needs by their own efforts.

In Catholic Church documents, the term "subsidiarity" is often used to refer to the principle under discussion. Subsidarity is derived from the Latin name for auxiliary or reserve military troops and hence it means "helpfulness." We prefer the more common term "participation," since the principle requires that every member of a community should participate as fully as possible in its common life and its benefits according to their abilities and needs. It elaborates the implications of the principle of human dignity in community by showing the respective roles of the individual, subgroups, and the total community, so that by this division of labor the dignity of every member of a community will be fully recognized and actively promoted. It has its source in our basic need for society.

The Christian specification of this principle is given by St. Paul in 1 Corinthians (12–13), where he shows that the Christian understanding of the person based on Jesus' concern for "the little ones," "the least brethren" (Mk 9:33–37), must be the principle that governs the Church, conceived as the Body of Christ, ensouled by the Holy Spirit, which is the model for the coming Kingdom of God. The Church is compared to the Body of Christ, in which, as in the human body, there must be a differentiation of organs in the service of the whole.

Now the body is not a single part but many. If the foot should say, "Because I am not a hand I do not belong to the body," it does not for this reason belong any less to the body. Or if an ear should say, "Because I am not an eye I do not belong to the body," it does not for this reason belong any less to the body. If the whole body were an eye, where would the hearing be? If the whole body were hearing, where would the sense of smell be? But as it is, God placed the parts, each one of them, in the body as he intended. . . . But God has constructed the body as to give greater honor to a part that is without it, so that there may be no division in the body, but that parts may have the same concern for one another. If one part suffers, all the parts suffer with it; if one part is honored, all the parts share its joy." (I Cor 12:14–18, 24b–26).

Recently in the United States and elsewhere a political reaction has set in not only against utopian communism and socialism but also against the liberal welfare state. It has become as popular to blame bureaucracy and "big government" for our social ills, as it was not long ago to blame the corporations and "big business" for them. The Church's social teaching has always tried to strike a balance between these ideological extremes (John Paul II, *Centesimus Annus,* 1991). Government is not of itself an evil, or selfish individualism a good. The principle of participation opposes an excessive centralization of social control, but it also favors concern for the common good and the care of neglected members of society. The notion that a competitive "free market" will automatically produce the common good has historically proved quite as utopian as communism. It is also unrealistic to believe that a good social order can operate without citizens being willing to sacrifice their opinions to political compromise and to make their contribution to the common good in needed taxes and public service.

Also, some authors have written as if all "hierarchy" is contradictory to the fundamental human equality on which the Gospel insists. This is the philosophical error of "anarchism," which asserts that in an ideal society there should be no leaders nor followers, no authority nor subjects of authority, but all decisions should be made by consensus, so that no one needs obey anybody else (Woodcock, 1962). It has been fostered by the formalistic ethics of Immanuel Kant which, as we showed in the previous chapter, exaggerates the individual autonomy and hence cannot adequately ground an ethics of human rights.

Anarchism has always proved a disastrous way to try to run any community, whether family, business, school, church, or state. It denies the plain fact that we are unique individuals with different gifts and experiences. Thus, even with the best good will, we cannot always come to a consensus on practical decisions in the way we sometimes can in theoretical judgments. In arithmetic, for example, there is one right answer to a problem and many wrong ones, while in practical matters there are not only many wrong answers but also very often many right but different answers—"many ways to skin a cat." Consequently, we may discuss the pros and cons of a practical decision forever and still not arrive at true consensus.

Thus every human community must have an organic structure, a differentiation of parts unified for common action by a hierarchy of offices and functions. Sometimes members of a community must obey authority, whether this be the authority of a leader, a committee, or the majority (Y. Simon, 1962). This does not necessarily imply inferiority in dignity on the part of the one who obeys, since the one who commands and the one who obeys both act for the common good in which all have equal rights. That Dr. A is chief of the medical staff does not prove he or she is a better person or even a better physician than Dr. B, but simply that someone had to be head if there was to be any unity in policy and effective cooperation among all members of the staff.

The specific Christian teaching on this point was given by Jesus, as the leader of the apostles who used his authority to appoint them as leaders and authorities in his Church. Jesus was no anarchist, and he founded a structured, hierarchical community of faith with a common mission to accomplish (Vatican Council II, 1964a), but he denounced leaders who abuse their office to serve their own interests instead of those of community.

> "You call me "teacher" and "master," and rightly so, for so indeed I am. If I, therefore, the master and teacher, have washed your feet, you ought to

wash one another's feet. I have given you a model to follow, so that as I have done for you, you should also do" (Jn 13:13–15).

"You know that the rulers of the Gentiles lord it over them, and the great ones make their authority over them felt. But it shall not be so among you. Rather, whoever wishes to be great among you shall be your servant, whoever wishes to be first among you shall be your slave. Just so, the Son of Man did not come to be served, but to serve and to give his life as a ransom for many" (Mt 20:25–28).

Thus the Gospel conception of social authority is service, not domination or exploitation (Mk 10:41–45). In a health care facility the CEO is indeed in authority, but for that very reason a CEO has the ethical obligation to be the servant of the whole staff and all those it serves. The principle of subsidiarity indicates how this service is to be performed, with concern for the dignity and special contributions of all.

Principle of Totality and Integrity

The basis for the *principle of totality and integrity* can be formulated as follows:

To promote human dignity in community, every person must develop, use, care for, and preserve all of his or her natural physical and psychic functions in such a way that:

1. Lower functions are never sacrificed except for the better functioning of the whole person, and even then with an effort to compensate for this sacrifice.
2. The basic capacities that define human personhood are never sacrificed unless this is necessary to preserve life itself.

This principle makes explicit another aspect of the principle of human dignity in community by requiring *self-respect* as well as respect for each other. Unless persons respect their own personal integrity, both physical and psychic, as children of God and seek to preserve and perfect their own gifts, they cannot expect the community's respect. One of the effects to be feared from the current drive to use technology to remake the human body by sterilizing it, genetically engineering it, or using it for experimentation is a gradual erosion of societal respect for human life.

A certain analogy exists between this principle and the principle of participation but it is only an analogy; i.e., they are more unlike than like. Both recognize that the community and the person are complex systems of mutual interdependence between the whole and its parts. They differ radically, however, because the human person is a natural, primary unit in which the parts completely depend on the whole and exist for its sake. On the contrary, the community is a system made up of primary units, that is, human persons. It exists for the sake of these persons, not merely as isolated individuals but as sharers in a common, profoundly interrelated life. To treat this analogy as univocal is the error of totalitarianism, which sacrifices the person to the communal state, as in communism and fascism.

Human wholeness consists in the interdependence of higher and lower spiritual and bodily functions. Consequently, the lower functions cannot, without qualification, be sacrificed to the higher functions. This sacrifice might be to the advantage of the higher function but will not be to the good of the whole person, since the good of a person is essentially complex, irreducible to the good of one part, even if that part is the highest.

To be a complete human being, therefore, is not merely to have the higher level of functions but to have all the different basic human functions in harmonious order. This order requires the subordination of the lower functions to the higher but also forbids their total sacrifice. For example, the feasibility of intravenous feeding does not justify elimination of the human alimentary system, nor does the ability to produce a baby in the laboratory justify the elimination of the human reproductive system. Human integrity requires us to eat and reproduce in a *human* manner. Human body functions contribute to higher functions by supplying what is needed for physiological brain functions, but they also supply part of the human experience that is essential to human intelligence and freedom. Bodily feelings (movement, eating, sexuality, and manipulation of the environment) develop one's self-awareness and relation to others in the community. Thus, if children were nourished only intravenously without ever enjoying a meal with others, or conceived in laboratories and raised by "experts" rather than parents, they would miss experiences essential to integral human development. The following norms pertain to human integrity:

1. Primarily, human health is not merely a matter of organs but of capacities to function humanly.
2. Generally speaking, any particular human functional capacity can be diminished when necessary for the good of the whole person; that is, so that the person can better exercise all other human functions.
3. Secondary functions can always be sacrificed to more basic ones. For example, a finger can be removed to save the use of the hand because the capacity of action given by one finger is secondary in relation to the capacity given by the hand as a whole.
4. Primary or basic functional capacities, however, cannot be destroyed to promote even more important capacities, except when it is necessary to preserve the life of the whole person.

It is sometimes permissible to sacrifice one of the basic human functions to preserve life but not to save another basic function because without the life of the whole, all functions of the parts are destroyed.

The great importance of the principle of totality and integrity for medical ethics is that it establishes a norm for setting priorities when one human value must be subordinated to another. Contrary to ethicists (Grisez, 1983, and others who hold that the basic human goods are incommensurable), we have argued for the more traditional view that there is a hierarchy of basic goods. In Chapter 1 we worked out this hierarchy of values in terms of the biological, psychological, social, and spiritual dimensions of human personality. The spiritual and social values have higher priority than the psychological and biological values, but such priority must not be understood dualistically as if the lower are merely means to the higher values. This was long ago settled in the Church by its disapproval of the action of Origen, the great third century theologian, who castrated himself hoping to free his study and teaching of sexual distractions. His well-intentioned error was repudiated by the Church as objectively a sin against God's gift of the human body, which ought not to be mistreated even when it gives us problems. In the human person there is a mutual interdependence of the body and the soul, the lower and the higher. Therefore, if we sacrifice one to the other, we injure both.

This principle of totality and integrity is rightly classified as one of the norms of love because it expresses the sense in which each person must have a proper self-love, without which the love of others is impossible and is a merely sentimental altruism. Did not Jesus command us to "love God and one's neighbor *as one's self*" (Mk 12:31)? Its specific Christian character arises from the Incarnation, in which the Word of God became flesh, lived a bodily life, died, and was truly resurrected. In order to prove his love for his enemies, Jesus, rather than fight back, permitted them to kill him. He did not, however, commit suicide but sought to avoid death as long as he could without abandoning his mission. "The Pharisees went out and took counsel against him to put him to death. When Jesus realized this, he withdrew from that place" (Mt 12:14–15).

Christian anthropology, therefore, admits a certain polarity with the human person between our share in the material world and in the spiritual world, but it rejects any form of dualism that would deny the dignity of the human body of Jesus or our resurrected bodies. As persons who are also bodies, we are "temples of the Holy Spirit" (1 Co 3:16). This principle is well expressed by the writer of Ephesians (5:21–33) when he makes the analogy between Christ's love for humankind, a man's love for his wife, and one's love for one's own body.

8.5 COORDINATION OF THE PRINCIPLES

The text by Beauchamp and Childress (1994) cited in 7.1 proposes four principles for bioethics: (1) autonomy, the right of persons to care for themselves; (2) nonmaleficence, that is, "do no harm"; (3) beneficence, or seeking the patient's benefit; and (4) justice to all concerned. These four principles relate to and foster the professional–patient relationship of trust. For their principle of "autonomy," we prefer the principle of informed consent, and for their concept of "trust," the principle of professional communication. Their principles of "nonmaleficence," "beneficence," and "justice" are similar to our principle of human dignity in community, principle of the common good, etc. As noted at the beginning of this chapter, Beauchamp and Childress ground these four principles only in "common morality," the prevailing customary morality of our culture, increasingly dominated by humanism, while we have looked for a deeper and more permanent grounding in human nature and Christian faith.

Why have we chosen to list thirteen principles rather than a few broad ones, as have Beauchamp and Childress? The main reason is that in the actual process of bioethical decision making, each of these thirteen principles plays a separate and important role. In fact, the thirteen could be still further multiplied by additional corollaries. Our list, however, can be coordinated and simplified by showing how it flows from the four basic needs of human persons:

1. *To preserve life* grounds the principles of totality, of inner freedom, and of growth through suffering.
2. *To procreate* grounds the principle of family-oriented sexuality.
3. *To know the truth* grounds the principles of well-formed conscience, free and informed consent, inner freedom, moral discrimination, double effect, legitimate cooperation, and professional communication, which provide the conditions for a prudent conscience.
4. *To live in society* grounds the principles of human dignity in community, the common good and subsidiarity, and also stewardship and creativity, which relates human society to the environment and to the use of all gifts for the common good.

Note that this coordination does not imply that each principle has only one source in human needs; for example, although the principle of family-oriented sexuality rises primitively from the human need to procreate, it is also closely related to the principles of inner freedom, of human dignity in community, of the common good, and of stewardship and creativity.

CONCLUSION

To sum up this discussion of the principles that govern bioethical decisions from a Christian point of view:

1. Faith requires persons to act with an informed conscience, which requires the intellectual effort of moral discrimination between right and wrong, even in complex cases in which moral actions involve evil side effects or material cooperation. Faith also requires a relation of trust between persons, especially between professional and client, in which there is an honest exchange of the information necessary for an informed conscience.
2. Hope requires persons to fulfill in a creative manner their stewardship of their own nature and the world God has given them. It frees them interiorly from enslavement to pleasures and fears so they can pursue

their true goals, accept growth through suffering, and continue the human community through the institution of the family.

3. Love, the most inclusive of all, requires a profound respect for human dignity, no matter what the condition of the person. Love also requires a proper love of self and a responsibility for one's own health. Finally, love requires persons to work for and share in the common good. One must accept the social responsibility of promoting the distribution of health care for all.

PART 4

Difficult Bioethical Decisions

Some of the specific ethical issues associated with health care have been considered in earlier chapters; for example, informed consent and confidentiality in Chapter 3. The main ethical issues concerned with patient-physician relationship and the preparation of men and women for service in health care professions we have presented in Chapters 4 and 5. Moreover, the ethical issues in health care arising from social organizations have been considered in Chapter six. There are several different ways in which the other ethical issues could be presented. We have chosen to cluster these issues around several key concepts; human generation and birth, integrity of the body/spirit composite and issues surrounding dying and death.

First of all then, in Chapter 9 we consider the ethical issues which can be clustered under the general title of ethical issues concerned with the beginning of life. In this section, we consider the scientific and philosophical evidence related to the question "When does human life begin?" Next we consider the various artificial reproductive technologies, testing for fetal anomalies, and abortion.

In Chapter 10 we continue to study ethical issues which follow upon human generation and birth; thus contraception, sterilization, and treatment for rape are considered here. Because many have difficulty accepting and following the teaching of the Church in regard to contraception and sterilization, we then consider the pastoral approach of the Church in regard to actions considered to be objectively evil. In other words, we consider subjective dispositions and how they sometimes mitigate the culpability which arises from non-observance of objective norms.

Various means of modifying the human body and the human personality are considered in Chapter 11. Insofar as they modify the body/spirit composite the ethics of genetic intervention and genetic screening are considered. Routine surgeries which affect the body such as appendectomies and hysterectomies have long been justified by means of the principle of double effect and the principle to totality (cf. p. 362; p. 412). Even though these surgeries injure the body and its capacities, the direct purpose of these procedures is the well-being of the body/person. Hence, the injury is an indirect effect and there is a sufficient good resulting from the surgery which justifies the unintended evil. Hence, there is no need to devote attention to the ethical import of standard surgeries. Some surgeries however do cause ethical concern. Thus the transplanting of organs and sexual reassignment are treated in this chapter. Finally, because research and experimentation upon persons more often than not involves the human body, we then consider the ethical norms for research.

After considering ethical issues arising from therapy concerned primarily with the body, we then consider therapy primarily designed to heal or alleviate mental pathologies. Of course, some of the therapies we study for the mind also have an effect upon the body, but their ultimate purpose is to treat mental illness. Hence, ethical issues associated with psychosurgery, electroconvulsive therapy, the use of pharmaceuticals to change behavior and insight psychotherapies are considered. Lastly we consider addiction and chemical dependency insofar as they affect emotional and mental activity.

The final chapter in this section considers the many ethical issues which surround the care for dying persons. The first and perhaps most serious ethical issue is fear of death. Hence, our first consideration is directed toward a sound theology of death. In addition to the more general issues concerning truth telling to the dying and care for the body after death, we consider the more difficult issues concerning the withdrawal of life support, euthanasia, and suicide.

9

Artificial Reproduction, Fetal Testing, Abortion

OVERVIEW

In Chapter 8 we discussed the various principles or norms for virtuous human action, describing how these principles are related to the fundamental virtues of faith, hope, and charity. As one norm relating to the virtue of hope, in Chapter 8 we discussed the principle of sexuality. In our times ethical questions regarding human sexual behavior are highly controversial, but we showed that according to Christian faith and the natural law the right use of our sexuality must accord with its intrinsic teleology; i.e., the purpose of the Creator and our present understanding of human nature as it has been refined by the life sciences. We then showed that the human race is divided into male and female in giving them a basic orientation and enabling people to join actively in forming family, the natural unit of human society, in which it is best ecologically for human persons to be born and reach maturity so as to be able to find their human fulfillment in families of their own. Hence, uses of sexuality which destabilize good family life or which fail to strengthen it are harmful to individuals and to society and may not ethically be promoted by the health care profession. On the contrary, the health care profession may make a very important contribution to a Christian expression of sexuality.

Since many of the medical problems associated with sexuality are connected with its reproductive aspect and depend on the judgement of "When does life begin?" in 9.1 we will deal with this question as preliminary to its ethical implications. Then in 9.2 we will treat of methods of artificial reproduction based on the advances in embryology, but which often incidentally involve the destruction of human embryos. In 9.3 we will examine methods of ascertaining the condition of the fetus in the womb, since these can be used for purposes of either therapy or termination of pregnancy. Finally, in 9.4 and 9.5 we will treat of the most serious violation of responsible parenthood, namely, the intentional destruction of a living human person before its birth. Other bioethical questions relating to human reproduction will be discussed in Chapter 10.

9.1 WHEN DOES HUMAN LIFE BEGIN?

Embryologists who are asked this question in a purely scientific context usually answer without hesitation, "A human organism, a member of the human species, comes into existence when a human ovum is fertilized by a human sper-matozoa and a one-celled zygote is produced." Nevertheless, the abortion con-troversy has led many people, even embryologists, to question the correctness of this answer or at least its ethical significance, especially when the term "human person, subject of human rights" is introduced into the discussion. They then opt for some theory of "delayed hominization" according to which human personhood does not begin until sometime after conception (Callahan, 1970; Lotstra, 1985; McCartney, 1986; Bole, 1989; Cahill, 1993). We will try to list and discuss the major theories of this type in an orderly sequence (cf. Gallagher, 1985; Grisez, 1990; Regan, 1992; Johnson vs. Porter, 1995).

Ancient and Modern Embryology

First, one very old difficulty originated in Greek thought with the Pythagoreans, who said that "the body is the tomb of the soul" and taught reincarnation. Adopting this conception, the Platonists believed the human spiritual soul had existed eternally in heaven, but as the result of some original sin it was "infused" at conception into a body alien to it. On the contrary, for Aristotle, a physician's son and a biologist, the human soul was not alien to the body but its natural form. Yet in view of his basic philosophical principle that "the matter and form of any substance must be mutually proportionate," he doubted that the human soul with its complex faculties could be present at conception, as his teacher Plato had thought, because he himself thought that at that moment the only matter available was the relatively formless menstrual blood. Hence Aristotle reasoned that it must take some time before the active power in the semen (which he supposed remained working for some weeks in the womb) could form the menses first to the level of physiological ("vegetative") life and then to the level of sentient ("animal") life. Only when the fetal body had reached this high state of formation could it receive its final organization which, because of our human spiritual intelligence, requires the direct action of the First Cause of the universe, the divine "Thought Thinking Itself" (B. Ashley, 1976). The Stoics were influenced by both Plato and Aristotle, but believed it was only at birth that a child breathed in the "vital spirit."

Aristotle's biology was authoritative for medieval theologians. The fact that it was accepted both by the Dominican Thomas of Aquinas (Taylor, 1982) and the great Franciscan theologian Duns Scotus led to the general supposition of Catholic theology until modern times that ensoulment takes place between one and two months of gestation, when the fetus has a definitely human form. Some Catholic philosophers have recently attempted to rehabilitate this theory of "delayed hominization" as proposed by Aquinas (Donceel, 1970, 1985; Pas-trana, 1977; Wallace 1989) or Scotus (Shannon and Wolter, 1990; critique by Arkes, 1992).

Officially the Catholic Church has never based its opposition to direct abortion on the claim that the human soul is created at conception. The *Declara-tion on Procured Abortion* (CDF, 1974), while affirming that from the time of conception direct abortion is always a grave sin, appended a note #19 saying,

"This declaration expressly leaves aside the question of the moment when the spiritual soul is infused. There is not a unanimous tradition on this point and authors are as yet in disagreement." The advances in embryology, however, have made the CDF more confident that the theories of delayed hominization are scientifically obsolete, so that its more recent *Instruction on Respect for Human Life* (1987) (I, 1, italics added) says:

> Certainly no experimental datum can be in itself sufficient to bring us to the recognition of a spiritual soul; nevertheless, *the conclusions of science regarding the human embryo provide a valuable indication for discerning by the use of reason a personal presence at the moment of this first appearance of a human life:* How could a human individual not be a human person? ... Thus the fruit of human generation from the first moment of its existence, that is to say, from the moment the zygote has formed, demands the unconditional respect that is morally due to the human being in his bodily and spiritual totality. The human being is to be respected and treated as a person from the moment of conception and therefore from that same moment its rights as a person must be recognized, among which in the first place is the inviolable right of every innocent human being to life.

Aristotle's view still has philosophical supporters because of the philosophical cogency of his principle that human ensoulment cannot take place until the body it substantially unifies is proximately organized for it. But he did not know that all the essential information needed to construct the human body is already present at conception in the zygote's nucleus. We now know that the sperm is haploid (has only half the human set of chromosomes) and ceases to exist once it has initiated fertilization by contributing its half of the genetic information. We know too that the ovum is already highly structured and contributes the other half of the genome, the bulk of the cytoplasm, and certain additional genetic factors in its cytoplasmic mitochondria. Since the zygote is thus already highly organized, the Aristotelian requirement for human ensoulment seems satisfied at conception.

This conclusion, however, is rejected by Bedate and Cefalo (1989; cf. answer by DeMarco, 1991) because the embryo in its interaction with the mother during pregnancy acquires additional information necessary for its normal development. This overlooks the fact that the first stages of embryo development can take place *in vitro,* entirely independent of the mother. Moreover, even after birth when it is obviously individuated, the child continues to receive from its food and environment information necessary for its development to adulthood. Any organism processes and assimilates all this additional information in the course of its normal functioning as a self-preserving and self-constructing unit. But what guides this developmental process as a consistent whole in which any step missed is disastrous? It certainly is not the information the organism assimilates during subsequent developmental phases, but the genome present from conception. It is odd that Bedate and Cefalo try to support their thesis by pointing to the existence of false pregnancies that produce only hydatidiform moles, masses of disorganized tissues or fragmentary organs, since it is well established that these are the result of radical genetic defect in the pseudozygote (Lejeune, 1989; Suarez, 1990; R. A. Fisher, 1991).

Continuity of Life

A second objection to saying that human life begins at conception is whether, in view of biological and cosmic evolution, it makes sense to speak of a "beginning" to human life at all. Before the zygote, the ovum and sperm were already alive, and they in turn had progenitors going back through evolution to early life on earth, and then on back through the chemical and physical processes of cosmic evolution to the Big Bang—and who knows what came before that!

But the question at hand is not the "beginning" of all life or of the cosmos, but the coming into existence of this individual organism, Ms. or Mr. Jones, a member of the human species. The ovum and sperm are indeed two living entities, but not complete organisms, since each has only half the human set of chromosomes and thus they are unable to reproduce themselves. Only when the two gametes unite to form one zygote does one complete new, unique human organism capable of self-development and reproduction come into existence. Nor is it true as pro-choice advocates used to claim that the embryo and fetus are not independent organisms but only cells of the mother's body (Wahlberg, 1971; Wasserstrom, 1975). The conceptus has a unique genome, distinct from its mother's, and its dependence on her in prepartum is not unlike its postpartum dependence on her for its nourishment and on a suitable environment for its warmth and protection.

Thus philosophers who insist that a definition of a human person cannot be merely "substantialist" are correct (Goldenring, 1985); it must be processive and developmental. The first step in medical procedure is to take a history of the patient. But not all processes are changes like a rise in temperature or an increase in size or velocity. As was shown by the process philosopher Alfred North Whitehead (1929), the essence of any process is genuine *novelty*. In the complex processes of becoming new, entities emerge that are materially continuous with the past but formally discontinuous with it in structure and function. Process is not always a mere reshuffling of what was already there, but the emergence of new realities radically distinct from those that previously existed. Therefore we still need to ask exactly when in the long process of biological reproduction is the critical point at which a new organism, which did not exist before, comes to exist so that where there was one organism, there are now two, or where there were two, there is now a unique third. During a lifetime any human person undergoes startling changes from childhood to old age, but we recognize the same person. Psychiatrists are also acquainted with aphasiacs who seem to have forgotten their past, and with patients with "multiple personalities." Nevertheless, therapy for such patients rightly assumes that each really remains an identifiable person whose healing will be the restoration of his or her sense of unitary identity as a person.

Development, Process, Potentiality

Third, because of this developmental, processive character of human life, some, notably Grobstein (1983, 1988), followed by Richard A. McCormick (1987, 1990, 1991a, 1991b; cf. Holbrook, 1985), refuse to admit that the identity of a human being is established at conception by its unique genome. Instead they urge a "developmental" rather than a "genetic" approach to embryology and claim that human identity is only gradually established through a series of phases. Others have expressed much the same idea by claiming that the embryo and fetus are only "potentially" a human being, or are "in the process of becoming human but are not yet human."

Thus we read in a current bioethics textbook (Engelhardt, Jr., 1986a) the following argument:

> If X is a potential Y, it follows that X is not a Y. If fetuses are potential persons, it follows clearly that fetuses are not persons. . . . Undoubtedly, the language of potentiality is itself misleading, for it is often taken to suggest that an X that is a potential Y in some mysterious fashion already possesses the being and significance of Y. It is therefore perhaps better to speak not of X's being a potential Y but rather of its having a certain probability of developing into Y (p. 111).

But is it accurate to describe the change of a fetus into an adult as X becoming Y? It is the identical organism P which is both X (a fetus) and Y (an adult), and it is this P which in ordinary language we call a "human being," "a member of the human species," or a "human person." To say a fetus is "potentially" an adult means it is in the process of becoming an adult, while continuously remaining a human being or person. That this potentiality is something real about the fetus itself is evident from the fact that a dog fetus is not potentially a human adult; nor is a zygote potentially any adult but only an adult with the same unique genome. It will not do to say, as Engelhardt suggests, that a fetus is "probably" an adult, rather than "potentially" an adult. The concept "potentiality" implies "real possibility" but says nothing about whether the realization of this possibility is certain, probable, or improbable.

The concept of "matter" so essential to science denotes some reality as it is potential, i.e., subject to change, either change of certain attributes (as a fetus changes into a teenager) while remaining the same identical individual, or a more radical change in which old individuals are destroyed and a new individual or individuals produced (as the sperm and ovum lose their individuality and by uniting produce a zygote). Potentiality, in this sense of "matter" or "stuff," is something *passive*, as clay in the sculptor's hands. But "potentiality" has also an *active* sense, as the power to mold and develop passively potential material. Thus the sculptor has active potential to form a variety of shapes out of clay, while the clay has passive potentiality for various figures. Organisms are "potential" in *both* these quite different and correlative senses. At any moment of its biography, an organism is made of matter, of cells, of organs which are passive stuff capable of being further organized and regulated. But the same organism also has inherent power to differentiate, develop, and regulate itself by its active functions (active potentialities). This capacity for self-development is the "life principle" that gives unity to the organism and guarantees its biographical identity. Thus the *X* that was *Z* (a person in its fetus phase) not only becomes *Y* (a person in its adult phase), but *X* is the *cause* of this change of *X* from *Z* to *Y*. As the early Christian theologian Tertullian said, "The one who will be a human being is already one" (Tertullian; d. 240).

This active potentiality for self-development, as with any function, presupposes some kind of organic structure, but it is necessarily a minimal structure, since on its relatively simple basic structure the organism is able to elaborate itself into its adult complexity. Modern embryology has shown clearly (I. Kaiser, 1986) that this minimal initial structure must be understood not in a preformist way as a miniature model of the completed structure, but *epigenetically,* as endowed with the information necessary to construct this total structure as well as the directing energy to build it. Thus, the potentiality of the zygote consists neither in a mock-up of the many-celled adult, nor even in just a blueprint of the adult, but in an *active potentiality for self-development and self-reproduction,* a potentiality based on the minimal actual structure of the zygote and residing principally in the chromosomes of its nucleus containing the information necessary to produce the maximally differentiated adult structure.

Some also question exactly how to pinpoint the time of "conception," since the fertilization process from the penetration of the sperm to *syngamy* (the fusion of the haploid nuclei of the ovum and the sperm into the single nucleus of the zygote) is not instantaneous, and the chromosomes and their maternal or paternal origin remain identifiable (Daly, 1987, 1988). More probably the new organism comes into existence at syngamy rather than at penetration, since only then a new, single nucleus with its complete set of chromosomes exists to unify the new organism and direct its orderly development. Certainly, the time between penetration and syngamy is much too brief to be of practical significance from an ethical perspective.

Between Syngamy and Implantation

Richard A. McCormick, SJ, 1991b (following Mahony, 1984, and Grobstein, 1988; see also Dedek, 1972; C. Curran, 1975; B. Brody, 1975; Häring, 1976; see critique Diamond, 1991; Irving 1993a, 1993b) argues that during the two weeks between fertilization and implantation, at which time twinning ceases to be possible, the conceptus, though deserving special respect, cannot be a human person for two reasons:

First, early events in mammalian development concern, above all, the formation of extraembryonic—rather than embryonic—structures. As the report by the Ethics Committee of the American Fertility Society (1986, p. 27) says, "This means that the zygote, cleavage and early blastocyst stages should be regarded as preembryonic rather than embryonic." . . .

Second, genetic individuality and developmental individuality do not coincide. As Grobstein has noted, at fertilization:

> uniqueness in the genetic sense has been realized, but, for example, unity or singleness has not. The zygote, with its unique genome, may give rise in either natural or induced twinning to two or more individuals with identical heredity. In some species this occurs naturally and regularly. Moreover in mice (and probably in most if not all mammals including humans) cells of two or more different genotypes can be combined to form one embryo which develops into an adult that is a mosaic of more than one genotype (Grobstein, 1988, p. 25).

A third similar objection was developed by the Catholic theologian Norman Ford (1988; answered by J. J. Billings, 1989; A. Fisher, 1991; Flaman, 1991) who argued that, though the zygote is an individuated organism, this individuality is lost when cleavage produces a loose collection of cells held together only by the jelly-like *zona pellucida*, each totipotential cell of which is capable of becoming a complete organism. Therefore, only when the possibility of twinning ceases does a new unified organism that can be hominized come into being.

The first of these objections, in spite of its support by the American Fertility Society and certain other embryologists (e.g., Austin, 1989), arises from a terminological confusion. It is misleading to speak of the inner cell mass as "embryonic," the trophoblast as "extraembryonic," and the two together as "preembryonic." In fact the blastocyst (embryo) is one living organism which has two differentiated parts: the temporary but necessary trophoblast formed from the outer cells of the blastocyst and the permanent but still very small inner cell mass. At this phase the inner cell mass consists of very few cells compared to the trophoblast because the permanent body of the child cannot grow until it has access to nourishment from its mother. For this, implantation in the uterus by means of the trophoblast is necessary (Lindenberg and Hytel, 1989). Once this is achieved, the inner cell mass grows rapidly and differentiates as the permanent body of the embryo, while at birth the placental apparatus derived from the trophoblast will be discarded. It should also be noted that some cells of the trophoblast become incorporated in the permanent body.

The second and third objection neglect much of the known detail of the embryological process. To distinguish, as Grobstein does, between "genetic" and "developmental" individuation is meaningless, since the genome guides the organism's own self-development. As we have already noted, the entire developmental sequence from zygote to mature adult is controlled by the genome, including the incorporation of new information from the environment (Ashley B, 1976; May, 1991; Moraczewski, 1990; Heaney, 1992; Ashley and Moraczewski, 1994). It is not surprising that a process so complex as human gestation sometimes fails; and in about 0.04 percent of births identical twins result (MacGillivray et al., 1988). For the human species, with its massive brain, multiple births are maladaptive. Hence, only one ovum normally matures at a time, and admits only one sperm, but sometimes two ova or more are fertilized almost simultaneously and heterozygous twins or multiple births are produced. Again, many species of animals normally produce multiple, genetically identical litters, but in the human species a zygote normally develops into a multicellular organism that retains its singleness to term. But in the first two weeks (and perhaps a little beyond) twinning (or triplets, etc.) may be produced either at the two-cell stage with two separate placentas, or in the blastocyst with one placenta, or very late with the risk of the formation of conjoined twins (cf. K. Moore, 1988, 1989; Thompson and Thompson, 1980; Sadler, 1990).

This abnormal separation of the two cells formed at the first cleavage or later of the inner cell mass of the blastocyst in probably about 30 percent of the cases is due to a genetic defect (Parisi et al., 1983) (This also happens in heterozygous twinning, Phillipe, 1985). The cause of this developmental accident in other cases is still not known. The fact that a group of cells is able after separation to develop independently into a second individuated organism in no way refutes the prior existence of an individuated organism, but confirms it. If twinning occurred at the first cleavage, then it was preceded immediately by the single-cell zygote. If it took place at some later point in the development of the blastocyst, then it was preceded by the blastocyst, which had developed normally up to that stage or its regular development would have been terminated.

Recently J. Porter, criticizing a refutation of delayed hominization by M. Johnson (Johnson vs. Porter, 1995), has argued that if an individuated human person existed before twinning, this person would have to split into two persons, neither identical with the previous single person. The embryological evidence suggests not that the original organism splits, but that it remains itself but loses one or more cells that become the twin. At this stage the abnormally separated cells are capable of developing as a distinct organism, in the manner of asexual reproduction in plants, because the expression of the whole genome still remains possible (totipotential) in all the cells of the organism, although later genomic expression is differentially limited as different groups of cells are destined to form different tissues and organs (Scott, 1991).

Nor is it true, as Ford supposed, that for a while after cleavage of the zygote only a loose collection of independent cells is present (Peredo and Coppo, 1985). Actually, after cleavage of the zygote begins the blastomeres (dividing cells forming the blastocyst) begin to compact, form interconnections, express the genome by protein synthesis (Braude et al., 1988) and, after the third cleavage, differentiate into outer and inner cells. Already in the first two cleavages the orientation of the division is genomically determined and the position of each cell in the whole is found to be significant for future differentiation (Sadler, 1990; Scott, 1991). At the first cell division, although the two cells have the same genome, they are not identical since they do not receive the same portion of cytoplasm; until implantation the total volume of cytoplasm is simply subdivided again and again. Significantly, at the second division one cell, evidently more active than the other, divides before it, so that for a time there are three (not four) cells. Even the dorsal–ventral and anterior–posterior axes on which the whole body plan of the organism is constructed are probably determined very early, perhaps even at conception. (Scott, 1991, p. 127; Gurdon, 1992).

"Infusion" of the Spiritual Soul

From a philosophical and theological viewpoint the fact of identical twinning is said to raise the question, "Since a spiritual entity is indivisible, if the zygote A was a human being with a spiritual soul, when part of its body became the twin B, where did the spiritual soul of B come from?" To answer this question we must first correct the impression given by the commonly used expression (originating in Platonic philosophy) "the infusion of the soul," meaning that God first creates the spiritual soul and then infuses it into the body.

On the contrary, the Catholic Church teaches that (a) because the soul is spiritual it cannot be produced by any material process, but can only be immediately created by God; (b) the human soul does *not* preexist its union with the human body; (c) therefore, God first creates the human body, using the human parents as his instruments, then completes this same continuous process by creating the human soul as the unifying form of the body He has prepared for it through its parents as his instruments, thus producing a unique human person. Hence God first produces and ensouls organism A designed to develop normally, but if through some genetic defect or chance some part of A, namely B, becomes separated from A at an early phase of A's development, God ensouls B just as he did A, since at this point the cells of B are still totipotential. The fact that the Creator, whose providence extends to abnormal, chance events as well as to normal, natural events, uses chance to produce individual B is no odder theologically than that he ensouls the child begotten of a sinful act just as he does one begotten in holy matrimony.

Miscarriages

Fourth, related to this last problem is the difficulty of some theologians (Häring, 1976) who are troubled by the high percentage of conceptions that never reach delivery. Some estimate this to be as high as 55 percent, although a recent study indicates this may be closer to 30 percent, as determined from the earliest stages of fertilization (Grudzinskas and Nysenbaum, 1985; Wilcox et al., 1988). They ask, "Is it possible that God could have created so many human souls, foreseeing that they will never reach the level of conscious human life?" In answer to this difficulty it should be recalled that through most of human history, at least 50 percent of all infants perished in infancy. Also, evidence suggests that syngamy frequently fails to be successfully completed (Diamond, 1975; Wilcox et al., 1988). Probably many of these imperfectly fertilized ova were never prepared for ensoulment. Although the ova were stimulated by the penetration of sperm to begin a certain number of cell divisions, these entities were never true human organisms. Thus this theological problem of apparent human wastage, which is only one facet of the general problem of God's permission of evil in the world and of miscarriages in particular, however it is to be answered, cannot be solved by a theory of delayed hominization.

Cerebration

Fifth, the basic principle on which Aristotelians based their theory of delayed hominization was that human ensoulment presupposed a highly organized body, but Aristotle gave this a still more concrete, empirical formulation. For him the criterion of this organization was the appearance in the matter of a "primary organ" through which the soul activated the organism, just as in a machine there must be a prime mover (e.g., the engine in an automobile). Therefore, a fetus could be activated not just with vegetative (physiological) life, but with animal (cognitive) life, only when its central organ of sensation with the minimal structure required for psychic functions had appeared. Mistakenly, Aristotle believed that this primary organ of sensation is the heart. Thus, on the evidence of his famous experiment in which on successive days he broke fertilized chicken eggs laid on the same day one by one to observe successive embryological phases, he concluded that the chick passed from the vegetative to the animal stage when the first signs of a heart appeared. Hence, Donceel (1970, 1985, 1986) and Pastrana (1977) argue that since in modern biology the "primary organ" is the central nervous system, especially the cerebrum which is first observable in the fetus at about three months, before this stage the embryo or fetus is not even an animal organism and *a fortiori* not human. Apart from any reference to Aristotle, others also argue that human life begins late in fetal development, at the beginning of sensation or thought (L. Sumner, 1981), brain activity (Goldenring, 1985; Shea, 1985, 1987), viability, birth, or even at one or two months of infancy.

The weakness of such arguments is evident when we take into account the fact, not known to Aristotle, that a sequence of primordial centers of organization in the embryo goes back continuously to the nucleus of the zygote, long before the brain appears as the final center. From the beginning of this developmental sequence the zygote's nucleus has contained all the information and active potentiality necessary eventually to develop the brain and bring it to the stage of adult functioning (Ashley, B., 1976). Thus, although it is true that the developing fetus first actively exhibits vegetative (physiological) and animal (psychological and motor) functions and finally, long after birth, specifically human functions, it possesses from conception the active potentiality to develop all these functional abilities. Only the minimal structure necessary for this active potentiality of self-development (even on the basis of Aristotle's philosophical principles) is required for an organism to be actually a human person, not the brain structures necessary for adult psychological activities (Australian Research Commission, 1985).

We should note here also the special problem of the anencephalic infant. "Anencephaly is a congenital absence of a major portion of the brain, skull, and scalp with its genesis in the first month of gestation" (Stumpf et al., 1990). We cannot conclude that such a child is not a human person, and certainly it must be given the "benefit of the doubt." In anencephalics the brain is seldom if ever wholly lacking, but the cerebral cortex has not developed normally and even after some development may have degenerated. "In some embryos, before degeneration has occurred, a laminated but abnormal cerebral cortex may exist. Late-gestation fetuses or infants with anencephaly may still have small foci of histologically normal cerebral cortex or olfactory tracts" (Stumpf et al., 1990). Such brain rudiments would not have developed at all unless the organism had the radical genetic capacity to produce a complete organism with a brain, as is evidenced by its otherwise often normal somatic development, but this capacity has been frustrated at some point by genetic or mechanical factors.

Personhood as Social or Legal Construct

Sixth, some proponents of delayed hominization simply bypass the whole biological analysis we have just sketched and maintain that the presence of a biologically defined human organism or "human being" does not settle the question of when the "human person," the subject of "human rights," comes into existence (Engelhardt, 1977, 1986a, pp. 104–35). The Vatican *On Respect for Human Life* (1987) asked, "How could a human individual not be a human person?" Yet J. Porter contends that "it is not *obvious* that a human organism is *ipso facto* a human person" (Johnson vs. Porter, 1995). It would seem that the reason some today argue that the terms "human being" and "human person" are not identical nor coextensive is that for them "human being" seems to be a biological term equivalent to "member of the human species," for which definite empirical criteria exist, just as for "elephant" or "pigeon." "Human person," however, seems to them to be a legal, philosophical, or theological term difficult to correlate with the biological "human organism" based on objective scientific facts. This doubt may reflect a dualistic notion of the human person, or for some it may express the conviction that the notion of "person" is not an objective datum of nature but a social construct relative to a particular culture or social system. Thus Engelhardt, Jr. (1986b) argues:

> Not all persons need be human, and not all humans are persons. In order to understand the geography of obligations in health care regarding fetuses, infants, the profoundly mentally retarded, and the severely brain damaged, one will need to determine the moral status of persons and of mere human biological life, and then develop criteria to distinguish between these classes of entities. Further, even if infants are not persons in the strict sense E.T. would be, there still may be important reasons for according special rights to infants. (p. 108)

Ethicists who hold this or similar views hasten to assure us that the social consensus on who (or what) is or is not a person should not be based on merely arbitrary criteria such as race or sex, but they insist it can never be absolute, since only adults capable of actually functioning as free citizens are unequivocally persons. Engelhardt tries to show that there can be good reasons for modern society to treat infants as persons, although, according to his criterion, they are not in fact such, while at the same time not to treat the unborn child as a person (p. 115–17). Yet he excludes seriously defective children from personhood (Engelhardt, 1986a; also Tooley, 1983).

This moral and cultural relativism rests on the assumption propagated by philosophical idealism and secular humanism that ethical values are simply human constructs relative to different cultures. But if our definition of the human person and thus of human rights is merely constructed, how is it possible to criticize the laws of the state as unjust or a culture as inhumane? We have already argued (p. 9), that personhood is not bestowed by society, but is rooted in human nature (O'Donovan, 1984). We are social beings because we are persons, not persons because society designates us as such. The criteria of personhood must transcend human laws and values, even if these are based on what appear in a given culture to be good, nonarbitrary reasons. This is why in the United States we have always appealed to the "inalienable rights of man," as does the *Universal Declaration of Human Rights* of the United Nations (1948). This need for a prophetic criticism of human laws and customs has always been the basis of the Christian theological insistence that the definition of personhood should be broad and should extend to the unborn (Dougherty, 1985; Noonan, 1985). We have also shown (p. 5) that human nature can be known, although not exhaustively, by empirical methods which can be appreciated by the scientifically trained health care professional.

Conscious and Unconscious Persons

Seventh, a final type of argument for delayed hominization probably is the underlying assumption of most of the others, namely that if the embryo or fetus is unconscious it is not really a person. How popular this notion is was vividly evidenced by the reactions to the film, "The Silent Scream." Pro-life people used this film to show that the fetus was capable of response to painful stimuli, and pro-choice people tried to refute this evidence. Thus both parties seem to think that the criterion for being a human person with rights is sensitivity to pain. The same assumption appears in the controversy over animal rights. If animals can feel pain, which is obvious, are they not persons? At least, do they not have rights that are same or similar to those of humans? Undoubtedly, a lack of respect for the life of animals and even of plants and the environment opens the way to ruthlessness toward human persons (Rodd, 1985; Mulvanney, 1986).

It is also true, however, that if the distinction between the kind of respect due to human rights and the kind due to subhuman nature is blurred, the value of both may be minimized. Some argue that, after all, experimentation on animal subjects and on human subjects is only a difference of degree (Singer, 1986). For reasons elaborated in Chapters 1 and 2, this book assumes that, although veterinary medicine is also an important profession to which general bioethics has applications, the health care profession deals with human persons whose rights are valued differently from the respect due to other forms of life.

We have already cited Tristram Engelhardt Jr.'s (1986) contention that human personhood is a social construct. In order to show that this social construction of personhood need not be arbitrary, Engelhardt supplies the following definition:

> . . . Persons are persons when they have the characteristics of persons, when they are self-conscious, rational, and in possession of a minimal moral sense. . . . [S]uch entities are *persons in the strict sense* (p. 109, italics in original).

This conception of personhood is derived from the tradition initiated by Descartes when he said, *"Cogito ergo sum"* ("I think, therefore I exist"), thus identifying his personhood with his thinking, not with himself as a thinking organism. This Cartesian assumption later became the basis of the idealism of Immanuel Kant, whose ethics, we have shown (p. 153), has greatly influenced current bioethics. It also underlies the legal positivism that makes personhood depend purely on a legislative or judicial decision. Engelhardt meets the obvious objection to identifying personhood with consciousness that even persons "in the strict sense" are not always conscious, but continue to exist while asleep or anesthetized, by arguing that their bodily continuity bridges the gaps in conscious experience since, "The body's capacities are the capacities of a person" (p. 122). But if the body's capacities are those of a person, why are not the capacities of the zygote which has the capacity (active potentiality) to develop itself into a self-conscious adult also a person and indeed the very same person as the adult into which it develops itself?

The nature of "consciousness" is highly debated in current literature (Dennett, 1995; Edlerman, 1995; Penrose, 1995; Rosenfield, 1995), but we must make a distinction between animal and human consciousness. Animals are conscious both of external objects and of internal states of pleasure, pain, fear, aggression, etc. Humans share this type of consciousness with animals, but also have the capacity for abstract thought and reflective self-consciousness, as is evident from the specifically human use of abstract and syntactic language. Once a totally unconscious fetus has developed a central nervous system it no doubt experiences a certain level of animal consciousness, but it is unlikely that even a child before the age of six or seven has more than moments of truly human, reflective self-consciousness. Are we then to say that personhood and human rights are only attributed to a child of four or five by social consensus?

Unless one is an idealist for whom the human self is nothing but thinking, a human person is an organism which sometimes sleeps, sometimes wakes, sometimes is comatose or anesthetized, and who becomes actually self-conscious only gradually and may become unconscious long before dying. But subhuman animals have no active potentiality ever to achieve such abstract and reflective thought, while the zygote has the capacity to develop itself into the human adult who thinks humanly. The ethical and political dangers in the idealistic identification of personhood with thinking on which Engelhardt's definition is based should be obvious. Because I alone am sure that I am authentically self-conscious, it is easy for me to explain the behavior of those who do not belong to my in-group as merely subhuman and animal, as slave owners once excused their treatment of black slaves.

Conclusion

We conclude this exploration of when human life begins by affirming that a bioethically adequate definition of human personhood must not only consider the person as a conscious, intelligent, free adult, but it must also include the entire biography of the unique organism, whose personhood is fully self-conscious and fully evident in morphology and behavior only at certain periods of that biography. This means that even if personhood is defined behavioristically, not only *actual,* here-and-now performance must be taken into account but the real potentiality for behavior. As embryologic research advances, the evidence that human life begins at fertilization has become overwhelming. Thus it seems difficult for a scientifically educated health care professional to doubt that he or she has been the same person with a continuous biography since that unique zygote began to develop itself into this adult who can look back over this personal history and acknowledge it as his or her own.

The medical profession, therefore, needs to work toward consensus on this issue of who is a person with human rights on the basis of what it knows best, namely, biology and psychology, plus its own professional self-understanding (Burtchaell, 1980). Such considerations may need to be tempered by legal, philosophical, or theological reflections, which in turn must take into full account and be consistent with direct professional experience. It would be a gross evasion of professional responsibility to follow the example of the Nazi physicians and leave it to demagogues to determine which human beings are persons and which are nonpersons (Lifton, 1986).

9.2 REPRODUCTIVE TECHNOLOGIES

We have dwelt at length on the question of when life begins because of its great relevance to a very ancient, practical, and heart-rending problem which physicians often meet today, infertility. We read in the Bible the story of Hannah, one of the two wives of Elkanah, father of the great prophet Samuel.

> Her rival [Penninah, who had several sons and daughters], to upset her, turned it into a constant reproach to her that the Lord had left her barren. This went on year after year; each time they made their pilgrimage to the sanctuary of the Lord, Penninah would reproach her, and Hannah would weep and refuse to eat (1 Sm 1:5–7).

The principle of personalized sexuality (p. 210) indicates that God made us sexual not only for the survival of our species, but for the complete expression of a married person's mutual self-giving love that finds its complete fulfillment not just in orgasm but in children. Yet in the United States (OTA, 1988, p. 3):

> Infertility, generally defined as the inability of a couple to conceive after 12 months of intercourse without contraception, affects an estimated 2.4 million married couples (data from 1982) and an unknown number of would-be parents among unmarried couples and singles.

Infertility has many causes: venereal infections (20 percent), hormonal disturbances, endometriosis, abortions, contraceptive practices, drugs, genetic and chromosomal abnormalities, "gametic interaction" (physiological incompatibility of the couple's gametes), cancer, iatrogenic and other factors. As high as 20 percent of the cases are simply unexplained by present diagnostic procedures, while explained infertility is attributed about equally to male and female partners (OTA, 1988, p. 61–82). The best remedy is the prevention of such conditions. Many cases also yield to relatively simple therapies, but physicians faced with the urgency of the existing problem have developed more ethically dubious methods of solving it, notably artificial insemination and laboratory reproduction.

Collection of Gametes

For diagnosis of male infertility, it is necessary to obtain semen to examine the presence of sperm cells, their number in a given volume of semen, and their motility. Diagnosticians generally prefer this to be obtained by masturbating, both because of convenience and because the ejaculate obtained is most indicative of what is present in intercourse. Other less preferred methods are to use residual semen in a perforated condom used during intercourse or to aspirate a sample from the testicles. Some physicians question whether such testing is even necessary, since it is generally satisfactory first to determine if the wife is infertile, and if she probably is not, then to assume male infertility and to deal with this by such remedies as are now available. Similar procedures are necessary if sperm is to be used in the various methods of artificial reproduction.

It has been argued that self-stimulation by a man whose aim is not to seek genital satisfaction but to obtain a semen sample for a legitimate purpose, for either testing or artificial reproduction, is not masturbation. This argument, however, seems mistaken, because the means used to obtain this legitimate end is in fact the production of a solitary orgasm and ejaculation. Thus this is the use of an evil means for a good end, since it violates the purpose of genital acts, which are essentially interpersonal as stated in the principle of personalized sexuality (p. 210).

For certain methods of artificial reproduction it is necessary that mature ova be collected from the female after medical stimulation of her ovaries to produce several mature ova at the same time. These are then removed either through the vagina by ultrasound guidance or surgically by a small laparoscopic incision. These procedures do not seem to violate the principle of totality and integrity, since the mature ova removed will be replaced by others. But there is a serious question about the use of "fertility drugs" to mature several ova at once, since this may very well result in a woman finding herself pregnant not only with twins but even with sextuplets! We have already pointed out why it is maladaptive for the human species to have multiple simultaneous pregnancies and births. Moreover, it is becoming common practice (Farrell, 1995) to solve this problem by "selective pregnancy reduction," i.e., abortion of the feebler fetuses in such a human litter.

Artificial Methods of Reproduction

Artificial insemination is any process by which fertilization of an ovum results directly not from the normal marital act, but as the result of sperm being introduced into the woman's vagina artificially. The sperm used in artificial insemination may be from the husband of the woman who wishes to conceive; if so, the process is referred to as *homologous insemination* or *artificial insemination by the husband* (AIH). If the semen is from a man other than the husband, it is known as *heterologous insemination* or *artificial insemination by a donor* (AID).

Although the feasibility of artificial insemination of human beings was known in the past century, it was not practiced to any significant extent until the 1930s and has now become common. People who have children in this way, however, usually do not care to reveal the fact, and thus it is difficult to collect accurate statistics. Judging from the number of scientific and popular articles written on the subject in the past few years in the United States and elsewhere, many thousands of children are conceived and born as a result of artificial insemination (Olshansky and Sammons, 1985).

The process of artificial insemination is comparatively simple (Strickler, 1975). Semen is collected, usually by masturbation, into a sterilized container. Sometimes the semen may be frozen and used at a later date, but more frequently it is used within a few hours. If the semen of a donor is used, some attempts are made to screen him in order to avoid transmitting a disease, especially AIDS, but recent surveys indicate that only one third of the donors are screened (Olshansky, 1985). The semen is introduced into the vagina as near as possible to the day of ovulation by means of a syringe or plastic cap placed at the cervix. Recent studies show that conception results in approximately 60 percent of the cases; a higher percentage results if insemination is repeated over a number of cycles.

In natural reproduction, one ovum is released into the fallopian tube each month at midmenstrual cycle. During intercourse, millions of spermatozoa are deposited in the vagina. Many of them swim through the uterus, but only a few dozen reach the ampullary end of the fallopian tube, and only one can successfully penetrate the ovum so that conception results. A recent study seems to show that normally fertilization takes place on the very day of ovulation, within no more than five or at most six days after intercourse (Wilcox et al., 1995). The resulting embryo remains in the fallopian tube for two or three days and then enters the uterus, where it implants in about a week.

The process of *in vitro* fertilization with embryo transfer (IVF–ET) was originally a remedy for infertility from blocked fallopian tubes, but it is now used for many types of infertility (Seppälä and R.G. Edwards, 1985, Seppälä and Hamberger, 1991; Cataldo, 1996). Several mature ova (oocytes) which have been obtained as already described are treated (capacitated) to improve the chances of sperm penetration. Sperm (usually obtained, as noted, by masturbation) is also prepared by various processes and placed with the oocytes *in vitro*, where fertilization of the oocytes takes place with the formation of several zygotes. After they have been cultivated for about forty hours, three to six zygotes that seem most normal are selected and transferred to the uterus. If there are "extra" embryos, either they are frozen (cryopreservation, CPE) with the intention of using them later for the same or another woman, or they are destroyed. Some countries allow research on "extra embryos" (Warnock Report, 1985).

According to the *New York Times* (Gabriel, 1996), there are now some thirty clinics in the United States performing some 40,000 IVFs a year at a total expense of some $350,000 million, with a 37 percent profit to the clinic and a cost to an individual couple from $11,000 to $25,000 or more. Success rates vary highly, from 0 percent for one clinic to 15 percent at the best clinics, and many are in the lower range. Another report (Cataldo, 1996) claims that for the United States success rates are 26 percent for pregnancy, 17 percent for delivery. Some couples repeat these procedures many times, and the strain, expense, and disappointment are often severe (Lauritzen, 1990; Farrell, 1995).

Other Methods

Among the other procedures which have been tried are low tubal ovum transfer (LTOT), which tries to bypass obstructions between ovary and uterus by removing one or more ova and then transferring them to the uterus to be fertilized by normal intercourse (McCarthy, 1983). Although LTOT was deemed acceptable by the Archbishop of Cincinnati (Griese, 1987), its success rate was very low, probably because conception normally takes place in a fallopian tube. Therefore, other methods use tubal transfer. In pronuclear stage tubal transfer (PROST) the oocyte is transferred before syngamy is complete so that conception takes place in the mother. In zygote intrafallopian tube transfer (ZIFT) a single zygote is transferred, thus avoiding the death of other zygotes or multiple pregnancy. The latter has produced about 29 percent pregnancy and 23 percent delivery (*ibid.*, p. 1124).

To increase the chances of successful fertilization when there is a low sperm count or unfavorable interaction of the gametes, intracytoplasmic sperm injection (ICSI) is used. In this method semen is collected and treated, and then single sperms are injected directly by microscopic needle into each of the oocytes. A procedure whose efficacy is still doubtful is intrauterine insemination (IUI), in which the sperm is inserted into the vagina, or near or within the cervix, to insure that access by a large number of sperm to the oocyte is increased. In natural cycle oocyte retrieval intravaginal fertilization (NORIF), an oocyte which has matured naturally is removed at the time of ovulation and placed with sperm in a culture medium in a special vial, which is then placed in the vagina for forty-eight hours for fertilization to occur. The embryo is then removed and transferred, with about 10 percent pregnancy resulting. In gamete intrafallopian tube transfer (GIFT), the process of IVF is commonly followed (although the semen may be collected not by masturbation but during sexual intercourse about two hours prior by the use of a perforated condom), except that the oocytes and sperm are not put together *in vitro* but injected into a fallopian tube at the end nearest the uterus, where about 34 percent pregnancies occur with about 26 percent successful deliveries.

Since only zygotes that appear normal are accepted for transfer, in these procedures birth defects seem no more frequent than those occurring in natural generation and it seems that the process itself is not the cause of the birth defects (Seibel, 1988). The success rates, as already indicated, are not high and are often achieved only after several attempts. Each attempt costs anywhere from $6,000 to $10,000 and the process is usually not covered by private health insurance or HMOs (*New York Times*, July 27, 1988).

From a legal point of view, the children resulting from artificial insemination and *in vitro* fertilization with embryo transfer have been in an ambiguous position. In some countries, laws considered heterologous insemination (AID) as a form of adultery, and thus the children would be considered illegitimate. At present in the United States, it seems that children born of gametes of the parents would be considered legitimate without question (Strasberg-Cohen, 1982).

Ethical Evaluation

In evaluating both artificial insemination and *in vitro* fertilization, the Church relies on the principle of personalized sexuality, which teaches that the family is the complete fulfillment of human sexuality and that the unitive and procreative aspects of the act of generation must not be separated by a deliberate human act. To act otherwise is to contradict the natural and moral order of human reproduction revealed by God and manifested in human experience (John Paul II, 1984b). This is the principle on which the CDF document *Instruction on Respect for Human Life* (1987) is based, and the diverse reactions of theologians to this document was due chiefly to their attitude to this principle (Shannon and Cahill, 1988).

Since the principle of stewardship and creativity (p. 207) favors technology if it ecologically perfects the natural order, artificial reproduction is not wrong because it is artificial, but because the particular set of techniques usually so named separate the procreative from the unitive purpose of the marital act, just as contraception separates its unitive teleology from its procreative purpose. The principle of moral discrimination requires that in judging the morality of an act one must first consider its moral object which, if it is intrinsically bad, cannot be justified by some further good purpose. "The desire for a child is a good intention, but the good intention is not sufficient reason for making a positive moral evaluation of *in vitro* fertilization between spouses" (CDF, 1987); i.e., the end does *not* justify the means.

Already Pope Pius XII (1956b) had condemned heterologous artificial insemination (i.e., from a donor not the husband, AID) and implied that homologous artificial insemination (from the husband, AIH) was also to be rejected. Some Catholic theologians, however, thought the pope's statement ambiguous and maintained that AIH would be acceptable, provided the semen was not obtained by masturbation (Griese, 1987; Häring, 1973). Hence, in the CDF (1987) *Instruction on Respect for Human Life* the teaching of the Church in regard to both AIH and AID, as well as IVF–ET, are summarized in four principles:

1. Human procreation must take place in marriage.
   The procreation of a new person, whereby the man and the woman collaborate with the power of the creator, must be the fruit and the sign of the mutual self-giving of the spouses, of their love, and of their fidelity. The fidelity of the spouses in the unity of marriage involves reciprocal respect of their right to become a father and mother only through each other (p. 23).
2. Using the sperm or ovum of a third party is not acceptable.
   Recourse to the gametes of a third person, in order to have sperm or ovum available, constitutes a violation of the reciprocal commitment of the spouses and a grave lack in regard to that essential property of marriage which is its unity. . . . Moreover, this form of generation violates the right of the child; it deprives him of this filial relationship with his parental origins and can hinder the maturing of his personal identity (p. 24).
3. Generation of the new person should occur only through an act of intercourse performed between husband and wife.
   Fertilization is licitly sought when it is the result of a conjugal act which is per se suitable for the generation of children, to which marriage is ordered by its nature and by which the spouses become one flesh. . . . Spouses mutually express their personal love in the language of the body which clearly involves both spouses' meaning and parental ones. . . . It is an act that is inseparably corporal and spiritual. It is in their bodies and through their bodies that the spouses consummate their marriage and are able to become father and mother (p. 27).
4. The fertilization of the new human person must not occur as the direct result of a technical process which substitutes for the marital act.
   Homologous artificial fertilization in seeking a procreation, which is not the fruit of a specific act of conjugal union, objectively effects an analogous separation between the goods and the meaning of marriage (p. 27).
   Conception *in vitro* is the result of the technical action which presides over fertilization. Such fertilization is neither in fact achieved nor positively willed as the expression and fruit of a specific act or the conjugal union (p. 30).

Some have questioned the statement in point 2 that IVF violates the rights of the child, saying, "How can a child have rights before it exists?" Yet, it is not odd to claim that it is unjust to illegitimate children to bring them into the world outside wedlock. Similarly, we can reasonably say that it is unjust to children to bring them into the world without the assurance that they originated in the natural marital act of their parents which is the natural expression, designed by God, of the couple's permanent union. As the number of these artificial births increases in our society, every child will wonder whether it really has the profound natural bond to its parents on which its security ultimately rests.

Unfortunately, in our opinion, *Ethical and Religious Directives* #41 is not very precisely stated:

> Homologous artificial fertilization (that is, any technique used to achieve conception using the gametes of the two spouses joined in marriage) is prohibited when it separates procreation from the marital act in its unitive significance (e.g., any technique used to achieve extracorporeal conception).

This should be interpreted in the light of the *Directives'* own reference (note 29) to the *Instruction on Respect for Human Life*, which more clearly rejects all forms of AIH. Hence, the example which Directive 41 gives in parentheses should not be understood as saying that AIH separates the unitive and procreative significance *only* when the conception is extracorporeal, that is, when IVF is used. Even if the conception takes place within the woman's body AIH is forbidden if the placement of the semen in the vagina is not the result of marital intercourse.

Thus, the Church has a very different view of what is ethical and what is not in human reproduction from that of many in the health care professions (cf. American Fertility Society, 1986; Alpern 1992). The *Instruction* makes very explicit the criterion by which unethical assistance can be judged from ethical, as follows:

> Homologous IVF and ET is brought about outside the bodies of the couple through actions of third parties whose competence and technical activity determine the success of the procedure. Such fertilization entrusts the life and identity of the embryo into the power of doctors and biologists and establishes the domination of technology over the origin and destiny of the human person. Such a relationship of domination is in itself contrary to the dignity and equality that must be common to parents and children (II. B., 5).

Unethical Modes of Reproduction

It seems clear, therefore, that IVF, PROST, ZIFT, and ICSI are all morally unacceptable because they "replace the conjugal act (even if the sperm is collected morally)" since "the immediate conditions of fertilization are created by the procedures themselves." Not only do these procedures have this essential defect, but the frantic efforts of couples to obtain a child by any means are leading to many abuses (Lauritzen, 1990; Farrell, 1995). "[E]xtra embryos are routinely frozen or used in experimentation" and such "practices constitute the moral equivalent of abortion. In these technologies the zygote and embryo are also externalized, placing their lives at additional risk" (Cataldo, 1996). NORIF is also unacceptable; even though fertilization takes place within the body, it is directly the result of the procedure and isolated from the body by the vial in which it takes place.

GIFT, which has the highest success rate of any of these methods, is defended as ethical by some Catholic moralists (McCarthy, 1988; Cataldo, 1996). It has not explicitly been rejected by official church teaching. Cataldo's argument is that, if masturbation is not employed, none of the seven or so required interventions by technicians in the reproductive process in themselves "violate the intrinsic link between the conjugal act and procreation." Thus, he argues, "The number of steps in between the conjugal act and fertilization is not morally decisive for the difference between assistance and replacement, but rather it is whether any one or more of those steps constitute the immediate conditions by which fertilization takes place." (Cataldo, 1995).

We agree, however, with DeMarco that even if fertilization is not extracorporeal, the ethical defect of GIFT is that fertilization is not directly the result of the marital act, since the semen used is not deposited by that act in the vagina, but by a technician's manipulation which substitutes for the marital act (DeMarco, 1988). Hence, "the immediate condition by which fertilization takes place" it seems to us is not the marital act but the technician's manipulations. Nor is it relevant to cite as a precedent the traditional statement of the moral manuals, for which also Pius XII made allowances, that it would permissible (if it were shown to be effective, which seems not to be the fact) for the husband to use some device to move semen higher into the vagina or uterus to enhance the possibility of conception. In that case it was supposed that the semen was deposited in the vagina of the woman by normal intercourse and remained within her.

Surrogate Motherhood

The Church certainly rejects "surrogate motherhood," understood as the agreement by a woman to carry a child for a married couple or for a person other than her spouse, because it involves the gamete of a third party. The CDF document states (1987):

> Surrogate motherhood represents an objective failure to meet the obligations of maternal love, of conjugal fidelity, and of responsible motherhood; it offends the dignity and the right of the child to be conceived, to be carried in the womb, to be brought into the world and to be brought up by his own parents; it sets up to the detriment of families a division between the physical, psychological, and moral elements which constitute those families (p. 25).

The Supreme Court of New Jersey determined in the famous "Baby M" case that surrogate contracts are not valid and that the mother should retain visitation rights, no matter what agreements were made before the birth of the baby (Hanley, 1988). Although the decision applies only to the state of New Jersey, it serves as a guide for decisions in other states. One commentator on the Baby M case remarked that surrogate motherhood calls on a woman to be everything a mother should not be (Callahan, 1987a).

Another form of surrogate motherhood is for a woman to donate ova to an infertile woman for use in some form of IVF (or even GIFT). This too falls under the ethical objections to both IVF and AID, producing a child who is not the offspring of the marital act of the couple, but of a technician using the ovum and sperm of two persons not united in marriage. It could be asked, however, whether a fetus already conceived might be transferred to the womb of another woman who would carry it to term? This might be compared to the old practice of the poor "wet nurse" who relieved upper-class women of the inconvenience of nursing their children. Catholic moralists condemned this latter practice except in cases of necessity to save the life of the infant or the mother, and it would seem similar reasoning could be applied to fetal transfer when necessary to save the child or the mother's life, but not otherwise.

Although some reactions (McCormick, 1987; Vacek, 1988) to the *Instruction on Respect for Human Life* (CDF, 1987) accused the Church of being behind the times, others welcomed it as a needed warning directed to the reproductive changes that science has introduced into human society without benefit of public discussion (NCR, 1987).

A variety of bizarre cases are reported in the press, some of which have reached the courts: IVF technicians using their own sperm without the knowledge of couples, a woman in South Africa who became pregnant by IVF with ova from her daughter and sperm from her son-in-law, a feminist sperm bank in California which supplies sperm for lesbians, another in the same state which supplies sperm donated by Nobel Prize winners, and a divorced man suing to have embryos destroyed which he and his former wife had produced by IVF and then put in cold storage!

9.3 AMNIOCENTESIS AND FETAL TESTING

Amniocentesis

The need to develop satisfactory therapies for gene defects is medically important, as is evident from the following statistics. There are approximately 3,000 different diseases which are known to involve single defective genes (Ngyan and Sahat, 1987). Today, 33 percent of infant deaths are related to genetic causes. More than 100 genetic conditions can be diagnosed prenatally. Parent carriers of defective genes may have as much as a 50 percent risk of generating offspring with a genetic defect. The polygenic conditions, such as diabetes mellitus, gout, and some allergies, occur in 1.7 to 2.6 percent of all live births. There seems to be approximately a 5 percent incidence of genetic disease in all live births (Kahn, 1987; Osmundsen, 1973; Taysi, 1983).

The medical specialty of diagnosing and attempting to treat these genetic defects, as well as the task of screening populations for them and counseling couples who are or may become parents of defective children, is developing rapidly (Capron, 1984; 1993b; Clark A., 1994). A technique frequently employed in diagnosing the genetic and sexual characteristics of unborn infants is *amniocentesis,* by which the genetic condition of the unborn child can be determined by examining the amniotic fluid in which the fetus floats in the womb. Another technique is *chorionic villi sampling,* in which a plastic catheter is inserted through the cervix to biopsy villi or hairlike projections of the placenta. This test may be performed about eight weeks earlier than amniocentesis, and the results of chromosome tests of these rapidly growing tissues are available in a few days (Holder, 1985; Kahn, 1987). Unfortunately, although some remedies for the consequences of genetic defects are being worked out, so far the prospect of methods for correcting the defective genes themselves by DNA recombination seem clouded and generally involve unethical IVF (Hendren and Lillehi, 1988; NIH, 1987). While there is some danger of an abortion accidentally resulting from amniocentesis or chorionic villi sampling, and while some use prenatal testing to determine whether or not they will seek an abortion, Pope John Paul II recently wrote in *The Gospel of Life* (1995), n. 63:

> Special attention must be given to evaluating the morality of prenatal diagnostic techniques which enable the early detection of possible anomalies in the unborn child. In view of the complexity of these techniques, an accurate and systematic moral judgment is necessary. When they do not involve disproportionate risks for the child and the mother, and are meant to make possible early therapy or even to favor a serene and informed acceptance of the child not yet born, these techniques are morally licit. But since the possibilities of prenatal therapy are today still limited, it not infrequently happens that these techniques are used with a eugenic intention which accepts selective abortion in order to prevent the birth of children affected by various types of anomalies. Such an attitude is shameful and utterly reprehensible, since it presumes to measure the value of a human life only within the parameters of "normality" and physical well-being, thus opening the way to legitimizing infanticide and euthanasia as well.

Some scientists, in the name of preventive medicine, advocate prenatal or postnatal *genetic screening* of the whole population for four purposes: (1) to advance scientific research, since such research is necessary to achieve full understanding and control over human inheritance; (2) to assist responsible parenthood so that carriers of genetic defects may not pass them on; (3) to make possible early therapy before the malfunctioning of defective genes has caused extensive damage; and (4) to give the parents the option of aborting the child when the defect is serious and no therapy is yet known (Macklin, 1985; Murray et al., 1984).

Later in this chapter we will discuss why this last purpose is ethically unacceptable, but the first three are certainly legitimate. They do, however, raise serious incidental questions (Capron, 1984). First, the research purposes of genetic screening must be regulated in the same way as any other type of research on human subjects (see p. 324). Although the risk of miscarriage as a result of amniocentesis has been reduced with the help of sonography to less than 1 percent, it cannot be used unless there are also proportionate benefits for the fetus and, as we have noted, therapeutic help for a genetically deficient fetus is at present limited. Some ethicists maintain that amniocentesis benefits the fetus because it helps the parents prepare more adequately for the birth (Dube, 1983). In sum, amniocentesis is indicated only when a pregnancy is thought to be at increased risk for a particular disorder (Kahn, 1987). Recently, Roy (1984) has pointed out a more profound ethical issue that may result from prenatal screening:

> Prenatal diagnosis delivers the knowledge required to exercise the kind of quality control over the unborn that amounts to a control over birth. . . . The earlier long-standing belief of a theocratic reproductive culture in the equality of all human beings based on the identity of their origin and destiny has given way to an emphasis on the empirical inequalities of human beings.

Most screening techniques used postnatally only involve the withdrawal of an insignificant amount of body fluid or tissue and are harmless. Nevertheless, informed consent is required in all such cases, and it is highly questionable to enact laws that require compulsory screening for research purposes alone. Even when consent is given, care must be taken about how the information is used (Crauford and Harris, 1986). If the results are made known to subjects, there is danger that they may misunderstand or exaggerate the seriousness and possible consequences of their condition or the condition of their children. If the results are known to others, there is danger of stigmatization, e.g., to label African-American carriers of the sickle cell trait or Jewish carriers of the Tay-Sachs syndrome as inferior or somehow dangerous to others.

Second, the use of screening to promote responsible parenthood is in general a laudable purpose, since couples undoubtedly should not bring into the world children for whom—with the reasonable assistance of society—they cannot adequately care, and since the care of defective children presents special burdens. Consequently, prospective parents have the duty to seek the scientific information useful to such decisions, and society has the duty to assist them in obtaining such information (John Fletcher, 1982). Moreover the right of married couples to beget children is conditioned by their capability to provide for them. (NCCB, 1973, p. 6)

Eugenics

Caution is necessary, however, in the face of programs of *negative* eugenics advocated by certain enthusiasts (Glass, 1975; Modell, 1982; Osmundsen, 1973) who argue that modern medicine has upset the ecological balance by saving the lives of more and more defective persons who formerly would have died before they could reproduce; and who claim that the load of defective genes in the gene pool is increasing so that a much higher level of genetic disease may soon occur in the population. But as Lappe (1972) has written:

> The consensus of the best medical and genetic opinion is that whatever genetic deterioration is occurring as a result of decreased natural selection is so slow as to be insignificant when contrasted to "environmental" changes, including those produced by medical innovation (p. 421).

If only those persons who themselves suffer from a particular genetic disease are prevented from reproducing, this still does not eliminate heterozygous carriers who will continue to transmit defects dependent on recessive genes (Thompson and Thompson, 1988). At present, technology is far from being able to detect all these carriers. Even if science had this ability, such elimination would extend to many people. This would probably also mean the elimination from the gene pool of many desirable traits because the same persons carry both good and bad traits, which sometimes are genetically linked in ways still very obscure (Andrews, 1994). Thus programs of negative eugenics based on present knowledge would achieve their goals only very slowly, over many generations, and might have side effects worse than the evils they would remedy. Moreover, as defective genes are eliminated from the gene pool, they are constantly being replaced by mutations caused by environmental factors.

It seems, therefore, that genetic information ought not be used to compel persons to refrain from reproduction, but it may be supplied to them to enable them to make responsible personal decisions. Even here, however, some public caution is needed. Some states have adopted compulsory screening of newborn infants to detect those afflicted with phenylketonuria (PKU), a genetically based metabolic disease that results in mental retardation and can be treated by diet (Andrews, 1985). After these programs were instituted, it was discovered that some persons who test positively do not develop mental retardation and that the dietary treatment to which they were subjected may even have been harmful (Barden et al., 1984). Thus genetic testing programs have to be carefully designed. The Research Group on Ethical, Social, and Legal Issues in Genetic Counseling and Genetic Engineering (Hastings Center Institute, 1972) has suggested guidelines, which can be summarized as follows:

1. The attainability of the program's aims should be pretested by pilot projects and other studies, and the program should be constantly evaluated and updated.
2. Community participation in planning and executing the program should be secured to educate the public as to the true significance and legitimate use of the information obtained.
3. The information obtained should be made available according to

clearly stated policies known to those participating before they consent, and their privacy should be carefully protected.

4. Screening programs should be voluntary. The rights of parents to make their own decisions about the use of the information in family planning should be protected and care taken to avoid stigmatizing them or their offspring.

5. Information about screening should be open and available to all, with priorities given to well-defined populations suffering from frequent defects.

6. Programs should not be instituted unless the tests used are able to give relatively unambiguous information, and this should be precisely recorded.

7. The general principles with regard to experimentation with human subjects, such as informed consent and protection from risks, should be observed.

8. Persons to be screened or who have their children screened should be informed before they consent about the nature and cost of therapy and its risks, or if no therapy is available.

9. Counseling to help the subjects understand and deal with the information should be provided.

We would also add that it is important to consider whether the cost in money and personnel in administering such programs give them high priority in view of the rarity of most of these conditions. It must be recognized, however, that in some cases (e.g., PKU) the testing per subject is quite inexpensive, whereas the cost of caring for even a few mentally retarded children in institutions may be very high.

9.4 ABORTION

In what follows, we assume the conclusion of 9.1 that it is at the least highly probable—and therefore in moral decisions *practically* certain—that from conception (syngamy) the human organism is a human person endowed with a spiritual soul and therefore endowed with the same human rights as any adult person. Its right cannot be placed in competition with those of the mother, because both have the same basis and are equally to be respected.

Some, however, who admit this conclusion, nevertheless still argue that no one but the mother has a right to decide whether she must carry the child to term. Thus Judith Jarvis Thomson (1971, 1983), in a widely quoted and anthologized article, argued that a woman has an abortion not to deprive the child of the right to life but only to defend her own right, in some circumstances at least, to refuse to lend her body for the child's support. The most plausible case is that of the rape victim who is forced to care for a child for whom she has never willingly taken responsibility. Consequently, we will discuss the abortion question and its legal consequences at some length (Grisez, 1970a; Callahan, 1970; Dworkin, 1993).

Direct and Indirect Termination of Pregnancy

Abortion is the termination of a pregnancy with resulting death of the human fetus. Abortion may occur spontaneously, in which case it is usually called a *miscarriage,* or it may be caused deliberately and is called an *induced* or *procured abortion.* Catholic theologians also distinguish between those procured abortions that are direct and indirect. A *direct abortion* is one in which the direct, immediate purpose of the procedure is to terminate the pregnancy by destroying the human fetus at any stage after conception or to expel it when it is not viable. Most procured abortions are direct in nature. An *indirect abortion* is one in which the direct, immediate purpose of the procedure is to treat the mother for some threatening pathology, but in which the death of the fetus is an inevitable result that would have been avoided had it been possible. Two examples of indirect abortion are surgery for ectopic pregnancy and surgery for a cancerous uterus when the woman is pregnant.

The *Ethical and Religious Directives* (United States Catholic Conference, 1995b, nn. 47, 49; cf. Connery, 1977) permit indirect abortion if the conditions for the application of the principle of double effect are met:

1. The procedure itself is directly for the purpose of treating the mother and is thus not intrinsically unethical.
2. The mother and physician do not have any evil circumstantial intention; that is, they would save the child if they could.
3. The death of the child is not the *means* by which the mother is treated, but only a result of the treatment; that is, it is not a cause but an effect of the act.
4. There is a proportionate reason if the treatment is necessary to save the life of the mother, especially since the child is doomed anyway.

While these norms are certainly correct, there remains debate among moralists over what standard medical procedures to save the mother from a tubal rupture and hemorrhage will only indirectly result in the death of the child and thus permit the application of the principle of double effect. William E. May (1994) has argued that while removal of a portion of the pathological tube along with the fetus is permitted, it is not permitted to use linear salpingostomy which only splits the tube so as to leave it intact, because in that case it is necessary to free the tube that the fetus be detached. To do this, in May's opinion, is to cause the child's death as a means to save the tube and protect the mother from serious harm. For the same reason he rejects the use of the drug methotrexate, which causes degeneration of the fetal implantation in the tube and hence frees the tube by killing the fetus (Carson and Buster, 1993).

Nevertheless, other moralists (deBlois, 1994; Moracewski, 1996), with whom we ourselves agree, have argued that while to detach a child from its *normal site* of implantation in the mother is clearly direct abortion, to detach it from an abnormal site in which it cannot live for long and in which it causes serious pathology in the mother is a different case altogether. In this latter case the moral object intended is not the death of the infant as a means but the treatment of the pathological condition in the mother by freeing her tube of an abnormal infiltration of the placental villi of the child. In doing so, of course, the physician has, at least theoretically, the responsibility to replace the fetus in a normal position (deBlois, 1994). Recent attempts to do this have not yet been successful but may be in the future. The fact that such a technique is not yet developed excuses physicians not engaged in research in the matter from even attempting it, but it illustrates that the intention of the procedures themselves do not aim at the death of the child as a means to treat the pathology of the woman. It would seem that *Directive* n. 47 (ERD, 1995) is phrased so as to leave this question open.

History of Abortion and Infanticide

The real area of difficulty, therefore, concerns *direct* abortion, of which many millions are now performed each year in the world. On this subject there is an age-old controversy (Brodie, 1994). Although in all human cultures people have valued, loved, and protected their children, and this care has been recognized as one of the most basic of ethical responsibilities, direct abortion has also been widely practiced. A study of primitive cultures (Devereux, 1955) shows that the motivation for abortion in these cultures is highly varied, including not only pragmatic reasons, but also religious and symbolic reasons arising from unconscious urges, such as hostility to male domination. This was also true of the ancient civilizations, although here economic and demographic factors came more and more to prevail. Thus, in the Greco-Roman world in which Christianity arose, abortion and infanticide in some places produced rates of reproduction below the level of zero growth (Noonan, 1967). For these cultures it can generally be said that abortion and infanticide were not strictly distinguished (Carrick, 1985). In Roman culture, for example, an infant did not have legal status until accepted by the *paterfamilias*. This gave rise to the tradition that illegitimate persons are, in effect, nonpersons.

In contrast to these views is the attitude in the Jewish Scriptures. For the Jews, all human life has as its author the One God, whose creative power produces the child in the mother's womb and brings it step-by-step to full life. The parents play only an instrumental role in this creative process, so that from the beginning a direct, personal I–Thou relation exists between the Creator and the human being whom he is creating, just as truly as he created Adam and Eve. Several of the prophets of Israel express the profound religious conviction that it was God who formed them in their mother's womb for a special purpose (e.g., Jdg 13:5; Is 49:1; Jer 1:5; Job 31:15; Ps 119:73). These texts led to later theological speculations among the more mystical or philosophical Jewish thinkers on the time of the "infusion of the human soul." These speculations joined with Greek philosophical tendencies that enhanced respect for the dignity of the unborn. In any case, Orthodox Jews are convinced that when the child of a Jewish mother becomes a "living soul," it is destined for the Kingdom of God, although this membership in the Chosen People requires for the male that it be sealed after birth by circumcision. Thus death in the womb does not exclude salvation (Feldman, 1986b).

Jewish thought in practical ethics, however, has been dominated by the legislation of the Torah, which in time was elaborated by the system of rabbinical interpretation that became normative for postbiblical Judaism. The Torah inculcates a high respect for human life, and the rabbis insisted that since the principle of justice is "an eye for an eye, a tooth for a tooth, a life for a life" (Ex 21:23–25; Rosner, 1986), one cannot sacrifice one human life for another unless that other is an aggressor or criminal in some way. Consequently, Judaism has resolutely opposed any form of infanticide and has required Jews even to accept martyrdom rather than to kill innocent persons. But the rabbis also held that in conflict situations where the life of the mother is endangered, the child can be considered an "unjust aggressor" or "pursuer" against whom the woman can defend herself. In such cases, therefore, for Jews induced abortion is permitted. Hence, a child is not considered to have a full right to life until birth, or "when the head emerges."

This rabbinical reasoning was confirmed by the fact that the law in Exodus 21:22 sets only a monetary fine for one who causes an abortion by striking a pregnant woman. Some rabbis, however, following the Septuagint translation of Exodus 21:11, drew the line before which abortion was permitted more strictly at the stage when the fetus assumed human form. Others wished to draw the line 30 days *after* birth if the delivery was premature. There were also wide differences on what degree of danger to the mother justified induced abortion, some even accepting psychological reasons as sufficient justification when they threatened the married life of the couple. Underlying all these debates, however, is the basic Jewish conviction of the high value of marriage and of children to preserve the Chosen People (Meier, 1986).

Jesus did not repudiate the Jewish Scriptures, nor even their rabbinical applications, but he gave them his own characteristic interpretation by stressing that God's care extends to every human being, no matter how sinful, ignorant, or ritually unclean. Jesus preached the good news of God's love for the "little ones," the outcasts rejected by secular and religious authorities, including powerless little children, whom he declared should be given special respect as privileged members in his Father's Kingdom (Mk 9:33–37). Far from being un-Jewish, Jesus' attitude represents the deepest prophetic spirituality of Israel.

Christian Rejection of Abortion

The Christian Church, confronted with the widespread Greek and Roman practices of infanticide and abortion, evaluated such customs in the light of this teaching of Jesus on the dignity of children. Luke, in his infancy narratives based on Judeo-Christian sources, takes up the Old Testament theme of the prophetic vocation and pictures John the Baptist as called to his mission by the Holy Spirit already in Elizabeth's womb (Lk 1). In striking parallel to this, Jesus as the new Adam is created by the overshadowing Spirit in the Virgin Mary's womb, where he is already Lord, the Holy One, the Son of God. Thus the Old Testament conviction that God is the creator of human life from the moment it begins, so that the human person is defined primarily by this unique I–Thou relation to its Creator rather than by the legal provisions of Exodus, has always guided Christian thinking about the unborn child.

The dignity of the child asserted by Jesus led to the practice of infant baptism in the Church, which made even more evident the wickedness of abortion. While the Catholic Church today does not teach that unbaptized children are excluded from salvation (Catechism, N.1261), it does insist on the grave responsibility of parents to have their children baptized in order to assure them of the graces Jesus intended for them.

The sacredness of human life is so fundamental to the practical moral exhortations of the New Testament that abortion is not even mentioned in the teaching on family life in the Epistles. In the *Didache*, however, a manual of Church discipline written in the Apostolic period, probably in Jewish–Christian circles, it is explicitly forbidden. Yet in conflict cases, Christian theologians, like the rabbis, sometimes engaged in casuistic controversy. As Connery (1977) has shown, a few Catholic theologians in the past favored the notion that when the mother's life is threatened, the child is an aggressor, as do some Protestant and Eastern Orthodox even at present (J. Davis, 1984). Recently some Catholic theologians have also attempted similar opinions (C. Curran, 1979; D. Maguire, 1986). Since as far back as 1679, however, the Catholic popes have repeatedly reaffirmed that the killing of one person could never be a means of therapy for another because such a practice seems utterly inconsistent with the equal dignity of human persons.

These controversies in Judaeo-Christian tradition will be examined here only briefly; readers may refer to the detailed studies of Noonan (1970a, b; 1985); Ramsey (1973); Connery (1977), Lotstra (1985), and McCartney (1987). It should be emphasized that this disagreement on how to deal with rare conflict cases does not negate the basic agreement among Jews and all the Christian churches (1) that abortion is contrary to the will of God, who creates each human person, and (2) that if abortion is ever permissible in a conflict situation (and this is denied not only by Catholics but by many Protestants), it can be justified only by the most serious reasons. This ought to be a basis for religious Jews, Protestants, Orthodox, and Catholics to work together to decrease the great number of abortions in our country which cannot reasonably be excused as "conflict cases," but are simply for convenience or to escape the consequences of irresponsible behavior.

Following the tradition of the early Church, Vatican II condemned procured abortion along with infanticide as an "unspeakable crime" (1965c, *Gaudium et Spes*, n. 51). This teaching was made even clearer in the *Declaration on Procured Abortion* (CDF, 1974) and subsequent documents. Finally in *The Gospel of Life* (1995), John Paul II has made clear that it is a doctrine pertaining to the Christian faith and can never be changed:

Therefore, by the authority which Christ conferred upon Peter and his successors, in communion with the bishops—who on various occasions have condemned abortion and who in the aforementioned consultation, albeit dispersed through the world, have shown unanimous agreement concerning this doctrine—I declare that direct abortion, that is abortion willed as an end or as a means, always constitutes a grave moral disorder, since it is the deliberate killing of an innocent human being. This doctrine is based upon the natural law and upon the written word of God, is transmitted by the church's tradition and taught by the ordinary and universal magisterium. No circumstance, no purpose, no law whatsoever can ever make licit an act which is intrinsically illicit, since it is contrary to the law of God which is written in every human heart, knowable by reason itself and proclaimed by the Church (n. 62).

Since Vatican II declared that doctrines taught by the ordinary and universal magisterium (the bishops and pope teaching in agreement on matters of faith, even when not assembled in an ecumenical council) are infallible, it is now evident that this is an infallible teaching based on the Word of God. Hence, acceptance of this teaching is required of all Catholics. Note that this authoritative Catholic position does *not* depend on the view argued in 9.1 that human personhood begins at conception, but rather on the following proposition stated in the *Declaration on Procured Abortion* (CDF, 1974):

> From a moral point of view it is certain that even if a doubt existed whether the fruit of conception is already a human person it is an objectively grave sin to dare to risk murder.

In view of these unequivocal statements of the Catholic Church, the proposals of Daniel Maguire (1986), Carol Tauer (1985), and others to apply the methodology of probabilism to cases of abortion because of remaining doubts about delayed hominization or conflict situations can no longer be defended, since even "solidly probable" moral opinions do not prevail against certain moral truth confirmed by the highest teaching authority in the Church. While proportionalists may still argue about how to define "direct abortion," it is difficult to see how this statement of John Paul II can be evaded.

Woman's Right to Decide

The teaching of the documents we have just quoted refers to the *objective* morality of abortion, i.e., to the *de facto* violation of human rights. *Subjectively*, of course, a pregnant woman may in good faith believe that not to have an abortion will do more harm (not only to herself but to others) than to have one. Pope John Paul II (1995) referred to the subjective element of decisions to have abortions and stated:

> Decisions against life sometimes arise from difficult or even tragic situations of profound suffering, loneliness, depression and anxiety about the future. Such circumstances can mitigate, even to a notable degree, subjec-

tive responsibility and the consequent culpability of those who make choices which in themselves are evil (n. 18).

Denes (1976), Francke (1978), and Reardon (1987) have documented subjective factors in a very sensitive way from actual interviews with women who have had, or are about to have, induced abortions. Some of the considerations frequently cited in favor of a woman's right to make this decision for herself are as follows:

1. A woman has to bear the risk and burden of pregnancy, delivery, and child care, which she will hardly be able to sustain unless to do so is her own choice.
2. Sometimes in the case of very young, inexperienced, or retarded women and in the case of incest or rape, a woman has little or no responsibility for the pregnancy, yet she must bear the consequences.
3. Even when she has shared in the responsibility for the pregnancy, the woman nevertheless has the right to a normal sex life, on which her marriage and care of other children also depends; however, contraception does not give her complete control over pregnancy. Therefore she has the right to use abortion as a last resort.
4. For a woman to bear an unwanted child is a disaster for the child as well as for herself, because no matter how the woman may try, she may not be able to provide the child with the necessary psychological atmosphere. As a result of her own psychological tensions, this may lead to child neglect or abuse.
5. A woman who discovers she has a defective child, especially a genetically defective child who may perpetuate the defect, has an obligation not to bring a child into the world whose life will be one of suffering and a burden to society (Clayton, 1994).
6. A woman cannot depend on help from society to care for her unwanted child, nor to provide for the child's adoption. Such help is often insufficient and given on degrading conditions.
7. A woman should not be forced to obtain an abortion from an illegal and probably dangerous abortionist, perhaps at the risk of death or of future sterility.
8. Modern women should be free to fulfill their duty of contributing to the solution of the very serious modern problem of population control by using abortion as a backup when contraception fails or is unavailable.
9. Women should not be inhibited in their use of this right of choice by suffering interference from others who attempt to impose their own religious value systems on others, or punish women for having sex, or arouse neurotic guilt feelings in those who choose abortion (Harrison, 1984). It is especially unfair that men, who do not experience pregnancy, should have the power to tell a woman what she should do with her own body.

Thus the apparent advantages of abortion for the woman and for society are very tangible. In a concrete situation, many may concur that the opposite disadvantages of pregnancy seem so overwhelming, especially if the woman is poor, already heavily burdened with children, and physically or psychologically ill, that the woman may believe that there is no other way out. As Wahlberg (1973) puts it, "Those who are not involved personally with an unwanted pregnancy tend to discuss the philosophical, medical, or moral questions. Those who face nine months of pregnancy and 15 to 20 years of child raising are more concerned with the immediate crisis."

Faced with a woman in such a dilemma, it may seem to a compassionate health care professional that it would be utterly cruel and inhumane to refuse the medical cooperation she requests. Physicians (and also pastoral counselors) dread this situation and find it extremely difficult to refuse to assist the woman in distress. This is especially difficult when they are convinced that the woman will have the abortion anyway from an illegal abortionist or by self-inflicted methods, or may even commit suicide, so that the physician's refusal to cooperate will still not save the child. Thus it may seem contrary to the command of Jesus, "Do not judge, and you will not be judged" (Mt 7:1), for Christians to condemn as murderers such women and the compassionate physicians who assist them. Yes, instead of judgment, Christians must seek ways to assist women to escape such anguishing dilemmas. The right of the mother to compassion, however, is based on the same grounds as the child's right to life, so that human sympathy and justice must be given to both. As John Paul II says in *The Gospel of Life* (1995, n. 57):

> As far as the right to life is concerned, every innocent human being is absolutely equal to all others. This equality is the basis of all authentic social relationships which, to be truly such, can only be founded on truth and justice, recognizing and protecting every man and woman as a person and not as an object to be used.

Right of the Unborn to Life

Thus some of the effects of permitting abortion must also be considered.

1. By choosing to abort the child, the mother seeks to defend her own rights by destroying another human being, an action that is radically unjust to another and contrary to her own moral dignity as a person. It is true that the continued existence of the child places a woman in a unique relation to another person existing within her own body, yet the harm she suffers from this is only a relative harm for which other remedies may be sought, even if her life is endangered. The fetus, however, suffers the absolute loss of the right to live, for which no remedy is possible (Krason, 1983). However tangible and certain are the rights of the mother, the evil consequences to the child are still more tangible, certain, and immediate. A woman who threatens to kill herself

or who may die in childbirth is still faced only with a *possibility* of death, which may never occur and which she may take other steps to prevent. Abortion, however, dooms the child irretrievably. Richard A. McCormick, SJ, arguing as a proportionalist, has concluded (1973, 1984b) that it is difficult to see what collection of values favoring putting to death an innocent human being could be proportionate to the one basic value of that person's right to live. How can even the rights of the mother or of society outbalance the right of an innocent human being to life?

2. Abortion of children in difficult cases encourages the widespread practice of abortion in much less justifiable cases because it becomes the easy way out. Thus the preponderance of evidence is that the social approval of abortion will imperil many more lives of children than social disapproval (about a million and a half a year in the United States), even taking into account the prevalence of illegal abortions. Furthermore, children raised in a society where it is known that abortion is permitted, or that their mothers have had an abortion, lack the important psychological assurance of unqualified parental acceptance if the child, once born, is found defective.

3. Women are encouraged and even forced by society to act in a way contradictory to their love and care for their own and others' children. It is risky to suppose that apparent social approval of abortion will do more than cover up the deep conflicts that this introduces in a woman's self-regard or in society's appreciation of the dignity of women as persons. Furthermore, the physical risks of abortion (including sterility) are not negligible, nor is the argument significant that the risks are less than those of childbirth, since maternal mortality with proper medical care today is very low.

4. Abortion policies also tend to exclude the father from his proper responsibility for pregnancy and for the child and from his role of supporting his wife and sharing her burdens. Thus he, too, is degraded as a person and burdened with deep conflicts.

5. Unmarried women, mentally retarded women, and victims of rape and incest deserve the protection and care of society, which is too likely to dispense itself from this obligation simply by providing abortion as a solution. The same is true of poor women, whose rights to raise a family are ignored by the encouragement of abortion to keep down welfare expenses.

6. The family institution, which is basic to society, is further weakened when the values of parenthood and of the child as a gift of God are undermined by the spreading practice of abortion, which today is an important element in the decline of the family in the United States. Little evidence suggests that such practices encourage an attitude of responsible parenthood; rather, they promote irresponsibility by providing an easy way to escape its consequences. Thus, although very effective in population control, abortion is not a sound long-term solution for a long-term global problem.

7. Easy abortion encourages in society and in individuals an attitude of low regard for the human person, as such, and favors a merely functional evaluation of persons in terms of their actual, present contribution to economic productivity and subjective well-being. This is contrary to the advance of the concept of the dignity of the person and of inalienable rights, on which modern democracy is based. The mother's rights have the same foundation as those of the child. That is, the human personhood that mother and child possess are equal, and it is this equality of rights that it is the prime purpose of society to protect. We Americans are horrified at the genocide practiced by the Nazis, Communists, and others, but have become complacent about the fact that we are guilty of our own holocaust of millions of children, more than were destroyed in the Nazi Holocaust (Arkes, 1994)!

It seems that what really lies behind the pro-choice position is the view that precisely because the problem is so complex and incapable of an objective solution, it must be left to the mother herself to decide because she is the one most affected. This is to forget the child, however, who is affected even more directly. Also, this abdicates society's responsibility to protect the child, even against the mother, a responsibility generally accepted without question when it concerns child abuse or infanticide (although even infanticide has its current defenders; Tooley, 1983). No one would argue today that a slave master should be left free to do with his slave what he thinks best because the slave is *his* property; yet the pro-choice position treats the child as the mother's property to dispose of as she wishes.

Why Norm Against Direct Abortion Is Absolute

Thus, John Paul II's *The Gospel of Life* (1995, n. 57) not only defined, against proportionalist contentions, that abortion is part of the infallible teaching of the Church but also that the direct killing of innocent human beings can never be ethically justifiable. Some have accused the Church of contradicting its own teaching by permitting killing in self-defense, in a just war, and in the punishment of criminals, but these are cases of aggressors who have forfeited their right to life by deliberately attacking the right of others to life. One obvious exception to this absolute norm against direct killing of the innocent, however, has been proposed by some critics of the authoritative Catholic teaching against direct abortion, which they believe reduces the position to absurdity, that is, the case where a physician can only save the mother by killing the child, but seems required by this rule to let both die. This theoretical criticism can be answered in several ways. O'Donnell (1976) provides a detailed analysis of the so-called medical indications for therapeutic abortion. He shows that today the medical profession has solved this dilemma by providing the physician with the means to save both mother and child, or at least to deal with the problems of both when both are at risk, without attempting to choose the life of the mother against that of the child. Grisez (1970a) and Joseph Boyle (1980), while maintaining firmly that direct abortion is always wrong, answer the problem of choosing between mother and child by a more careful formulation of the principle of double effect, which they believe permits the physician in extreme situations to kill the child *indirectly* in saving the mother.

Related Issues

Since direct abortions are intrinsically evil, it is hardly necessary to discuss in detail the various methods used to produce them. The later the stage of pregnancy, the greater danger to the mother. This was recognized even in *Roe v. Wade,* although subsequent judicial decisions favoring the so-called "right of the woman to decide" in effect have made restrictions on late pregnancies difficult. Recently there has been controversy over "partial birth" abortions, in which very late in the pregnancy the brain of the child is sucked out in order to make removal of the body easier. The cruelty of abortion has become more evident to some who previously had not recognized it due to this process.

But surgical abortion at any stage, whether it be by suction, destruction by a saline solution, or dissection of the fetus, is a brutal business. Hence, there is a demand for supposedly less violent methods and especially for an "abortion pill" that a woman can take at home to terminate her pregnancy at the earliest possible stage. Such drugs are now becoming available, notoriously RU-486 (Crooij et al., 1988). The purpose of RU-486 (mifepristone) has sometimes been disguised by calling it not a contraceptive but a "contragestant" (Baulieu, 1989; 1991), or it has been advocated as "an abortifacient to prevent abortion" (Grimes and Cook, 1992) or its legislation has been urged on the grounds it may have other therapeutic uses. In spite of the enthusiastic promotion given such highly profitable drugs, it is not true that they make possible "safe, private" termination of pregnancy (Nathanson, 1992a). To be relatively safe and effective, RH-486 requires at least four visits to a physician. No doubt in the future, however, methods of abortion will be found which will make any legal regulation as difficult as the control of narcotics has proved.

Three of the *Ethical and Religious Directives* (ERD, 1994) relate to questions sometimes raised in relation to abortion:

D.47. Operations, treatments, and medications that have as their direct purpose the cure of a proportionately serious pathological condition of a pregnant woman are permitted when they cannot be safely postponed until the unborn child is viable, even if they will result in the death of the unborn child.

D.48. In case of extrauterine pregnancy, no intervention which constitutes a direct abortion is morally licit.

D.49. For a proportionate reason, labor may be induced after the fetus is viable.

These are all applications of the principle of double effect and should be interpreted with careful attention to all the conditions required by that principle

(p. 196). Thus No. 47 distinguishes truly necessary treatment for serious pathologies of the mother, which happen to produce an *unintended* side effect injurious to the child, from direct abortion, in which the death of the child is an *intended* means used to treat the mother. Examples of such pathologies might be uterine cancer demanding hysterectomy, or other cancers requiring radiation harmful to the fetus, or fulminating infection which has spread from the fetus to the mother. As we have already noted, No. 48 is stated in such a way as to leave open the possibility for the development of effective techniques by which the abnormally located fetus can be removed to the woman's uterus so as to save its life and correct the tubal pathology of the woman. It also seems to leave open the debated question as to what surgical technique is permitted in treating the tubal pathology (Moraczewski, 1996). The cases of anencephalic infants and others with genetic disabilities pose a question: May infants with these abnormalities be delivered early? If the infant is human, delivering it before viability constitutes an abortion because the early delivery *ipso facto* kills the baby. Some authors believe early delivery would be ethical before viability (Bole, 1992) and ethical after viability (Drane, 1992). However, these opinions seems to use the term viability in an equivocal manner. Viability is not a general characteristic which all infants acquire at the same time. An anencephalic infant, to whom no aggressive care will be given, cannot be declared viable at the same time of pregnancy as a nomal child, to whom aggressive care will be given to prolong its life. It seems the *finis operis* of the early delivery of an anencephalic infant is to hasten or cause death. Thus, we believe the anencephalic infant should be allowed to go to term, be baptized, and be allowed to die (O'Rourke, 1996).

What practical conclusions for health care professionals can be drawn from this discussion? The following norms are drawn from a pastoral document issued by the National Conference of Catholic Bishops (NCCB, 1974) and are helpful in determining what to do in particular situations.

Conclusion

1. Catholic hospitals cannot comply with laws requiring them to provide abortion services, even on the ground of material cooperation (NCCB, 1994, D. 45).
2. Catholic physicians, nurses, and health care workers who work in facilities that provide abortion services may not take part in such procedures in good conscience. Their rights of conscience in this regard are recognized by federal law (E. Rubin, 1987).
3. Physicians, nurses, and health care workers should give public witness to their belief in the sanctity of life, the integrity of every person, and the value of human life at every stage of its existence by their compassion and care for their patients.
4. Physicians, nurses, and health care workers who work in facilities that provide abortion services should notify the institution in writing of their conscientious refusal to participate in such actions.
5. Abortion is a serious and immoral action. Catholics who perform or

obtain an abortion, or persuade others to do so, are doing grave harm to another human being against the Christian commandment of love of neighbor. All who willingly and deliberately assist in abortion procedures share the sinfulness of this destructive act. This is particularly true of the attending surgeon and the health care personnel who administer abortifacient drugs or other abortion procedures.

6. Cooperation in the sinful act of abortion would not ordinarily extend to preparing patients for the procedure or providing aftercare. Christian witness, however, may well require Catholic nurses to avoid even those actions, which (although not necessarily evil in themselves) may be interpreted as a compromise of Christian values.

7. Under Church law, those who perform or obtain an abortion or deliberately persuade others to do so incur an automatic excommunication. The purpose of this severe penalty is to reinforce the Christian tradition that the Second Vatican Council (Vatican Council II, 1965c) repeated when it declared, "Abortion and infanticide are unspeakable crimes." Of course, it must be understood that this automatic excommunication applies only to those who know that they are incurring it, yet freely choose to do so, understanding that they are committing a serious sin. This excommunication, as with all others, can be removed by sincere repentance and confession, with the purpose of trying to make amends to others for the harm done, insofar as this is possible. The tragedy of at least a million lives a year destroyed in the United States by the medical profession through abortion can only be contemplated with profound sorrow and the determination to work to educate people about its great injustice in the same way as to work against racism and war.

9.5 THE LAW AND ABORTION

Abortion in a Pluralistic Society

In 9.1 we discussed the biological facts concerning human personhood and the ethical norms that follow from these facts. Worthwhile laws are built on relevant facts and are based on ethical norms. Have the legislators and courts in the United States who have made statements about human personhood and the rights deriving from it been consistent with biological fact and ethical reasoning? This is the consideration of the following discussion.

Since the very nature of a profession involves a certain autonomy, as recognized by the principle of participation (p. 222), it is understandable that health care professionals are very reluctant to permit laypersons, including legislators, to prescribe limits for professional activities. The autonomy of the profession, however, is relative to its purpose of serving the health not only of individual patients, but also of the community. Laws have to be made to restrain lawyers, and even the clergy have had to submit to some government regulation of their activities (e.g., the clergy may not perform marriages between parties who do not have a license). The medical profession has generally accepted such regulations as those relating to dispensing narcotic drugs and to issuing death certificates.

Far more important is the question of the legal definition of the human person, which necessarily determines who are the subjects whose rights must be respected in every medical decision. Defining the human person affects the question of abortion and also concerns many of the problems concerning death, as discussed in Chapters 11 and 13. It would seem obvious that laws should supply such a definition, yet historically it has been assumed that the matter is so obvious as to require no definition (St. John-Stevas, 1961, 1971). Yet our American legal tradition has always been ambiguous on this question (Horan et al., 1987; Shaw and Doudera, 1983; Brodie, 1994), as is evident from the history of slavery and racial discrimination in the United States, where there has been a long struggle to have members of the racial minorities recognized as full persons with rights equal to those of the majority.

Medieval and British common law regarded abortion as a serious crime, although the courts were not always clear as to whether or at what stage of pregnancy abortion was to be punished as homicide. In 1803, the first statute law in the United States on the subject declared abortion to be a crime punishable by death if the child had "quickened" and by lesser but serious penalties if the child had not. Throughout the nineteenth century in England and in the United States, increasingly strict laws were passed against abortion, but with exceptions for therapeutic abortion to save the mother's life. Such legislation was strongly supported by the American medical profession, partly because the medical risks for the mother in abortion were still high, but also because the advance in embryology had convinced physicians of the humanity of the fetus (Mohr, 1978).

A number of factors, however, were at work in the opposite direction. First, in Europe and the United States, the value systems of humanism, Marxism, and Fascism, with their emphasis on human technological control over life, came to dominate the profession. Hence, as abortion became medically safer, it seemed to many just another effective method of controlling human destiny. Second, the antiabortion laws proved increasingly difficult to enforce equitably, since women of means could obtain an abortion on therapeutic pretexts, whereas poorer women could not. This reason seems to have greatly influenced many clergymen and physicians who worked with the poor, as has Dr. Bernard Nathanson (1983; Nathanson and Ostling, 1979). Nathanson recounts his change of mind to an antiabortion position after seeing the enormous increase in abortions, which he and his associates had not anticipated when they worked for permissive legalization. Third, the increasing concern over the population explosion and the growing tax burden for social welfare suggested that abortion was a very effective method of reducing the birth rate, at least as a backup to contraception. Fourth, the feminist movement, which originally opposed abortion, began to favor it as giving women more control over their own lives and greater equality with men. Fifth, the emphasis on the right of privacy in sexual matters increased with the spread of new contraceptive methods and the "sexual revolution."

The Supreme Court Decision

New York, Colorado, and California adopted very permissive laws with regard to abortion in the 1960s. Finally, on Jan. 22, 1973, the U.S. Supreme Court, in *Roe v. Wade* and *Doe v. Bolton*, came to the decision that it is unconstitutional for any law to infringe on the right of privacy, by which a woman has the sole power of decision as to whether to have an abortion, just as couples have the same right to the practice of contraception (Krason, 1983). The great ethical difference between contraception and abortion was ignored. Perhaps, however, this confusion indicates, as we have noted elsewhere, that the contraceptive mentality is intimately related to the abortion mentality (John Paul II, 1995, n. 13). Although some laws regulating medical procedures, especially after the first trimester of pregnancy and even more restrictively after the second trimester, were not automatically excluded by the court as having possible constitutional validity, the right of the woman to decide was stated unequivocally. Also, the court reinforced this in later cases by declaring that a woman did not need the consent of the child's father to have an abortion, nor did a minor need the consent of her parents. Surprisingly, in *Maher v. Roe* (1977), the Supreme Court ruled that this right of the woman to have an abortion does not imply that she has the right to have assistance for such an abortion from state or federal funds, since the government as a matter of public policy can favor childbirth over abortion, provided that it does not infringe on the woman's freedom. Several states have sought to limit the practice of elective abortions by specifying requirements in regard to informed consent or parental permission, but for the most part the courts have declared this legislation unconstitutional (Haas-Wilson, 1993). Critics point out that this decision again introduces the factor of inequity, which had been one of the strongest arguments for liberalization; that is, under previous laws poor women could not have an abortion, but well-to-do women could.

The main complaint, however, that can be brought against the present stance of the Supreme Court is not that it has moved to protect the woman's rights, which is entirely in accord with its main historical effort to strengthen and extend human rights. Rather, the primary criticism is that the court has simply evaded the question of the rights of children, unborn as well as born, on the very flimsy pretext that it is a speculative question on which there is no general agreement (Dellapenna, 1987; Noonan, 1979). One may well ask when there has been more than a verbal general agreement on the issue of rights for racial minorities or for women. It is just because such issues are highly controversial and "speculative" that the Supreme Court has the duty to face them squarely. In fact, the court has decided that the unborn child is not a human being with human rights, but it has not done so honestly nor persuasively, as will be evident to anyone who checks the unscholarly history of the controversy with which it documented its decision (Ely, 1973). As Callahan (1973a) has said:

> It is often thought that when the State withdraws from resolving "speculative" questions (by definition those which command no consensus?) then freedom is somehow served; that was the gist of all those arguments

which would leave abortion decisions up to individual choice and conscience. I have always found that an odd kind of contention, one which, if followed rigorously, would leave all decisions bearing on concepts of "justice," "equality," "the general welfare," and the like up to individual consciences as well. For what notions could be more speculative in their final meaning and implications, to judge from all the disagreement they provoke (p. 7)?

Some who favor the Supreme Court's stand have tried to blunt this issue by arguing that the court has not only considered the mother's rights, but has in effect also protected the right of the unborn child not to be born into a world where the child is unwanted and may suffer from physical or psychological disabilities. If a child does have such a paradoxical right, however, then the child has the right to choose to live or not live, just as the mother has the right to choose to abort or not. This right of the child to choose to live is denied when the mother exercises her right to abort. Thus the question of conflict of rights cannot be evaded (Garfield and Hennessey, 1984). Either the rights in question are not truly rights, or some way to balance them must be found. The Court has simply confused this question.

Abortion and Public Policy

Supreme Court's evading of the fundamental issue of whether the child as well as the mother is the subject of human rights has led to a vigorous pro-life movement whose membership includes not only Catholics but a large number of those of other faiths (J. Davis, 1985; McClendon, 1986; Wilson, 1994). In fact, evangelical and fundamentalist Christians seem more militant on this issue than do Catholics. The Catholic bishops have expressed support for some type of antiabortion amendment, leaving the choice of its exact form to public discussion, and have launched a campaign of education on the "respect life" question, but have not entered directly into the political arena.

After the failure in the 1980s to pass a constitutional amendment against abortion, hopes were raised for a reversal of *Roe v. Wade* due to the appointment of conservative Supreme Court justices, but this also soon failed. At present the Democratic Party officially backs "a woman's right to choose," while the Republican Party claims to be "pro-life," but only its "religious right" wing unequivocally opposes abortion. Some efforts at the state level are being made to restrict certain forms of abortion, but whether these will pass the constitutional test before the present Supreme Court is very doubtful. As for public opinion in the United States, it would seem that the majority would permit abortion in hardship cases but would probably not support "abortion on demand" (Cook et al., 1992).

The pro-life movement, however, is severely criticized by some groups in the United States who in other matters have been strong supporters of human rights and social justice. These proponents of civil liberties charge that the pro-life members focus all their interest in human rights on the unborn, while showing little concern for the social injustices suffered by those already born (Jackson, 1988). One might ask if social justice and civil rights enthusiasts are not equally inconsistent when they hail *Roe v. Wade* as a triumph for civil liberty and connect abortion with the cause of women's rights. Both sides need to realize that human rights can only be furthered by a broad and consistent effort to extend legal protection for every human being regardless of race, sex, religion, and age, from conception to death. Moreover, the debate about how best to protect human rights must not be clouded by accusing this or that party to the debate with imposing their religious values on others, when in all such debates every side, religious or secularist, is necessarily advocating a particular value system with which others will differ.

American pluralism demands that minority groups have a right to advocate their own values and to attempt to assign these values an influential role in public decisions. Catholics begin to wonder what will happen to their values if the courts, in the name of women's rights, seek to require Catholic hospitals and Catholic health care professionals to cooperate in abortion. So far, the law and the courts have been rather careful to protect the consciences of health care professionals in such matters, but this protection may break down as Catholics become integrated into a national comprehensive health care program or enter into joint ventures with non-Catholic hospitals, especially those run for profit. Recently a professional accrediting agency for physicians studying in obstetrics and gynecology attempted to force medical residents to be trained in abortion procedures, without regard to conscientious objections, but widespread protest made them retreat from this demand (ACGME, 1995).

Despite the U.S. bishops' advocacy of pro-life, some Catholics are hesitant to support legal restrictions of abortion. They argue that Catholics should work to educate the public to the evils of abortion but should not favor laws against it, since in a pluralistic society this can only be divisive and ineffectual (Cuomo, 1985; Donceel, 1985). But what, then, of the rights of the powerless unborn? John Paul II in *The Gospel of Life* (1995) points out that the evil of abortion is not only a matter of the individual conscience, but a grave social evil, the responsibility for which belongs to legislators and judges who have promoted abortion, to those who have encouraged "the spread of an attitude of sexual permissiveness and a lack of respect for motherhood," and finally to "the network of complicity which reaches out to include international institutions, foundations and associations which systematically campaign for the legalization and spread of abortion in the world (n. 59)." Later in the same encyclical, however, he says (n. 90):

> The church well knows that it is difficult to mount an effective legal defense of life in pluralistic democracies because of the presence of strong cultural currents with differing outlooks. At the same time, certain that moral truth cannot fail to make its presence deeply felt in every conscience, the church encourages political leaders, starting with those who are Christians, not to give in, but to make those choices which, taking into account what is realistically attainable, will lead to the reestablishment of a just order in the defense and promotion of the value of life. Here it must be

noted that it is not enough to remove unjust laws. The underlying causes of attacks on life have to be eliminated, especially by ensuring proper support for families and motherhood.

Pro-Life Education and Health Care Professionals

Catholics, therefore, if they are to be true to their belief in the advocacy of helpless and neglected persons, need to work vigorously for practical legislation—ultimately a constitutional amendment correctly defining the subject of human rights, but at least for positive efforts to reduce the number of abortions. It is certainly not enough for a politician to say, "I personally disapprove of abortion, but I do not believe in imposing my private views on the public," since that amounts to a public official saying, "I personally abhor racism, but do not want to impose my private opinions on others." Reading the materials prepared by the American bishops on the respect-life issue will show that Church leadership in the United States is making a great effort to propose a consistent program of social justice in accordance with papal teaching, of which the defense of the unborn is only one part (Bernadin, 1986; NCCB, 1974, 1986). The problem is that this consistent peace-and-justice stand is little noticed in the public media, nor well-communicated from the pulpit, nor emphasized in Catholic religious education. Nor is much money spent to educate the public in the most effective way of getting public notice, TV advertising.

Undoubtedly, the task of Catholics as a community should first and last be educational rather than merely political. Jesus has taught trust in the power of truth, love, and forgiveness rather than in the power of law or law enforcement. Political action cannot be neglected, but it must be supported by a more transformative educational effort. In this struggle to promote respect for the rights of the human person, the battle over abortion is only one element, although the primary issue since it involves the very definition of personhood and the most fundamental of rights (Hitchcock, 1984). What confronts Catholics is the religion of humanism, with its own value system supported by the economic, cultural, and political power of the elites who dominate modern life (Hitchcock, 1982; Hittinger, 1996).

The health care professional and Catholic health care institutions have crucial roles to play in this educational effort regarding all medical–ethical issues and their social impact. They have the biological and medical information necessary to understand such issues, and they have the professional prestige and influence to be heard. Above all, they deal with the concrete situations in which a respect for life can be most clearly witnessed. In using this legitimate power, they need not think that they are imposing their religious views on others, provided they seek to listen to and respect the conscientious convictions of others in the debate, without un-Christian attitudes of judgment and labeling.

Undoubtedly, the outcome of all the struggles over laws that affect the medical profession will be various forms of compromise that shift and change in each generation. Nothing is wrong with compromise when required to achieve common action in a society. It is wrong, however, when the form this compromise takes is determined by the cowardice of those who should have spoken up for persons who cannot speak for themselves.

CONCLUSION

Catholic tradition in regard to the generation and birth of children is based upon the firm conviction, drawn from Sacred Scripture and reason, that the family is the God-given entity for cocreating human life. Moreover, the acts of love and unity proper to married couples are the only human acts worthy of bringing new life into the world. The family is not only the proper source of life, but also the proper setting for education in virture for the young. Closely allied with the teaching in regard to family and reproduction is the teaching in regard to the sanctity of each human person. Thus, the teaching of the Church in regard to abortion and fetal testing are also of great importance in contemporary society. But unfortunately, contemporary society is blind to the meaning of sanctity of life, especially for the weak, and the meaning of family as the only proper site for reproduction. In a word, the teaching of the Church in this regard is counter-culture. The task of the Catholic society is not only to live the teachings of the Church but also to defend and explain the teaching, using the science and language of contemporary society.

10

Conception Control, Contraception, and Natural Family Planning

OVERVIEW

In the previous chapter we dealt with abortion, the destruction of human life already conceived, and with artificial reproduction which, though it seeks to overcome infertility, often does so by means which also involve the destruction of newly conceived human life. Our principle concern in this chapter is with the ethical and medical problems in the responsible regulation of conception itself. We will deal first with ethically questionable means of regulating conception, contraception (10.1) and sterilization (10.2), and then with ethically acceptable methods (10.3). In 10.4 we will also deal with women's right to protect themselves against pregnancy by rape. Finally, in 10.5 we will explore the question of the pastoral care of those who are struggling with the sexual and reproductive problems treated in this and the previous chapter.

10.1 CONTRACEPTION

A Crisis in Ethical Thinking

The ethical issues related to contraception, although less serious than those of abortion which we discussed in the last chapter, nevertheless are intimately connected to abortion, as is evident from the following statement from a report on RU-486, the "abortion pill" (Gervais and Miles, 1990):

> Abortion will continue to be a large part of women's reproductive choices. Two-thirds of all women have unintended pregnancies, half from contraceptive failure. Half of all unintended pregnancies are electively terminated. Contraceptive research and family planning education remain controversial and disrupted public activities. Abortion is and will remain a fact of American life.

Moreover, a study of the controversy over contraception is of wider significance for bioethics than the particular issue itself, because it is in many ways typical of the struggle of the Church to bring the light of the Gospel and its rich tradition of moral reflection to bear on current medical problems. The Church's fidelity to its tradition and mission is too often represented as intransigent conservatism or as a power struggle by reactionary clergy to control the progressive laity. Hence, we will devote what may seem a disproportionate amount of space to the history of the contraceptive controversy.

Our approach to this topic recognizes the painful fact that today the Catholic community is profoundly divided on the issue. Such divisions over ethical questions are not rare in Church history. One has only to think of how issues of ethnicity, racism, slavery, and economics have all produced widespread dissent from papal and episcopal guidance. In many countries there is a deep gap between the ways in which this teaching is presented and interpreted by priests and theologians, and between this teaching itself and the actual lives of Catholics.

Some Catholics are convinced that the outcome of this debate can only be the ultimate reversal of the present official teaching; others look for its ultimate vindication. Evidently a process of discernment is still going on within the Christian community. Our aim is to present the different aspects of the question as fairly as we can and correctly convey the definitive official teaching, since this is essential information for the well-informed Christian conscience (p. 49).

The rise of a new value system, in the form of the humanism of the Enlightenment in the eighteenth century and of the immense social changes brought on by the Industrial Revolution in the nineteenth century, led to a renewed Christian concern for the family as an institution in society. In the twentieth century this concern has been intensified by the rapid rise in the divorce rate and the decline of the birthrate in "advanced" countries toward zero growth. Humanists generally accept these changes as an inevitable part of technological progress, to which social mores must be adjusted by what is often called "the sexual revolution" (Greer, 1984).

Christians have reacted in different ways. Some reassert traditional norms (Quay, 1988). Others attempt to rethink these norms (Shannon and Cahill, 1988). The chief point of controversy among Christians, however, has been whether the practice of contraception will further weaken marriage or can be used to strengthen it (J. Kelly, 1986).

The Christian Tradition Against Contraception

Contraception is the performance of sexual intercourse with the deliberate intention of rendering infertile an act which could be fertile. The practice of contraception is very ancient (Noonan, 1965; Riddle, 1992). The Bible tells the story of how Onan, grandson of Jacob, evaded the Levirate law (Dt 25:5–10; Ru 4:7–12) requiring him to beget with Er's widow an heir for his dead brother. So that he would not have to share inheritance with an heir, he "wasted his seed on the ground" (*coitus interruptus*) and "What he did greatly offended the Lord, and the Lord took his life" (38:9–10). Some recent exegetes think Onan was punished not for his contraceptive act, but for violating the Levirate law. But, as a Jewish scholar has pointed out, such a violation was not a capital offense and was easily compensated (Dt 25:9). Hence what so gravely offended God could not have been Onan's evasion of the Levirate law, but the contraceptive means he used to do so (Sacks, 1990).

In New Testament times contraception and, when this failed, abortion and infanticide were common pagan practices, abhorred by the Jews and even denounced by the Greek philosophers. The Christian biblical understanding of God's purposes in creating us sexual, as we have formulated it in the principle of personalized sexuality (p. 210), maintains the ethical inseparability of the unitive and procreative purposes of sexual acts. From this biblical principle it is obvious why Christians from the very beginning rejected contraception. Since all genital sex outside marriage was considered sinful, contraception outside marriage was condemned because it facilitated sin. Within marriage contraception was also rejected, because it separated the unitive and procreative meanings of marriage which the Creator had inseparably joined in creating us sexual, and thus devalued family life.

Although contraception continued to be practiced both in and outside marriage by some Christians, its sinfulness was never questioned in any of the major Christian churches until the present century, when new methods of "birth control" became readily available. These more effective methods and the "sexual revolution" (p. 211) greatly encouraged contraceptive practices; but at first these were seen by Christians as a facilitation of extramarital sex and as such were condemned. A basic change of attitude among the Protestant churches was finally initiated by the Anglican Church when at its Lambeth Conference in 1930 it declared that contraception in marriage might be morally justified for economic or health reasons (Gallagher, 1981). In defense of the traditional Christian view, Pope Pius XI reacted sharply in the encyclical *Casti Connubii* (1930) in which he declared:

> . . . any use of marriage, whatever, in the exercise of which the act is deprived through human industry of its natural power of procreating life, violates the law of God and of nature, and those who do anything of this nature are marked with the stain of grave sin.

Pius XI's teaching was frequently repeated with greater precision by Pius XII. For example, in 1951 in an "Allocution to Italian Midwives," Pius XII said:

> Matrimony obliges to a state of life which, while carrying with it certain rights, also imposes the fulfillment of a positive work concerning the state of life itself. . . . On married partners who engage in the specific act of their state, nature and the Creator impose the responsibility of providing for the conservation of the human race. This is the characteristic service from which their state of life derives its peculiar value, the *bonum prolis* (good of children).

By this Pius XII did not imply that every couple has a duty to propagate the race, nor that the use of sex always entails such an obligation, but simply that marriage finds its proper completion in begetting and raising a family (John Paul II, 1981b; Caffara, 1985).

Debates on the Use of Fertility Cycle and Antiovulants

On the whole, this official teaching was received without much public protest by Catholic married couples, but soon medical discoveries raised new questions. About the same year as *Casti Connubii* was published, 1930, Kyusaky Ogino of Japan and Hermann Knaus, working at Prague, Czechoslovakia, announced their discovery of a method to predict the infertile period of a woman's menstrual cycle, thus making possible the regulation of conception by the exclusive use of this period for sexual intercourse—the *rhythm method*, or more accurately *calendar rhythm*, since its use depends on the monthly regularity of the cycle (Griese, 1987)

At first theologians disagreed as to whether this method of limiting pregnancies was contraception, although as early as 1853 there was official recognition that it was not (Sacred Penitentiary, 1853, 1880). Pius XII ended this controversy in the 1951 address just quoted, in which he said that methods of controlling conception by restricting intercourse to the infertile period, even for the whole duration of a marriage, were ethical when justified by serious medical, eugenic, economic, or social reasons. Thus, for the first time, clear papal authority was given to the principle of responsible parenthood and to the use of scientific methods to control conception. The Church thus showed its openness to new reproductive technologies, provided they are conformed to basic ethical principles. Pius XII's declaration was consistent with *Casti Connubii* because the use of the infertile period, as we will explain later, does not involve any positive alteration of the essential meaning of marital acts. Many Catholics, therefore, hailed and promoted calendar rhythm as a modern pastoral solution to the practical dilemmas faced by married couples in our present economy. Enthusiasm began to wane, however, when it became evident that even normal irregularities in the menstrual cycle may invalidate the prediction of the infertile period, and when many couples reported that the necessary abstention and uncertainty could be a source of marital tension.

Soon after this papal approval of the use of the infertile period, in 1952, the first progesterone drug ("the pill," as it became known) which prevents conception by preventing ovulation, became available. This new method led to another theological debate that, as William Shannon (1970; see also Valsecchi, 1968) has observed, went through two different phases. In the first of these phases a number of theologians, of whom Louis Janssens of the University of Louvain was the most prominent (Swift, 1966), argued that the use of progesterones is not contraception as defined by *Casti Connubii*, since it can be used simply as an aid to the use of the infertile period by extending this period under effective control.

The lack of consensus on the validity of this interpretation, however, and especially the discovery that progesterones not only suppress ovulation but also sometimes may be abortifacient since they can prevent implantation of the fertilized ovum after conception (Hume, 1983), led to a second phase of the debate. Some theologians now began to question the whole interpretation of the Bible and of natural law on which the teaching of *Casti Connubii* was grounded. They argued that most contraceptive methods (provided they were not aborti-facient), since they are not really different in ethical purpose from the use that the Church approves of the infertile period (Birmingham, 1964) should also be approved under the same circumstances. It was noted too that Church documents (probably in deference to the exegetical opinion which we have mentioned), had ceased to appeal to the story of Onan to give biblical support to their rejection of contraception as older documents had done.

The Papal Commission on Birth Control

In view of the publicity given to the number and prominence of theologians favoring the notion that "the pill" was not contraceptive, many Catholics began to use contraceptive pills and many confessors tolerated or even advised this practice. Many Catholic health care professionals and educated, conscientious Catholic couples who had followed this theological debate with great attention believed this new view confirmed their own experience and reasoning. Thus it began to appear that this discernment process going on in the Church might lead to a modification of the previous teaching (Cavanaugh, 1964).

At the same time, as the Second Vatican Council approached, the social problems of world poverty greatly concerned Pope John XXIII and led him to organize a Pontifical Study Commission on Family, Population, and Birth Problems to examine the population policies of the United Nations and to recommend a course of action for the Church. This commission met once in 1963 and twice in 1964, but as the Second Vatican Council continued, Pope Paul VI enlarged it to 58 members, including three married couples, five laywomen, moral theologians, physicians, psychologists, demographers, sociologists, and pastoral marriage counselors. Its fourth session was held March 25–28, 1965, in Rome (Hoyt, 1969). The council itself concluded with the issuance of the document *The Church in the Modern World* (Vatican Council II, *Gaudium et Spes*, 1965c), which contained the very important section "Fostering the Nobility of Marriage" (nn. 47–52), in which for the first time (but not without some anticipation in the writings of Pius XII) a new, fully personalistic formulation of the traditional Christian view of marriage was proposed, along with a renewed condemnation of abortion. The "duty of responsible parenthood" was affirmed and the possible dangers of prolonged sexual abstinence in marriage referred to, but the question of licit and illicit methods of birth regulation was reserved by Paul VI until the completion of the commission's work. At the same time the council (Vatican Council II, 1965) insisted on the familial orientation of sexuality, saying that:

> Marriage and conjugal love are by their nature ordained toward the begetting and education of children. Children are really the supreme gift of marriage and contribute very substantially to the welfare of their parents (n. 50).

After the close of the council, a fifth and final session of the commission, again enlarged to include 16 bishops as an executive committee, was held in Rome for two months in the spring of 1966. The commission was simply consultative and never published any documents. Its discussions centered on two questions: (1) Is contraception intrinsically evil? (2) Can the Church change its teaching? The final majority report, "An Outline for a Document on Responsible Parenthood," written by six members of the theological subsection of the commission, was approved by nine of the bishops in attendance, opposed by three, with three abstentions, and was sent to the pope on June 23, 1966. It argued that the pope might use his authority to approve at least some form of contraception within marriage. It was accompanied by a separate document called "Pastoral Approaches," along with a minority report and a rebuttal by those favoring the final report (Valsecchi, 1968; Hoyt, 1969; Murphy, 1981; Kaiser, 1985; J. E. Smith, 1991).

One of the leading theologians of the commission was Fr. Josef Fuchs, SJ, a professor at the Roman Gregorian University who afterwards became the leading proponent of proportionalism, which holds that an act cannot be evil by reason of its moral object alone, but only when taken with its intention and circumstances. His influence seems evident in the majority report, "which the minority report rejected on the grounds that contraception is *intrinsically evil by reason of its object*, apart from its intention and circumstances." Thus the two reports disagreed not just on the special issue of contraception, or even on the principle of family-oriented sexuality, but on the much more general and fundamental principle of moral discernment underlying all moral judgments (p. 192).

The Encyclical *Humanae Vitae*

Paul VI, who according to some never had doubts about the evil of contraception but only about whether the use of antiovulants was contraceptive, then took almost two years of further study, apparently through private consultation of bishops and theologians, before publishing the encyclical *Humanae Vitae* (afterwards HV) on July 29, 1968. In explaining why he did not accept the commission's conclusions, Paul VI writes (n. 6), "This was all the more necessary because certain approaches and criteria for a solution to this question had emerged which were at variance with the moral doctrines on marriage constantly taught by the Magisterium of the Church." It seems probable that "certain approaches" refers to proportionalism, which was later decisively rejected by John Paul II in *The Splendor of Truth* (*Veritatis Splendor*, 1993, afterwards VS).

Because four years of waiting had produced widespread expectation of change, and because many had already adopted practices contrary to the traditional teaching, the encyclical provoked still further controversy (C. E. Curran, 1975, 1978; C. E. Curran and Hunt, 1969). Many Catholics who had accepted Vatican II without difficulty were alienated by it (Greeley, 1976). The national bishops' conferences of many countries issued pastoral letters attempting to explain the encyclical in terms acceptable to their people and to indicate how it might be pastorally applied, several of them emphasizing the rights of personal conscience and even the ambiguous notion of "the lesser evil" (Flannery, 1969; McGrath, 1976; Garcia de Haro, 1993).

Yet HV's condemnation of contraception was not a new teaching, but simply reaffirmed in a very definitive way a consistent position of previous popes. Moreover, the World Synod of Bishops, meeting in 1980 to discuss the problems of the Christian family in today's world, after very frank and realistic discussion of these difficulties (Murphy, 1981) unanimously reaffirmed the teaching of HV in agreement with John Paul II, who had already repeatedly confirmed it. The apostolic instruction issued after the synod of 1980, *On the Human Family (Familiaris Consortio)* John Paul II, (1981b), affirmed and developed the same traditional teaching. Even more decisively, after consultation with all the bishops of the Church it has now been reaffirmed in the *Catechism of the Catholic Church* (#2369–2371).

Hence some theologians (Ford and Grisez, 1978) have argued that the teaching of HV is infallible since it pertains to the ordinary and universal magisterium which Vatican I and II declared to be infallible and unchangeable (p. 53). For this criterion to be certainly met, however, a doctrine must be taught not only universally but precisely as a matter of faith or as so intimately connected with the faith that to deny it is equivalent to denying some doctrine of faith (p. 54). What is now indisputable is that the teaching of HV, whether infallible or not, is at least a teaching of the ordinary magisterium (p. 53) and as such, according to Vatican II (Vatican Council II, 1964a, n. 25) requires from all Catholics "obedience of intellect and will".

This continuing controversy has also broadened its scope to extend to all the issues of traditional sexual morality, as evidenced by the action of the Congregation for the Doctrine of the Faith (CDF) in its *Declaration on Certain Problems of Sexual Ethics* (1975a), its critique of the study on *Human Sexuality* (Kosnick et al., 1977) commissioned by The Catholic Theological Society of America, and its instructions on *The Pastoral Care of Homosexual Persons* (1986) and *On Respect for Human Life* (1987).

The Church's continued opposition to contraception has been vigorously defended by many American theologians, philosophers, and physicians (R. Connell, 1970; Ford and Kelly, 1964; Grisez, 1964; Kippley, 1974; W. E. May, 1977, 1983; Ratner, 1981; J. Smith, 1991; Hilgers, 1995) as solidly grounded in Scripture, tradition, and natural law. On the twentieth anniversary of the document, as the result of the research and experience of those years, national and international meetings of theologians supported its conclusions (e.g., International Congress of Moral Theology, 1988).

Arguments Against *Humanae Vitae*

Although the position of the Church on this matter seems clear and consistent with its historical tradition, many Catholics continue to suppose that this position can and should be modified. We will present the principal arguments to this effect, which dissenting theologians have presented since the publication of HV, and show why we believe that they are without solid foundation.

First, some attack HV on the grounds that since it is based on natural law reasoning rather than on the Scriptures, the Church, whose authority, it is claimed, concerns matters of faith and not reason, has no right to settle such a question. This argument ignores the statement in HV n. 4:

> Let no Catholic be heard to assert that the interpretation of the natural moral law is outside the competence of the Church's Magisterium. It is in fact indisputable, as our Predecessors have many times declared [reference is made to documents of Pius X, Pius XI, Pius XII, and John XXIII], that Jesus Christ, when he communicated his divine power to Peter and the other apostles and sent them to teach all nations his commandments, constituted them as the authentic guardians and interpreters of the whole moral law, not only, that is, of the law of the gospel but also of the natural law, the reason being that the natural law declares the will of God, and its faithful observance is necessary for men's eternal salvation. The Church in carrying out this mandate, has always provided consistent teaching on the nature of marriage, on the correct use of conjugal rights, and on all the duties of husband and wife.

The last sentence is especially significant, since it implies the principle of the inseparability of the unitive and procreative meanings of marriage, on which the judgment of HV against contraception is based, is not only derived from the natural law but from the "nature of marriage" as this is taught in the Bible and Tradition and hence is grounded in revelation, as we have shown in discussing the principle of personalized sexuality (p. 210).

Second, most of the theological critics of HV are also proponents of the ethical methodology of proportionalism, now definitively condemned by John Paul II in VS. Yet they have often claimed that Paul VI rejected the reasoning of the "Majority Report" simply out of concern to defend papal authority (Kaiser, 1985). Some have even attributed it to celibate male clerical bias against women. As we, however, have mentioned, quite independent of his concern for papal authority or any androcentrism, Paul VI must have been aware that acceptance of the advice of the majority of the commission implied acceptance of proportionalism. Proportionalism in fact seems to have been developed and to have become popular largely because it appeared to provide a theoretical rationale for the dissent from HV. We have already shown in p. 159 why proportionalism fails as a methodology of moral judgment.

Third, some (Curran 1968, 1977b, 1979, 1985, 1988) reject HV on the grounds that its evaluation of contraceptive acts as intrinsically evil is based on "physicalism" or "biologism." Thus F. X. Murphy (1981), under the pseudonym of "Xavier Rynne," one of the sources of the famous reports on Vatican II in the *New Yorker*, writes in an historical assessment of HV:

> Pope Paul's argument was based on an obsolete concept of biology that attributes to every act of coitus a possibility that happens only relatively rarely, namely, the transmission of life. The encyclical admitted that coital acts during infertile periods are legitimate. But, by their very nature, such

coital acts are not directed toward procreation, and thus they do actually separate the unitive meaning of conjugal intimacy from the possible transmission of life. This means that at one point the encyclical itself unwittingly accepts a factual separation of the unitive and generative aspects of coital acts—those that occur during the woman's infertile periods. The second great difficulty pointed out by theological opponents of the encyclical is that it measures the meaning of the human act by examining its physiological structure. In a number of places in the document, biological organisms and the processes of nature are accepted as the determinants of moral meaning. They are said to represent God's plan and therefore to be morally normative (p. 24).

Nevertheless, Gustave Martelet (1969, 1981), reputed to be one of the drafters of the encyclical (W. Shannon, 1970), has shown that Paul VI clearly intended to avoid basing his teaching merely on biological structures. Hence, in HV he stressed that the human *meaning*, not merely the physical facticity of the sexual act, is primary. Although it is not the material but the formal aspect of a human act (i.e., its immediate intention as a means to the end) that gives an act its formally moral character, this immediate intention cannot rectify physical structures if these, by their own intrinsic teleology, imply something contradictory to basic human needs.

In VS (1993), nn. 49–50, John Paul II points out that the unity of the human person, body and soul, requires that to evaluate the morality of human acts we must consider not only the good intentions of the acting person, but also the bodily character of the actions performed to accomplish these intentions. For example, a mature person cannot reasonably perform acts of masturbation as if these really satisfied the true meaning of human sexuality; nor can married persons perform acts of *coitus interruptus*, sodomy, or mutual masturbation as if these really expressed the true meaning of sexual love. The question, therefore, is not whether the physical character of the act can be determinative of its morality, but whether contraception contradicts the true human purpose of the act, as do some of the perverse acts just cited. In the context of personalism also, John Paul II (1984b) has commented extensively on HV in a series of biblical–theological allocutions explaining the traditional doctrine as an expression of the teaching "on redemption of the body and sacramentality of marriage."

More Arguments Against *Humanae Vitae*

Fourthly, it is often charged (Kosnick, 1977) that HV did not remain true to the "spirit" of Vatican II. As F. X. Murphy (1981) claims:

> Insisting that the moral aspects of any procedure to be used in regulating the transmission of life depended on objective standards, the council refrained from entering the debate over contraceptive methods, deferring to the decision of the pope whose commission was studying this matter. But the council declared that moral evaluation of sexual conduct should be based on consideration of "man's person and his acts." In *Humanae Vitae*

Pope Paul chose to ignore this innovation and returned to the traditional basis of "marriage and its acts" (p. 23).

Paul VI in fact, however, begins the doctrinal part of the encyclical by saying:

The question of human procreation, like every other question which touches human life, involves more than the limited aspects specific to such disciplines as biology, psychology, demography or sociology. It is the whole person and the whole mission to which the person is called that must be considered: both its natural earthly aspects and its supernatural, eternal aspects. And since in the attempt to justify artificial methods of birth control many appeal to the demands of married love or responsible parenthood, these two important realities of married life must be accurately defined and analyzed. This is what we mean to do, with special reference to what the Second Vatican Council taught with the highest authority in its *Pastoral Constitution on the Church in the World Today* (n. 7).

Vatican II itself had said in *The Church in the Modern World* (n. 51):

Therefore when there is question of harmonizing conjugal love with the responsible transmission of life, the moral aspect of any procedure does not depend solely on sincere intentions or an evaluation of motives. It must be determined by objective standards. These, based on the nature of the human person and his or her acts, preserve the full sense of mutual self-giving and human procreation in the context of true love. Such a goal cannot be achieved unless the virtue of conjugal chastity is sincerely practiced.

Consequently, Paul VI very explicitly attempted in HV to treat the question of contraception in terms of "human person and his or her acts." Thus the council had left for the pope to decide what the "objective standards" for the marital act might be, based on the "nature of the human person and his or her acts," and it is just this that Pope Paul VI tried to do. To find any contradiction between HV and the *Church in the Modern World*, one must show they present different views of the "nature of the human person and his or her acts," which is far from evident. What is evident is that Paul VI tried to write his encyclical with the same dynamic and personalistic approach to Christian anthropology that the council itself had taken. Although it said, "Marriage to be sure is not instituted solely for procreation," the council also strongly stressed in n. 50 that "marriage and conjugal love are by their nature ordained toward the begetting and educating of children."

We admitted in our discussion of the ends of marriage in p. 214 that HV did not explain as precisely as might be desired what is the positive relation of the unitive and procreative ends, but limited itself to treating them as *correlative and hence inseparable*. But it is not true that HV denies married love to be an end in itself or treats it as a means. In our own discussion in p. 217 we showed that married love is generically an intimate friendship and specifically family-oriented or procreative, so that together its unitive and procreative purposes form one unified end. Neither end, therefore, is a mere means to the other.

The real difficulty of the critics is indicated by Murphy's (1981) charge against HV: "They [biological processes] are said to represent God's plan and therefore to be morally normative." HV, however, does not limit "God's plan" to the body. The Christian vision is that the whole universe, including the human person as a soul–body unity, is the purposeful expression of the Creator's wise love. Thus it stands in stark contrast to the humanist view that finds no teleology in nature but only blind evolutionary forces. The Christian vision of the nature of the human person, as we have shown in discussing the principle of stewardship and creativity (8.3), also reveals that by our gift of reason we are cocreative with God. Persons have the right and duty to perfect their bodies. Hence artificial contraception is not wrong because it is artificial, but because this art is misused not to perfect nature but to thwart and misdirect it.

Is *Humanae Vitae* Self-Contradictory?

Fifth, even more frequently HV is charged with contradicting itself by declaring that the intention not to incur pregnancy is moral when intercourse is limited to the woman's infertile period, but immoral when contraception is used for the same purpose (Murphy, 1981). Certainly many Catholics have great difficulty with this distinction. The point is not, as Murphy wrongly claims, that "Pope Paul's argument was based on an obsolete concept of biology" (since the CDF documents demonstrate that it takes great care to be properly informed on such scientific and medical matters), but whether it makes sense to say that acts deliberately chosen during the infertile period are "open to the transmission of life" in some morally significant sense that contraceptive acts are not. HV explained the difference briefly in this way:

> In reality, these two cases differ greatly from each other. For in the former case, the married couple use an opportunity given them by nature; but in the other, the couple prevent the order of generation from having its natural processes. (*In priore, coniuges legitime facultate utuntur sibia natura data; in altera vero, iidem impediunt, quominus enerationis ordo suos habeat naturae processus.*) If it is undeniable that in both cases the married couple by mutual and certain agreement for plausible reasons desire to avoid offspring and seek the certainty that offspring will not be born, nevertheless it must also be admitted that in the former case only does it occur that the couple are able to abstain from marital intercourse in the fertile periods, when for just motives the procreation of children is not desired [authors' translation].

In *On the Human Family*, n. 32, Pope John Paul II (1981) elaborated this distinction in a more personalistic way:

> When couples, by means of recourse to contraception, separate these two meanings that God the creator has inscribed in the being of man and

woman and in the dynamism of their sexual communion, they act as "arbiters" of the divine plan and they "manipulate" and degrade human sexuality and with it themselves and their married partner by altering its value of "total" self-giving. Thus the innate language that expresses the total reciprocal self-giving of husband and wife is overlaid, through contraception, by an objectively contradictory language, namely, that of not giving oneself totally to the other. This leads not only to a positive refusal to be open to life, but also to a falsification of the inner truth of conjugal love, which is called upon to give itself in personal totality.

When, instead, by means of recourse to periods of infertility, the couple respect the inseparable connection between the unitive and procreative meanings of human sexuality, they are acting as "ministers" of God's plan and they "benefit from" their sexuality according to the original dynamism of "total" self-giving, without manipulation or alteration.

In the light of the experience of many couples and of the data provided by the different human sciences, theological reflection is able to perceive and is called to study further the difference, both anthropological and moral, between contraception and recourse to the rhythm of the cycle: It is a difference which is much wider and deeper than is usually thought, one which involves in the final analysis two irreconcilable concepts of the human person and of human sexuality. The choice of accepting the cycle of natural fertility–infertility of the woman thereby involves accepting dialogue, reciprocal respect, shared responsibility, and self-control. To accept the cycle and to enter into dialogue means to recognize both the spiritual and corporal character of conjugal communion and to live personal love with its requirement of fidelity. In this context the couple comes to experience how conjugal communion is enriched with those values of tenderness and affection which constitute the inner soul of human sexuality in its physical dimension also. In this way sexuality is respected and promoted in its truly and fully human dimension and is never "used" as an "object." (n. 32)

Thus it is ethically possible for a couple to perform the marital act in an infertile phase of the natural cycle with the aim of achieving three values: (1) the expression of mutual love through total self-giving (the unitive meaning), (2) rational family planning (the procreative meaning), and (3) freedom from sexual compulsion through the discipline of periodic abstention. On the other hand, when they perform a contraceptive act, they positively exclude the procreative meaning and distort the unitive meaning, which, because it is separate from its essential relation to procreation, no longer has the character of total self-giving. They also lose the ascetical growth in the freedom of self-control. It must be emphasized, however, that while the exclusive use of the infertile period is a *means* of family limitation which is not intrinsically evil, it must also be for a good *end*. If practiced merely for hedonistic purposes, to have money to spend on luxuries, or because of a selfish or cowardly reluctance to accept family responsibilities, it is not ethically justified.

To summarize: *The intention (finis operis) to use the infertile period to achieve responsible parenthood differs morally from the intention to do so by contraception because in the former case fertile acts are not deliberately rendered infertile, while in the latter case this is precisely what is intended.* They differ ethically, therefore, in that the former practice seeks to achieve a good end by a means which is not intrinsically contrary to human nature, while the latter seeks to achieve a good end by a means which is intrinsically contrary to human nature.

The Single Contraceptive Act

Sixth, it is argued that the error in HV is not its condemnation of contraception as a general pattern of action, since it must be admitted that normally a couple who loves each other desires to have children, but its insistence that a single contraceptive act is wrong, even when performed by a couple with the intention of responsible parenthood and the strengthening of family bonds. Since the teleology of marital acts in the infertile period is only *remotely* ordered to procreation, do not contraceptive acts performed to strengthen the family retain at least this remote ordination? The majority-approved final report of the Pontifical Commission (Hoyt, 1969), attempting to make use of the principle of stewardship and creativity, asked and tried to answer this question as follows:

> What are the limits of the dominion of man (*sic*) with regard to the rational determination of his fecundity? The *general principle* can be formulated in this matter: It is the duty of man to perfect nature (or to order it to the human good expressed in matrimony) but not to destroy it. Even if the absolute untouchability of the fertile period cannot be maintained, neither can complete domination be affirmed. Besides, when man intervenes in the procreative process, he does this with the intention of regulating and not excluding fertility. Thus he unites the material finality toward fecundity which exists in intercourse with the formal finality of the person and renders the entire process "human."

The report did not explain how in each contraceptive act the deliberate suppression of an act's natural fertility "regulates" it, or how the "material" and "formal finality" of the act can be united when the "material finality" is completely inhibited.

What the report really claims is that there is no ethical difference between a couple who use only the cycle's naturally infertile periods and a couple who use only periods they have made infertile. But while both have the same good end and act intelligently to accomplish it, are the means they choose ethically the same? Or is there an ethical difference between using acts which are naturally infertile and using acts one has made infertile? The encyclical claims there is an essential difference because the naturally infertile acts "remain open to the transmission of life," at least in the remote sense that they form part of the natural cycle whose ultimate teleology is procreative, but in contraceptive acts this remote teleology is deliberately suppressed so that the single act totally separates any procreative meaning from its unitive meaning. The fact that the pattern of marital acts as a whole is motivated by a good purpose does not justify occasional perverse acts, any more than a man's genuine love for his wife can excuse occasional acts of adultery or a general inclination to tell the truth can justify occasional lies.

Is Marital Abstinence Moral?

Seventh, advocates of contraception also appeal to St. Paul's warning to married couples, "Do not deprive each other, except perhaps by mutual consent for a time, to be free for prayer, but then return to one another, so that Satan may not tempt your lack of self-control" (1 Cor 7:5). Hence, if it is not wrong for good reasons to limit intercourse to the infertile periods, or to abstain altogether in order to limit procreation—as HV itself admits—then are not couples justified in resorting to contraception to maintain their marriage bond by frequent expressions of their love? To this we reply that St. Paul was warning against an exaggerated asceticism, not against marital abstinence when this is necessary for other reasons. Many couples who practice the moderate abstinence required by natural family planning testify that this discipline can strengthen rather than weaken marital love (Cubb, 1990).

Eighth, it has been argued that the practice even of the moderate abstinence required by responsible parenthood presupposes the possession of the virtue of chastity, but according to Thomas Aquinas (*Summa Theologiae*, I–II, q. 100, a. 1, a. 3), only the primary precepts of the natural law and those easily deduced from them—i.e., the precepts of justice contained in the Decalogue, such as that against adultery—are "absolute natural law" known to all and hence obligatory on all. Other precepts, including that of chastity and hence that against contraception, are known only by reason to "the wise" or by divine revelation. Hence, it is argued, people are morally guilty only for sexual practices which sin against justice, unless they live in a society which teaches these more refined or revealed precepts, which is certainly not true of our society.

We agree with Aquinas' analysis of how natural law is known and have tried to follow it in this book. He also held, however, that these refined natural and revealed moral truths are accessible to all Christians through the teaching authority of the Church and that therefore they are obliged by faith to follow this teaching even when it is not supported by the culture in which they live. Moreover, Christians have access to the grace of the other sacraments, which makes possible for us what would otherwise be impossible, namely, to observe the law of Christ. Certainly, Catholics are often ignorant of the scope the Church's moral authority and its moral doctrines, and are limited in their moral responsibility by many social determinisms, which undoubtedly lessens their culpability if they violate the norms of the Gospel and natural law. But this does not lessen the objective obligation of those norms, nor the duty of the Church to promulgate them to all, any more than similar factors which impede people from living healthy lives excuses the health care profession from promoting the scientific truth about health and disease to the public.

The *Sensus Fidelium* Argument

Ninth, the weakness of the foregoing objections to HV have become so evident in the course of the lively debates that have taken place since 1968 that most critics of HV no longer say much about them. Rather, they rely chiefly on the argument from the *sensus fidelium,* according to which the apparent fact that HV has not been "received" in practice by most Catholic couples in the "advanced" countries, even those otherwise devout, is evidence that this teaching is not from the Holy Spirit who guides all Christians (Birmingham, 1964; Bromley, 1965). Archbishop John Quinn of San Francisco at the 1980 synod stated that 76.5 percent of Catholic women of childbearing age in the United States use contraception and that only 29 percent of American priests regard this as sinful (Murphy, 1981). Note, however, that there is also a minority report of those couples, especially those practicing natural family planning, who strongly reject contraception and must be heard (Kippley, 1974; Zimmerman, 1981).

To respond to this line of argument, we note first of all that in discussing the principle of well-formed conscience (p. 51) we explained that the *sensus fidelium,* or more properly *sensus fidei* ("sense of the faith"), is not popular opinion or practice. In fact, the *sensus fidei* or "faith intuition" of Catholics is their corporate witness as members of the Church to the faith transmitted to them through the Church, which they have grown to understand and accept in their prayers and Christian living through the enlightenment of the Holy Spirit. Does the acclaimed "new insight into the nature of human sexuality" that approves contraception have its source in the Gospel and reverence for the work of the Creator? Or is its source the influence of the humanism that dominates the contemporary "free world" and teaches that technology is the answer to every human problem? An early Christian community received the inspired biblical advice, "Beloved, do not trust every spirit, but put the spirits to a test to see if they belong to God, because many false prophets have appeared in the world" (1 Jn 4:1; see also John Paul II, 1981b, n. 5).

Of course, the witness of married Catholics can by no means be denied; it is a very important voice in the theological effort to advance our understanding of the full God-given meaning of sexuality. Some polls, however, show that 50 percent of Catholics in the United States are pro-life and 50 percent pro-choice. Which is the *sensus fidelium?* If this rise in the practice of contraception had resulted in an increased stability of Catholic marriages, we might feel more confident that it is in conformity with the Gospel, but the divorce rate among Catholics is about the national average. It is doubtful, therefore, that *sensus fidei* of the Catholic faithful has yet been clearly heard, not because the bishops turn a deaf ear, but because as yet no adequate process exists by which this witness of faithful married couples can be expressed.

The history of the Church shows that only gradually have the Christian people come to see the moral truth of the Gospel preached to them, at least as regards certain difficult problems. For example, it took centuries for the Gospel teaching on human equality to lead the members of the Church living in a Roman culture built on slavery to recognize that slavery is incompatible with human dignity. That there can even be historical regression in Christian understanding is evidenced by the record of how, although the Church strongly opposed the use of government power to suppress heresy during its early period, in medieval times and until recently it came to accept it.

The fact, therefore, that in our century contraception, which throughout the history of the Church was considered perverse, has now, under the pressure of modern economy and the sexual revolution, become acceptable to many Christians is no proof that HV is wrong. Rather, the serious crisis of the family which confronts us may well be in part due to the change in attitudes toward human sexuality which the practice of contraception has spawned. Moreover, Vatican II confirmed the solemn declaration of Vatican I that papal definitions:

> need no approval of others, nor do they allow an appeal to any other judgment. . . . To the resultant definitions the assent of the Church can never be wanting, on account of the activity of that same Holy Spirit, whereby the whole flock of Christ is preserved and progresses in unity of faith (*The Church*, 1984, n. 25).

While this does not apply directly to HV, which does not have the form of a solemn definition, it does apply to the ordinary and universal magisterium to which, as we have seen, the teaching of HV probably belongs.

Tenth, many have argued that the problem of the world population explosion, the very problem that led John XXIII to set up the famous commissions, makes the practice of either contraception or abortion imperative for the survival of the human race. Hence, since contraception is surely a lesser evil than abortion, to prevent abortion it is justifiable. This argument—which we will treat later in more detail in 10.3—overlooks the principle that one may not do something that is morally intrinsically evil to avoid a greater physical evil, such as overpopulation would be. Since this problem pertains more to the social teaching of the Church than to its sexual teaching, it is sufficient here to point out that the former alarmist predictions on this subject are now seriously questioned. It has become clear that world poverty is not so much the result of overpopulation as its cause. Consequently, although many still advocate contraception and even abortion (Byers, 1995) it is far from certain that these will solve the population problem, which instead requires a radical correction of the economic imbalance between the poor countries and the rich. It is an illusion of the rich countries, whose birthrate is already very low, that they can impose population controls on the poor without helping them to share in prosperity (Simon, 1994).

Thus none of the arguments favoring a change in the Church's traditional rejection of contraception are conclusive. We have argued for the view of sexuality presented by HV already in our discussion of the principle of personalized sexuality. We will here only briefly recapitulate that argument.

1. The Old Testament in *Genesis* 1–2 makes clear that God created us as sexual beings in view of marriage, which has both unitive and procreative purposes so mutually related as to be morally inseparable.

2. In the New Testament Jesus confirms this teaching and perfects it by teaching (a) that marriage is a monogamous and permanent covenant; (b) that children possess full human dignity; and (c) that married love is sanctifying.

3. The Tradition of the Church has consistently opposed contraception as contrary to the will of the Creator revealed in the Scriptures and the natural law.

4. Human reason also tells us that (a) the teleology of the human sexual act has both unitive and procreative functions best fulfilled in the permanent, monogamous family; (b) these values are morally inseparable; and (c) support for them is essential for a good society.

5. Practices that deliberately render fertile genital acts infertile are contradictory to this natural teleology and are thus contrary to natural moral law, harmful to the family and society, and intrinsically evil no matter what the circumstances or purposes for which they are performed.

6. Although the commission majority arguing for contraception in 1966 vehemently rejected the charge of the minority that this would lead to accepting masturbation, homosexual acts, and extramarital intercourse, in fact many Catholic theologians (Curran, 1982; Curran and McCormick, 1988; Kosnik et al., 1977) found that once they had accepted contraception they were logically forced to accept, at least in some circumstances, these same behaviors. Indeed, our actual experience of the effects of widespread contraception on family stability and sexual morality in this century, foretold by Paul VI in HV, are one of the "signs of our times" that must be honestly heeded.

Thus HV is a "sign of contradiction" not only to humanists who deny its basic assumptions, but also to many Christians of goodwill to whom it seems far-fetched and hopelessly unrealistic. But may this not be because the contemporary mind has accepted as "realistic" a social system based on an unlimited and antiecological manipulation of the natural order that is surrealistic and ultimately self-destructive?

10.2 STERILIZATION AND OTHER METHODS OF CONTRACEPTION

Sterilization

Humanae Vitae accepts the ethical concept of responsible parenthood through use of the infertile period but rejects as unethical other methods of family limitation that are widely accepted today:

Therefore in conformity to these principles of a human and Christian teaching on marriage, we must again declare that the direct interruption of generation already begun as a legitimate way of regulating the number of children, and especially abortion, even for therapeutic motives, are to be altogether rejected. Equally to be excluded, as the teaching authority of the Church has frequently declared, is direct sterilization of a man or a woman, whether this be temporary or permanent. Likewise is every act to be rejected which, either in anticipation of the conjugal act, or in its accomplishment or in the development of its natural consequences, proposes, whether as an end or a means, to render procreation impossible (n. 14).

In *On The Human Family* (1981b), John Paul II states that it is "a grave offense against human dignity and justice for governments or public authorities to attempt to limit the freedom of couples in deciding about children. Consequently, any coercion applied by such authorities in favor of contraception, or still worse, of sterilization and procured abortion, must be altogether condemned and forcefully rejected." *The Catechism of the Catholic Church*, n. 2287, says the same.

For some, however, the birth control issue is a purely technical matter of calculating the evident advantages and disadvantages of particular methods, since they disregard the considerations that have occupied Catholic thinking. For example, a pioneering theologian in bioethics, Joseph Fletcher (1954), concluded that if persons have the right to control parenthood, they have the right to use any means that assists to this end unless it has serious medical disadvantages.

From this point of view, the most effective and apparently the least dangerous method of preventing pregnancy is permanent sterilization of the man through vasectomy or of the woman by ligation of the fallopian tubes (Population Crisis Committee, 1985). However, "the risk of sterilization failure is higher than generally reported." (Peterson, et al, 1996). This is termed *direct* sterilization because its direct purpose is contraceptive. Rather than a treatment for pathology, it is intended to render the subject sterile but not impotent. The latest figures state that 16.6 million adults have been sterilized in the United States (Hatcher et al., 1987).

When sterility results merely as a side effect of a medical treatment directly aimed at a specific pathology, it is said to be *indirect* and can be justified by the principle of totality and integrity (p. 224) because the direct purpose of the procedure is to restore health as Directive 53 (ERD, 1994) states:

> Procedures that induce sterility are permitted when the indirect effect is the cure and alleviation of a present pathology and a simpler treatment is not available.

Thus diseased sex organs can be removed surgically or can be treated by drugs or radiation therapy, even if treatment results in sterility (Lawler et al., 1995).

Direct sterilization is intrinsically unethical because it is contrary both to the principle of personalized sexuality as a form of contraception and to the principle of totality and integrity because it sacrifices a basic human function without the necessity of preserving life (*Catechism of the Catholic Church*, n. 2399).

Sterilization is less risky to health than oral contraception and intrauterine devices. Although surgeons are having increasing success in repairing both vasectomies and tubal ligations for people who change their minds, the risk that such attempts will fail remains high. An increasing number of both men and women, especially those who have been sterilized at an early age or those planning to remarry, now wish to have children.

Involuntary Sterilization

As a form of birth regulation, the chief disadvantage of sterilization is that it deprives the human person of a basic human capacity (W. E. May, 1987). Individuals so deprived do not at the time want any more children and often report subjective satisfaction with the results. Nevertheless, the ability to reproduce, even when not actually used, relates the individual to the community and its future. The sense of power, of life, and of belonging that this engenders is reflected in the religions and philosophies of all cultures, as the Old Testament testifies by treating sterility in man or woman as a curse (Ho 9:14). It is also manifest, as we have seen (p. 215) in the anguish that infertile couples often feel in their disability. The efforts of Indira Ghandi, politically disastrous to her regime, to enforce a sterilization program on a people of ancient culture illustrate both how tempting this method is to governments seeking a simple and permanent solution to the problem of population control and how deeply it is resented and feared where this sense of the human meaning of complete sexual power is still alive among the otherwise powerless.

Involuntary sterilization is an obvious violation of the principle of free and informed consent (John Paul II, 1981b). In 1979 the U.S. Department of Health, Education, and Welfare issued guidelines for federally funded institutions that ensured such consent for any sterilization of persons confined to these facilities. These rules include a moratorium on the sterilization of all mentally incompetent persons under the age of 21 and a 30-day waiting period for all others. Nevertheless, there clearly can be considerable pressure for sterilization of even mildly retarded persons and of the poor, especially blacks and Hispanics, allegedly for eugenic reasons, but really to reduce the costs and trouble to parents and the public of "unwanted children" (Varga, 1984).

Sterilization Is Mutilation

The highly technological culture of the United States is singularly insensitive to deep human needs, which are unconscious or suppressed by cultural influences. Simply because most sterilized persons claim to experience only a feeling of relief and freedom as a result of their surgery is not necessarily a reliable indication of its deeper consequences. Social and psychological research on such effects is still very superficial, and the present ecological crisis warns of the gradual long-term risks of what at first appeared to be harmless and effective technologies.

The National Conference of Catholic Bishops (NCCB, 1994) in the *Ethical and Religious Directives for Catholic Health Services* has the following directive, n. 53:

Direct sterilization of either men or women, whether permanent or temporary, is not permitted in a Catholic health care institution when its sole immediate effect is to prevent conception. Procedures that induce sterility are permitted when their direct effect is the care or alleviation of a present pathology and simpler treatment is not available.

The content of this directive is essentially the same as that of Directive n. 20 in the 1971 edition of the *Directives*, which gave rise to controversy concerning its interpretation. To solve the debate concerning the meaning of Directive 20, the Holy See was questioned by the National Conference of Catholic Bishops (NCCB) whether "medical sterilizations," that is, sterilizations desired because the woman would experience some physiological difficulty after she became pregnant, were to be considered direct or indirect sterilizations. For example, a woman with nephritis might suffer from uremic poisoning if she became pregnant. The result of this dialogue between the Holy See and the U.S. bishops was a clarification of Directive 20. The response of the Holy See (CDF, 1975b) was followed by two statements of the NCCB (1977, 1980) offering greater clarification of the issue. In regard to the nature of the act in question, the document of the Holy See distinguished between direct sterilization and indirect sterilization:

> Any sterilization which of itself, that is, of its own nature and condition, has the sole immediate effect of rendering the generative faculty incapable of procreation, is to be considered direct sterilization, as the term is understood in the declarations of the pontifical Magisterium, especially of Pius XII. Therefore notwithstanding any subjectively right intention of those whose actions are prompted by the care or prevention of physiological or mental illness which is foreseen or feared as a result of pregnancy, such sterilization remains absolutely forbidden according to the doctrine of the Church (CDF, 1975b). Thus sterilization may not be used as a means of contraception nor may it be used as a means for the care or prevention of a physical or mental illness which is foreseen as a result of pregnancy (CDF, 1975b, n. 1).

The Congregation for the Doctrine of the Faith also commented specifically on the reasons that had been put forward to allow direct sterilizations in Catholic hospitals. These reasons invoked (1) the common good, (2) the principle of totality and integrity, and (3) dissent (CDF, 1975b). Hence, the documents explained:

1. Neither can any mandate of public authority, which would seek to impose direct sterilization as necessary for the common good, be invoked, for such sterilization damages the dignity and inviolability of the human person.
2. Likewise, neither can one invoke the principle of totality in this case, in virtue of which principal interference with organs is justified for the greater good of the person; sterility intended in itself is not oriented to the integral good of the person . . . inasmuch as it damages the ethical

good of the person, which is the highest good, since it deliberately deprives foreseen and freely chosen sexual activity of an essential element.

3. The congregation, while it confirms this traditional doctrine of the Church, is not unaware of the dissent against this teaching from many theologians. The congregation, however, denies that doctrinal significance can be attributed to this fact as such, so as to constitute a "theological source" which the faithful might invoke, and thereby abandon the authentic magisterium to follow the opinions of private theologians which dissent from it.

Sterilization and the "Principle of Totality"

Thus according to the consistent application of the principle of totality and integrity, surgery may not be used to excise or damage a part of the body unless (1) the continued presence or functioning of a particular organ causes serious damage to the whole body or threatens life; (2) the harm to the whole body cannot be avoided except by the surgery, which gives promise of being effective; and (3) one can reasonably expect that the negative effect will be offset by the positive effect (Pius XII, 1952).

Some theologians (Nolan, 1968; Häring, 1973; Curran, 1973) have proposed a "principle of totality" (omitting the correlative of "integrity," which we include in our formulation, cf. p. 224) which would justify the sacrifice of bodily integrity by sterilization not merely as a side effect of treatment for a physical pathology but for the "good of the total person." Thus they would permit a woman to be sterilized in order that she might not again conceive while continuing to engage in intercourse even during her fertile periods because, considering her physical or mental health, or her economic or family circumstances, this would be for her total good. But how can it be for the total good of a person to solve a behavioral or social problem by mutilating her body? In our formulation of the principle of totality and integrity we showed that the total human good requires respect for *all* the essential human functions—physical, psychological, social, and spiritual—so that it is not right to sacrifice one to the other unless this is necessary to preserve life, without which none of the other goods can be achieved.

Therefore, although by the principle of double effect it is ethical to remove a cancerous uterus to save a woman's life though this also sterilizes her, it is not ethical to remove a healthy uterus to sterilize a woman on the grounds that it is for her total good as a person not to have another child. It may indeed be better for her not to have another child, but she must solve this problem by changing her behavior, not by mutilating her body.

Sterilization and Hospital Policy

Concerning contraceptive sterilizations in Catholic health care facilities in the United States, the NCCB (1977) declared:

Freely approving direct sterilization constitutes formal cooperation in evil and would be "totally unbecoming the mission" of the hospital as well as "contrary to the necessary proclamation and defense of the moral order." The Catholic health facility has the moral responsibility (and this is legally recognized) to decide what medical procedures it will provide services for. Ordinarily, then, there will be no need or reason to provide services for objectively immoral procedures (n. 1, 2, 6–7).

Although the documents declared that formal cooperation was not allowed, material cooperation might be allowed under certain conditions with regard to sterilization (CDF, 1975):

> The traditional doctrine regarding material cooperation, with the proper distinctions between necessary and free, proximate and remote, remains valid, to be applied with the utmost prudence, if the case warrants. In the application of the principle of material cooperation, if the case warrants, great care must be taken against scandal and the danger of any misunderstanding by an appropriate explanation of what is really being done (n. 3, 6).

Specific criteria for the use of material cooperation were set forth in the statements of the NCCB in 1977 and 1980:

1. If the cooperation is to remain material, the reason for the cooperation must be something over and above the reason for the sterilization itself. Since, as mentioned, the hospital has authority over its own decisions, this should not happen with any frequency (1977) (n. 4).
2. In making judgments about the morality of cooperation, each case must be decided on its own merits. Since hospital situations, and even individual cases, differ so much, it would not be prudent to apply automatically a decision made in one hospital, or even in one case, to another (1977) (n. 5).
3. The local Ordinary has responsibility for assuring that the moral teachings of the Church be taught and followed in health care facilities which are to be recognized as Catholic. In this important matter there should be increased and continuing collaboration between the bishop, health care facilities, and their sponsoring religious communities. Local conditions will suggest the practical structures necessary to insure this collaboration (NCCB, 1980) (n. 5).

The Catholic health care facility must take every precaution to avoid creating misunderstanding or causing scandal for its staff, patients, or the general public and must offer a proper explanation when necessary. It should be made clear that the facility disapproves of direct sterilization and that material cooperation in no way implies approval. Consequently, it is not proper for a hospital to propose in its ethical code a list of "medical indications for which sterilization is permitted," since this amounts to an approval of elective sterilization.

Material Cooperation in Sterilization

While the possibility of justifying material cooperation in performing contraceptive sterilizations is mentioned in the documents issued by the Holy See and the NCCB (1980), it is considered as an "unlikely and extraordinary" occurrence. Moreover, before allowing it on these grounds, the Catholic hospital should consult with the bishop or his delegate. The traditional norms of moral theology in regard to cooperation are explained on page 199. Although formal cooperation with ethically wrong actions is never permissible, material cooperation in actions that are objectively evil is not only permitted but may be even ethically required in a world where, without such cooperation, many good actions would be frustrated or eliminated altogether. If Catholic hospitals are to carry out their ministry, they cannot avoid cooperating in some activities with evil but unintended effects. Some of these will involve working with persons who choose to perform acts that the hospital would not be ethically justified in doing on its own behalf, but that must be tolerated for the sake of the primarily good results of the cooperation. Thus, by paying dues to state hospital associations, Catholic hospitals give support and recognition to some hospitals in which abortions are performed. Their failure to belong to the association, however, would endanger their own ability to pursue their mission and would also weaken the work of the association to uphold medical and ethical standards. In belonging to the association, Catholic hospitals perform a good moral action, and their support of hospitals performing abortions is remote mediate material cooperation.

What type of situation in the United States might warrant material cooperation of Catholic health care facilities with persons wishing to perform or who have performed direct sterilizations? Some thought that the failure of the 1971 *Ethical and Religious Directives* to allow for a liberal use of material cooperation in regard to sterilizations was a serious mistake, if not an injustice (Bayley and McCormick, 1980). What are Catholic hospitals to do when staff physicians believe a sterilization is justified and they have a responsibility to perform it? Or when it might be possible to reduce the risk of two separate surgeries (e.g., Caesarean birth and tubal ligation) by performing both at the same time?

It was hoped, therefore, that the 1994 revision of the *Directives* would clarify this point, and on the advice of the Holy See an Appendix, "Principles Governing Cooperation," was added in an effort to do this. The Appendix looked especially to the problems now arising from joint ventures between Catholic and non-Catholic hospitals and to government and HMO pressures to provide "standard treatment," often defined so as to include sterilizations. We have already explained on p. 203 why we believe the Appendix of the ERD is itself in need of caution as regards its statement:

Immediate material cooperation is wrong, except in some instances of duress. The matter of duress distinguishes immediate material cooperation from implicit formal cooperation.

In fact, duress cannot justify immediate cooperation in actions which are intrinsically evil, since that makes the cooperator freely and deliberately choose to be an instrument of the wrongdoer's evil act. Duress, although it restricts freedom, usually does not deprive the cooperator of all freedom. If, however, the duress were so great as to deprive the cooperator of the freedom to choose, the act would not be a human act, and the norms for legitimate cooperation refer only to human acts. Thus it is not correct to say that under duress one may immediately cooperate with evil. Hence, the statement in the *Directives* may not be understood to justify a Catholic hospital, pressured by the threat of its physicians to leave or the need to form a joint venture with a non-Catholic hospital, in accepting the responsibility to furnish sterilization services on the excuse that its cooperation was immediate but under duress. To do so would be equivalent to formal cooperation in intrinsically evil acts.

Because of the many difficulties involved in this issue of cooperation, William Smith (1977) has argued that cooperation by a Catholic hospital in direct sterilizations would never be sufficiently remote to be justified, even if the patient and physician's actions were in good faith. Some recent articles by theologians writing on the issue of cooperation allow leeway in this regard, especially if there is some duress involved (Keenan and Kopensteiner, 1995). In light of the allowance for material cooperation mentioned in the documents of the magisterium quoted earlier, we believe that exceptional cases may occur in which material cooperation of the Catholic hospital would be justified if it is mediate cooperation only. Consider the following example.

The declining birthrate in the United States has led to a strong movement for hospitals to consolidate obstetrical departments so that a single center located in one of the hospitals can afford the highest quality care. Catholic hospitals cooperating in such an effort would not be allowed, as we have already noted, to cooperate in a center that performed abortions, but would they be allowed to cooperate in forming a common obstetrical unit where contraceptive sterilizations were performed under the auspices of a non-Catholic hospital? Would this be mediate material cooperation?

It seems this type of cooperation would be mediate and legitimate if the medical personnel and operating rooms of the Catholic hospital did not assume responsibility to provide the direct sterilizations, made it clear that it did not approve them and would end them if it could, and took steps to correct any scandal that might ensue. Moreover, the Catholic hospital should not profit significantly from their performance; if it did, it would signify formal cooperation. If Catholic hospitals do not cooperate in such joint ventures, they will be accused of wasting health care resources and frustrating an effort to provide quality health care in the local community. If a Catholic hospital or health care corporation is involved in setting up a prepaid health maintenance organization (HMO), the same reasoning would apply; the ethical issue is who accepts responsibility to provide and who profits from the unethical acts. The contract for membership in such ventures should clearly state that the services the Catholic hospital provides will not include direct abortions or sterilizations, regardless of services performed by other members of the HMO, nor will it receive any payment for them. Such restrictions are legal and have not rendered Catholic HMOs less marketable.

Other Contraceptive Methods

Sterilization is the most radical form of contraception because it is permanent, but other methods also raise questions. *Oral contraception* in its various forms also is used extensively in the United States (Hatcher et al., 1987). As already noted, some theologians believe that oral contraception approximates natural methods because (1) it is not permanent, (2) it operates by artificially extending the natural period of sterility by suppressing ovulation, (3) it does not alter the sexual act psychologically or aesthetically, and (4) it seems simple to use in a pill-consuming culture. The teaching of the Church, however, clearly states that hormonal pills used as a means of contraception separate the unitive and generative purposes of the marital act. On the other hand, if honestly used to treat a pathology in the generative organs, they are not unethical. The following ethical questions must be asked in evaluating oral contraceptives: Is there true pathology? Are the drugs really being used to correct this pathology, or is the resultant sterility really the direct aim of the medication?

Oral contraceptives have two very serious drawbacks. Early evidence of undesirable side effects were reported (Mann et al., 1975; Ory, 1977). Some are dangerous or even fatal to those suffering from circulatory disease, especially for women past 35 years of age who smoke. While the risk of pathology has subsided somewhat due to the development of oral contraceptives with less estrogen (Petitti et al., 1996) use of oral contraceptives is not a problem free practice. Despite apparent ease of use, therefore, contraceptive drugs have to be taken under medical supervision. The potential harm is offset in some physicians' opinion by the statistical evidence that these risks are considerably less than the risks of the pregnancies which the method prevents. A statistical comparison of the risks of pregnancy for all women (including, for example, minority women, who in the United States do not receive adequate maternity care) does not tell us much about the comparative risks for a woman given high-quality care. In any case, to risk death to bring a child into the world and to risk death to avoid one are not easily compared. Although many scientists seek to allay fears by comparing risk and benefit (Ory et al., 1983), the risks of oral contraceptives remain very real. Hence the reluctance of manufacturers of contraceptive drugs and devices to expend money on research for new methods because of their increasing liability to legal action for the damage caused by such products. For example, the maker of Norplant, a contraceptive device by which antiovulant drugs are administered continuously through an implant in a woman's arm, is now deluged by damage suits which often result from efforts to remove the device (Hilgers, 1993).

The second and much more serious drawback of oral contraceptives is that they may not act as a contraceptive that suppresses ovulation but rather as abortifacients by altering the uterine lining so that it will not receive a fertilized ovum (Hume, 1983; Speroff et al., 1983). The abortifacient action is more likely to occur with the present-day "minipill" contraceptives than with the original pills, which used estrogen as well as synthetic progesterone compounds (Hilgers, 1980).

Several other methods are used for contraceptive purposes: intrauterine device, intrauterine diaphragm with cream or contraceptive jelly, condom, and reduced-dosage hormonal drugs (Hatcher et al., 1987). The Food and Drug Administration requires that the following information be issued with *intrauterine devices* (IUDs; cf. Hume, 1983): "IUD's seem to interfere in some manner with the implantation of the fertilized egg in the lining of the uterine cavity. The IUD does not prevent ovulation" (*Physician's Desk Reference,* 1986); i.e., its action is not contraceptive but abortifacient. The incidence of uterine perforation and pelvic inflammatory disease (PID) also make the use of an IUD a serious health risk (Hatcher et al., 1987). For this reason, malpractice risks associated with their manufacture and insertion have resulted in virtual abandonment of IUDs in the United States (D. Edelman, 1987). Moreover, as high as 20 to 25 percent of women using IUDs were involuntarily infertile after removal (Cramer et al., 1985; Daling et al., 1985).

Barrier devices such as the *diaphragm* with spermicidal jelly and the *condom* (female condoms are now available) are probably medically safe and are contraceptives in the strict sense; that is, they prevent conception rather than destroy the conceptus. Similar to the diaphragm are the contraceptive *vaginal sponge* and the *cervical cap.* The use of these "barrier" methods is not without physical difficulties (Kelagham et al., 1982), and their effectiveness varies depending on the consistency of use (D. Edelman et al., 1984). The vaginal sponge is no longer marketed in the United States (Blaskiewicz, 1996). Users also complain that they are inconvenient and reduce sexual pleasure. Ethically evaluated, just as the sterilizing methods suppress the generative significance of the sexual act, these methods diminish its *unitive* significance. They resemble, to a degree, *coitus interruptus* (withdrawal before ejaculation), which all would admit cannot express total self-giving. Other contraceptive methods such as *vaginal foams and jellies, coitus interruptus,* and *postcoital douche* are generally rated as ineffective (Shirm et al., 1982).

The AIDS epidemic raises the question whether a married person should use a condom to protect the healthy partner from infection. Is it not evident that it is seriously wrong for someone to subject a sexual partner to a significant risk of what is at present a fatal disease? And can the healthy partner responsibly accept such a risk of life itself? That intercourse, especially regular intercourse with a condom, is not "safe" is evident from the significant rate of contraceptive failure when condoms are used. Thus, while the condom will reduce the risks, it still subjects the life of the partner to a grave danger, not to mention the possibility of transmitting this danger to any children that may be conceived.

In our opinion, therefore, those with HIV must cease genital sexual relations until a vaccine or cure is discovered or until it becomes evident that the partner is already infected. They must also practice periodic abstinence to avoid pregnancy. Yet we do not exclude the possibility that as formerly couples, of whom one was a leper, might continue marital relationships by free, mutual consent; so now a couple, one of whom has AIDS, might by free, mutual consent continue marital relationships in order to preserve their marriage during the brief life remaining to them, abstaining, of course, during times of fertility so as not to transmit the virus to a child. Nevertheless, the infected party has no right to demand this sacrifice of the other; nor is the healthy party obliged to it by the marriage vow. HIV is not the only condition which might affect the baby; for example, persons who are known carriers for genetic diseases such as trisomy 21 should refrain from generating offspring.

All these problems of birth regulation raise complex pastoral problems which we will treat later in this chapter (10.4).

10.3 RESPONSIBLE PARENTHOOD THROUGH NATURAL FAMILY PLANNING

The Second Vatican Council, HV, and *The Role of the Christian Family* all emphasize that to be truly human and moral, sexuality must express the freedom and responsibility of mutual love, including the intelligent planning of parenthood, so as to provide for the proper care and education of the children. The primary responsibility for such care belongs to the parents. Families, however, have the right to community assistance in this task, according to the principle of participation (6.1, 8.2), both because the right to marry and have children is a basic human right and because a family makes a fundamental contribution to the common good of the community (John Paul II, 1981b).

Catholics, especially health care professionals, therefore cannot be indifferent to the population explosion and the ethical problems it raises. Also, they cannot solve such problems by blind trust in God's providence, since according to the principle of stewardship and creativity, God gave us our intelligence to use in perfecting his creation. All recent papal documents dealing with social problems address these issues (Paul VI, 1967; John Paul II, 1991b; PCJP, 1996) and papal representatives have become involved in the work of the United Nations and other international organizations in an effort to plan for the global future, as in the 1995 Beijing Conference on Women's Rights. The popes generally have favored a position that, although it is not popular in the United States, is probably the majority opinion in the world at present (Byers, 1996; Gelbard, 1996).

Briefly, this view can be summarized as follows.

1. The growth rate in developed countries, including those with a high percentage of Catholics, has steadily declined for many years and will soon reach zero.
2. This crisis results from the ecological imbalance produced when developed countries introduced modern medicine into their colonies or

dependencies without at the same time raising the standard of living proportionately.

3. The Malthusian view that population growth must exceed growth in food production has been proved false, and modern technology should be able to supply food for all, provided that the present abnormal population growth can be slowed.

4. The most effective program of responsible parenthood will have two features:

   a. It will be supported by strong economic development.

   b. It will promote those methods of birth regulation most acceptable to the value systems of a people, including methods acceptable for Catholics (John Paul II, 1987b).

Thus the popes, in disapproving some methods of birth regulation, have not neglected to promote a definite social program that includes a reasonable answer to the population problem. Even those who would not agree with that answer should admit that it is more realistic than the two solutions most popular in the United States: (1) "lifeboat" ethics (Hardin, 1974, 1980) according to which the United States should maintain its own standard of living and let the rest of the world starve; and (2) the Planned Parenthood solution, which relies on promoting the use of contraceptives and abortion by the poor, while ignoring the need for a radical global economic readjustment. (Population Crisis Community, 1985). Both these solutions rest on the unrealistic assumption that the United States and the other developed countries can indefinitely continue their present style of life, based in large measure on the exploitation of underdeveloped countries.

If one accepts the view that population control has to be achieved by profound social changes rather than by the use of particular methods of birth regulation, then what methods are ethically acceptable in view of the Catholic and other value systems which emphasize the intimate relation between sexuality and procreation? How can couples limit the size of their families and still achieve the genital expression of their love in a way that will strengthen their permanent commitment to each other, give joy to their life together, and provide a healthy model of sexual love for their maturing children?

The Second Vatican Council (Vatican Council II, 1965c) in the *Modern World* (n. 51), HV (Paul VI, 1968), and *The Role of the Christian Family* (John Paul II, 1981b) affirm the Christian value of periodic abstinence and the acceptability of natural family planning methods, that is, those making use of naturally infertile periods. The council, however, also recalled the pastoral advice of St. Paul (1 Co 7:5), already mentioned, that while a married couple by mutual consent may abstain from sexual relations for a time, especially for spiritual and ascetic reasons, prolonged abstinence can be dangerous to the marriage.

Historically, as we have related, such periodic abstinence first began to be practiced scientifically by the calendar rhythm method, which depends on the regularity of a woman's menstrual cycle. Because this cycle varies considerably in different women and for some is quite irregular, this method could not be practiced effectively by many couples. It is said sometimes to have led to insecurity and tension in married life, and hence it gave the whole theory of birth regulation through natural methods a poor reputation, with the result that many physicians are still not well-informed on the whole issue. Today, however, new techniques for detecting ovulation have been discovered, so that the irregularity of a woman's cycle, which was a difficulty for the success of calendar rhythm, has become less of a problem (E. Billings and Westmore, 1985; Gross, 1987; Ryder, 1993). Moreover, knowledge of the cycle of fertility can not only help couples limit pregnancy; it can also help them to overcome infertility (World Health Organization [WHO], 1984).

Modern Methods

Two modern and well-tested methods of determining the time of ovulation and the periods of fertility and infertility are the sympto-thermal method and the ovulation method (often called the Billings method after the physicians who developed it). The *sympto-thermal method* uses several criteria for determining the time of ovulation: changes in cervical mucus, changes in the position and softness of the cervix and the dilation of its opening, and a shift in temperature, all of which are caused by a rise in blood estrogen as a result of the ovulation process in order to prepare the woman naturally to receive a possible conception. Some sympto-thermal methods add a calendar calculation as in the older calendar rhythm method. Those who prefer this method believe the concurrence of these signs ensures greater certitude in regard to ovulation (Flynn, 1991).

The *ovulation* or *Billings method,* on the other hand, uses only the appearance of mucus at the vulva, determined by the woman herself on the basis of a sensation of wetness and the color and elasticity of the secretion. This alkaline mucus of an appropriate viscosity provides a kind of natural valve that facilitates the movement of the sperm into the uterus and fallopian tubes at precisely the time when ovulation has produced a mature ovum ready for fertilization, while at other times its absence leaves the sperm to be destroyed by the normal acidity of the vagina (Billings, 1983; Hilgers, 1994). In the presence of this facilitating mucus, the sperm can survive for several days, but probably not for more than six (Hilgers, 1980; Klaus and Brennan, 1981). Recent studies seem to show that pregnancy usually takes place on the very day of ovulation (Wilcox, 1995). Hence conception is possible only when intercourse has taken place during the five or six days before and including ovulation, when the sperm is still available and active. Scientific studies show that the Billings method is as effective in judging the time of ovulation for many couples as the more complex sympto-thermal method (WHO, 1987).

Breast-feeding, which affects the hormonal balance of the mother and seems to be intended by nature to space human births, can also be a useful element in natural family planning, but it is not always effective for the individual mother (Hatcher, 1987). Nevertheless, it should be strongly encouraged for both the health of the child (it can provide proper nourishment and increase immunity to disease) and the full development of the mother–child bonding, which is important for the child's psychological growth and the mother's personal fulfillment.

Other scientific natural family planning studies (WHO, 1984) report 97 percent *use* effectiveness and 98 percent *method* effectiveness, the latter figure taking into account those pregnancies that could be explained by a failure of the couple to abstain at a time when they knew by the method they might be fertile. Thus the method effectiveness rate is as good as or better than any known contraceptive method except sterilization. User failures occur in all forms of contraception but in fact are not always failures, since interviews often reveal both conscious and unconscious motivation by couples to achieve pregnancy (WHO, 1987).

Recently, another method to identify fertility in women has been discovered. Ovarian and pituitary hormone production shows characteristic patterns during the fertility cycle. Urinary estrogen and pregnanediol measurements detect the beginning, peak, and end of the fertile period. Economical enzyme immunoassays and other tests that measure the luteinizing hormones have been developed. Seemingly, this will enhance the effectiveness of the ovulation method (Brown et al., 1987).

Proponents of these methods insist that while they are not difficult to teach any couple, their effectiveness depends on accurate instruction and the competence of well-instructed teachers (WHO, 1981). Learning the method from books is discouraged unless competent teachers are unavailable. Unfortunately, these methods have not yet won serious support among many physicians in the United States (Kambic, 1994). Several reasons are put forward for this lack of acceptance, the most prominent being that U.S. physicians tend to have excessive confidence in pharmaceuticals and too little respect for the natural "wisdom of the body."

Advantages of Natural Family Planning

No methods of birth regulation are without some serious disadvantages (Peterson et al., 1996), and natural methods have been criticized on several grounds. First, although they are highly effective under ideal conditions, natural methods, since they make no money for drug companies and risk no damage litigation, have not been as widely tested scientifically as have progesterones and intrauterine devices. It has been shown, however, that the Billings method can be used with excellent success even by uneducated women (WHO, 1981). Second, some (Guerrero, 1973) have theorized that natural family planning may produce genetic defects, since if a pregnancy does occur, it is more likely to be at a time when the ovum or sperm are somewhat aged. Hilgers (1977) has shown that not only is there little evidence for such a theory, but strong reason to regard it as false, and a recent study (Brown et al., 1987; Wilcox et al., 1995) again disproves this theory. Third, and much more important, natural methods require a period of abstinence, which if they are to equal hormones and intrauterine devices in effectiveness, may be as long as half the cycle, which may seem too difficult for many people, (WHO, 1984, 1987).

In answer to this last and most serious difficulty, proponents of natural family planning first point out that because of improved methods, abstinence can often be reduced with safety to five or six days in a cycle. Second, they emphasize that contraceptive methods also have strong psychological drawbacks. Thirdly, the same studies from WHO that set forth the difficulties of NFP also reported overall satisfaction with the method, even though it required greater self-discipline to follow.

Positively, proponents of natural methods (Kippley, 1974; Zimmerman, 1981; Ryder, 1993) argue that:

1. Such methods place responsibility on *both* partners, not merely on the woman, as do most methods, or on the man, as does vasectomy.
2. Many women who use such methods have reported an enhanced sense of personal dignity resulting from an awareness of their own body and its rhythms.
3. Abstinence from intercourse can help a couple learn to have confidence in the strength of their love for each other and to express it in a variety of ways, without that preoccupation with "total orgasm" which is proving to be a source of tension for many men and women today.
4. Periodic abstinence removes something of the sexual routine and enhances the experience when it is actually decided on.

Although spontaneity is an element of lovemaking, a truly mature notion of spontaneity is not just being able to have intercourse at any time. Rather, it is knowing how to give oneself to another at the *appropriate* time, a time necessarily determined by the rhythm of any couple's particular relationship and lifestyle. The principle of inner freedom, which as we have shown (p. 208) has both a sound biblical and psychological basis, indicates that self-control in sexual matters as in all matters of pleasure is difficult but is necessary for moral maturity. This is one of the reasons that chastity before marriage is so important as a preparation for a successful marriage.

Besides these possible subjective psychological advantages, natural family planning has several definite objective merits.

1. When properly practiced, it can be as effective as any method except sterilization and does not have the obvious disadvantages of a sterilizing procedure.
2. Unlike other comparably effective methods, namely, progesterones and intrauterine devices, it has no medical risks.
3. It is never abortifacient, as progesterones and intrauterine devices almost certainly are.
4. It is inexpensive, does not require regular medical checkups to avoid side effects, and can be effectively taught by simple practical instruction.

Finally, the mechanistic tendencies of our society are evidenced in reaction to natural family planning. The tendency is to evaluate methods of family limitation only from statistical efficiency, instead of questioning which methods result in greater marital love between husband and wife. The attitude that says that it is impossible for people to learn to control their sexual appetites even when given adequate social support is an offense to the principle of human dignity in community and is like saying that since many people are sick it is unrealistic to try to prevent or control disease.

Health care professionals need to be well-informed on natural family planning and have a serious professional obligation to promote it as a method indubitably in keeping with Christian values, as well as having important medical advantages for couples who use it consistently and satisfactorily. Catholic health care facilities and physicians should provide instruction in this method honestly and objectively. Also, they should give correct information about other methods so that couples will not think they are being treated as guinea pigs but have free and informed consent in trying to use natural methods for responsible parenthood. It is especially essential that Catholic scientists advance research on natural methods so as to overcome the crisis of conscience among Catholics. They also must provide others with a method of responsible parenthood and population control that does not tend to separate sexuality from family life, as has the spread of contraceptive practices.

10.4 CARE OF RAPE VICTIMS

Sensitivity to Rape Trauma

Rape is one of the more common social crimes. Because many rape victims hesitate to expose themselves to shame and notoriety, and because false charges of rape are possible, it is difficult to ascertain with any degree of accuracy the number of rapes committed in the United States each year. When crimes of violence are tabulated, however, the percentage of rapes increases each year. There is evidence that rape is motivated by hostile impulses—a desire to assert the aggressive power of the rapist and to humiliate the victim—more than a desire for sexual pleasure (Lifshitz, 1986). Furthermore, many rapists force the victim to engage in perverse sexual acts. To perform even natural sexual acts, outside or even within marriage, against the will of the partner is contrary to the meaning of sexuality as an expression of mutual love (E. Bayer, 1982). Pope John Paul II (1980c) pointed out the sinfulness of the husband who even in thought considers the wife a mere sexual object, without regard for her free personhood. Such behavior is wife abuse, which is at last being exposed to public concern.

A victim of rape should be given the most sensitive and charitable care possible. Such victims often complain justifiably that they are treated by the police and medical personnel alike as though they were responsible for provoking the attack, thus compounding the grave injustice from which the woman has suffered. Possible imprudence on the woman's part does not make her the criminal. Many cities now have formed rape treatment task forces, not only to help educate police and medical personnel concerning humane treatment of rape victims, but also to prevent the crime by alerting the public to the signs of impending attack and to the measures that might ward it off (Hampton, 1995). After the police, the responsibility for care of the victim of rape generally falls on the health care profession, although the clergy and especially the family of the victim have important roles as well. Hospital procedures developed by such task forces are designed to accomplish four things:

1. To offer the psychological support and counseling that the woman needs to work through the trauma of the attack and its aftermath. Often this will require follow-up treatment with a counselor or psychologist.
2. To provide medical care for injuries or abrasions that might have occurred.
3. To gather evidence to be used if the rapist is apprehended and prosecuted. This usually consists of a rather extensive examination of the vagina, pelvic area, and clothing.
4. To provide treatment to prevent possible venereal disease and pregnancy.

Prevention of Conception from Rape

This last point, preventing pregnancy, raises special ethical problems. Since more probably the woman is in an infertile portion of her cycle and because the trauma of rape may have an antiovulatory effect (Mahkorn and Dolan, 1981), the chances of conception after rape statistically are very low. In a recent article, Harriette Hampton (1995) states that the risk of pregnancy is estimated at 2–4 percent but no proof is given for this statement. Moreover, a small survey in the midwest found that 50 percent of women treated for rape were using contraceptives (Piccione, 1995). Becoming pregnant is naturally a very serious concern to the victim, however, and she deserves every help that medical professionals can give her, provided that help is ethical. Of course, in many cases, it will be possible to ascertain that conception is not at all likely, for example, if the woman is taking contraceptive drugs or if an examination of cervical mucus shows she is not in a fertile phase. If pregnancy is a possibility, since the victim is in no way responsible for the possible pregnancy, she has the right to avoid it if this is ethically possible. A woman who has consented to intercourse takes responsibility as a free person to use the sexual act in keeping with its intrinsic significance of love and procreation. On this responsibility the arguments of *Humanae Vitae* against contraception are based. The rape victim, however, has no such responsibility because she has not consented to the sexual act. Thus she has assumed no responsibility to give proper meaning to the sexual act that has been unjustly forced on her.

Therefore, most Catholic moralists today admit that a woman who is in real danger of rape may, before the attack and if the danger is real, take a drug to prevent conception or even insert a diaphragm (Perico, 1993). After the rape, through her own action or that of a medical person, she may do what is possible to render the sperm inoperative, to prevent it from joining the ovum, or to delay the production of ova. The Ethical and Religious Directives (n. 36) confirm this approach:

> A female who has been raped should be able to defend herself against a potential conception from the sexual assault. If, after appropriate testing, there is no evidence that conception has occurred already, she may be treated with medications that would prevent ovulation, sperm capacitation or fertilization. It is not permissible, however, to initiate or to recommend treatments that have as their purpose or direct effect the removal, destruction or interference with the implantation of a fertilized ovum.

From the discussion of abortion in 9.2, however, it follows that once the woman has conceived, she cannot take any action that would abort or destroy a fertilized ovum directly or request others to do so, nor may they cooperate with her in doing so. Although she has the right to protect herself from the effects of the aggression, she does not have the right to do so at the expense of the life of a fetus who is in no way an aggressor. There is no proportion between the fetus' right to life and her right to be free of the injury done to her, overwhelming as this is. A woman does not restore her personal dignity and integrity by destroying the life of another person who is biologically her own child, but rather by caring for that child and thus demonstrating to herself and others her great dignity as a human person, a strong woman, and a caring mother.

Problems arise, however, when methods to prevent conception are proposed that not only prevent conception, but that also may be abortifacient. As already noted, even though a woman is protecting her rights, it is wrong for her to do so at the expense of the rights of a child already in existence. This is true even in the period before the implantation of the fertilized ovum in the uterus because, as 9.2 argues, most probably the zygote is truly human even before implantation, and this probability requires that fetal rights be respected. Thus to use a method that not only prevents ovulation but also inhibits implantation of the embryo after the sperm is no longer active (72 hours) cannot prevent conception and would have no purpose except as an abortifacient. On the other hand, when honest *doubt* exists as to whether conception has in fact taken place, and the sperm is still active the probability should favor the certain rights of the woman. This means, therefore, that as long as it is truly doubtful that the woman has conceived, she can take means to prevent conception, even if these means might in some cases actually be abortifacient if conception has taken place unrecognized. Once it becomes certain or highly probable that conception has occurred, however, she must then recognize the rights of the fetus to life and avoid any serious risk of abortion.

Formerly, when discussing licit methods of attacking the sperm before conception, Catholic moralists recommended (with some limitations as to time) dilation and curettage (D & C), vaginal douche, or intrauterine douche (O'Donnell, 1957). Today, from both the medical and moral points of view, none of these methods seems to be acceptable. The vaginal douche may be used for cleansing but is unlikely to prevent conception. Conception takes place ordinarily in one of the fallopian tubes, not in the vagina or uterus, and studies show the sperm enters the tubes 5 to 30 minutes after intercourse (Fordney-Settlage et al., 1973). Thus, the vaginal spermicidal douche might attack some of the sperm remaining in the vagina but would be ineffective for most of them. The intrauterine douche is considered too dangerous because the fluid it introduces could flow through the fallopian tubes into the peritoneal cavity and perhaps cause serious infection. Competent gynecologists do not employ this procedure today.

The theologians who formerly allowed D & C realized that the scraping of the womb made it impossible for an already implanted zygote to survive or for a fertilized ovum to be implanted. They argued, however, that the principle purpose of this action was to eliminate the sperm, and if this were done soon enough after the attack, the principle of double effect could be used (Healy, 1956). Given the new evidence of the motility of the sperm, it is no longer reasonable to say that D & C is a specific remedy to remove the sperm when the effective sperm is probably already out of the uterus.

Use of Antifertility Drugs

Most rape treatment protocols recommend that antifertility drugs be administered orally or by injection over a few days. At one time diethylstilbestrol (DES) was a favored drug for treating rape victims. Because of acute side effects for the woman and possible birth defects in the fetus if the treatment is not successful, this treatment is no longer utilized (Stenchever, 1987). At present, the recommended pharmaceutical treatment is marketed in the United States as Ovral; a dosage of 100 micrograms is given within 72 hours of rape, with the same dosage repeated 12 hours later. The rape protocols state that Ovral or other hormones should not be administered until a pregnancy test is administered. At present, there is no test that would be effective shortly after the attack has taken place. Hence, if the test is positive, it is a sign that the pregnancy began before the attack occured. If the test is positive, then the rights of the conception must be respected. If it is not positive, "then medication to prevent ovulation, sperm capitation, or fertilization" may be used.

What if pregnancy tests are not available? Then medications may be used as long as there is reasonable doubt that ovulation has occured in the current cycle (Pennsylvania Catholic Conference, 1993). The Committee for Bioethical Issues of the Bishops of Great Britain and Ireland, after medical consultation and applying the principle of double effect to the respective rights of the woman and child, considered the treatment for rape victims and stated (GBI, 1986a):

> Catholics may seek and administer hormonal postcoital contraception after insemination by sexual assault, provided *(i)* that there are no grounds for judging that ovulation preceded or will coincide with the administration of postcoital contraception, and *(ii)* that the postcoital contraceptive is administered urgently.

In an effort to establish without doubt the occurence of ovulation, or lack of same, and thus insure that the medication is truly contraceptive, the use of an ovukit is recommended (Piccione, 1995). While this is certainly worthwhile, the ovukit may not be available at all health care facilities.

Rape Protocol

In conclusion, we would summarize the responsibilities of Catholic health care facilities when caring for rape victims in the following manner:

1. Catholic health care facilities should prepare and carefully observe a protocol for the treatment of rape victims in which the first concern is respect for the dignity of the woman, regardless of her character or socioeconomic condition (Gregorek, 1988). This should include both medical and counseling help, including the offer of pastoral counseling, to reduce the harm she has unjustly suffered, and should shield her as much as possible from embarrassment.

2. The protocol should provide for the collecting of adequate and accurate information for the police so that the aggressor can be brought to trial and conviction.

3. The protocol should also include medical tests to determine if the woman is pregnant. If the tests are positive, nothing should be done that would cause harm to the embryo.

4. If it is determined that the woman is not pregnant and not using contraceptive medications or devices, the following norms are offered as guidance in administering antifertility medications.

   a. Antifertility medications should not be administered if the sperm are probably no longer active. Otherwise, the purpose of the action would be abortifacient. Thus, the antifertility medication must be used within two to three days of the attack.

   b. If ovulation has not occurred within a current menstrual cycle, antifertility medications may be administered to prevent ovulation.

   c. If it is certain ovulation has occurred within the menstrual cycle, antifertility drugs may not be used because their effect could only be to inhibit implantation.

   d. If there is doubt as to whether ovulation has occurred or not within the present menstrual cycle, antifertility drugs may be used with the purpose of preventing ovulation. The doubt in question concerns the fact of ovulation, not the fact of conception.

Under these guidelines, the woman is not attacking another person but prudently seeking to avoid conception. Although there is remote risk that implantation might be affected, the risk is not substantial (GBI, 1987b). If physicians or rape victims wish to avoid even this small risk to a potential third party and thus would not wish to administer or receive antifertility hormones, their consciences should be respected by the Catholic health care facility.

5. Facilities should be aware that, depending on state laws, they may be liable to legal suit if they fail to provide a rape victim with the opportunity to avoid pregnancy. Consequently, if a Catholic facility believes in conscience that it is unable to provide treatment that can be established as adequate in the local courts, it should make sure that victims can be promptly referred to their own physicians for whatever anti-pregnancy treatment they themselves choose.

10.5 PASTORAL APPROACH TO MEDICAL SEXUAL PROBLEMS

The "Morality Gap"

As everyone is aware, some of the more difficult moral issues in the life of Catholics arise from the Church's teaching on sexual ethics. Health care professionals are not expert moral or spiritual counselors in regard to the decisions concerning sexual behavior. Yet it is important that health care professionals seek to understand the pastoral practice of the Church, because the teaching of the Church may have great impact upon their practice of medicine.

Above all, it should be emphasized that the purpose of pastoral counseling is not to deny or mitigate the objective teaching of the Church in regard to the norms for a beneficial practice of sexuality. Just as the medical profession does not "make rules" about how to be healthy and avoid sickness, the Church does not "make rules" about what is helpful and harmful behavior as regards sexual or other kinds of behavior. When they state norms for healthy or moral behavior, both the medical profession and the Church are striving to give true and practical advice. The Church does not seek to "impose guilt." It only strives in the light of the Gospel to help people achieve a realistic understanding of the consequences of their actions and to help them to find forgiveness and healing for the harm these actions may knowingly or unknowingly have caused, as well as to help them forgive and repair the harm done to themselves knowingly or unknowingly by others.

History shows that a "morality gap" between Church teaching and the moral understanding of many Catholics is by no means unusual. Indeed, like the gap between medical knowledge and human health habits, it has always in various degrees prevailed and is immensely difficult to overcome. To cite only one notorious example in United States church history: for many years—and even now in some places—priests did not preach against racism or question white penitents about racist attitudes and practices. They justified this pastorally on the grounds that given the racist milieu in which many whites had been educated, such admonitions would only drive penitents from the sacraments and even out of the Church without actually improving their conduct. When we look back on this pastoral policy, we see that on the one hand it was intended to be compassionate and realistic in regard to the subjective culpability of most white individuals. On the other hand, objectively it perpetuated a grave social injustice that disregarded the equal dignity of blacks.

Doubts and Certainty of Church Teaching

The best contemporary example of the conflict which may arise in regard to objective teaching of the Church and subjective culpability occurs in regard to the teaching of the Church about antiovulant pills, contained in the encyclical letter of Paul VI, *Humane Vitae* (HV). Before the controversy over the use of antiovulants, the general Catholic pastoral practice was to refuse sacramental absolution and communion to those who would not promise to abandon contraceptive practices. In the United States this policy was surprisingly successful, as shown for a long time by a Catholic birthrate significantly above the national average. We have told the story in Chapter 10 of the controversy over whether "the pill" was was "contraception" and how this debate finally led to the encyclical HV. In the pastoral conclusion of that encyclical, Paul VI wrote:

> We do not at all intend to hide the sometimes serious difficulties inherent in the life of Christian married persons; for them, as for everyone else, "the gate is narrow and the way is hard, that leads to life." . . . Let married couples, then, face up to the efforts needed, supported by the faith and hope which "do not disappoint . . . because God's love has been poured into our hearts through the Holy Spirit, who has been given to us"; let them implore divine assistance by persevering prayer; above all, let them draw from the source of grace and charity in the Eucharist. And if sin should still keep its hold over them, let them not be discouraged, but rather have recourse with humble perseverance to the mercy of God, which is poured forth in the Sacrament of Penance. In this way they will be enabled to achieve the fullness of conjugal life . . . (n. 25).

And to priests:

> To diminish in no way the saving teaching of Christ constitutes an eminent form of charity for souls. But this must ever be accompanied by patience and goodness, such as the Lord himself gave example of in dealing with men and women. Having come not to condemn but to save, he was indeed intransigent with evil, but merciful towards individuals. In their difficulties, many married couples always find, in the words and in the heart of a priest, the echo of the voice and the love of the Redeemer (nn. 28–29).

In promulgating HV, some national episcopal conferences (Delhaye, 1970; Flannery, 1969; Horgan and Flannery, 1972) simply urged their people to obey the encyclical (India, Ceylon, Philippines, Mexico, Spain, Scotland, and Ireland). Others (Italy, Switzerland, Germany, England, Japan, and the United States) urged confessors to deal with those practicing contraception in a very compassionate way and to avoid anything that might make these couples give up the regular use of the sacraments. The French, Belgian, Dutch, Austrian, Scandinavian, and Canadian bishops raised the question as to what attitude the confessors should take toward those who believed that it would be morally wrong to give up the practice of contraception in their present circumstances, concluding in guarded and sometimes obscure terms that it was not always necessary for the confessor to refuse absolution (Delhaye, 1970; O'Callaghan, 1970; Horgan and Flannery, 1972). Certainly, however, the subsequent interpretations of HV by John Paul II and the bishops as expressed in the *Catechism of the Catholic Church* (#2371) have left no doubt that contraception is intrinsically a moral evil which does serious harm and is therefore always *objectively* a mortal sin.

No doubt one of the chief reasons that so many today cannot see how genital acts with oneself or between consenting adults can be a serious sin is because in our individualistic culture it is supposed these are purely private acts. But *private* acts can have public effects, as drug addiction of individuals has had such disastrous social consequences. Sex acts, if they become addictive, distort the integrity of personal character, undermine family life, do great injustice to children, often transmit venereal disease, and thus are of inevitable concern to society as a whole. More positively, sexual acts as intended by God to express intimate committed love and to share in God's creation of unique new persons are of immense importance to human happiness, so that their abuse cannot be trivial.

Many of the critics of *Humanae Vitae* (Paul VI, 1968), the subsequent *Declaration on Certain Problems of Sexual Ethics* (CDF, 1975a), and the *Pastoral Care of Homosexual Persons* (CDF, 1986) issued by the Congregation for the Doctrine of the Faith have complained that the pastors of the Church seem content to pronounce moral judgments without providing much pastoral help for dealing with problems Christians experience in everyday life. Did not Jesus denounce the religious teachers of his day "who tie up heavy burdens, hard to carry, and lay them on people's shoulders, but will not lift a finger to move them" (Mt 23:4)? Yet if we carefully read HV and *The Role of the Christian Family,* as well as the pastoral letters of the various national episcopal conferences explaining HV (Horgan and Flannery, 1972), we will begin to understand that the Church is trying to steer a pastoral middle way between the one extreme of harsh, punitive discipline and the other extreme of permissive neglect, in order to help people to a more Christ-like and truly fulfilling life and successful marriages.

Pastoral Gradualness

In a response to a paper written by theologians criticizing *Humanae Vitae,* the official Vatican newspaper, *L'Osservatore Romano,* stated:

> [The] Christian moral tradition has always maintained the distinction—not the separation from, much less the contraposition—between objective disorder and subjective guilt. For this reason when it becomes a matter of

judging subjective moral behavior, within the unavoidable framework of the norm which prohibits the intrinsic disorder of contraception, *it is perfectly legitimate to give due consideration to actions of individuals, not only to their intentions and motivations, but also to the various circumstances of their lives, and above all, to the causes that might impair their conscience and free will.* This subjective situation, which can never change into "order" what is intrinsically "disorder," can have some bearing on the responsibility of the individual's behavior. As we know, this is a general principle which is applicable therefore to the issue of contraception (italics added).

This distinction (cf. p. 49) between *objective* morality, i.e., what is in fact helpful or harmful to human persons, and *subjective* culpability, i.e., their own understanding and responsibility for good or ill, is fundamental to pastoral care, which is directed to helping people overcome the gap that exists between moral truth and sincere but often inadequate moral sensitivity. In 1980, after reaffirming the teaching of HV, the Synod of Bishops wrote to married people:

> We wish to say to you, brothers and sisters, that we are fully aware of the frailty of our common human condition. In no way do we ignore the very difficult and trying situations of many Christian couples who, although they sincerely want to observe the moral norms taught by the Church, find themselves unequal to the task because of weakness in the face of difficulties. All of us need to grow in appreciation of the importance of Christ's teaching and his grace and to live by them. Accompanied and assisted by the whole Church, these couples continue along the difficult way toward a more complete fidelity to the commands of the Lord (n. 20).

Among the propositions adopted by the synod as the basis of a future pastoral document to be issued by the Holy See, the bishops suggested that priests should use the "law of gradualness," recognizing a need frequently for "patience, sympathy, and time" in educating couples to an understanding of the papal teaching, but at the same time insisting on the normative nature of this teaching. John Paul II (1981b), acknowledging that "persons who have been called to live God's wise and loving design in a reasonable manner, are historical beings, and so they know, love, and *accomplish moral good by stages of growth*" (italics added) in his encyclical *On the Human Family* (1981), commented on the synod's statement by saying:

> Really, the "process of gradualness," as it is called, cannot be applied unless someone accepts the divine law with a sincere heart and seeks those goods which are protected and promoted by the same law. Thus, the so-called *lex gradualitatis* (law of gradualness) or gradual progress cannot be the same as *gradualitas legis* (the gradualness of the law), as if there were in the divine law various levels or forms of precept for various persons and conditions (n. 34).

And he also wrote in *Evangelium Vitae* (1995):

In fact, while the climate of widespread moral uncertainty can in some way be explained by the multiplicity and gravity of today's social problems *and these can sometimes mitigate the subjective responsibility of individuals,* it is no less true that we are confronted by an even larger reality, which can be described as a veritable structure of sin . . . (n. 12).

Decisions that go against life sometimes arise from difficult or even tragic situations of profound suffering, loneliness, a total lack of economic prospects, depression and anxiety about the future. *Such circumstances can mitigate even to a notable degree subjective responsibility and the consequent culpability of those who make these choices, which in themselves are evil* (n. 18, italics added).

Patience Leads to Conversion

Health care professionals, we believe, can sympathize with this pastoral dilemma from the analogy of their own experiences in dealing with real-life patients. We live in a very unhealthy society which makes it difficult for persons to understand healthy living or practice it, and often they have lost trust in their physicians because of what they have heard of malpractice or alternative theories of medicine. Should, then, a physician refuse to treat patients who do not seem to understand or cooperate with what they are told about what they cannot do and what they must do if they are to be healthy? Physicians are often tempted to give such patients a prescription to satisfy them and let them go. Surely, however, the right policy is for physicians to tell patients the truth about what they are doing to themselves, to persuade and encourage them to better living, and to be patient with them in hopes the good advice may gradually sink in, while the physician avoids driving the discouraged patient to some quack. They must also build up the patient's confidence and trust in them and their disinterested concern for the patient, so that cooperation with therapy becomes easier.

Similarly, the Church must be patient with people who have become confused about fundamental Christian values and about the Church's trustworthy authority to guide them, whether it be about social justice or married chastity, and sincerely see no other solution for their problems than ways plausibly promoted in their secular milieu but which are in fact morally harmful. As we said at the beginning of this chapter, the sexual revolution and the well-meant but sometimes mistaken advice of priests influenced by specious theological opinions has shaken the confidence of many Catholics in the pastoral guidance of the Church (Kosnick et al., 1977). On the other hand, the Church must not lack the courage to keep trying to educate its members concerning what God and sound ethics tell us makes for good family life. In this balanced, pedagogic effort we must first of all educate people about God's purpose in making us sexual. Only in that context of God's creative and loving purpose will the harmfulness of the practices against which the Church warns become credible. The Catholic health care professional and health care facility can make a great contribution to this educative process.

Personal Responsibility for Moral Decisions

In order to understand the pastoral process of the Church, a final few words concerning personal responsiblity are in order. The Second Vatican Council stated in regard to the formation of personal conscience:

> For guidance and spiritual strength let people turn to the clergy; but let them realize that their pastors will not always be so expert as to have a ready answer to every problem (even every grave problem) that arises; this is not the role of the clergy: it is rather *up to the laymen to shoulder their responsibilities under the guidance of Christian wisdom and with eager attention to the teaching authority of the Church* (GS, 1965c, n. 43).

In Chapter 3, p. 47 ff, on personal responsibility for health and in Chapter 8, p. 184 on the principles of moral decision making, we have already explained how individuals must form and act on their own well-formed consciences and take responsibility for their own decisions. Here we need only recall the following points:

1. No one is a fair judge in his or her own case. Thus, when making decisions of conscience, consulting people of knowledge and objective viewpoint is mandatory.
2. Simply because a teaching of the Church is difficult to follow does not mean that one may disregard that teaching (Dulles 1991), any more than one ought to disregard a physician's advice about dieting or surgery because it is hard to take.
3. Even if one's subjective responsibility for objectively wrong sexual behavior is diminished by various factors, the harm caused by intrinsically wrong sexual acts, just as by other wrong acts, is still real and objectively harmful.
4. With the help of modern medical knowledge, there are better, ethical solutions to sexual and reproductive problems than contraception, sterilization, and abortion. Yet, as in all matters of health and morals, to use these good alternatives to bad ones, one must become well-informed and with the grace of God grow in self-discipline.

Health Care Facilities and Sexual Ethics

Catholic-sponsored institutions, including recognized Catholic health care facilities, are not in the same position in regard to pastoral decisions as are individuals. Institutions sponsored by the Church are responsible for the mission of witness and evangelization committed to the Church by Christ. Thus it is of their very nature to accept this teaching, especially as outlined in the *Ethical and Religious Directives* (NCCB, 1994) and to communicate it to others. In extreme cases of violation of these directives, the bishop may be forced to withdraw the Church's recognition of the facility as a Catholic institution, with the consequent loss of its role in the mission of the Church.

Following these *Directives,* and seeking to help others, whether Catholic or not, to understand them, is an important responsibility of every health care facility sponsored by the Church. If the administration and staff of these facilities are themselves ignorant of the Church's ethical teaching and the reasons for it, they will either seek to evade this teaching or conform in a half-hearted way that undermines it. Just as we have done much in our time to promote Christian views opposing racism and sexism, so we can do much to promote the Christian views on the right use of sexuality.

Education in Chastity

The sexual revolution projects a future in which the Christian vision of human sexuality will appear ridiculous and unrealizable. For Christians, however, human sexuality is governed by norms of *hope,* a hope on which a truly human future must be built. To build a healthier future it is essential to help Christians develop a fully human understanding of their sexuality (CDF, 1975a). We suggest three contributions for which there is urgent need.

First, the chief of these responsibilities is to promote and cooperate with sound programs of education for chastity. Effective sex education is primarily spiritual and ethical, not medical, but health care professionals make an essential contribution to sex education because of its close connection with bodily life. Although many sex education programs today provide excellent biological and psychological information, they also promote the value system of a secular humanism that Christians find quite inadequate to help people attain personal freedom, moral integrity, and self-esteem. Such programs, however, can hardly be criticized without providing superior ones. A Christian program should begin by helping parents succeed in their natural role as the principal sex educators (Council for the Family, 1996).

Today many parents suffer from (a) the predominant influence of a hedonistic and individualistic secularism and (b) incorrect, distorted views of Christian values that stress negative, repressive aspects of sexual morality based on fear, rather than a positive but realistic view based on a true understanding of God's gifts and their own stewardship. A program of Christian education for chastity should provide the following types of instruction (Council for the Family, 1996):

a. Understanding of the unitive–procreative meaning of sexuality in sacramental marriage;
b. Knowledge of mental hygiene and essential biological knowledge about sexual differences and equality, lovemaking, intercourse, pregnancy, and birth;
c. Information on why people have a need for children and on the problems of sterility, adoption, and limits on the right to have children;
d. Information on the problems of responsible parenthood in today's society, natural family planning methods, and the medical and ethical evaluation of all birth regulation methods;

 e. Explanation of the rights of the unborn child;

 f. Discussion of the problems of genetic defects and the Christian attitude toward defective persons; and

 g. Consideration of the problem of homosexuality and similar difficulties in psychosocial development.

Such programs are an important factor in preventive medicine since they can go a long way to reducing the frequency or severity of many of the problems described in this chapter. However, they will not have a widespread effect unless they are also joined to social programs aimed at improving the climate of society.

Second, sound education for chastity must be based on continuing research and open discussion. When sexual issues are involved, such objectivity is difficult to achieve. Some physicians and nurses have had to struggle to obtain a hearing for natural methods of delivery and breast-feeding, since such an approach appears to be a conservative attack on medical progress. Similarly, in ethical questions dealing with sexual matters, modern culture has a strong bias toward voices announcing the coming of new "freedoms" or accepting sexual misconduct as inevitable. Many are prejudiced against any attempt to retain and strengthen traditional values of modesty and chastity and the disciplined restraint these values require. To arrive at an atmosphere in which both sides can be fairly heard when discussing sexual issues is extremely difficult.

Third, Catholic health care professionals who play a role in public and social agencies that deal with sexual problems should take care that these agencies do not content themselves merely with promoting contraception with an abortion backup. Responsible parenthood must be an important objective of any such agency, but this objective should not be merely negative. Rather, the principal goal of all such work should be to strengthen and promote the family as the basic institution of society. Only in an atmosphere of good family life based on faithful love can the next generation develop toward a mature, fully human sexuality for all, whether married or single.

CONCLUSION

Unfortunately, when writing about human sexuality it is often necessary to discuss actions which fall short of ethical norms of chastity, rather than the actions which fulfill this dimension of the human personality. Friendship and marital love are actions which fulfill the social potential of our personality which we designate as sexuality. As any other dimension of our personality, sexuality is exposed to the frailty experienced today in many sociocultural concepts. Nevertheless, the redemption by Christ extends to our sexuality, as to all other dimensions of creation. By living the virtue of chastity, whether a married or single person, one can experience the joy of chastity. Thus chastity in sexuality is not a repressive attitude. On the contrary, it should be understood as the spiritual energy capable of defending love from the perils of selfishness and aggressiveness and able to advance human beings to their full realization.

The person who is capable of a higher expression of sexuality, which sees beyond merely satisfying one's appetites, is capable of friendship and self-giving, with the capacity to recognize and love persons for themselves. Controlling sexuality in this manner enables one to truly love others. Such love generates communion between persons because each considers the good of the other as his or her own good. Each person is called to love as friendship and self-giving.

11
Reconstructing and Modifying the Functions of the Human Body

OVERVIEW

In recent years, medical technology has moved from the mere capability of repairing the human body to new capabilities of remodeling the body through surgical reconstruction, and even by genetic intervention, which will alter not only individuals, but also all their descendants. Some of these new capabilities are already practical, others still futuristic. This chapter deals in some detail with certain present problems associated with modifying the human person, but also touches on the futuristic ones for purposes of illustration.

After discussing briefly the theological norms guiding the development of the human body (11.1), this chapter then considers the potential of changing the human body through genetic intervention (11.2) and the need to counsel and screen those who have genetic defects (11.3). Next the methods of reconstructing the human body through organ transplantation (11.4) and transsexual surgery (11.5) are examined. Finally, ethical norms for research upon human subjects, a form of manipulating and improving the function of the human body, are formulated (11.6).

11.1 MODIFYING THE HUMAN BODY

Can We Re-create Ourselves?

A basic axiom of medicine has always been the Greek dictum, *art perfects nature,* which implies that human persons can be healed (or patched up) and helped to develop to maturity, but they cannot be essentially remade. Today, however, the situation has changed. We must face the questions: Is it right for persons to become their own creators? Can and should human nature be remade? Can genetic engineering hasten the processes of evolution by eliminating troublesome wisdom teeth or appendices, or at least can we remove the problem by some type of surgery at a very early age, before trouble arises? Might the technology of the future greatly reduce the complexities of the digestive system, which so often becomes diseased? Can human beings be fed in some simpler way, perhaps by a more effective intravenous method? Might all human beings be sterilized and reproduce artificially? Francoeur (1972) has answered that because "we can, we must" and calls this the "technological imperative." Jonas (1979, 1984), however, cautions against the tendency to accept scientific progress as an unalleged benefit.

The first steps toward remaking the human body have already been taken (L. Shapiro et al., 1986; Gustafson, 1994). Three levels of physical remaking seem possible:

1. Surgical procedures which would replace existing organs with transplants, biological constructs, or artificial organs that are not mere substitutes for natural organs but which expand old functions or insert new ones into the body as suggested.

2. Embryological development might be influenced by drugs or surgery so as to mold the development of the phenotype (the actual body) while not changing the genotype (inherited characteristics). Thus the phenotypic sex of a child could be determined at will, despite the genotype, by altering the course of development very early in embryonic life (Frenkiel, 1993). There are possibilities of expanding the human senses to extend our sight or hearing beyond their present ranges or to enhance their power to resolve colors or pitches, etc.

3. Ultimately genetic engineering might be employed to produce any gene combination in the fertilized ovum, thus creating human beings by "recipe" (Anderson, 1994). Already the development of the technique of "recombinant DNA" (deoxyribonucleic acid) has made it possible to produce new species of bacteria with useful (and perhaps dangerous) combinations of genetic traits. Related to this is the production of clones from the somatic cells of a parent or artificial reproduction of multiple individuals all having the same genetic composition (Cohen, 1994).

The basic ethical issue here is seen by some theologians to be how great is the extent of human dominion over nature. This is a classical way of posing the issue, but it is perhaps too much influenced by the Greek image of God as a jealous monarch who becomes angry when Prometheus infringes on his prerogatives. Others would see such attempts to improve on human beings as an insult to the work of the Creator, whose masterpiece is humankind, or at least as a fatal temptation to pride (Ellul, 1965, 1980).

Today, however, in considering radical human development, two theological points must be stressed. First, God is a generous Creator, who in creating human beings also called them, giving them intelligence to share in his creative power. Consequently, God does not want human beings to leave fallow the talents he has given them, but encourages them to improve on the universe he has made. Second, such improvement is possible because Christian theology can assimilate the scientific view of an evolutionary universe in which the human race has been created through a still-continuing evolutionary process, if God is acknowledged as the ultimate cause of that process. Thus God has called us to join with him in bringing the universe to its completion, and in doing this, he has not made us merely workers to execute his orders or to add trifling original touches on our own. Rather, God has made us his genuine co-workers and encourages us to exercise real creativity (Ashley, 1995).

Granted such a theology, however, it is not so clear that the remaking of the human body on new lines is really the appropriate focus for our creativity. Remolding the environment and creating human culture takes time enough. No doubt with greater knowledge some of the business of evolution may be tidied up by removing such vestiges as wisdom teeth or appendices if, indeed, this would be a real improvement. Someday genetic disease may also be eliminated and even human health advanced eugenically. Yet before technology attempts to produce Superman, it needs to heed the paradox proposed by MacIntyre (1979), who first imagines what types of human beings he would like to produce. They would have the ability to live with uncertainty; to keep rooted in the particularity of everyday life; to form nonmanipulative relations with others; to find their fulfillment in their work; to accept death; to keep hopeful; and be willing to die for their freedom. He then concludes, "The project of designing our descendants would, if successful, result in descendants that would reject that project."

Cooperation in Creation

It is important to remember, however, that human creativity depends on a human brain. Any alteration that would injure the brain and thus a person's very creativity would indeed be disastrous mutilation, especially if this were to be transmitted genetically, thus further polluting the gene pool with defects that might be hidden and incalculable.

It is generally admitted that knowledge of this wonderful brain is still in its beginnings (ITEST, 1975; Edelman, 1987, 1995; Harrington, 1992; Penrose, 1995). The complexity of the brain is beyond any other system imaginable, and this complexity is reduced to a relatively very small organ capable of self-development from the embryo and of self-maintenance, but not of self-restoration. The human brain may be near the limit of complexity and integration possible in organic, living systems (Ashley, 1995). In this case any radical improvement may be illusory, whereas even slight alterations may be very damaging. Thus, to say the least, radical attempts to alter the structure of the human brain must be viewed with the utmost caution, since the risk of producing only persons of lowered intelligence is very high.

This is certainly not so true of other organ systems, and it is possible to imagine that someday in other environments it might become necessary, for example, to replace the human lungs with other ways of obtaining oxygen. In principle it would seem that such changes would be ethical (1) if they gave support to human intelligence by helping the life of the brain and (2) if they did not suppress any of the fundamental human functions that integrate the human personality. Thus alterations that would make it impossible for a human being to directly sense the external world at least as effectively as he or she now does with "five senses" would be contrary to the principle of totality and integrity (p. 224), as would alterations that would make it impossible for human beings to experience the basic emotions, since emotional life is closely related to human intelligence and creativity. Again, alterations that would make human beings sexless and incapable of parenthood would also be antihuman. The power to procreate through intercourse, and to form families for holistic development of children and parents are functions that pertain to the very essence of being human. Hence the following conclusions can be drawn:

1. The use of surgery and genetic manipulation to improve human bodies is ethically good, provided that they take full account of such risks and are not carried away by a false ambition to work technical miracles without regard to their real meaning for human living. In particular, Christians should be concerned that such innovations do not weaken the fundamental relations within the family or the sense of the child as a unique gift of God.

2. Genetic engineering and less radical transformations of the present normal human body would be permissible if it improves rather than mutilates the basic human functions, especially as they relate to supporting human intelligence and creativity. Transformation would be forbidden, however, (a) if human intelligence and creativity are endangered and (b) if the fundamental functions that constitute human integrity are suppressed. Experimental efforts of this radical type must be undertaken with great caution and only on the basis of existing knowledge, not with high risks to the subjects or to the gene pool. In this regard we need not draw a firm line between somatic cell genetic intervention and germ-line cell intervention. Surely, somatic cell intervention is more problem-free, but if germ-line cell intervention could be perfected, it could ethically be utilized if the goals of such intervention were in accord with the norms already mentioned.

3. The principle of stewardship and creativity throws light on many of the problems of human reconstruction. Natural law should not be conceived of as a fixed pattern of human life to which human beings are forever confined. Rather, the Creator has made human beings free and intelligent, and it is precisely this intelligent freedom that is human nature and the foundation of natural moral law. Human intelligence, however, is not disembodied; it depends on a brain and a body that have a specific structure and purpose. In caring for their total health, persons have not only the right but the obligation to understand their psychological and biological structure and to improve themselves even in ways that may seem novel to past generations. Such improvement is good stewardship of the share in divine creativity with which God has endowed humankind, provided it perfect, not destroy, what He has given us already.

11.2 GENETIC INTERVENTION

Ordering a Child?

The most ambitious scientific project, as extensive in its implications as the Manhattan Project which made possible the release of atomic and nuclear energy, is the Human Genome Project. Utilizing the resources and skills of the scientific community throughout the world, the Human Genome Project seeks to identify the activity of all human genes and locate the place of each gene on the human chromosome.

Eventually this knowledge, it is hoped, will be used to modify the effect of deteriorative genes and to introduce into the human genotype genes which will improve the structure and behavior of human persons. To date, astounding progress has been made in regard to identifying the location and activity of human genes (Collins, 1995). Efforts to modify the activity of the human genotype by eliminating from or introducing genes into the human genotype have not been as successful as yet. But indicators for future success in manipulating genetic activity should not be discounted (Kolata, 1995).

The issue of the parents' need and right to have children or even to "order" the sort of child they want is also at the base of many new problems that loom on the horizon concerning genetic engineering, or to use an expression with less pejorative connotations, "genetic intervention." This is the effort to repair genetic defects at their genotypic source in the genes and chromosomes rather than in their phenotypic effects and, further, to control and produce at will new combinations of genetic traits in offspring (Anderson, 1985; Glover, 1985).

One of the simplest forms of such engineering would be to determine at will the sex of the fetus by selecting sperm that do or do not have the Y chromosome that determines maleness and then using selected sperm for artificial insemination or in vitro fertilization and implantation. Even if a technique could be invented that would promote or suppress the production of one or the other type of sperm in the male parent without interfering with the normal process of sexual intercourse, the social and ecological consequences of such intervention could be counterproductive.

Biologists are convinced that evolutionary selection has developed the process of sexual differentiation by a genetic mechanism of the sort we find in the human species because this ensures an approximate 50/50 distribution of the sexes. Some additional mechanism not fully understood even produces a slightly higher number of male zygotes to offset the higher mortality of males. Studies made in the United States (Holmes, 1985) show that most young couples now want two children, preferring a boy first, but once the boy is assured, then a girl. Although this preference is probably cultural and subject to cultural modification, it possibly also has a sociobiological foundation in the greater mortality of males. These studies predict that if sex selection was widely adopted, there would first be a marked rise in male births, but then a leveling to a 50/50 distribution. It seems, therefore, that the promotion of sexual selection might not be seriously deleterious to society, although it certainly would have risks and would have few, if any, social advantages over leaving it to nature. Its only advantage would be that parents would have freedom of choice, provided that overall they use this choice to have equal numbers of boys and girls.

Ethically speaking, is this free choice of a boy or a girl an advantage to the *child?* After all, parents should not let their subjective preferences operate at the expense of their children in this matter, just as it is unethical for them to insist that the child be a doctor or a lawyer if this is not truly for the best interests of the child. It might be argued that it is somewhat advantageous for a boy to have a sister, and vice versa, rather than a sibling of his or her own sex, but it would be difficult to prove that such an advantage, if it exists, is of major significance. On the other hand, Christian teaching shows that it is highly significant to children that they be accepted by their parents as a divine gift to be loved for what they uniquely are and not merely because they conform to the parents' hopes or expectations. At present, society is becoming more aware of the immense injustice and harm done to women by cultural patterns and structures that constantly say to a girl, "You should have been a boy." Sex selection by the parents either will reinforce this male preference pattern or, if parents can be reeducated to equal preference, will still say to the individual child, "You are loved because you conform to your parents' preferences." This seems an injustice to the child and further reinforces the cultural message that children exist primarily to fulfill the needs of the parents rather than for their own sake. This implication is already built into many cultural structures, and people have an ethical responsibility to fight against it. The health care profession should discourage such attitudes, not promote techniques to further them.

Complex Forms of Intervention

The same consideration applies to more complex forms of genetic intervention. Although some progress has already been made in genetic recombination at the level of simple organisms, the possibility of using such methods to correct genetic defects or to create new genetic structures in human zygotes or embryos is still remote (Leiden, 1995).

If the purpose of such techniques is therapy for an individual fetus, the only ethical issue is the proportion of probable benefit to risk. The issues already discussed, however, concerning in vitro fertilization and artificial insemination and implantation arise if these techniques can be used to produce a healthy embryo only at the expense of creating several embryos from which one will be selected and the others allowed to perish (see p. 244) (Lejeune et al., 1984).

What if the purpose is not therapy of an existing fetus, but the production of superior human beings through germ-line therapy? Two methods have been proposed. One is to replicate many genetically identical individuals by cloning. In such a process, nuclei from the somatic cells of a "superior" individual would be transplanted into a denucleated ovum, which would then develop into an identical twin of the donor. This would require in vitro fertilization and implantation into a foster mother's womb (Bashim, 1984; Watson, 1971). Another method is to recombine genes in the nucleus of a zygote, for example, by using viruses that have the capability of incorporating a section of a chromosome derived from one nucleus and fixing it in a chromosome of another (*transduction*) (Fackleman, 1994). Theoretically, it may become possible to synthesize chemically new genes that have never existed in the gene pool or to produce them by artificial, controlled mutation. Thus it might also be possible to produce a human being according to "recipe," with the height, complexion, physiological traits, and mental abilities desired. Although this is still very remote (Kass, 1985), we would not rule it out ethically merely on the grounds that it would be usurpation of God's creative power, since God wishes to share this creative power with human persons if we use it well (principle of stewardship and creativity, 8.3).

Grave ethical difficulties, however, do arise over whether society has either the knowledge or the virtue to take the responsibility for creating these superior members of the race (Callahan, 1981; John Fletcher, 1985; Kass, 1987). Attempts to define *superior* eugenically are so ambiguous as to be arbitrary (Rifkin, 1984). Because human beings are evolutionary and historical beings, *superior* does not mean a being superior in one age and culture, but rather a being with capabilities of meeting the challenges of new and unpredictable situations. Genetic variation assists this flexibility, whereas the production of many identical human beings or favoring certain supposedly superior types amounts to a restriction on this genetic variability. At most, a eugenic policy would have to be content with introducing into the gene pool some new, apparently valuable traits or increasing somewhat the percentage of their presence. Furthermore, all the difficulties already raised about the way in which such techniques tend to separate the child from its relations to parents and family arise once more.

The following conclusions can be drawn:

1. It is more feasible, technically and ethically, to improve the human condition by improving the environment and development of the individual, that is, the *phenotype*, than by modifying genetic endowment, that is, the *genotype*. Priority in research and investment of medical resources should be given to the former effort. Genetic research is extremely important, however, to understand the interactions of genotype and phenotype.

2. Presently proposed methods of genetic reconstruction of human beings involve in vitro fertilization and other procedures that are ethically objectionable because they separate reproduction from its parental context and involve the production of human beings, some of whom will be defective because of experimental failure and who probably will be destroyed. This contravenes the basic principles of ethical experimentation with human subjects (see 9.5; Ramsey, 1970; CDF, 1987).

3. Proposals to improve the human race by sex selection, cloning, or genetic reconstruction are ethically unacceptable in the present state of knowledge. Unless limited to very modest interventions, they would

restrict the genetic variability important to human survival, and they would separate reproduction from its parental context.

4. If the foregoing problems can be overcome, it will be ethically desirable to develop and use genetic methods for therapy of genetic defects in existing embryos, keeping in view the risk–benefit proportion (OTA, 1984).

Because the ethical questions arising from genetic research are so important for our society, the Human Genome Organization has issued a statement of principles to guide genetic research (Hugo, 1996).

Ecology and New Life Forms

In addition to discussion about efforts to manipulate human genes, much discussion has focused recently on the possible effects on the ecological balance and the possible medical and commercial uses of experiments with and large-scale production of new life forms by the technique of *recombinant DNA* (deoxyribonucleic acid). This involves the modification of the genetic code of existing life forms by introducing into their chromosomes fragments derived from the chromosomes of other life forms, thus producing organisms with combinations of genetic and inheritable traits never before found in nature. For example, it is possible to produce food plants that can directly utilize atmospheric nitrogen and thus eliminate the use of fertilizers, or to produce rather inexpensively the heretofore extremely scarce interferon, a natural substance believed to have many important medical uses, including cancer therapy. The U.S. Supreme Court, in *Diamond v. Chakrabarty*, held that a live, synthetic microorganism is patentable, thus opening the way to its commercial development (Ehrman et al., 1980).

Those who favor patenting such biological inventions argue that this will promote research, as it has for drugs. The analogy, however, also suggests the possibility of serious abuses for profit. The same basic ethical principles that govern any form of research apply here (11.6), with the additional precautions that what is involved are not merely individual human subjects, but the total environment, and that possible widespread epidemics could result if something goes wrong (NIH, 1987). The greatest worry, but one which should not be exaggerated, is whether some new life form, against which there is no existent immunity in the human, animal, or plant ecosystem, may multiply beyond bounds, as has so often occurred when alien species are introduced into an ecosystem already in balance (Crespi, 1993).

11.3 GENETIC SCREENING AND COUNSELING

The medical specialty of diagnosing inherited or genetic defects and their treatment, as well as the task of screening populations for these defects and counseling couples who are or may become parents of defective children, is developing rapidly. Special clinics dedicated to this are being founded throughout the United States.

Three basic discoveries have made it possible at times to predict inherited traits of a child before birth (Reed, 1980; Carmi, 1983; Watson et al., 1987): (1) Gregor Mendel's theory of the laws of the combinations of units of inheritance, (2) these units or *genes* being located in the chromosomes of the nucleus of every cell, and (3) genetic code consisting in variations in a fundamental substance, DNA, out of which the genes are composed. Techniques of diagnosing these defects at early stages of child development are being perfected. These include *amniocentesis,* by which the genetic condition of the unborn child can be determined in some respects by examining the amniotic fluid in which the fetus floats in the womb. Another technique is *chorionic villi sampling,* in which a plastic catheter is inserted through the cervix to biopsy villi, the hairlike projections in the placenta. This is rapidly growing tissue, and results of chromosome tests are available in a few days (Kahn, 1987). The chorionic villi test may be performed about eight weeks earlier than amniocentesis. Also, techniques to counteract some of the deleterious consequences of genetic defects are being worked out, and there is even the prospect of methods for correcting the defective genes themselves by DNA recombination (Anderson, 1985), although so far these have not succeeded.

Why such advances are medically important is evident from the following statistics. There are approximately 3,000 different diseases in the single-gene disorder group, all of which are caused by different abnormal genes (Ngyan and Sahat, 1987). Today 33 percent of infant deaths are related to genetic causes. More than 100 genetic conditions can be diagnosed prenatally. Parent carriers of defective genes may have as much as a 50 percent risk of generating offspring with a genetic defect. The polygenic conditions, such as diabetes mellitus, gout, and some allergies, occur in 1.7 to 2.6 percent of all live births. There seems to be approximately a 5 percent incidence of genetic disease in all live births (Kahn, 1987)

In view of these facts, some scientists, in the name of preventive medicine, advocate prenatal or postnatal *genetic screening* of the whole population for four purposes: (1) to advance scientific research, since such research is necessary to achieve full understanding and control over human inheritance; (2) to assist responsible parenthood so that carriers of genetic defects may not pass them on; (3) to make possible early therapy before the malfunctioning of defective genes has caused extensive damage; and (4) to give the parents the option of aborting the child when the defect is serious and no therapy is yet known (Macklin, 1985; Murray et al., 1984).

We have already given reasons why this last purpose is ethically unacceptable, but the first three are certainly legitimate. They do, however, raise serious questions. First, the research purposes of genetic screening must be regulated in the same way as any other type of research on human subjects (see p. 348 ff). Thus, since amniocentesis involves risk of spontaneous abortion (although the risk has been reduced with the help of sonography to less than 1 percent), it cannot be used unless there are also proportionate benefits for the fetus. At present, therapeutic help for a genetically deficient fetus is limited, but more progress in this field is noted each year. Some ethicists maintain that amniocentesis benefits the fetus because it helps the parents prepare more adequately for the birth. This thought has been confirmed by a recent statement of John Paul II (1995): "Prenatal diagnosis presents no moral objection if carried out in order to identify the medical treatment which may be needed by the child in the womb" (n. 14, Cataldo, 1996). In sum, amniocentesis is indicated only when a pregnancy is thought to be at increased risk for a particular disorder. A few years ago, David Roy (1984) pointed out a more profound ethical issue that may result from prenatal screening:

> Prenatal diagnosis delivers the knowledge required to exercise the kind of quality control over the unborn that amounts to a control over birth. . . . The earlier long-standing belief of a theocratic reproductive culture in the equality of all human beings based on the identity of their origin and destiny has given way to an emphasis on the empirical inequalities of human beings (p. 18).

Screening for Genetic Defects

Most screening techniques used postnatally only involve the withdrawal of an insignificant amount of body fluid or tissue and are harmless. Nevertheless, informed consent is required in all such cases, and it is highly questionable that it is legitimate to enact laws that require compulsory screening for research purposes alone. Even when consent is given, care must be taken about how the information is used (Wertz, 1995). If the results are made known to subjects, there is danger that they may misunderstand or exaggerate the seriousness and possible consequences of their condition or the condition of their children. If the results are known to others, there is danger of stigmatization, that is, that victims will be regarded by others as humanly inferior or dangerous. For example, it is unfair to label those blacks who are carriers of the sickle cell trait or those Jews who are carriers of the Tay–Sachs syndrome as diseased or defective.

Caution is necessary, however, in the face of programs of *negative* eugenics advocated by certain enthusiasts (Glass, 1975; Modell, 1982) who argue that modern medicine has upset the ecological balance by saving the lives of more and more defective persons who formerly would have died before they could reproduce. Thus the load of defective genes in the gene pool is increasing, and a much higher level of genetic disease may soon occur in the population. As Lappé (1972) has written:

> The consensus of the best medical and genetic opinion is that whatever genetic deterioration is occurring as a result of decreased natural selection is so slow as to be insignificant when contrasted to "environmental" changes, including those produced by medical innovation (p. 421).

If only those persons who themselves suffer from a particular genetic disease are prevented from reproducing, this still does not eliminate heterozygous carriers who will continue to transmit defects dependent on recessive genes (Thompson and Thompson, 1988). At present, technology is far from being able to detect all these carriers. Even if science had this ability, such elimination would extend to many people. This would probably also mean the elimination from the gene pool of many desirable traits because the same persons carry both good and bad traits, which sometimes are genetically linked in ways still very obscure. Thus programs of negative eugenics based on present knowledge would achieve their goals only very slowly, over many generations, and might have side effects worse than the evils they remedy. Moreover, as defective genes are eliminated from the gene pool, they are constantly being replaced by mutations caused by environmental factors.

It seems, therefore, that such information cannot be used to compel persons to refrain from reproduction, but it may be supplied to them to enable them to make responsible personal decisions. Even here, however, some public caution is needed. Some states have adopted compulsory screening of newborn infants to detect those afflicted with phenylketonuria (PKU), a genetically based metabolic disease that results in mental retardation and can be treated by diet (Andrews, 1985). After these programs were instituted, it was discovered that some persons who test positively do not develop mental retardation, and that the dietary treatment to which they were subjected may even have been harmful (Modell, 1992). Thus genetic testing programs have to be carefully designed. The Research Group on Ethical, Social, and Legal Issues in Genetic Counseling and Genetic Engineering (Hastings Center Institute, 1972) has suggested guidelines, which can be summarized as follows:

1. The attainability of the program's aims should be pretested by pilot projects and other studies, and the program should be constantly evaluated and updated.
2. Community participation in planning and executing the program should be secured to educate the public as to the true significance and legitimate use of the information obtained.
3. The information obtained should be made available according to clearly stated policies known to those participating before they consent, and their privacy should be carefully protected.
4. Screening programs should be voluntary. The rights of parents to make their own decisions about the use of the information in family planning should be protected and care taken to avoid stigmatizing them or their offspring.
5. Information about screening should be open and available to all, with priorities given to well-defined populations suffering from frequent defects.
6. Programs should not be instituted unless the tests used are able to give relatively unambiguous information, and this should be precisely recorded.
7. The general principles with regard to experimentation with human

subjects, such as informed consent and protection from risks, should be observed.

8. Persons to be screened or who have their children screened should be informed before they consent about the nature and cost of therapy and its risks or if no therapy is available.

9. Counseling to help the subjects understand and deal with the information should be provided.

We would also add that it is important to consider whether the cost in money and personnel in administering such programs give them high priority in view of the rarity of most of these conditions. It must be recognized, however, that in some cases (e.g., PKU) the testing per subject is quite inexpensive, whereas the cost of caring for even a few mentally retarded children in institutions may be very high.

Genetic Counseling

If such screening programs are to be voluntary, the main concern is to counsel parents as they attempt to decide how to use this information in planning their families (Parker, 1994)

Genetic counseling may be characterized as a process of communication that attempts to deal with the human problems associated with the occurrence, or the risk of occurrence, of a genetic disorder in an individual or family (Atkinson and Moraczewski, 1980). This process involves an attempt by one or more appropriately trained persons to help an individual, couple, or family do the following:

1. Comprehend the medical facts, such as the risk of occurrence or recurrence of a disorder, the possibilities for diagnosis, the probable course of the disorder, and the available therapies.

2. Appreciate the ways in which hereditary and environmental factors contribute to the disorder, and the extent to which specified relatives are at risk for being affected or for producing an affected child.

3. Understand the options for dealing with a positive diagnosis, such as methods of contraception or sterilization, abortion, institutionalization, adoption agencies, and other social services.

4. Choose the course of action that seems appropriate to the clients in view of their own values and goals, and act in accordance with that decision.

5. Make the best possible adjustment to the disorder in an affected member of the family or to the risk of a recurrence of the disorder.

A family comes to a genetic counselor because of fears about possible defects in children already in existence or about their responsibilities for future pregnancies. These fears may have arisen because of positive test results in mass screening, or because of a record of genetic disease in parents, previous children, or close relatives.

Some argue that if serious reasons exist to believe a fetus is gravely defective, the parents should be persuaded to agree to abort the child if this suspicion is confirmed by amniocentesis (Silber, 1981). Otherwise, they argue, it is difficult to justify the risks of the amniocentesis procedure. If abortion is ethically unacceptable, the counselor should not recommend prenatal screening that is potentially dangerous to the infant unless this is justified by the possibility of intrauterine therapy proportionate to the risks or of some benefit to the infant because the parents will be better prepared to care for the child. A recent survey of fetal surgery expresses that the main value of antenatal diagnosis lies in prompt postnatal treatment of major malformations before complications develop (Hendren and Lillehi, 1988). The desire to satisfy the parents' curiosity concerning the sex of the child does not seem to be a sufficient reason for subjecting the infant to even minimal risk of harm.

Again, some counselors would suggest that even when amniocentesis cannot determine genetic defect with certainty, the parents are free to decide whether they wish to take the risks or to abort; the law seems to suggest this option (Dickens, 1986). This means that if parents decide to abort, they are also risking the destruction of a normal child because such tests are not infallible, nor do they perfectly predict the degree of phenotypic impairment. We believe that counselors should not recommend abortion as a solution. If the parents declare a firm intention to abort, the counselor should not cooperate in any way with them. The reason is that the rights of the fetus to life should be protected by counselors—exactly as they would protect the rights of a child already born—against the infringement of these rights by the parents, no matter how well-intentioned they may be. A counselor, however, in doing whatever possible to avoid abortion, should exercise great prudence, avoiding threats, pressures, and recriminations, since these will only aggravate the situation. Indeed, undue persuasion may lead to a malpractice claim (Annas, 1985a; Holder, 1985). In sum, if abortion is in question, the counselor should respect the conscience of the parents while doing everything possible to protect the child.

Is it permissible for a counselor to give information to parents whom the counselor only suspects may resort to abortion? In the present ethical climate this suspicion always exists, and it has deterred Catholic health care facilities from instituting genetic counseling centers. Parents, however, have a right to such information, which has good as well as bad uses, and the counselor who supplies it cooperates only materially and remotely if the parents use it for a purpose the counselor considers unethical. Moreover, counselors may be legally liable if they do not inform parents that an unborn child may be suffering from a genetic defect and that it is possible in some cases to make sure of this by amniocentesis or other prenatal tests (Annas, 1979), even though parents might use this information to obtain an abortion. In our opinion, Catholic health care facilities have a duty to provide such counseling in accordance with Christian moral standards, since otherwise parents will be forced to obtain information from centers where abortion will be an accepted and even encouraged solution (McCormick, 1984a).

It certainly is a right for a child to be free of every defect that medicine has the power to prevent or correct. It is paradoxical, however, to believe that this right is protected by destroying the child who has not been saved from defect. Parents may have the responsibility not to generate such children, but having generated them, they also have the duty to care for them. They cannot lighten their burden by destroying an unborn child any more than an infant or adolescent. Underlying such arguments is the basic conviction that it is better never to be a defective person. This is an assumption of some humanists, but it is not consistent with a Christian view of the value of a person or the true meaning of human life.

It is also true, however, that couples have the duty of responsible parenthood, and society has a legitimate concern to support and encourage this responsibility. The genetic counselor, therefore, has the function of helping prospective parents prepare themselves for the possibility that a fetus will be defective and to plan ways to provide for this eventuality. The counselor also has the task of helping them decide whether they will or will not generate children.

Parental Responsibility

In the past, some would have argued that a person or a couple at risk of begetting a defective child or children, or of transmitting defective genes to future generations, should fatalistically marry and beget children and "leave it to God." This fatalism, as already pointed out, has not been as damaging to society as some eugenic enthusiasts have thought, since it does not upset the ecological balance established by evolutionary selection. Even today, when medical advances have upset this balance by counteracting this selective process, such fatalism can only very slowly increase the social burden. Nevertheless, Christian teaching does not favor fatalistic attitudes, but rather advocates parental responsibility.

Prospective parents, therefore, have to consider these factors: (1) their own need to have children as the completion of their mutual love, (2) their own capacity to care for these children, and (3) the risk that each particular child may suffer from grave handicaps requiring special care, including the possibility that this child will be faced in turn with the question as to whether he or she should pass on defective genes to the next generation. Some significant risks of defect exist for *every* child and could not be eliminated even by the most radical use of abortion. Thus in all cases parents must decide whether they have the capacity to care for a potentially defective child. Furthermore, the counselor and society have the duty to assist the parents in accepting and meeting reasonable risks. For counselors or society at large to encourage in parents the attitude that they should not have children unless the children are perfect and require the least care possible is as reprehensible as to encourage parents to reproduce fatalistically.

Certainly, the correct professional attitude for genetic counselors is to give the parents reliable, objective information as to the probabilities of defect and its consequences and the type of therapy and care that will be required. Counselors should also help them (directly or by referral to others professionally competent) to deal with personal, economic, and social factors that determine the parents' capacity to meet the demands of care if a child has a particular defect. They should also inform the parents about the social resources that may be available to help. On the basis of this objective information and counseling support, the individual or couple must make their own decision about whether their need for children justifies taking the risks involved. Such decisions must be made not merely by some persons, but by all prospective parents, since begetting new life is essentially a risky business. The reason that genetic counselors are needed today is that now more information is available about the risks involved in reproduction and more help is needed in dealing with the complexities this information discloses.

As already argued in 10.5, the need and right of a couple to have children is not absolute. Thus, if the risks are high, such as 25 percent, of begetting a child so defective as to require care that the parents cannot supply, even with reasonable and available social assistance, then they have the responsibility to consider not begetting children. Genetic counselors, therefore, while respecting the consciences and psychological freedom of their clients, will help persons at high risk to make this difficult decision. Moreover, these parents should be informed properly about the various methods of birth regulation, especially natural family planning, and the ethical evaluation of these methods (10.3).

Problems also arise with regard to adults who have a genetic defect that will eventually become a serious handicap or lead to early death, for example, Huntington's chorea, which in middle life results in progressive neurological degeneration (Quaid, 1993). On the one hand is the responsibility of the person not to pass this defect on to children, and on the other, the personal difficulty of living under a sense of doom. Undoubtedly, as people become more aware of the existence of genetic defects, it will become impossible to keep such knowledge from them. It would seem that all individuals should have the freedom to decide whether they wish a diagnosis. Nevertheless, we would argue that individuals who seriously suspect they have such serious defects would be wise to have the matter settled by a reliable test and to adjust their life plans accordingly (Rice and Doherty, 1982).

At the same time, the right of persons to make decisions about reproducing genetic defects should be respected both by the church and by society, and they should not be stigmatized because of their decision. The reasons are these:

1. The balance of factors cannot be reduced to objective certitude, especially because weighing of personal needs and capacities is involved.
2. The value of personal responsibility in the use of sex and living of family life greatly outweigh the damage done society by the increased genetic load, which cannot be significantly lightened in the short run

and about which insufficient information exists to lighten significantly in the long run.

3. If the parents prove mistaken in their decision, society can and should assume the responsibility for adequate care of the children, a burden that is not great compared to many other health problems.

Clearly, if society promotes adequate education about genetic hazards, in a population where the birthrate is low and falling, it is probable that negative voluntary eugenics will become a part of the general social pattern. Genetic counseling will promote this. Catholic genetic counseling will also promote it without encouraging abortion or neglecting the parents' freedom of decision, while actively promoting a more optimistic and life-affirming attitude toward the inevitable risks of parenthood.

11.4 ORGAN TRANSPLANTATION

Transplants from Deceased Donors

Any surgical procedure involves some reconstruction of the human body, but there is a striking difference between procedures such as setting a broken bone or sewing up a wound or removing a tumor, which assist a natural healing process or remove a diseased part, and a procedure by which an organ originally belonging to another is transplanted into the human body in place of one of its own parts that has become dysfunctional. The latter procedure involves the rights not of one person but of two and thus raises a new moral question.

Two types of organ transplants are possible, one involving an organ or tissue taken from a dead person and given to a living person and the other involving an organ taken from one living person and given to another living person. Transplanting an organ or tissue from a dead person to a living person in itself presents no ethical problem. With few exceptions, religious groups as well as humanistic ethicists have recognized the worth and ethical validity of such transplants (Jonsen, 1985; John Paul II, 1984d, 1995). If some serious question arises concerning transplant from a dead person to a living person, it stems from factors other than the transplant itself. For example, concern was expressed at first about the worth of heart transplants, most of it arising either from the great expense of money and personnel involved in a medical procedure that brings little substantive value to human society in general (Ramsey, 1970; Thorup et al., 1985) or from fear that in some cases the organ donor had not actually expired (P. Williams et al., 1973). These concerns are no longer prominent, however, because of better survival rates in recipients of heart transplants and from greater ability to ascertain the criteria for total brain death (Black, 1984). John Paul II (1995) echoing the thought of Pius XII (1956a), summed up Catholic teaching on transplants involving an organ from a dead person:

> The Gospel of Life is celebrated above all else in the daily living of life which should be filled with selfgiving for others ... A particular praise-

worthy example of such gestures is the donation of organs performed in an ethically acceptable manner, with a view to offering a chance of health and even life itself to the sick who sometimes have no other hope (n. 86).

Transplants from Living Donors

Far more difficulties arise, however, with organ transplants between living persons. Before 1950, the morality of transplanting an organ from one living person to another was discussed by Catholic theologians from a theoretical point of view (Cunningham, 1944). Although an interesting question, it was somewhat impractical because transplants between living persons generally were not yet technically feasible. Many theologians who considered the subject did not approve of it. These theologians argued that the principle of totality and integrity would justify mutilation or injury to one part of the body only if it was done to preserve the person's own health or human life. The principle would not justify a transplant to another person, however, because one person is not related to another person as means to end or as part to whole. Thus one person's bodily integrity could not be sacrificed for another.

Whatever the theoretical discussions, organ transplants from living donors began to be performed in the early 1950s. Because of genetic similarity, identical twins were the first subjects of kidney transplants. Many early transplants were not successful because the transplanted organ often was rejected by the reaction of the recipient's immune system (Murray, 1986). Yet as some succeeded, scientists began to argue that unless there was freedom to undertake such experiments, medical progress would be hampered (Fox and Swazy, 1978). Thus, ethicists and moralists gave the problem closer scrutiny.

Gerald Kelly (1956), a leader in this development, wrote:

> It may come as a surprise to physicians that theologians should have any difficulty about mutilations and other procedures which are performed with the consent of the subject but which have as their purpose the helping of others. By a sort of instinctive judgment we consider that the giving of a part of one's body to help a sick man is not only morally justifiable, but, in some instances, actually heroic (p. 246).

In developing the rationale for a more liberal opinion, Kelly maintained, "It is clear from reason and papal teaching that the principle of totality cannot be used to justify the donating of a part of one's body to another person. Moreover, since man is only the administrator of his life and bodily members and functions, his power to dispose of these things is limited." Kelly, however, sought to delineate as clearly as possible the limits of this dominion, especially concerning organ transplants. Further, he asked whether there is any other way in which this seemingly worthwhile and Christian action can be justified. He suggested that the principle of fraternal love, or charity, would justify the transplant, provided that there was only limited harm to the donor. Although it was not unanimously accepted, some theologians agreed with this opinion and developed it more clearly. Distinguishing between anatomical integrity and functional integrity, they stated that the latter, not the former, was necessary to ensure human or bodily integrity (McFadden, 1976).

Anatomical integrity refers to the material or physical integrity of the human body. *Functional integrity* refers to the systematic efficiency of the human body. For example, if one kidney were missing from a person's body, there would be a lack of anatomical integrity, but if one healthy kidney were present and working, there would be functional integrity because one healthy kidney is more than able to provide systematic efficiency. If a cornea were to be taken from the eye of one living person and given to another, however, the case would be different. Not only would anatomical integrity be destroyed, but functional integrity would be destroyed as well. The loss of sight in one eye severely damages vision, especially depth perception. Thus in this case, more than anatomical integrity is involved. For the most part, the transplant of a cornea from living persons is no longer a problem because transplanting corneas from dead persons has been perfected.

This distinction between anatomical and functional integrity that we have incorporated in our formulation of the principle of totality and integrity (2.4) explains why blood transfusions and skin grafts are acceptable and why theologians have approved elective appendectomy if the abdominal cavity is open for another legitimate reason. In these situations loss of anatomical integrity may occur through loss of blood, skin tissue, or an internal organ, but no loss of functional integrity occurs.

Thus the concept of functional integrity is the key factor in addressing the morality of transplants between living persons. Certainly, a risk is involved if a donor surrenders an organ to another person, even if the donor has two of them. Aside from the risk involved in the surgical procedure, such donors take the risk of serious illness themselves if the one remaining organ becomes damaged or diseased. The risk, however, although serious, is deemed to be justified by the fact that donors share in the common good of the community to which they contribute by helping another, that is, by love (Ramsey, 1970).

Clearly, organ donation is not an obligation; rather, it is something chosen in the freedom of charity. Motivated by the same charity, one could decide not to offer an organ. Such a decision would not be unethical. For this reason, it is imperative that a donor's free and informed consent be obtained. Given the fact that the more successful transplants are between members of the same family, familial or social pressure to offer oneself as a donor may at times be severe but the courts (rightly, we believe) refuse to compel such donations (Hartman, 1993). Because of the motivation that should underlie the donation of an organ by a living person, it is clear that selling organs is unethical. The federal government has prohibited the sale of all organs in the United States, but sale of organs by living donors in some countries is a common practice (Barnett and Kaserman, 1993).

Kelly was certainly right in holding that organ transplants between two living persons are licit if the donor's functional integrity is maintained, but we would caution that great care should be taken in weighing the merely potential benefit against the actual risks. Consent should not be given unless the prognosis for both the donor and the recipient is good. In some cases it is necessary to weigh the value of a brief prolongation of life for the recipient against the lifelong risk to the donor.

In addition to the rationale put forward by Kelly and others to justify transplants between living persons, some theologians go a step further and seek to justify these procedures either by expanding the principle of totality and integrity or by treating the whole process as a curative action, even though two people are involved and one will be injured (Nolan, 1968). In so doing, they destroy the limits so carefully delineated by Kelly and others to protect human integrity. According to these theories, the human unity predicated on body and soul is destroyed, and the body becomes something merely used by the person, part of which, at least, is at the disposal or "over against" the person and thus may be sacrificed by the person for any higher good. Falling heir to Cartesian dualism that renders appreciation of the body–soul unity of human nature impossible, one author even concludes that both eyes may be donated "for the good of another person." Section 2.4 lists the reasons why we believe such views do not do justice to the Christian view of the integrity of the human person (Ramsey, 1970).

The development in the past 40 years of the moral teaching of theologians concerning organ transplants between the living is of more than antiquarian interest. First, it shows clearly that the opinion of theologians can evolve. Second, it shows that by refining accepted principles, and not denying them, new conclusions can be drawn from long-established principles. Third, it demonstrates that many ethical problems are solved by starting with intuitive judgments and then examining the principles in light of the solution proposed in the intuitive judgment.

In summary, the transplanting of organs or tissues from a dead person to a living person does not offer any intrinsic ethical problem. Transplanting organs from one living person to another is also ethically acceptable, provided that the following criteria are met:

1. There is a serious need on the part of the recipient that cannot be fulfilled in any other way.
2. The functional integrity of the donor as a human person will not be impaired, even though anatomical integrity may suffer.
3. The risk taken by the donor as an act of charity is proportionate to the good resulting for the recipient.
4. The donor's consent is free and informed.

Allocation of Organs for Transplantation

Other issues connected with organ transplantation can also be solved by reference to the principles of totality and integrity and of common good and community. The success of organ transplantation, largely due to the use of cyclosporin and other drugs that suppress the activity of the recipient's immune system (Purviance, 1993), has produced the following new problems:

First, "How can we fairly allot available organs to recipients?" Because so many different organs and tissues are now subject to transplant—not only heart and kidneys, but lungs, liver, pancreas, spleen, skin, and bone marrow as well—there is a continual shortage of suitable organs and tissue for transplant. At present, the system of obtaining organs and allotting them is not well-defined. Regional transplant centers, funded in part by the federal government, publicize the need for organ donations; maintain waiting lists of who those need transplants and of possible donors; and assist physicians in allotting the available organs. Federal legislation has set guidelines for national sharing of available organs based on genetic matching between donor and recipient (McDonald, 1988). In general, the organs are allotted to those in most grave need who at the same time have some chance of survival if the transplant is successful. Thus medical criteria are the basis for allotment. Because all potential recipients are registered, a "first come, first served" allotment is followed in theory.

Surely, the buying and selling of organs as commercial products ought to be judged unethical because of the motivation of charity that alone justifies the transplant in the first place. The federal government has supported this ethical principle by prohibiting the sale of organs for transplant. In many other countries, however, their sale is neither prohibited nor unusual (Blumstein, 1993). Should available organs in the United States be allotted only to U.S. citizens, or should aliens be allowed to benefit from the transplantation program? Congressional hearings reveal that approximately 8,000 Americans await treatment for kidney transplants because wealthy citizens of other countries are able to pay to receive a transplant (U.S. Congress, 1984).

Since "Charity begins at home" is a sound ethical maxim, the Task Force on Organ Transplantation of the Department of Health and Human Services (DHHS, 1986) recommended that a quota system be established to place foreign nationals on a waiting list. To date, this has not been done, and many transplant centers look on foreign nationals as a source of profit. Thus, if foreign nationals can pay, they are usually accepted as candidates for transplant. This issue illustrates the problems that arise because the United States does not have any adequate national health policies to handle such problems. Although we do not maintain that foreign nationals should be totally excluded from transplant programs in the United States, there should be norms, or even federal regulations if necessary, that eliminate monetary factors as the major criterion for transplant candidacy and that strengthen medical need as the basic factor for candidacy.

Financing Transplantation

A second ethical question flowing from the success of the organ transplant program is "Who finances organ transplants?" Should organs be made available to all citizens of the United States, or only to those who can afford the procedure? And if the federal government is to fund all organ transplants, must any limits be set on the program? The medical, hospital, and postoperative costs for transplants are well above the means of the average family (Benjamin, 1988). At present, the federal government funds most of the costs of kidney transplants and funds heart transplants if the potential recipient qualifies for the Medicare program (DHHS, 1986), which, however, not many do. Some private health insurance plans fund heart transplants, but the tendency is to limit this type of benefit. At present, for liver transplants and other procedures that are still considered experimental, the recipients or their families are required often to raise funds themselves through public appeals, which sometimes are not successful. Some private insurance companies are beginning to fund liver transplants at selected medical centers. Many states limit Medicaid expenditures to "basic" health care benefits and will not fund such procedures as liver or bone marrow transplants (Welch and Larson, 1988). In response to the growing desire for organ transplants and the need to have some public policy in regard to funding of organ transplants, Callahan (1987b) suggests that consideration be given to limiting access for the elderly to transplants and other life-prolonging procedures.

Although there are no easy solutions to the funding issues that arise from the success of organ transplants, two points should be kept in mind as we seek ethical criteria for a solution: (1) Are we as a nation devoting enough resources to health care? Although the present expenditures exceed 15 percent of the gross domestic product (GDP), is there any indication that this sum represents the limit that should be devoted to health care? Clearly, although the percentage of the GDP devoted to health care in the past 30 years has increased dramatically, so has the complexity and sophistication of medicine and health care. (2) An overall health care policy must be formulated if we are to have a just and fair access to health care for all citizens. As Callahan (1987b) points out, at present no national policy deals with access to health care, but decisions are made as though our policy is to keep everyone alive as long as possible. In the immediate future, some policies must be determined for the United States that not only will afford basic care to all people who at present do not have adequate care, but that will also establish some equitable limits to public funding of sophisticated technology and innovative therapies (Fox and Swazey, 1992).

The difficult part of framing new policy in this regard is that some people will not live as long as they would if no new policy existed. For example, if Callahan's ideas were followed, some elderly people would not live as long because they would not be eligible for organ transplants financed through public funds. On the other hand, some people now are dying sooner than they would because our present policies are inequitable (Lurie et al., 1986).

Increasing the Supply of Organs for Transplantation

A third question arising from the success of transplant surgery is "How may we increase the supply of organs suitable for transplant?" As organ transplantation has become more successful, the issue of organ supply has become more of a national priority (GAO, 1993). How can organs be procured without violating the rights of families and dying patients? In addition to increased public appeals made by voluntary groups, the Joint Commission for the Accreditation of Health Care Organizations has requested each hospital to frame a policy that stipulates the procedure for requesting organ donations from the family of a dying or deceased person (AHA, 1986b). At present, the Anatomical Gift Act has been approved in each state (Sadler et al., 1968); this allows a person to sign his or her driver's license and indicate the desire to donate organs after death. However, the custom in most states requires the family to confirm such a donation; if the family were to disagree with the statement the patient made before death, it is unlikely that physicians or hospital administrators would approve surgery to remove organs for fear of ensuing malpractice litigation.

Basing their arguments on the common good and that a transplant after death would not harm the donor in any way, Boyle and O'Rourke (1986) maintain that a presumption in favor of organ donation should be established. In the Boyle/O'Rourke proposal, those who have religious or other reasons for denying the donation of organs could make their desires known before death, in much the same way people now reveal their desires to donate organs. If no objections are verified, however, the organs could be removed for transplant, even if no positive statement granting this permission was made beforehand by the deceased person. Although changing the presumption in regard to organ donation by the deceased may seem rather radical, it corresponds to the practice in some other countries (Roels et al., 1991). This proposal would not only increase the supply of organs for transplant, but it would impress on the public the need to emphasize community needs in the provision of health care.

Another effort to increase the supply of organs has been made by some who challenge the present *criteria for brain death*. Must the person's total brain be dead before organs are removed? In the case of anencephalic infants, for example, the higher brain (cortex) will never develop, but the brain stem is still functioning. Although these infants will die shortly after birth, some maintain they are not "alive" and thus have their vital organs removed, causing the death of debilitated infants (Holzgreve et al., 1987). The Ethical and Judicial Council of the AMA stated in 1994 that it would be ethical to transplant organs from anencephalic infants, even though the infant would die as a result of the transplant (AMA, 1994). The council later withdrew this opinion, mainly because of the criticism offered by ethicists and physicians (*N.Y. Times*, 1996). The physical evidence clearly shows that the development of the cerebral cortex of any infant does not constitute a "marker event" between prehuman and human development (Australian Research Commission, 1985). Moreover, absence of the higher brain alone would not constitute death. For example, the President's Commission for the Study of Ethical Problems in Medicine and Biomedical and Behavioral Research (PCEMR, 1981) stated:

> First … it is not known which portions of the brain are responsible for cognition and consciousness; what little is known points to substantial interconnections among brainstem, subcortical structures, and the neocortex. Thus, the "higher brain" may well exist only as a metaphorical concept, not in reality. Second, even when the sites or certain aspects of consciousness can be found, their cessation often cannot be assessed with the certainty that would be required in applying a statutory definition (p. 40).

This statement has recently been challenged, but still holds true for those who look to the body as a vital part of personality (Veatch, 1993).

Therefore, although the anencephalic infant may not develop in a manner that fulfills the full potential usually associated with "person," there is no scientific justification to consider anencephalic infants as dead (O'Rourke, 1996a). Rather, they should be considered living human beings until total brain death occurs. True, an anencephalic infant is a severely debilitated human being and a human being who will not live for long. Because there is no effective means of overcoming the pathology from which the anencephalic infant suffers, therapeutic care may be withheld. A real and dramatic difference exists, however, between allowing a person to die because a serious pathology cannot be overcome and directly killing an innocent human being. As death approaches, an anencephalic infant may be placed on a respirator to ensure that blood will continue perfusing the organs even after death so that the organs will be apt for transplant, as is done in the treatment of an adult who will be an organ donor. Thus anticipating the death of infants and keeping their body fluids flowing after brain death through use of a ventilator would not be unethical. However, no organs should be removed until brain death has been certified from clinical signs, as difficult as this might be if the infant is on life-support systems.

Research with Fetal Tissue

A different but related question is "May the tissue taken from fetuses be used for transplant or research purposes?" (Bauer, 1994). For example, people with Alzheimer's disease and Parkinson's disease have received transplants of brain tissue from recently aborted fetuses (Garry, 1993). Fetal tissue is more adaptable for research, and perhaps for therapy, because fetuses do not have a well-developed immune system. Thus the tissue garnered from fetuses is less likely to be rejected in another person's body and seems to grow faster than tissue taken from other sources. The best material for research seems to come from fetuses in the second trimester of life. Many scientists and other citizens have expressed concern about ethical issues involved in this form of research because the raw material for research comes from fetuses killed in elective abortions (Andrusko and Bond, 1988; Wolinsky, 1988).

Clearly, abortion was not legalized in order to obtain fetal tissue for research. One and one-half million abortions per year were being performed in the United States well before such research began. Nevertheless, such research may have the effect of encouraging abortion or at least justifying it ethically. Hence, those doing such research must take responsibility for avoiding this effect, or they become cooperators in the great social evil of elective abortion.

To fulfill this responsibility, it is necessary that the following measures be instituted (Cataldo and Moraczewski, 1994):

1. No commercial traffic in fetal tissue taken from aborted fetuses should be legal. There are federal laws against the sale of organs for transplan-

tation (McDonald, 1988); it also seems federal laws should prohibit the sale of fetal tissue for research as well.

2. Fetal tissue banks derived from the many miscarriages which regularly occur in hospitals should be instituted, along with a hospital network to identify and collect such material. While not all tissue obtained is suitable for research, neither is that obtained from elective abortions (Michjeda, 1994).

3. Fetal tissue derived from miscarriages should be cultivated by methods of cell culture which are already available and capable of further development.

Some ethicists and scientists compare fetal research to organ transplants from cadavers (Mahowald et al., 1987). Thus they maintain that the use of aborted fetuses is acceptable if the mother gives consent. However, further consideration disproves this assumption. When through proxy consent a family surrenders organs from a cadaver for heart or liver transplant, they have not been involved in causing the death of the person in question. Thus, although there is no direct connection between researchers and abortion, one must not assume that informed consent solves the ethical issues resulting from the use of tissue from aborted fetuses. At present, the federal government will subsidize research using fetal tissue, but some states have prohibited this type of research. Finally, the revised Ethical and Religious Directives (NCCB, 1994) prohibit the use of human tissue obtained by direct abortion even for research and therapeutic purposes (n. 66).

11.5 SEXUAL REASSIGNMENT

Reconstructive and Cosmetic Surgery

Without resorting to transplants, modern surgery is capable of remarkable feats of repairing bodily defects and injuries. Sometimes accidentally severed fingers or hands have been successfully reconnected to the body and restored at least to partial function. Self-transplants such as skinplants and the transfer of blood vessels from the limbs to be used as bypasses in heart surgery have become common. Recently there have been advances in restoring severed nerves, etc. Such reconstructive surgery raises no special ethical questions, other than general ones such as free and informed consent and cost/benefit, as long as the purpose is clearly one of restoring or improving normal function. Questions may be raised, however, in at least two types of cases.

What if the purpose of the surgery is not normal function but the destruction or inhibition of certain normal functions? We have already discussed contraceptive sterilization, whose purpose is the destruction of normal human fertility. We have also mentioned the castration of sex offenders. Other types of deterrent mutilation of criminals have been and are used even now in some countries, such as blinding criminals, cutting off their hands, or excising their tongues. Such procedures violate both the principle of human dignity and that of totality and integrity. What, however, about such a procedure as controlling obesity by surgically constricting the size of the stomach, etc.? In such procedures, as in contraception, the purpose is to solve a behavioral problem by a mechanical mutilation. If the cause of the obesity were a malfunction of the digestive system which could be remedied by surgery (for example, vagotomy or section of the vagus nerve, formerly used to treat ulcers by inhibiting an excessive stimulation of acid secretion in the stomach), then such an operation could be ethically justified. We are of the opinion, however, that when obesity or any such order is caused by lack of control of behavior, such surgery is not consistent with the principle of totality and integrity.

On the other hand, cosmetic surgery is not directed at restoring normal function, but at improving *appearance*. While human appearance can hardly be called a "function" of the body, yet it is certainly very important in human life, both with regard to sexual attraction and with regard to all our social relationships and sense of personal worth. We can, therefore, grant that it is ethically justified if the purpose is to acquire, when lacking, what is generally regarded as a normal, attractive appearance for one's gender or even to enhance it. Certainly when the defect in question is real and serious, and especially when it is associated with some functional defect, such as cleft palate, deformation of facial features, unsightly birthmarks, etc., such surgery is wholly reasonable.

When, however, the purpose is simply the enhancement of sexual attractiveness or the concealment of normal aging, such as face lifting, breast enhancement, liposuction, etc., now very popular among women, and even men's concern about baldness, obesity, lack of muscularity, etc., it is pertinent to ask whether the expense, the risks, and rationale of such procedures can really be justified. Society and style often promote stereotypes of youth and beauty which are illusory and harmful. It is to be feared also that some physicians promote such expensive procedures simply for their own profit and not for the real welfare of the patient. The fact that people request such procedures and are willing to pay for them is not a sufficient ethical justification for physicians to cooperate. While this is not one of the major problems of bioethics, it is symptomatic of mistaken priorities in the promotion of human health. The Christian attitude, from New Testament times, has always been that it is wrong to promote the idea that human worth is to be measured by appearances rather than by character. Certainly it is unjust for a society to devote so much of its resources to vanity when the poor lack necessities.

Sexual Reassignment

Since, as we have just argued, surgical and hormonal alteration of the human body to solve behavioral rather than functional problems is ethically very dubious, the issue of "sex change" as it is popularly called, or "sexual reassignment" as it is technically termed, is even more questionable. Sexual reassignment is a type of reconstructive surgery by which the sexual phenotype of a male is altered to resemble that of a female, or vice versa (Meyer, 1974; Cole et al., 1994). Such surgery, along with hormonal treatment and psychotherapy, is often used to treat transsexualism when psychiatric treatment fails. Transsexualism is described in the *Diagnostic and Statistical Manual of Mental Disorders* (DSM IV) as involving the following five criteria (APA, 1990):

1. Sense of discomfort and inappropriateness about one's anatomical sex;
2. Wish to be rid of one's own genitals and to live as a member of the other sex;
3. The disturbance has been continuous (not limited to periods of stress) for at least two years;
4. Absence of physical intersex or genetic abnormality; and
5. Not caused by another mental disorder, such as schizophrenia.

Transsexual surgery involves radical mutilation: castration and construction of a pseudovagina for the male, mastectomy and hysterectomy (sometimes also the construction of a nonfunctional pseudopenis and testes) for the female, along with hormonal treatments with possible serious side effects (Huang, 1995). This raises the ethical question of whether the attempt to change a person's biological sex is ever a legitimate aim of medical care (B. Brody et al., 1981).

Catholic moralists have always admitted that in cases where a child is born with ambiguous genitalia, the parents should raise the child as belonging to that sex in which the person is most likely to be able to function best. Also, there seems to be no objection to the use of surgery or hormones to improve the normal appearance or function of such persons in accordance with the sex in which they are to be or have been raised. The reasoning behind this traditional position is that a person must "live according to nature" insofar as this is humanly knowable.

Recently, however, knowledge of sexual development has vastly increased, and sexual ambiguity is seen as far more complex and common than formerly thought (Monteleone, 1981). The biological determination of sex depends on the presence or absence of the Y chromosome in the one-cell zygote, which in the beginning constitutes the human person (see 9.1). When present, the Y chromosome produces TDY (testicular determinant Y) as early as the eight-cell stage of development and the person begins to move toward maleness; otherwise all zygotes develop as females. All embryos originally have undifferentiated gonads and two sets of sexual ducts, the Wolffian and Müllerian, but at seven weeks the male gonads differentiate and begin to produce hormones that destroy the Müllerian ducts and cause the development of the male genitalia. Otherwise, the Wolffian ducts are absorbed and the gonads and the Müllerian ducts develop into the female sexual system. At the same time, the differing hormonal balance in the two sexes causes certain differences in the male and female brain, in particular preparing the female brain to regulate the menstrual cycle. It has been established for some animals, but not certainly for human beings, that these neurological differences also result in behavioral differences in the two sexes (Gemuth, 1988).

All these biological determinations are at work before birth. After birth it is probable, but not yet proved, that there are *biophysical* events at the unconscious level, similar to the imprinting demonstrated in animals, that also promote sexual differentiation, such as the way the mother cares differently for a female than for a male child. Finally, at the conscious *environmental* level, the person learns his or her own *gender identity* and assumes a *gender role* in society. In this long and complicated process many things can go wrong at each stage, with the result that in the human population a whole spectrum of conditions exists between the normal masculine and feminine conditions, both physical and psychological. "Normal" here means a condition determined by that sexual teleology designed by God to culminate in successful heterosexual marriage (see p. 210).

Among these possible abnormalities, *homosexuality* is a highly varied condition, probably having many etiological factors. In this case a person who is phenotypically unambiguously male or female and in no doubt about his or her gender is conscious of greater sexual attraction to those of his or her own sex than to others and who, consequently, is unable to enter into a satisfactory marriage. *Transvestism* is a condition in which a person, usually heterosexual in orientation, is more comfortable sexually while wearing clothing symbolic of the opposite sex (Levine, 1993). *Transsexualism* differs from these because of *gender dysphoria syndrome,* that is, an anxiety, sometimes reaching suicidal depression, as the result of the obsessive feeling that one's "real" sex is the opposite of one's phenotypic sex.

Pros and Cons of Sexual Reassignment

The argument of psychotherapists and surgeons who undertake sexual reassignment as a remedy for this syndrome is that the victims find no relief in other therapies, are insistent on surgery even to the point of threatening suicide, and are generally satisfied with its results (Springer, 1987). Ethicists who follow a utilitarian or proportionalist methodology can approve such surgery if they are convinced that the good effects outweigh the bad. The methodology used in this book (see Chapter 8) can approve of it only if this can be shown to be simply an extension of the classical position that, in cases of sexual ambiguity, it is permissible to choose the more probable sex, as already explained. Can this be demonstrated?

At present, we do not believe this case can be demonstrated for several reasons. First, it has not yet been established that the cause of gender dysphoria syndrome is biological (Hage, 1995), although this theory has been suggested by some (Monteleone, 1981; Peterson, 1981). No such cause is evident at the genotypic or phenotypic level, and as yet the evidence is tenuous that the reason transsexuals believe from early in their lives that they have "a soul different from my body" is caused by some developmental accident in the central nervous or hormonal systems. At present, it remains more probable that the determining causes are at the psychological level of development, although there may be some biological predispositions (Sugar, 1995). Consequently, the gender ambiguity in question is primarily psychological and should be treated psychotherapeutically. A recent study of the problem (Lothstein, 1982) shows that the condition is much more common in males than females and that of those males applying for sexual reassignment surgery, only about 10 to 25 percent can be diagnosed as having *primary* gender dysphoria, that is, of the type that "has an obvious, documentable, lifelong, profound disturbance of core gender identity." J. K. Meyer (1974) went so far as to state, "I have seen any number of men who would like to live as females and vice versa; I have not seen one with a reversal of core gender identity." Other candidates for surgery can only be diagnosed as suffering from *secondary* gender dysphoria, which is stress-related and results from "failures of other gender identity adaptations, such as transvestism, effeminate homosexuality, gender ambiguity." Thus the arguments for biological rather than a psychological etiology of this syndrome will hold (if at all) only for a very restricted group of patients.

Second, contrary to what is often stated, when candidates for surgery are required to undergo psychotherapy in preparation for surgery, many are found to be ambiguous about really wanting it and in the end decide against it. Moreover, most transsexuals who have been carefully diagnosed appear to be suffering from serious psychological problems, sometimes subtle and not immediately recognized, other than their gender dysphoria (Bodlung, 1993). Even after surgery they continue to need at least some psychotherapeutic support, although their frequent difficulty in forming stable personal relationships makes this follow-up difficult.

Third, although when this type of surgery was first introduced there were enthusiastic reports of its success, as experience accumulates there is less agreement that it does much good. The latest survey of studies evaluating the outcome of transsexual surgery concludes that previous studies have indicated more people being satisfied with the overall results of the surgery by a 2 to 1 margin (Cole et al., 1994). However, the surveys that offer the previous favorable reports are criticized for their lack of objectivity, and "the paucity of control groups make attribution of either improvement or deterioration to the surgical intervention scientifically untenable" (Abramowitz, 1986). Johns Hopkins University, noted for its leadership in research in this field, announced the suspension of its program for further reassessment as a result of a report by J. K. Meyer and Reter (1979), which concluded that this type of surgery offers no advantage over psychotherapy. Another study in regard to Medicaid funding of sex-reassignment surgery affirms this conclusion (Jacobs, 1980).

Fourth, from a theological point of view, it is clear that surgery does not really solve these persons' life problem because it does not enable them to achieve sexual normality or to enter into a valid Christian marriage and have children. Since many of these individuals are somewhat asexual (Snaith, 1994a) their problem is not primarily sexual satisfaction but the relief of the burden of anxiety, which can usually be at least considerably lightened by psychotherapy. Some (Lavin, 1987) raise the question of whether in severe cases the possible relief of anxiety might outweigh the other disvalues involved. Yet we would invoke the principle of totality and integrity (2.4, 8.2) to show that the good of the person cannot be achieved at the expense of the destruction of a basic human function, in this case the sterilization of the person, except to save the person's life. Furthermore, the studies reported by no means give assurance that sexual reassignment solves the more general characterological problems from which most of these victims suffer.

We conclude that, based on the present state of knowledge, Catholic hospitals or health care professionals are not justified in recommending or engaging in this type of surgery. Certainly compassion should be extended to this small but greatly suffering group of human beings, but it should take the practical form of psychotherapy and pastoral guidance. It is unfortunate that the widespread publicity given to sex-change surgery and the exaggerated reports of its success have created an increasing demand among troubled people, most of whom would not be accepted for such surgery by any reputable clinic.

How should such cases be dealt with pastorally? The fundamental aim of the therapist, as well as of the pastoral counselor, in these cases should be to restore the patient's sense of personal self-worth. He or she must be helped to see, as should homosexuals and those having other sexual problems, that today's culture is grievously mistaken in its exaggerated stress on sexual identity and activity as a primary determinant of human worth. They must be assisted to find interests—spiritual, intellectual, and social—that will enable them to escape their preoccupation with their sexual identity and discover their more fundamental value as human persons. As for persons who have already undergone surgery, we believe they should be counseled not to attempt marriage and should be supported in their efforts to live chastely with the assistance of the sacraments and the respect and fellowship of the Christian community.

11.6 EXPERIMENTATION AND RESEARCH ON HUMAN SUBJECTS

The Importance of Research on Human Persons

> When science takes man as its subject, tensions arise between two values basic to Western Society: freedom of scientific inquiry and protection of individual inviolability (p. 1).

These words introduce a major study by Katz et al. (1972) on the legal and ethical issues involved in research on human subjects, which may be defined as seeking generalizable knowledge concerning human function or behavior through empirical studies (Belmont Report, 1978). Katz' observations continue:

> Human experimentation in the practice of medicine is as old as the practice of medicine itself, but only during the last hundred years, since the age of Pasteur, has medicine become aware of the need for deliberate and well-planned experimentation (p. 1)

Since 1947, close to half a million projects involving human subjects have been carried out, about one third of which have been supported by the government (NIH, 1996). Thus human experimentation not only affects the rights of human persons now and in the future, but may also condition and change the very core of human nature itself (Shapiro et al., 1986).

That this growing research on human beings is often useful and often necessary for the common good is undeniable. Many beneficial vaccines and other therapies, such as smallpox and poliomyelitis vaccines, open-heart surgery, and successful treatment of certain birth defects, could not have been developed without research with human subjects, and the whole world attests to their value. At the same time, research on humans undoubtedly has also been abused. The world should never forget the horrors of the human research experimentation carried out on innocent human beings in the name of scientific progress in Nazi concentration camps (Lifton, 1982; Katz, 1993). Aside from such atrocities, other egregious violations of human rights have occurred in the United States, such as the withholding of newly discovered penicillin from patients in the Tuskegee syphilis study (Jones, 1982); the Willowbrook experiments, in which retarded children were used as experimental subjects (Krugman, 1986); and the injection of live cancer cells in unknowing subjects in the Jewish Chronic Disease Hospital case (Faden and Beauchamp, 1986).

Psychological experimentation has also given rise to serious debate about behavior control (Macklin, 1982). Such abuses are not always the product of demented or perverted minds; rather, they result from lack of care and ethical sensitivity on the part of well-motivated researchers who overlook the rights of human beings in an effort to ensure scientific progress or academic advancement (Shapiro and Charron, 1984). Today, in an effort to obviate excesses and facilitate progress, the federal government requires that every institution that carries on research projects with public funds establish an institutional review board (IRB) (PCEMR, 1983e). The federal government will not fund research projects unless they have been first approved by an IRB. In addition, the National Institutes of Health (NIH) requires that all persons receiving NIH training grants must complete a course in the ethics of research (DHHS, 1995).

Research and Therapy

Several categories of human subjects may be involved in research programs: (1) normal healthy adults, including the investigator, and elderly persons; (2) sick adults, including the acutely and terminally ill; (3) prisoners, soldiers, and students living in highly controlled situations; (4) children, both healthy and ill; (5) mentally incompetent adults and children; (6) unborn children or still-living aborted fetuses; and (7) the aging. Each of these categories presents special problems as shown in the various studies of the National Commission for the Protection of Human Subjects of Biomedical and Behavioral Research (DHEW, 1975).

Experimental research on human subjects should be sharply distinguished from therapy, since the primary purpose of research is not to heal but to learn (Applebaum et al., 1987). Yet it has become customary to classify research as either therapeutic or nontherapeutic. *Therapeutic research* studies the effects of using diagnostic, prophylactic, or therapeutic methods that depart from standard medical practice but hold out a reasonable expectation of success. Such research may actually give greater benefit to the human subject than standard treatment. Thus what begins as human research may later become standard medical practice. *Nontherapeutic research,* on the other hand, is not designed to improve the health of the research subject; rather, it seeks to gain knowledge or develop techniques that may benefit people other than the subject in the future (Belmont Report, 1978).

The proper manner of conducting these types of research on the various categories of human subjects has become one of the most discussed bioethical questions of recent years (Levine, 1981, 1983; PCEMR, 1983b; Katz, 1993). Through seminars, studies, and the work of the various federal commissions, some ethical principles have been developed to serve as a guide for researchers and for those who support research. As a result of such studies by legal, medical, and ethical groups throughout the world, especially in the generation after World War II, these principles have become widely accepted, even though there may be disagreement concerning their applications in particular cases. Interestingly, the norms produced by medical and legal experts of the World Health Organization (WHO), such as the Nuremberg Code (1946) and Helsinki statements (1964), are largely in harmony with the teaching of the Catholic Church on human dignity in that they propose exceptionless ethical norms which protect persons from exploitation and moral and physical harm. Subsequent statements of research groups, such as the Warnock Committee, however, are not in accord with Church teaching because they follow a proportionalist method of reasoning (O'Rourke, 1988b).

Principles of Research on Human Subjects

The basic norms for research on human subjects that are formulated and discussed here derive chiefly from three ethical principles: the principle of totality and integrity, which is especially relevant to therapeutic experimentation; the principle of human dignity in community, which relates to the limits of nontherapeutic experimentation; and the principle of free and informed consent, a corollary of the principle of well-formed conscience, which relates to the capacity of the various categories of human subjects to participate freely in research programs.

1. The knowledge sought through research must be important and obtainable by no other means, and the research must be carried on by qualified people.
2. Appropriate experimentation on animals and cadavers must precede human experimentation.
3. The risk of suffering or injury must be proportionate to the good to be gained.
4. Subjects should be selected so that risks and benefits will not fall unequally on one group in society.

5. To protect the integrity of the human person, free and informed (voluntary) consent must be obtained.

6. At any time during the course of research, the subject (or the guardian who has given proxy consent) must be free to terminate the subject's participation in the experiment.

The first three of these norms are necessary if human subjects are to be used at all. Because the principle of double effect (8.1) is used to justify the possible ill effects of human experimentation, the relation between risk and potential benefit is most important (Gillon, 1986a). Of course, predicting the degree of risk with certitude is seldom possible. Moreover, sometimes—as in the case of poliomyelitis inoculation in 1954 when the use of some poorly prepared live vaccine resulted in the death of children, or in the 1980 swine flu inoculation disaster—some risks were far greater than predicted. Thus absolute certainty in regard to the nature and degree of the risk cannot be required. To demand such certitude would paralyze all scientific research and would very often be detrimental to the patient. Care must be taken, however, to predict as accurately as possible the nature and magnitude of risk from any particular human experiment, and the bias of enthusiastic researchers in favor of the promise of some new procedure must be subject to review by an institutional review board (IRB) (Levine, 1985).

When determining the degree of risk that a person might undergo, one must also keep in mind the difference between therapeutic and nontherapeutic research. If research is therapeutic, persons may undergo greater risk and possibly even death from the illness or malady that the researcher is trying to cure. The principle of totality and integrity (p. 224) is especially relevant to therapeutic experimentation. The same principle of totality cannot be invoked in the case of nontherapeutic experimentation because one person is not related to another person or to society simply as part of the whole. Each individual person is an end in herself or himself and cannot be sacrificed for another, although all share in one common good. This is the basic reason why the public authority has no right to sacrifice individuals for "the interest of the state or for scientific progress" (Pius XII, 1952; John Paul II, 1986). Experiments carried out for the good of the state or for scientific progress may provide new knowledge or medical techniques and thus seem beneficial, but they do so and are so at the expense of human rights and human dignity and therefore are immoral.

Although it is sometimes fitting that researchers themselves participate in experiments, they are bound by the same restrictions as other subjects (Altman, 1987). The Nuremberg Code (WHO, 1946) is rather unclear about this stipulation, implying that researchers may take greater risks than others (n. 5). Pope Pius XII (1952) expresses a more accurate view:

He (the doctor or researcher) is subject to the same broad moral and juridical principles as govern other men. He has no right, consequently, to permit scientific or practical experiments which entail serious injury or which threaten to impair his health to be performed on his person, and even to a lesser extent is he authorized to attempt an operation of experimental nature which, according to authoritative opinion, could conceivably result in mutilation or even suicide (n. 545).

Experimental Controls

A special ethical issue arises in "double-blind" research (Koppleman, 1986; Marquis, 1986). The objectivity of scientific research depends largely on the use of controlled experimentation in which a group of subjects is divided into two subgroups, one of which receives the experimental therapy while the other, the control group, receives the standard therapy or a placebo. Sometimes three groups are used, one group receiving the experimental therapy, one receiving a placebo, and one receiving standard therapy or no treatment at all. This sometimes is called a *randomized* clinical trial. To ensure even greater objectivity, *double-blind* control may be used: not only are subjects not informed as to which form of treatment they are receiving, but even those researchers who evaluate the effects of the treatments do not know which subjects have received which therapy. Only the double-blind technique can eliminate the *placebo effect,* that is, the improvement frequently experienced by patients who expect it and the effect of bias on the part of scientists. Double-blind studies raise questions of justice, however, since it may be (1) that those subjects who do not receive the new therapy are at a therapeutic disadvantage and (2) that they may not have given free and informed consent to receive only placebo treatment (Marquis, 1986; Rothman, 1994). Thus in double-blind experiments the subjects should be informed that, if they consent to the experiment, some will receive the new treatment and others will not, but that none of the subjects will know. The potential subjects will then be free to consent to these experimental conditions or to refuse to participate.

If the clinical trial involves a placebo for the control group and the project aims at finding an agent that will mitigate or cure a lethal or disabling disease, a special ethical issue arises, because the control group may not be receiving adequate therapy for their illness or disease (Koppleman, 1986). This is especially true if there is some justification for thinking that the new therapy might be much more effective than previous ones. Thus the same protocol may be therapeutic for some and nontherapeutic for others. Researchers and review boards therefore must be doubly cautious when a double-blind placebo protocol is being designed or reviewed. If the new therapy proves to be effective, the protocol must be modified and the new therapy made available to all. Of course, a rush to judgment concerning the efficacy of a new therapy must be avoided.

Impartiality and Consent in Selecting Subjects

The fourth and fifth of the norms listed require that experimental subjects not be selected if they are subject to social or other pressures that limit their freedom of consent, since justice demands that the burdens associated with human progress be shared equitably. In recent years the poor of the world, especially in the United States, have borne an unequal burden in relation to medical research (Belmont Report, 1978). The causes of this situation are psychological as well as economic. Research protocols must be designed to offset this imbalance and ensure that when the poor take part in an experiment, their human rights are respected and they are given the freedom that their human dignity demands. While it may often be easier to obtain subjects from the poor than from other groups, for this very reason special care must be taken to protect their rights. The same consideration holds for those categories of subjects who are chosen because they live in restricted and controlled circumstances where the researcher has easy access to them, such as prisoners, soldiers, or those confined to rest homes or mental institutions (Wicclair, 1993; Candilis et al., 1993). Such persons are in need of advocacy lest they be too easily persuaded to join in experiments by group pressures or by rewards that their situation make excessively attractive. Prisoners, offered parole in return for participation in a dangerous experiment, may find this one hope of freedom too compelling to resist (*Scott v. Casey*, 1983).

The fifth norm requiring truly free and informed consent by the experimental human subject is perhaps the most important and the most debated of all the principles involved in human research and is also related to the principle of well-formed conscience (3.4), the very basis of all ethical decisions. According to one of the more astute statements on the subject (Applebaum et al., 1987), free and informed consent means the following:

> The idea of informed consent is the notion that decisions about medical care a person will receive, if any, are to be made in a collaborative manner between patient and physician. The concept also implies that the physician must be prepared to engage in—indeed to initiate—a discussion with the patient about the available therapeutic options and to provide relevant information on them (p. 12).

The Belmont Report (1978) states that the elements of informed consent on the part of the patient are knowledge, understanding, and freedom. Despite extensive descriptions of informed consent published in ethical literature, serious discussions and disputes still arise concerning the concept and its application. Many question, for example, whether prisoners can ever give *free* consent because of their situation. Others question whether double-blind procedures, an integral part of some experiments, can ever be employed. We believe, however, that both experimentation on prisoners and double-blind procedures can be performed if extra care is taken in obtaining consent (Pellegrino, 1981; Sachs et al., 1993).

Proxy or Vicarious Consent

The most difficult problems, however, occur in situations in which one person gives consent for another for whom the first is morally responsible. The need for such consent occurs when unconscious people are dying, as well as in research programs (Blank, 1993). Such substitute consent is usually called *proxy consent,* an unfortunate term because properly speaking a legal proxy is an agent acting on behalf of another by the other's consent, which is precisely what is often lacking in proxy consent. It would be better to call it *vicarious consent* because a vicar fulfills a duty for another irrespective of whether the other has authorized it.

Vicarious consent should be distinguished also from *implicit* consent and *presumed* consent. Persons consent implicitly when they actually consent to some general line of action, which implies more detailed permissions, as when a patient consents to surgery without specifying what anesthetic is to be used. Consent is presumed when it is highly probable that someone who is not able to give consent because he or she is absent or unconscious would have given it if present or conscious, as when a surgeon presumes a patient would expect the physician to remove a diseased appendix that the patient was unaware of but that the surgeon notes in the course of other abdominal surgery. Proxy or vicarious consent, according to some, is a form of presumed consent, but other explanations are possible. As such, it simply means that one person who represents the interests of another by some legitimate title gives consent for the experiment in place of the subject because that subject is incompetent at the time to do so (John Paul II, 1980b; M. Shannon, 1985).

Children and retarded, infirm, and dying persons are often considered as subjects for human research (Warren et al., 1986; Nilstan, 1992). It is sometimes argued that this gives them an opportunity that they might not otherwise have of contributing to the common good. Since they are not competent, or at least not fully competent, to act freely and with full understanding, consent can be given in their case only by the proxy or vicarious consent of a parent or guardian. Decisions of proxy consent must be made in view of the good of the individual person, not for a higher good, for a class good, or for the good of another person, which would amount to manipulation of the person as a mere means. Thus, if the experiment is therapeutic, there would be reason for the proxy to allow risk in proportion to the person's best interest. If nontherapeutic experimentation is involved, however, the decision is more difficult.

In recent years the responsibility of a proxy in regard to children has been hotly argued. Some authors (Ramsey, 1970; W. E. May, 1976) maintain that the person issuing proxy consent has no right to expose a ward to *any* risk. The justification for this position is that a proxy should make a decision in accord with the best interests of the subject. In nontherapeutic experimentation the interests of the subject are not clearly evident, however, and since the subject does not have the capacity to make a free choice about the matter, the proxy (guardian) has no right to presume or say anything on behalf of the ward.

Other authors (Ackerman, 1979; McCormick, 1976; Edwards, 1993) allow for exposing children and others who cannot consent for themselves to "minimal risk." Thus proxy consent is interpreted as a form of presumed consent. The argument for this position is that there are some things a child as a human being *ought* to do for others, for example, to take part in research when hope exists of "general benefit" and only minimal risk. The U.S. Commission for the Protection of Human Subjects, when determining the norms for fetal experimentation, followed the minimal risk theory (O'Rourke, 1975).

We follow the former, more protective opinion, maintaining that proxy consent is not licit in nontherapeutic experimentation, even when the risk is minimal. Guardians have responsibility for wards who cannot care for themselves because of the principle of human dignity in community, which affirms that no person can achieve fulfillment without sharing in the common good and contributing to it. But when a guardian or proxy consents to subject a ward to experimentation, they cannot do so on the grounds of the presumed consent of the ward, which is merely hypothetical, but rather must do so on the grounds of the actual need of the ward for care. Therefore theories of presumed consent based on what the ward *ought* to do if the ward *could* consent are weak.

It may be granted, however, that if a guardian in a concrete case gives proxy consent because the guardian is sure that the ward will suffer no more than minimal risk, the guardian does not fail in his or her responsibility to care for the ward, since "little counts for nothing," as the maxim of classical moral theology goes. In other words, a guardian should be an advocate, jealous of the rights of the ward, not ready to yield these rights for the sake of others who cannot act for themselves, nor for the merely hypothetical rights of future generations of other children.

Unborn Human Subjects

Another group of humans who have been subjected to research protocols are living human embryos (C. Baron, 1985; Polkinghorne, 1992; Fumento, 1992). Some study groups have approved of this type of research (DHEW, 1978; Warnock Report, 1985; NIH, 1994). Other commissions have disapproved such research (Australian Research Commission, 1985; Council of Europe, 1985; Dickson, 1988). But the approval of an NIH committee on embryo research led President Clinton to approve the use of federal funds for such research even though prior administrations had disapproved such funding. President Clinton did prohibit "created" embryos for experimentation (Gianelli, 1994). Many scientists and ethicists criticized the decision of the NIH Committee (1994) to approve such research (*Washington Post*, 1994). Committees and ethicists who approve of embryo research often assume a pragmatic, short-range view of the situation and usually proceed from proportionalist or pragmatic theories.

The Catholic Church issued a strong statement rejecting any form of research on human embryos that is nontherapeutic, but left the door open to therapeutic research, which is only now beginning (Hendren and Lillehi, 1988). The reasoning of the Congregation for the Doctrine of the Faith (CDF, 1987) was as follows:

> The fruit of human generation from the first moment of its existence, that is to say, from the moment the zygote has formed, demands the unconditional respect that is morally due to the human being in his bodily and spiritual totality. The human being is to be respected and treated as a

person from the moment of conception; and therefore from the same moment his rights as a person must be recognized, among which in the first place is the inviolable right of every innocent human being to life (p. 11).

John Paul confirmed this statement in the encyclical *Evangelium Vitae*:

Although one must uphold as licit procedures carried out on the human embryo which respect its life and integrity and do not involve disproportionate risks, . . . it must nonetheless be stated that the use of human embryos or fetuses as an object of experimentation constitutes a crime against their dignity as human beings who have a right to the same respect owed to a child once born, just as to every person. (n. 63)

Termination of Experimentation

The reason for this sixth guideline, which requires that human subjects be permitted to withdraw from the experiment at any time in spite of their initial consent, is that the consenting subject or proxy may not have been able to anticipate correctly the subjective factors involved, the amount of suffering, or the anxiety or depression until these began to be actually experienced. Also, the subject or proxy may even discover the information given was inadequate or deceptive or imperfectly communicated; or the subject or proxy may have second thoughts about his or her own understanding or freedom when the consent was given. The subject or guardian cannot consent to give away the primary responsibility for defending the subject's own health and integrity, since this is an inherent right and obligation. Consequently, if during the course of the experimentation the subject or proxy begins to see that serious risks to the subject's well-being may be involved, the subject or proxy is ethically obliged to stop participation.

Psychological Experimentation

Special problems are involved in psychological research (Webb, 1988). To discuss these problems more fully, we defer the topic to Chapter 12, after the nature of psychotherapy and its distinctions from medical therapy are more thoroughly explained. At this point, however, we can state that in such research all the precautions necessary in medical experiments must be preserved, especially informed consent, careful calculation of risks and benefits, and precautions against the bias of researchers in favor of their own freedom. We must also add the following three special rules for psychological research:

1. In psychological research, which shades imperceptibly into social research, the researcher should work *with* rather than *on* the human subject (Goldner, 1993).

That is, the researcher must gain the cooperation of the subject in the experiment so that subjects will participate with the purpose of gaining greater insight into themselves as persons in order to become freer and more realistic in coping with life's problems and also with the purpose of sharing this knowledge and freedom with others.

This principle is based on the fact that psychological experiments with a human subject are also psychological *experiences* for the subject that can be either healthy and psychologically therapeutic or traumatizing reinforcement of bad behavior patterns. In very few cases can such experiences be merely neutral. Even the experience of filling out a questionnaire can be educational or terrifying. Any experience in which the patient is treated as a passive object rather than as a person cannot be a beneficial experience. It is questionable whether such treatment can even be experimentally useful, since in such a situation the human person is no longer acting humanly, but subhumanly. Thus persons should not permit themselves to be treated in this way because those who seek to reduce them to objects are violating their human rights. Psychological experimentation must involve the human, active cooperation of the subject and produce some learning and growth benefits.

2. The researcher must avoid breaking down human trust by lying or manipulation, although subjects can give free and informed consent to experiments in which they have to learn to interpret ambiguous communications or meet puzzling situations.

In many psychological experiments, the experimentalist does not seem to have any qualms about lying to subjects. Not only is lying (in our opinion) intrinsically wrong and contrary to professional ethics (5.2), it is also psychologically harmful to the subject because it breaks down the social trust on which human relations are built. Commonsense proof of this is that those who have been subjected to such manipulation often react indignantly when they discover the deception and believe they have been treated unfairly (Cupples and Cochnauer, 1985). This is especially true when dealing with mentally disturbed patients, since elements of distrust, withdrawal, and paranoia present in most forms of emotional disturbance can only be reinforced by deception from professionals who claim to be especially trustworthy and authoritative (Dresser and Whitehouse, 1994)

This rule against lying, however, does not prohibit experiments in which previous warning is given that the experiment may involve games or tests with ambiguous clues and the subject's possible embarrassment and defeat. These are risks of the experiment to which the subject must have a chance to give free and informed consent or refusal. Deception in such a case is not what moral theologians define as a "lie," because traditional moral theology has always insisted that it is permissible to use ambiguous clues or language in situations where others are forewarned either explicitly or by the very nature of the situation.

Such games do not usually break down trust if the experimenter sticks to the rules. Moreover, they may be highly educational for the participant, since through them the subject gains insight as to how important it is to base one's interpretation of reality on solid evidence, rather than on ambiguous evidence or subjective feelings.

> 3. Researchers must not take serious risks of reducing the subjects' ability to perceive reality as it is or to make free choices except as a temporary experience through which the subjects can learn to cope with distortions of truth and attacks on their freedom.

This rule states more exactly the special risks involved in psychological experimentation. It excludes permission for any more than temporary damage to patients' ability to remain or become free in managing their own lives. Thus an experiment would be forbidden if it might cause organic brain damage or induce drug addiction. This also applies to experiments that might make the subject unduly liable to hypnotic control or to compulsive patterns of behavior or that might create recurrent hallucinations. A special case of psychological research that may involve risks to freedom is research in dealing with human sexuality. This issue is discussed in Chapter 12 in connection with therapy for inadequate or perverted sexual behavior.

These nine norms for ethical research are founded in the Christian concept of respect for persons and in the concept of responsibility that individuals have toward human community. On the part of researchers they require that their laudable desire to advance the cause of science and of the medical art should not tempt them to forget the interests here and now of the unique and irreplaceable human persons they are studying.

CONCLUSION

For many centuries, medical restructuring of the human body was confined to surgical procedures. Though surgical procedures would wound or impair the human body, whether temporarily or permanently, it was rather simple to determine the morality of such procedures. Would it help the person strive more effectively for the goods and goals of human life, and will it help the person do this without imposing a grave burden on the person or society?

In contemporary medicine, however, there are novel ways of modifying the human body. One may receive organs which at one time functioned in the body of other persons. The possibility of using animal organs to replace human organs is on the horizon. One's body may be changed through genetic intervention, either before or after conception.

Whatever the new methods of manipulating the body of the human person, the ethical norms to evaluate these new methods are the same as in the past: Does the procedure help the person strive for the goods and goals of human life, and does it do so without imposing a serious burden upon the person or society?

12

Neurological and Psychological Therapy of Mental Illness

OVERVIEW

Many ethical issues surround the topic of mental health and the methods used to promote and restore it. Such topics concern that borderline, difficult to draw, among the four dimensions of the human person—*physical, psychological, ethical (or social),* and *spiritual*—outlined in Chapter 1.4. In this chapter we discuss the concept of mental health, which has been much confused by lack of an adequate model of the human person (12.1). Then we consider the two main therapeutic models for treating mental illness: (a) the medical, neurological model that employs neurosurgery, electroconvulsive therapy, and pharmacotherapy (12.2); and (b) the psychotherapeutic model that employs psychoanalysis, cognitional reeducation, behavior modification, etc., (12.3) and the many ethical issues arising from these different therapies (12.4). Finally, we consider the special issues involved in chemical dependency (12.5) and sexual dysfunction (12.6).

12.1 THE CONCEPT OF MENTAL ILLNESS

The Freudian Models of the Human Person

In dealing with ethical problems in psychiatric medicine we must ask, "What is the difference between mental illness and ordinary physical illness?" In Chapter 1 a four-dimensional model of human personality (see diagram in 1.4) was proposed. We contrasted the *biological* level with which most of medicine deals to the *psychological* level with which psychiatry deals, but indicated the intimate interrelationship of body and psyche (soul).

We also pointed out that the term "psychological" as compared to "biological" can be taken in a broad sense to include not only the psychological (in a narrow sense) level, but also the ethical and the spiritual levels. Consequently, in this chapter we must first analyze in greater detail these three dimensions that stand in a certain contrast to the biological level. For this analysis it is helpful to compare two related models of the human person which have originated and

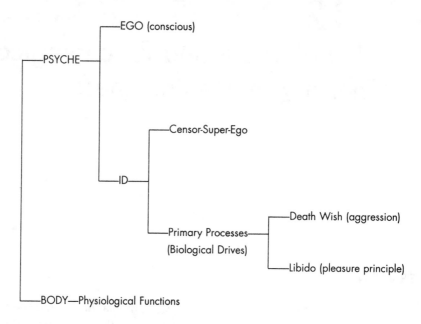

DIAGRAM 1. Freudian Model

been used in two very different but very influential traditions of thinking about human behavior and its ethical problems.

The first, more recent and more familiar to psychiatrists, is the *Freudian model*. The brilliant work of Sigmund Freud (d. 1939) is today under severe criticism for its lack of scientific verification, yet it has profoundly influenced modern psychology and psychiatry (Crews, 1994; Webster, 1995). It can be simplified in Diagram 1.

For Freud the "ego" (above the horizontal line in the diagram) is the conscious self of ordinary practical life in touch with the "real world," whose thought and feelings can be verbalized and communicated. But it has developed in a body whose physiological functions produce certain primary psychic processes or drives which Freud first identified with our desire for pleasure (libido). These pleasure drives are focused on the infant's mouth and its hunger for food and then spread to the erogenous zones of the body. Later Freud distinguished a second basic drive which, rather misleadingly, he called the "death wish" and which his disciples later identified as "aggression," the drive to attack obstacles to obtaining satisfaction of the pleasure drive (Freud, 1920; Menninger, 1938). These two drives—and the fantasies and memories manifested in our day and night dreaming which stimulate and express them—are irrational and contradictory and hence can never be fully satisfied in reality. Society, beginning with our parents, must impose order on these conflicting drives, which it does by rewards and punishments which create within the child's psyche the "superego." This superego or "conscience" inhibits the socially disapproved satisfaction of our drives and produces feelings of anxiety and guilt, but cannot prevent the energy of these drives from continuing to seek fulfillment.

Since the tension produced by this suppression of primary drives is painful, the superego also acts as a "censor" which prevents these forbidden drives from emerging into consciousness except in the form of neurotic behavioral symptoms which partially—but only partially—reduce this anxiety by satisfying these desires in a merely symbolic form. This neurotic way of dealing with desire or aggression, however, tends ultimately to break down and produce panic or other bizarre behaviors that demand therapeutic attention. Psychoanalytic therapy, therefore, consists in raising these unconscious desires to the level of the conscious ego (abreaction) where the sufferers can compare the unrealistic superego standards imposed on them in early childhood with their real situation in life and thus come to deal with them in a manner less neurotic and more realistic. Freud believed, therefore, that civilization of primitive human nature is inevitably painful and hoped that psychoanalysis might assist people to attain a realistic compromise between our biological drives and social demands (Freud, 1930).

The Aristotelian Model of the Human Person

The other tradition which we will consider is much older and goes back to Greek philosophy, later adopted in Christian theology and ethics. Neither it nor Freud's model has received strict scientific verification, but while Freud's theory was based on a quite limited (and not always very accurately reported) clinical experience, the Aristotelian model has been tested by hundreds of years of pastoral experience. The reason for considering it here, however, is that it is presupposed by the Catholic tradition of moral analysis and pastoral counseling. Hence, to bring these two traditions of life therapy together, the old and the new, the ethical and the medical, as we have tried to do in this book, it is necessary to attempt to relate the Freudian to the Aristotelian model, which can be diagrammed as in Diagram 2.

In this Aristotelian model the conscious self consists only in the *cognitional* functions, although the sense memory stores images and the intellect stores abstract knowledge, both of which remain unconscious until recalled. The rest of the human person is unconscious in itself but produces effects in the body which are sensed and then reflected on by the intellect. Thus the drives for pleasure and aggression are not themselves conscious, but they stimulate the body and thus produce "feelings" which are conscious sensations. Similarly, the acts of the will are not directly conscious but issue in conscious thoughts and sensed actions. Thus in this model, as in the Freudian one, much of the human person remains hidden to us and must be raised to consciousness. It should be noted also that in this model the sense appetites are divided as Freud finally did into a drive for pleasure and an aggressive drive.

Relations of the Two Models

Three important differences between the two models should be noted. First, Freud, because of his materialism and scientism, did not very clearly distinguish

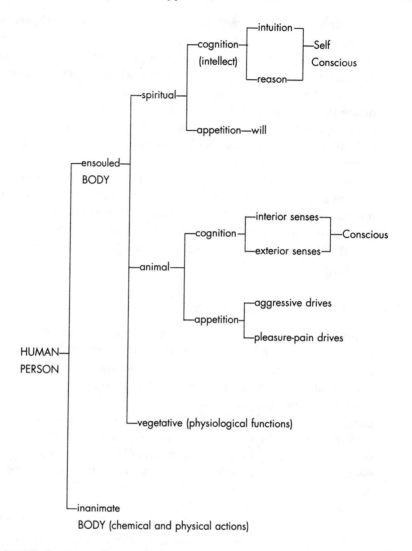

DIAGRAM 2. Aristotelian Model

between the animal level of sensation and appetition and the intellectual level of abstract cognition and free will. Yet as scientist and a realist he was forced to admit the objectivity of scientific knowledge and of pragmatic realism. He identified these with a strong ego and mental health in contrast to the illusory, self-contradictory, irrational character of the id. Second, Freud did not distinguish clearly between intellectual reason and intuition, and this led him to identify reason with the ego and to attribute the work of intuition to the unconscious. Thus for him the creativity of the arts and the religious commitment to ultimate goals in life had to be unconscious, irrational activities (Zika and Chamberlain, 1993). But how could that which is most human, creative, and free, the seat of what Maslow calls "peak experiences," have its source in what is most animal, instinctual, and deterministic in human nature? Freud himself had to admit that his view might explain certain features of a work of art but could not explain why some works of art are of high creative quality and others are not.

In Freud's model, therefore, intuitive intellection, on which scientific, artistic, ethical, and religious thinking is based, has to be attributed to the irrational id, and nothing is left for conscious intellection except scientific reasoning and pragmatic calculation. In an Aristotelian model, however, intuitive activities, such as scientific and artistic creativity and religious faith, find a place as the highest of human abilities and are attributed to a superconsciousness (not to be confused with the superego, which is really part of the id; [Arieti, 1967; Ashley, 1972, 1996]). The reason that Freud could confuse the superconsciousness with the unconscious is that both are outside the verbalizable consciousness of the ego: the id because it is more primitive than the ego, the superconsciousness because intuitive, creative truths and fundamental commitments are difficult to express in words. Thus the Aristotelian model makes room for the *ethical* and the *spiritual* levels of the human person which Freud, himself a very intuitive and creative person, so paradoxically reduced to the animal level!

Third, Freud does not give any place to the free will which the intellect makes possible by its intuition of ends (goals) and its reasoning about means in relation to ends. Thus, although psychoanalytic therapy is supposed to work by helping clients come to a realistic self-understanding and a free control over their lives, Freud did not provide an adequate model for such understanding. What he did contribute, and what must be integrated into the Aristotelian model, is a deeper insight into how the unconscious part of our psyche can interfere with the working of our conscious thought.

The Biological–Psychological Interface

Beginning in the 1950s and rapidly advancing after 1970, the Freudian or psychoanalytic theories of mental illness and the various psychotherapies to which it had given rise began to decline in favor, because of both their lack of scientific rigor and the greater success of pharmacotherapeutic drugs (Cohen, 1995). Moreover, research made it evident that certain psychoses, schizophrenia and bipolar psychosis, were probably due to genetic physiological defects (Malaspina et al., 1992). Psychoanalytic therapy had confined itself mainly to treating neuroses and had found these psychoses beyond its reach.

Obviously there is a danger of reductionism in this pharmacotherapeutic approach to mental illness. While it is very plausible that malfunction of the central nervous system due to organic or physiological defects should be the cause of the most disruptive forms of mental disease, it is improbable that they are its total cause, any more than, for example, obesity which is the result of lack of exercise or cancer of the lungs resulting from smoking can be explained simply by their physical causes. They are also the result of culture, behavior, education, etc., and cannot be prevented or healed without considering the lifestyle of the victim. Thus even the most enthusiastic advocate of pharmacotherapy recognizes that psychotherapeutic counseling still remains necessary in treating mental illness. We will discuss how pharmacotherapy and psycho-therapy can complement each other in the next section.

Here it is sufficient to point out by way of example that alcoholism, which can be considered a mental illness, is on the one hand a physiological condition which probably has a genetic basis that sensitizes some people to the action of alcohol, and on the other hand that alcoholism develops in individuals only in circumstances where drinking is socially acceptable and is also favored by traumatic experiences, poverty, etc. A holistic therapy, therefore, must consider both aspects of the condition.

The Psychological–Ethical Interface

The problem of defining mental disease is also involved in the current problem of penology (H. Schwartz et al., 1984; L. Schwartz, 1982). Crime seems to imply ethical responsibility on the part of the criminal who violates the rights of others. That is why criminals are brought before "the bar of justice" and why they are punished for their antisocial behavior. Our legal system was based on the assumption that a crime, unless committed by persons so mentally disturbed that they did not know they were breaking a law, was the agent's responsibility. The proper way to deal with crime was by death, corporal punishment, or imprisonment. These sanctions were considered both punishments for past crime and *deterrents* to future crime for both the criminal and others because fear of punishment for the crime would be an element in the rational calculation of anyone tempted to commit it.

In our century, however, the line between criminality and mental illness has tended to blur. The more criminologists have learned about those who commit antisocial acts, the more the perpetrators appear to be victims to be rehabilitated rather than criminals to be punished (Menninger, 1968). Those charged with crimes are found to be:

1. Victims as children or adolescents of abuse or neglect;
2. Victims of deep psychological maladjustments whose roots are unconscious and uncontrollable; and
3. Victims of social injustices, conditioned by the subculture in which they live to follow standards of behavior different from the laws of the dominant culture.

Thus it has been contended that many "criminals" are not ethically culpable at all and the proper means of social control of their behavior is not punishment, but therapy and reeducation.

This notion of crime as mental illness and social maladjustment, formerly popular, today is again under attack (Holmes, 1991). The rising level of crime in our country, aggravated by prevalence of drug abuse, the crisis of the family, and the conflict between racial and ethnic groups, has raised popular demand for more jails and stiffer sentences. The plea of "not guilty by reason of insanity" is often rejected as an invention of well-paid defense lawyers. Even persons who are admittedly mentally defective or suffering from paranoid delusions are executed with popular approval.

Moreover, the line between therapy and punishment and rehabilitation has become questionable. Criminals are incarcerated not to make them fear loss of freedom if they commit crimes again, but to cure them of mental illnesses and to educate them to conformity with accepted social standards of behavior, sometimes with little protection of their basic human rights (Many, 1980). On the other hand, the patients in mental institutions, even those who at first voluntarily accept confinement, come to believe that their condition is no different from that of prisoners, since they are subjected to treatment they do not understand and over which they can make no real choice (Fulford and Hope, 1994).

The controversy over ethical responsibility and mental illness has led to the denial by some that there is even such a thing as "mental illness." A group of "antipsychiatry psychiatrists" has made a strong, if exaggerated, case against the whole concept of mental disease and the medical model of psychiatry. Thus, the failure in the history of medicine to distinguish and properly interrelate these diverse facets of human personality has been a source of vast confusion and controversy (Elliott, 1991). Richard M. Restak in *Pre-Meditated Man* (1975) claimed that most of the problems of bioethics are not really ethical in the ordinary sense, but *political,* that is, questions of power as to whose will concerning human behavior is to prevail. The line between normal behavior and abnormal behavior thus turns out to be only a question of who is deciding what *they* want *us* to do.

Similarly, in *The Myth of Mental Illness* (1961, 1974), Thomas Szasz argued that the concept of mental illness is completely invalid and that the greater number of psychiatric illnesses are really social maladjustments between the behavior of a nonconformist individual and the demands of a social system. The cause of these maladjustments is found in the modern social system, which is unable to deal with individual differences. Szasz has even compared modern psychiatry and mental hospitals to the medieval religious inquisition, that is, to an institution whose purpose supposedly was to enforce conformity of more highly individualized personalities to a rigid and oppressive social system through a cruel process of interrogation and torture (Szasz, 1987). One group of psychiatrists call themselves "radicals" and see the whole mental health establishment as an instrument of oppression.

Evidence that these accusations are not without serious foundation is shown in the actions of some governments like the former Communist regimes (Stover and Nightengale, 1985) that have confined dissidents to mental institutions under the pretext that anyone who criticized the regime must be insane. Even the American Psychiatric Association (APA), by appointing a task force to study the use of seclusion and restraint in psychiatric therapy (APA, 1985), has admitted that such ethical problems can arise. The novel of Ken Kesey (and even more the classic movie based on it) *One Flew Over the Cuckoo's Nest* dramatized the way in which patients, even those self-committed to a mental institution, can be reduced to robotlike conformity by the "system." The tragedy of this story was that the "monster" Nurse Ratchett was in fact a dedicated, well-meaning, and highly professional person who quite unconsciously had become a manipulator of people. Clearly in such cases it is not the individuals who are sick, but a system that fits both patients and health care professionals into a mutually destructive gestalt.

This accusation is further strengthened by realization of the effect of the "total institution" on human beings (Goffman, 1962; Rothman, 1980), which shows the dangers of a closed social system where people so live within a rigid set of determined ideas and behaviors that they are cut off from contact with a reality beyond and different from their limited perception. This often leads to a distorted, *paranoid* way of perceiving and interpreting the world. But no asylum, prison, monastery, or hospital can become a "total institution." Only modern society itself, with its technological organization, its mass media of brainwashing, and its all-seeing surveillance, can act as a total institution, so that there is no escape except (as in Kesey's novel) to sail out to sea in a boat.

The Interface of the Ethical and the Spiritual

The term "religion" is often used to include both the ethical and the spiritual level of human personality, which our diagram distinguishes. It indicates that the spiritual level deals with the ultimate goals of human existence, and the ethical with the choice of means appropriate to these goals. Indeed, "religion" includes not only the ethical level of human personality, but also the whole human person in all its dimensions. Yet what is most proper to religion is the spiritual dimension of human existence. At this level intellectual intuition provides a vision of ultimate values, the realities that constitute the goals of authentic human living, while the will commits and moves the person to seek these goals.

Two mistakes are often made with regard to spirituality. First, Freud, a nineteenth century materialist who, without being very scientific himself, put his ultimate faith in science, argued in *Totem and Taboo* and *Civilization and its Discontents* that religion is a neurotic regression to the peace and security the child once experienced in its mother's womb. The mature, mentally healthy person, on the other hand, is ready to accept harsh reality in stoic resignation. While Freud's great disciple Carl Gustav Jung (d. 1961) was able to give a more informed and positive psychoanalytical analysis of religion, he too confused intuitive knowledge with what he called the "Collective Unconscious." Many psychotherapists, both because of their narrowly scientific education and because they have often seen religion playing a sinister part in their patient's mental ailments, share with Freud this same prejudice against it (Bergin, 1991).

Since sexuality is such a big factor in many people's mental problems, is sex a neurosis? Because spirituality relates to the ultimate goals that are central to human life, it is not at all surprising that mental illness often infects this life center with a neurotic, distorted religiosity. The schizophrenic, for example, who thinks he is God, probably does not do so because he is deeply religious, but because he is deeply religious his schizophrenic illusions take a religious form, just as a schizophrenic soldier claims to be Napoleon. In particular it is a mistake to think that the overwhelming guilt, scrupulosity, or anxiety that are frequently involved in neuroses is a genuine religious guilt. As Freud himself showed, neurotic guilt arises from the irrational superego, not from the mature, realistic ethics of a religious person who has achieved an objective self-understanding in terms of the ultimate goals of life. After all, who is more in touch with reality than maturely religious persons who live in the constant presence of ethical responsibility to their neighbors, of death, of judgment, and of the Creator?

Psychological studies of the Catholic saints often fall into either the error of reducing everything remarkable in their lives to mental illness, or the other extreme of supposing everything in their lives was a sign of holiness. For example, we cannot be sure whether the inability to eat of the great St. Catherine of Siena was *anorexia nervosa* or a miracle of sustenance by the Eucharist alone. Perhaps it was both! St. Therese of Lisieux seems to have suffered as a child from an hysteric illness, but as a young woman she faced death from very real tuberculosis with great courage and profound self-understanding. The scrupulosity St. Alphonsus Ligouri suffered to his dying day was perhaps due to an anxiety disorder, but he was a great church leader, scholar, and a very prudent counselor of others. Considering the complexity of human personality, mental mental disease is no less compatible with true human maturity than is physical disease. While mental disease is often a great obstacle to maturation, or to exercising one's maturity once attained, it can also become a source of maturation as a person struggles to overcome limitations. The biographies of great personalities often recount their struggles not only with physical disease, but with emotional problems that today we identify as mental illnesses (Levin, 1994).

The Reality of Mental Illness

From this discussion of the nature of mental illness, the following four conclusions can be drawn: First, mental illness in the strict and proper sense results from faulty development and use of human cognitive and affective capacities. Physical and physiological impairments may contribute to this faulty development and function because they inhibit the adaptive capacity of the person (Sider, 1983).

Second, it is necessary to hold firmly to the fact that dysfunctional forms of human behavior caused by organic and physiological defects do exist (Neppe and Tucker, 1992). Lesions of the central nervous system, as well as a wide variety of physiological disorders, can make it difficult or impossible for human beings to sense and perceive the world correctly, to live in a state of emotional balance and sensitivity, to think clearly, and to make decisions free from uncontrollable impulses (Tranel, 1992). Moreover, increasing evidence suggests that there is a genetic basis for some mental illnesses (Talbott, 1988; Michels and Marzyh, 1993). Yet the tendency to consider genetic causes as the source of all mental illness must also be resisted (Lewontin et al., 1984).

Third, it is essential to keep in mind that these physical disabilities (except in the most severe cases) do not automatically lead to highly abnormal behavior. Rather, it is a matter of tension between the innate capacities of the individual and the demands of the environment. For example, a patient with a respiratory disorder may be relatively comfortable under some atmospheric conditions and intensely uncomfortable under others that would not greatly distress a normal person. This disparity may also prevail among people with an inadequate or impaired capacity to adjust to certain environmental and social stresses. Clearly this suggests that the mental health of a society is to be achieved not only by treatment of the individual, but also by political and social readjustment of the environment to more adaptive lifestyles. It would seem that modern society should have enough social control to be able tolerate varied human capacities.

Fourth, prolonged hospitalization of the mentally ill is not only costly, but often bad therapy. Nevertheless, it is a serious injustice to dismiss them to wander, distressed and distressing, perhaps suicidal or dangerous, homeless in the streets. While those with mental illness need an environment that is as normal and open as possible, they also desperately need care, support, and guidance to cope with reality. A large number of people in society require psychiatric care that is impossible without hospitalization. Extreme caution must also be taken within practical limits to protect the human rights of mental patients, especially as to both voluntary and involuntary commitments and retention, the right of treatment during the patient's stay (Helmchen, 1994), and even the right to refuse some forms of treatment.

Thus psychiatric care must include an effort to help patients develop skills to cope with the social situation in which they must live after leaving the hospital, a situation they ordinarily cannot much alter. The patient's family must share in this process to assist in the patient's reentry into normal living, or a halfway house should be available to facilitate this difficult transition. It is essential, moreover, that Christians recognize and respond to the need for a profound social transformation of culture so that it will be able to meet the needs of so-called deviants, who are among the "little ones" for whom Jesus taught us to be advocates.

12.2 PSYCHOSURGERY, ELECTROCONVULSIVE THERAPY, AND PHARMACOTHERAPY

Psychosurgery

Since organic defects and malfunctions underlie many forms of mental illness, their healing requires the correction of these defects. Klerman and Beitman (1991) write:

> In the 1970s and 1980, the focus [of psychiatric training] changed dramatically. With the growing volume of double-blind, randomized studies on the efficacy of various forms of pharmacotherapy and the revaluation of ECT, scientific judgment increasingly questioned the nature of the evidence for the value of psychotherapy. The discrepancy between ideology and evidence in psychotherapy has now become the subject of professional and public debate. These ideological differences are reflected in clinical practice. Within psychiatry, there is divergence based on theoretical alliance (p. 9ff).

The theoretical alliance or "schools of psychiatry" are listed by the same work: biological, psychoanalytic, interpersonal, social, and behavioral/cognitive. Before treating this new dominance of pharmacotherapy, we will discuss two other modes of treating mental illness, much less often indicated, that seek to correct organic causes of such disorders: namely psychosurgery and electroconvulsive therapy (ECT).

Nerve cells do not regenerate like other parts of the body, perhaps because they need to endure for a lifetime to retain the record of learning experiences. Hence formerly it was thought that to repair them surgically in the ways we are used to doing with other body parts was out of the question. Recent research, however, gives hope that in the future we may be able to stimulate the nervous system to repair itself and may even be able to transplant portions of the brain. At present, however, brain surgery is largely a matter of relieving destructive pressures on the brain or removing benign or malignant tumors. It can be called psychosurgery only when its purpose is to treat conditions that are diagnosed in the regular categories of mental illness (Hay, 1993).

Arguments on the ethics and merits of psychosurgery vary from severe condemnation to considerable enthusiasm (Black and Szasz, 1977; Valenstein, 1992). The psychosurgical procedure that attracted the most attention was the *prefrontal lobotomy* performed in the 1930s and 1940s on people with severe psychotic disorders. In a recent article Dorman recounts the early days of psychosurgery, the factors responsible for its inception, and the different techniques used through the years (Dorman, 1995). This procedure, which in some cases could be done under local anesthesia, consists essentially in severing the white nerve fibers that connect the frontal lobes of the brain with the thalamus. It tended to result in a blunting of human emotional responses and thus calming antisocial behavior.

Because lobotomy is an irreversible and drastic procedure, it was performed only on persons with severe behavior problems such as acute aggression or severe despondency. According to some experts, the emotional responses leveled by lobotomy could be normalized to some degree, especially if proper treatment were given after the procedure. Nevertheless, lobotomized patients generally have inhibited, strangely one-dimensional, personalities. Because of the dramatic effect of this form of behavior modification, the procedure fell into disuse when psychoactive drugs became more effective for the treatment of severe psychosis. In recent years, psychosurgery has once again become more common throughout the world (Snaith, 1994b). Modern procedures using, for example, ultrasound, electrical coagulation, or implanted radium seeds are more localized and less destructive.

Electroconvulsive Therapy

In the 1930s vonMeduna (APA, 1978) working in Budapest and Vienna, developed the treatment of mental disorders not by surgery but by "shock treatment," in which the patient was caused by injections of metrazol, insulin, or other drugs to go into convulsions somewhat like those of epilepsy. A few years later, in 1938, Cereletti, working in Rome, utilized electric current to induce shock (McDonald,

1978). The theory was that this violent stimulation of the brain would cause the readjustment of disordered neural patterns. While shock therapy was sometimes effective, it could be dangerous, causing broken bones or heart attacks, and when used repeatedly it was said to leave the patient in much the same condition as lobotomy. It was also greatly dreaded by some patients who were frightened by its violence, risks, and aftereffects. Though vonMeduna's theory was never confirmed, the sometimes dramatic efficacy of the procedure led to further research. Thus, the way was opened for electroconvulsive therapy (ECT), defined as "the utilization of electrically induced repetitive firings of the neurons in the central nervous system . . . to treat psychiatric illnesses such as the affective disorders of depression and mania or psychiatric symptoms such as psychosis or catatonia" (Talbott et al., 1988 p. 836).

For some time after ECT began to be widely used, it was regarded as more destructive than therapeutic by some scientists and physicians. Chief among these critics has been Peter Breggin (1972, 1979), a practicing psychiatrist whose scathing denunciation, based mainly on ethical considerations, reprinted in the *Congressional Register* (March 30, 1972), gave rise to national debates. Today ECT is generally accepted as the preferred treatment for severe depression which has not yielded to drugs, where the patient cannot tolerate drugs, or where the patient's condition is very difficult to manage without a quick improvement (NIH, 1985). The reasons for its efficacy are still unknown conclusively. What is most certain is that these procedures produce temporarily a severe loss of memory and general state of psychic disorganization. Apparently this makes it possible for some patients to break out of fixed patterns of fantasy and feeling and to begin to respond in a more normal way.

Pharmacotherapy

A drug is psychoactive when it has some psychological effect: alters thoughts, imagination, perception, or emotions; causes alertness, drowsiness, or feelings of anger; and so forth. Such drugs, often called medications or pharmaceuticals to avoid negative connotations, are also called *psychotropic,* and the study of these drugs is called psychopharmacology. Some forms of psychoactive agents have been used since the beginning of civilization. Alcoholic beverages were invented at the same time as cereal agriculture. Opium in one form or another has been used as a pain reliever for centuries. Aspirin, the first of the wonder drugs, has been used for more than 100 years to treat pain and anxiety. But the use of modern medications which affect the brain has been dramatic. "This new medical approach to psychiatry has led to a vigorous pursuit of diagnostic systems that have greater precision, reliability and validity; to the delineation of genetic, neurodevelopmental, chemical, immunologic, endocrinologic and ideotrophysiologic aspects of specific disorders; and to the development of more disorder specific and pharmacologically specific treatments" (Michiels and Marzuk, 1993).

Hence, the treatment of major psychiatric disorders has become more pharmacologic and less psychotherapeutic.

Although the psychotropic drugs available for behavior control at present comprise an impressive array, the potential for the future is even more awesome (Baldessarini, 1985). Klerman states: "As knowledge of the relationship between brain and behavior increases, it is likely we will develop knowledge of the neurochemical and neuropharmacological bases of memory, learning, mood, aggression, appetite, and sexual lust." Thus, not only must psychoactive drugs be evaluated as therapeutic agents, but also future ethical evaluation must consider their potential to improve capabilities and enhance personal pleasure and enjoyment of life (Klerman, 1991).

Extreme ethical concerns over the use of psychoactive drugs, however, did not develop until recently after several pharmacological compounds were developed or synthesized that alter mental and emotional functioning (Snyder, 1986). Some of these drugs, which are readily available to the public at large, have demonstrated value to treat specific mental illness, but others such as lysergic acid diethylamide (LSD) are not associated with therapeutic use (Stevens, 1987). Given the wide range of known drugs, there seems to be one available to suppress or evoke any emotional state or symptom.

Psychotropic drugs have proved highly effective in psychotherapy in (1) tranquilizing patients in manic states or in uncontrollable anxiety; (2) reducing the condition of mental confusion and dissociation, especially in schizophrenia; and (3) lifting certain types of depression (J. Silver and Yudofsky, 1988; Klerman and Beitman, 1991). These effects may be symptomatic, rather than truly curative, but they raise the hope that as these underlying organic causes are understood, more successful therapies and preventives for mental illness can be developed. It is also clear, however, that drugs can never be the total answer to the problems of mental health, which also involve the factors of social environment and psychological development (Lewontia et al., 1984).

The possible clinical effects of the shift from psychotherapy to pharmacotherapy are as follows:

Negatively, the introduction of drugs into psychotherapy may:

1. Make both therapist and patient too dependent on faith in the "magic" of drugs, rather than seeking genuine insight into psychological processes (Coleman, 1995);
2. Reduce the patient's anxiety and tension and therefore the patient's motivation to seek help and change;
3. Reduce the patient's symptoms only to generate new symptoms in their place; and
4. Make patients feel they are being given drugs because they do not have the capacity to attain self-understanding through psychotherapy.

Positively, the use of drugs may:

1. Make patients more accessible to psychotherapy;
2. Improve "ego function," that is, "influence verbal skill, improve cognitive functioning, improve memory, reduce distraction, and promote

concentration," so that the client is better able to cooperate in psychotherapy;

3. Promote "abreaction," a basic element in psychotherapy, the ability to relive and confront past traumas and fixations; and

4. Replace the feelings of despair and stigmatization associated with mental illness, with the optimism and normality of getting medical help.

On the other hand, psychotherapy can have both negative and positive effects on drug therapy.

Negative effects may be:

1. If the illness is the result of a single physiological factor correctable by drugs, psychotherapy is irrelevant; and

2. Psychotherapy may disturb the patient and aggravate symptoms.

Positive effects may be:

1. Rehabilitation of the patient after drugs have done their work; and

2. Psychotherapy helps the patient accept and be consistent in use of the drugs.

Thus pharmacotherapy is based on the hypothesis that the mental disorder is the result of a neurophysiological malfunction which may or may not have a genetic basis and that the administration of drugs will correct this imbalance or at least mitigate its symptoms. Psychotherapy cannot correct this underlying problem, although it may assist in enabling the patient to cope with its disturbing effects in daily life. If this is the case, then to subject the patient to extensive psychotherapy is not only a waste of time and money but is unethical, since it must be motivated either by prejudices against the use of drugs, ideological attachment to unproven psychological theories, or simply an exploitative desire on the part of the psychotherapist to keep control of patients and the fees they pay.

In summary, from an ethical point of view the increasing reliance on pharmacotherapy seems justified by its results, but requires on the part of physicians that they:

1. Not succumb to the temptation to give pills, rather than to carefully diagnose and monitor the patient;

2. Not let prejudices in favor of the "medical model" of therapy lead them to neglect psychotherapy as indicated;

3. Not neglect assessing and monitoring possible side effects of the drugs to be used and observing the principle of free and informed consent before prescribing them; and

4. Promote and keep informed of continuing research to determine sci-

entifically the value of the drugs in question and to continue to improve them and increase their safety.

12.3 PSYCOTHERAPEUTIC MEANS OF THERAPY

Pharmacotherapy, psychosurgery, and ECT fit easily into the "medical model" by which physical diseases are usually treated, but psychotherapy as such is a strikingly different mode of therapy. To treat patients by talking with them or guiding them in recalling and reenacting past experiences or changing unreal ways of solving life's problems is very different from giving them a pill, cutting out a tumor, regulating their diet, or even directing their physical exercise. It is more similar to education or reeducation (Ursano and Silberman, 1988), if "education" means not the mere acquisition of information but rather the learner's own growth toward self-understanding and control, which the therapist facilitates but cannot originate. Psychotherapy is based on the assumption that the mentally disturbed person has at least some capacities for normal mental life, but that these capacities have not been properly developed, are malfunctioning, or are being poorly used. In other words, the mentally sick person has to a degree the capacity to cope with situations satisfactorily, but he or she has not learned how to use this capacity effectively or is inhibited from such use by abnormal fears and faulty perceptions of reality.

There is, however, an important difference between psychotherapeutic or mental health education and other types of education. *Education,* in the usual sense as a function of an academic institution, is the development of human capacities at the rational or conscious level. Psychotherapy deals with psychic processes less conscious and less free than rational thought, just as education at the spiritual level deals with psychic processes that transcend the level of discursive rational thought (Mack, 1994).

At present, there is a plethora of psychotherapeutic methods (Petrila, 1986; Ursano and Silberman, 1988); but two very different conceptions of human psychological development are reflected in the two main current schools of psychotherapy. Perry London, in *Behavior Control* (1969), named these "insight therapy" and "action therapy." In practice these therapies overlap, but they have different theoretical and clinical sources. The *insight therapies* derive largely from Freud and the psychoanalytical school, although they have now moved on to include a great variety of therapeutic methods other than psychoanalysis, especially to include the social group aspect of behavioral disorders (Engel, 1981). What characterizes these therapies is that they aim at helping individuals *understand* ("have insight into," "get in touch with") their own behavior and its affective sources and thus learn how to deal with life situations in an effective way.

Insight therapies assume that mental disorder means simply that (1) patients lack this insight or the skill to deal with their emotions and interpersonal relations; or (2) as with the obsessive person, they have much insight and little skill; or (3) as with the psychopathic person, they have much skill and little insight because during the course of their psychosocial development they have been traumatized or wrongly guided. Thus psychotherapy of this type deals with lack of coordination between the rational level, and in the case of the therapy of Jung et al. (1964), perhaps also with the spiritual level (Moore and Mockel, 1990); and the psychological level of the personality. Normal persons coordinate their rational and subrational processes satisfactorily, whereas neurotic or psychotic persons do not.

On the other hand, *action therapy* is the outcome of the behaviorist school of psychology, which rejects or bypasses the whole notion of the subconscious because it does not consider the notion of consciousness to be of any great help in psychological theory (Agras and Berkowitz, 1988). While most action therapists do not go in theory to this behavioralist extreme, they do seek to understand human behavior primarily in terms of *operant conditioning*. Human beings behave as they do because they live in a physical and social environment that has educated them to behave in a certain way. This education consists in an ordered series of rewards and punishments (positive and negative reinforcements) that favor some forms of behavior and eliminate others.

In such a view, mental illness is behavior that is unacceptable to society and that also may be internally so self-inconsistent as to cause painful conflict in the organism. Action therapy, therefore, is a process of reconditioning the person to a more self-consistent and socially acceptable type of behavior. Its methods do not depend on growth in insight from subjects, who need not know how their malconditioning has arisen or even how the therapy works; these methods are aimed simply at removing undesirable behavior patterns and developing new ones.

It should be noted, however, that action therapies include not only reeducation by means of external rewards and punishments (e.g., by administering painful electric shocks), but also extend to reeducation of the person's fantasy life by desensitization, as when a patient overcomes a phobia by imagining painful situations and gradually comes to feel less anxious about them. Thus methods that rely on suggestion are considered action therapy, although they may appear similar to methods in insight therapy (Valliant and Antonowicz, 1991).

More related to the insight therapies, yet sharing with action therapy a reluctance to explain behavior by unconscious processes is *cognitive therapy*, which tries to reeducate the way clients reason about themselves and their problems. For example, depressed persons think about reality in a pessimistic, defeatist way that fails to give attention to the options open to them, among which they can select more positive creative ways of acting. As long as they continue to live in a defeatist mental atmosphere, failure is inevitable. Cognitive therapy aims to enable such persons to recognize that this hopeless round of thought can be broken through and new thought patterns can be learned. Other persons habitually live, like Dickens' Mister Micawber, in a rosy but merely fanciful future, ignoring their real possibilities of decision and action. This daydreaming too is a sure recipe for failure, and cognitive therapy aims to bring the dreamer down to earth. Its technique is to help clients analyze the ways of thinking that have caused them to fail in living and to reeducate them to think logically and realistically (Joseph, 1995).

The controversy between these insight and action therapies still continues and is often obscured by bitter polemics, but it reflects two aspects of human psychology that are not necessarily contradictory (Clark, D. M., 1994). Action therapy reflects the fact that human behavior, which at first may be conscious and deliberate, quickly takes on a pattern and becomes automatic and subconscious. Thus when a person is learning to drive a car or play the piano, each motion is conscious and deliberate, but once the habit is acquired, these actions can be performed without conscious attention. This applies also to motivation because in general it is easier and more pleasant to perform in a habitual manner, and more difficult and even painful to go against a habit or routine response. The advantage of such automatization of behavior is obvious; it frees one's attention from the details of routine behavior and permits concentration on decisions about new or unusual situations, problems to be solved, and new skills to be acquired. Without this capacity to form habits, a person's energies would be wasted on routine acts rather than concentrated on the adaptive and creative ones.

Furthermore, in psychosocial development the formation of such habits in the child precedes the time when the human person is mature enough to have full self-consciousness and control. No wonder, then, that children who have been badly trained by their social environment arrive at the stage of self-control with many faulty, and perhaps disastrously restricted or inconsistent and conflictual, patterns of behavior whose origin and even existence they do not understand. These may operate in both the conscious and the unconscious levels of the psyche. Thus children may have developed irrational fears by associating fear reactions with harmless stimuli, but they no longer understand why they are afraid. Or the extreme pessimist or optimist may, at the conscious level, have developed patterns of noticing only the dark or the light side of situations.

The action therapies, based on a highly developed theory of learning through conditioning, seek to reeducate the patient by extinguishing undesirable patterns of behavior and establishing or strengthening desirable ones. Included are not only external behaviors, but also undesirable emotional reactions, especially the hampering and disorganizing type of fear called *neurotic anxiety*.

The insight therapies agree that the human being has many automatisms and that aberrant adult behavior is often rooted in faulty conditioning in early childhood, when the organism is highly impressionable and the power of the ego to resist environmental influences is low. The emphasis of insight therapies, including cognitive therapy, is on the emergence of the ego or self as controlling behavior in an adaptive manner in the face of the natural and social environments. Consequently, if the therapist simply corrects faulty habits in the client, this only treats the symptoms. The real problem is to help patients develop a strong ego and to understand how they came to have faulty habits of thinking and acting so they will be able under their own choice to form better ones. Thus it requires at least some measure of exploration of the past and a growing insight into one's own personality structure.

Apparently, therefore, the two therapies can complement each other. In fact, the latest behavioral theories go beyond Skinner and postulate an interaction between environment, behavior, and cognition processes to explain human behavior (Bandura, 1986). Moreover, clients who have acquired insight into their own behavior and unconscious motivation may still need to be taught how to recondition themselves and to be aided by others in so doing. Freud and the psychoanalytical school too quickly assumed that a person who understands why he or she acts irrationally will then spontaneously be free to act rationally. This failed to take into account that psychological restructuring in the form of breaking old habits and forming new ones is a complex task. In this case cognitive and learning theory is extremely important. On the other hand, the goals of action therapy seem too limited because they are based on a narrow, behavioristic conception of human life. Such learning theories have been developed from animal experimentation and have proved themselves most practical in dealing with subnormal intelligences, just as insight therapies are most successful with highly intelligent, verbal, and creative personalities. Learning good habits is not all there is to having an integrated personality. It is also necessary to develop an autonomous ego.

Thus, insofar as it is distinct from medical therapy, psychotherapy is not so much a process of healing a defective organic structure as of reeducation, not at the level of fully rational behavior, but at the level of automatic, conditioned, or subconscious behavior. Its purpose is to free the individual from undesirable patterns of behavior, especially those that are inconsistent, so that rational free life becomes more possible.

Goals of Psychotherapy

This definition of psychotherapy, however, raises a serious question: What is "normal" behavior when mental health is concerned (Truant and Lohrenz, 1993; Brenner, 1994)? The action therapist Joseph Wolpe (1966) quotes R. P. Knight (1966) with approval, saying that the criteria of successful psychotherapy of any type can be summarized as follows:

1. Relief of undesirable symptoms (e.g., excessive anxiety);
2. Increased productivity in the person's work;
3. Adjustment and satisfaction in sexual relations;
4. Better interpersonal relations; and
5. Increased ability to endure the stresses of life.

Robert Harper (1959), after surveying the bewildering array of therapies then current (the situation has not altered much since that time; see Petrila, 1986), concludes that most therapies have to settle for the following results to consider themselves successful:

1. The weak ego of the patient is supported by the stronger ego of the therapist.

2. The lack of realism of the patient is corrected by the more realistic attitude of the therapist.

3. The patient learns to see that many things he or she fears are not so terrible.

4. The patient learns to be more patient in solving problems, less impulsive and panicky.

5. The patient acquires a greater or new faith or "life-myth" from the example of the therapist, who represents a hope for health.

6. The patient gets a more objective perspective on his or her problems from discussing them with the therapist or therapy group.

7. The patient focuses his or her floating anxieties on the outcome of the therapy process, so that he or she feels less isolated and helpless.

At present, psychotherapeutic methods do not have a clear record of effectiveness (Hatfield and Lefley, 1993). Psychoanalytical methods are extremely time-consuming and expensive. Hence, there is increasing reluctance of HMOs and government agencies to pay for such extended treatment whose outcome is difficult to evaluate. The action therapists have argued that the insight therapists have very little objective proof that their methods succeed better than natural processes; furthermore, the success they have seems largely independent of the mode of therapy and mainly dependent on the personal relation with a therapist who is a sensitive, realistic, and caring person.

The action therapists claim to have a better and more demonstrable record of success, but on examination this success mainly appears in rather restricted areas of neuroses, and its permanence is often questioned. Furthermore, action therapy fails to achieve the ultimate aim of developing a strong autonomy in the patient. At present, it must be concluded that this type of problem is very complex, and knowledge about it and ability to cure it still very limited. Nevertheless, therapy usually produces moderate improvement and sometimes is very successful. Perhaps this is not so different from any other area of medical care, or of ethical and spiritual guidance. It can never be stressed too much that all modes of therapy are only of service to facilitate the inherent power of human beings as organisms and persons to heal themselves.

Clearly, the goals listed by Wolpe and Harper are rather modest. Other therapists speak in terms of "the mature personality." These terms, however, as well as the popular "autonomous person," are ambiguous. If *mature personality* means that therapy extends to total development of the human person—that is, to the development of what once was called "the virtuous person," who is morally excellent and also spiritually profound and creative—this clearly goes beyond the psychological level and touches on the ethical and spiritual level. It is true that some therapists, particularly those of the Jungian and existentialist schools (R. May, 1983), have come to be not only therapists in the usual sense, but also something similar to gurus or spiritual guides. Their work more closely resembles that of a philosopher, educator, or spiritual director than that of a health care professional. Although not denying the great value of the work of some of these persons, it seems that some limit must be put on the task of psychotherapy. Its work is complete when the person becomes psychologically normal (i.e., in a state of normal adult health). After this form of normality is attained, the individual should achieve even more growth in all the dimensions of human nature; however, guidance of this growth seems to exceed the work of psychotherapy and to demand ethical and spiritual counselors.

How, then, can this line be drawn? A look at the insight therapies provides the answer. Psychoanalysis, for example, is terminated when patients are sufficiently *free* to manage their own lives realistically, independent of the therapist, and are no longer hampered by unconscious motivations or self-deluding excuses that would prevent them from perceiving the world as it is; they can make free choices and carry them out effectively (Menninger, 1958). In short, the patient now has a self-determining ego, which realistically recognizes its own emotional complexity, its innate needs, and its limitations. It also realistically recognizes the practical and human situations of life to which it must accommodate itself to satisfy its needs. This does not mean that all clients who terminate therapy will live their lives well in an ethical sense. A psychologically healthy person can, theoretically at least, also be an ethically bad person and a spiritually undeveloped person, but this is caused by his or her own free choices, not from compulsions imposed by personal background or social situation. At the point when the client can live by free choice, he or she no longer needs the therapist or therapy. Of course, a client may later regress under new stresses and have to return to treatment.

This notion of autonomy or freedom as defining the term *therapy* is not so acceptable to action therapists. Influenced by behaviorism, they often reject the notion of freedom altogether. Thus B. F. Skinner and his followers carry on systematic war against the whole notion of human free will (Skinner, 1971, 1976, 1985). As many critics (Gaylin, 1973; Machan, 1974) have pointed out, however, Skinner and other behaviorists unconsciously contradict themselves. They assert that the therapist can assist the client to behave more realistically, that is, as the therapist behaves. This makes sense if the therapist is *free* to choose between alternative modes of behavior for himself or herself and for the client, whereas the client, although still *not* yet free, wants to become free. This makes no sense, however, if both are equally unfree and merely conditioned by their environment.

Therefore, even extreme behavioristic therapy really aims at freeing the patient. It does not merely substitute one determinism for another. Rather, it substitutes a type of determinism that is instrumentally consistent with self-determination at a higher level for a type of determinism (neurosis) that is incompatible with such self-determination. Thus skill in typing is a conditioning consistent with the freedom of the writer to create an original composition and is preferable to a neurotic compulsion to repeat a fixed pattern of words, which would be incompatible with creative writing.

Therefore, mental health is psychological freedom based on a realistic perception and understanding of the world, and it involves self-understanding, self-consistency, and self-control. By *self-control*, however, we mean a *realistic* self-control, that is, one based on a realistic recognition and practical provision for one's intrinsic needs as a human being. *Mental health must be considered before the ethical questions of moral right and wrong, since only when a person is free can there be a question of moral choice and moral responsibility.*

In view of the multidimensional and integral character of human personality, however, it is important to emphasize that no human being is *totally* free. Human freedom is limited (1) by innate biological structure, determined genetically, and by various accidents of development, with its innate needs or drives; (2) by unconscious conditioning of the sort already described and that therapy deals with; and (3) by one's knowledge of the world and self, set largely by the culture in which one lives and the scope of one's experiences and education. Psychotherapy deals principally, but not exclusively, with limitations of human freedom that arise from the level of unconscious conditioning.

It is best to conceive this limited freedom in terms of the *area* in which a given individual is free. Thus studies on members of extremist groups such as the Ku Klux Klan began with the assumption that racists are people of authoritarian personality type. To the surprise of the researchers, it turned out that these people, who appear to be imprisoned by political views that approach a paranoid view of reality, were on the average perfectly normal from a psychological perspective. Perhaps determinism here was more at the level of socialization rather than of unconscious conditioning and can be corrected only by ethical education, not by psychotherapy.

At the psychological level, the area of freedom is very limited in the psychotic person who is out of touch with reality. Most psychotic persons, however, probably have some areas of freedom, at least sometimes; this is why they can be reached by psychotherapy or chemotherapy (as the case may be), which aims to gradually extend these free areas. Neurotic persons are decidedly more free but have some areas of unfreedom that do not occur in normal persons. The normal person also has a limited area of freedom, but its limits lie near the level of the necessary determinisms of automatic and routine behavior that are compatible with normal freedom.

Also, the areas of freedom among normal individuals undoubtedly differ widely. Highly creative and adaptive persons have much greater freedom in their lifestyle than normal but limited, unimaginative, rigid people who operate best only in routine situations. Even here there is a question of whether therapy (e.g., of the Jungian type) may lead such people to greater freedom. Modern therapy has tended to move from the treatment of sexual neuroses, common as a result of the Victorian refusal to recognize basic biological needs, to the treatment of anxiety, common in this century as a result of excessive demands on a work-oriented society, which fails to recognize human needs for leisure and human intimacy (Masters and Johnson, 1976; Masters et al., 1986). Thus therapy deals more and more with neuroses of emptiness or lack of meaning as a result of society's failure to recognize the creative and spiritual sides of personhood. In all these cases, psychological therapy can only go so far to awaken the person's full capacity for freedom.

Freedom demands trust not only among persons but also within social groups. Recently, methods of *group* therapy are becoming common, not only because of the shortage of therapists but because mental illness is partly a disturbance of social relations and can be adequately treated only through learning social communication skills. In particular, family therapy, in which a family is treated as a dynamic system whose malfunction is reflected in the psychological problems of individual members, gives promise of a radically effective approach to many mental problems that originated in the family.

Such methods raise some special ethical issues, chiefly those of confidentiality and of adequate professional control. The frank communication required within the group can easily lead to an abuse of the privacy of individual members; if the therapist does not remain fully in charge and sufficiently sensitive to the needs of every member, some especially fragile participants may be more hurt than healed by the experience (Green, 1995). The therapist has the responsibility not to permit the psychological condition of any member of the group to be destabilized to a degree that the therapist is not willing or not able to see that it is worked out before the process is terminated, even if this means additional one-to-one sessions with the disturbed patient or at least proper referral for further therapy.

12.4 ETHICAL PROBLEMS IN TREATING THE MENTALLY ILL

Behavior Control

Behavior control might be described as "getting people to do someone else's bidding." In this sense, behavior control has existed since the beginning of time. In the more restricted sense, however, the sense in which we use the term in this section, behavior control is any *medically indicated* treatment, procedure, or process that is intended, with or without a person's consent, to cause a person to discontinue a personally or socially undesirable activity (Agras and Berkowitz, 1988). As this description indicates, behavior control is not necessarily contrary to a person's intention or desires, but it signifies that some force over and above internal human motivation has been used in the interest of changing an activity pattern. The purpose of this control may be therapeutic (e.g., the use of drugs can sometimes actually correct a physiological malfunction producing abnormal behavior), or it may simply be aimed at controlling antisocial actions.

For example, a person trying to overcome the habit of alcoholism may use Antabuse (disulfiram) to help conquer the habit. Although the use of this drug is in accord with this person's desire, it is still a form of behavior control. From an ethical point of view, behavior control has become a serious problem because of the increased efficacy of surgical procedures in controlling behavior, the vastly increased panoply of psychoactive drugs that modify emotional responses, and the increased tendency to impose conforming societal norms. These procedures are not only comparatively new; they are swift and efficient, and their effect on a human person can be deep and lasting. Thus they have greater potential for good or evil than many of the techniques of scientists and physicians in the past centuries. Also, a temptation exists to attempt the solution of problems by altering the person rather than attempting to transform the social environment. Given these examples of behavior control and modification methods that are prevalent and becoming more common every day, we suggest several ethical principles that should govern their use, all of which are applications of the more general principle of human dignity in community (p. 228), which requires that social control enhance the dignity of the members of the community, not reduce them to mere means of political manipulation.

1. No form of treatment may be used that will destroy human freedom. Pius XII (1952) stated this well when he wrote:

   In exercising his right to dispose of himself or his faculties and organs, the individual must observe the hierarchy of the scale of values and within an identical order of values the hierarchy of individual goods to the extent demanded by the laws of morality, so, for example, man cannot perform upon himself or allow medical operations, either physical or somatic, which beyond doubt do remove serious defects or physical or psychic weaknesses, but which entail at the same time permanent destruction of or a considerable lasting lessening of freedom, that is to say, of the human personality in its particular and characteristic functions (n. 361).

   Thus any form of psychosurgery, personality manipulation, and use of psychoactive drugs that would remove or severely limit human freedom or destroy human personality could not be permitted and may need legal control (NIH, 1985).

2. If the purpose of the behavior control is therapeutic, the benefit to the patient must be the purpose of the action and the damage or risk must be accidental to the therapeutic action. A frontal lobotomy, for example, should be performed only as a last resort and with some indication that there will be an overall benefit for the patient. Above all, lobotomy and ECT should not be considered as ordinary treatments for prisoners and others who have displayed antisocial behavior (Martin and Bean, 1992). As a general rule, signs of organic brain pathology should be present before psychosurgery is approved.

3. If the purpose of the treatment is therapeutic, the long-range effect of the treatment must be considered as well as the short-range alleviation of some particular difficulty. Simply because a particular therapy alleviates or eliminates a symptom does not mean that it is ethically acceptable. Most of the drugs currently available for the relief of anxiety and tension carry some danger of dependency, habituation, and addiction. Such dependency diminishes human freedom and dignity and thus is to be avoided. Therefore the very theory prevalent in the United States of using psychoactive drugs to treat psychological difficulties when the disorder lacks a physiological or organic basis must be questioned. Would it not be better to treat the causes of anxiety or depression through counseling or increased self-awareness rather than

to depend on pills, which merely treat the symptoms? Questions such as this are fundamental in developing a philosophy of health care, and they are too often neglected in search of easier, but less beneficial, solutions.

4. If behavior controls are used, the rules of free and informed consent apply, including the right to refuse treatment (Cournos et al., 1993). Thus operant conditioning, psychoactive drugs, and psychotherapy should not be inflicted on competent people or imposed on them. If they are incompetent, the norms for proxy consent for therapeutic treatment should be followed. Moreover, children, prisoners, and people with a limited sense of awareness should not be subjected to experimental behavioral control, nor should proxy consent be given unless the treatment is truly therapeutic for them.

5. The principle of professional communication (5.2) regarding confidentiality must be applied with special care in psychotherapy, since the trust of the patient in the therapist is of fundamental importance, even in group therapy or where peer review of the psychiatrist's performance is necessary (Smith-Bell and Winslade, 1994).

6. Experimental research on behavioral control should conform to the norms explained previously in the section on human experimentation (9.5).

7. Use of behavioral control procedures to improve human capabilities such as memory, intelligence, and sexual abilities would seem to be licit if free consent is given, if there is no other way to achieve the same goal, and if the action is in accord with the integrity of the human person. In itself, human betterment, or human improvement, is ethically acceptable and beneficial. Care must be exercised, however, to make sure that the basic integrity of the human person is not violated and that addiction does not result in the course of seeking self-improvement.

8. Using alcoholic beverages or even psychoactive drugs for relaxation or pleasure is not in itself ethically wrong, provided that freedom is not notably restricted. Such substances used moderately might provide needed and legitimate relief from the everyday strain and tension of life. Because there is a great tendency to abuse the use of drugs, however, even to become dependent on or addicted to them, and because of the potential bodily harm resulting from some drugs, great care is required in the use of any behavior-modifying substance for recreational purposes.

Given these general norms of respect for the human freedom of the mentally distressed, certain special ethical issues required attention in what follows.

Punishment

On the basis of the distinctions just made, it is obvious that any use of psychotherapy as *punishment* (although it must be admitted that the neurotic patient may at first perceive it as punishment no matter what the therapist intends) is wholly unethical. Punishment and reward (in the proper sense of the terms) belong only to *ethical* acts, that is, free, responsible acts. This, of course, requires penological reforms by which the courts decide first on the facts of a criminal action and then separately on the *moral* responsibility of the person who has committed the act. In this second decision, expert testimony from psychiatrists should be admitted, but it should be directed toward determining whether the defendant's freedom was so limited by psychological factors as to remove his or her freedom with regard to this particular class of acts. This expert testimony should be fully subject to the adversary process so that the lay jury can determine whether there are solid grounds to doubt the freedom of the defendant (Berlin, 1983; Fingarette and Hasse, 1979).

Therefore, psychiatrists called on in court for expert testimony, insofar as the present confusion of the law permits them, should be primarily concerned to make clear to the jury why in their expert opinion the chronic or temporary psychological condition of the accused person did or did not render him or her so unfree that the accused cannot be held responsible for the act he or she is accused of; or if the accused is partially or remotely responsible for the act, then in what degree or in what respect (Simon, 1993).

Much controversy surrounds proposals to rehabilitate prisoners by behavior control programs, which in effect are action therapies designed to recondition the criminal to social behavior by a planned series of rewards and punishment (Pincus, 1984). This can be conceived in three ways: (1) as voluntary education, in which case it is certainly ethical to give prisoners an opportunity to engage in it as they would in any type of socially acceptable education program; (2) as therapy; and (3) as part of prison discipline. In the last case, it is part of the prisoner's punishment and should have some supervision from the courts, which should not permit cruel and unusual punishment, that is, something other than prescribed by law as appropriate to the crime. Any therapy which the prisoner must undergo involuntarily should not be permitted without a court order committing the prisoner to such treatment.

In actual practice today, these matters are greatly confused. The psychiatric profession, however, has a responsibility to clear them up and to refuse cooperation with gross violations of the distinction between therapy and punishment, just as physicians have refused to act as executioners by administering capital punishment by lethal injections (W. Curran and Cassells, 1980; Malone, 1979). This is even more true if therapy is used as a means of suppression of political or social dissent, which amounts to a punishment for political crimes (Aviram and Shnit, 1984).

Confinement of the Mentally III

Patients self-committed to a hospital may find themselves in a situation where in fact freedom to withdraw from highly traumatizing treatment is no longer practically possible. Every psychiatric institution, however, must be dedicated to the proposition that it is therapeutic only to the degree that it really respects and seeks to enlarge the patient's capacity for freedom. If it lessens this capacity, it is countertherapeutic; it is making the patient mentally more ill than well.

On the other hand, when it is rightly judged that free consent, at least in the area of treatment, is impossible, then commitment must be made by the patient's guardian, with scrupulous observance of due legal process. The guardian (usually a member of the family) may be biased because of selfishness, ignorance, and more often through unconscious factors, which may very well be part of the client's own breakdown (Mossman and Hart, 1993).

Codependency

For patients whose psychosis is less all-embracing and for neurotic patients, not only action therapies but also the insight therapies are feasible. The use of insight therapies, however, raises a whole series of ethical problems. The first of these is the process of *transference* (Menninger, 1958). Psychoanalytic therapy depends in some measure on the dependence of the patient on the therapist for the duration of treatment. This dependency mirrors the child–parent relationship and involves not only trust but, at least sometimes, also an element of erotic love. Without this profound dependency, patients are not freed from their anxieties and inhibitions sufficiently to let themselves become conscious of their true motivations. The termination of therapy is indicated when the patient becomes sufficiently autonomous and under self-control that he or she no longer needs the therapist. They have become healthy adults who still love their parents (therapists) but no longer need them (Salvendy, 1992).

This vulnerability of patients obviously invests therapists with special ethical responsibilities. The first of these is that therapists must not violate the trust placed in them (Moffic et al., 1991). This requires that a therapist carefully maintain professional secrecy, be truly concerned for the patient, prompt in appointments, and reasonably available for consultation. It means also that therapists are honest with patients and do not lie to them or break promises. Furthermore, the therapist must avoid all manipulation of the patient in the sense of seeking personal gratification from the treatment rather than seeking the patient's benefit. The therapeutic relation requires dependency of the patient but not codependency of therapist and patient. This does not demand that the therapist have a superhuman objectivity; rather, it simply means that the therapist is worthy of trust (Ryle, 1995).

Clearly, this excludes the therapist from having sexual relations with the client, although some have defended this as possibly therapeutic (Lazurus, 1992). The idea that the therapist could engage in such relations merely for the patient's sake seems unrealistic, and the risk that the patient will then or later view it as exploitation is all too real. The principles of ethics adapted by the APA are clear in specifying that sexual relations between psychiatrists and their patients are unethical (section 2.1) (APA, 1981, 1986a, b).

Changing the Patient's Value System

Perhaps the most controversial issue of all regarding psychotherapy is whether the therapist is permitted to change the patient's value system (Block and Chodoff, 1981). The common answer is that a therapist should not change this system but should try to adjust the patient to the system. This answer, however, is somewhat disingenuous. As the existentialist psychoanalysts have pointed out, distortions in the patient's value system often underlie the disorder. Furthermore, the source of many problems is the patient's superego, which is the value system of the parents or society that has been incorporated in the child's unconsciousness. Here is the source of all the issues raised by the antipsychiatrists. Is therapy simply the adjustment of patients to the disordered value system of the society in which they live? On the other hand, if the psychological and ethical dimensions of human personality are distinct, as we have argued, it clearly cannot be the role of the therapist to indoctrinate the patient in the therapist's value system.

In answer to this difficulty, we must say that there are certain values on which the very relation of client to therapist depend, and these must be reinforced by therapy (Clements, 1983). Thus, the therapist must help the client to become more trustful, more honest, more hopeful, more courageous, more patient, and more realistic. Such values are common to most recognized ethical systems, whether religious or philosophical. The therapist must adhere to these values and should not be reluctant to strengthen them in the client. If clients submit voluntarily to therapy, they *freely* accept these values no matter how unfree they may be in other respects. This small area of mental health and moral virtue must become the basis of recovery. Therapists teach these values primarily by their *example* in their relations to clients as they attempt to establish satisfactory therapeutic transferences. Consequently, the importance of a genuinely personalist education for psychiatrists is even more important than for other physicians (Light, 1980; see also 4.3).

The effort of the therapist is thus to extend the area of freedom for patients. As patients become freer, they must make some free ethical decisions and will do so according to their own *conscious*, rational system of values. At this point, the therapist is nondirective in the sense that it is not the therapist's task to give the patient ethical advice, but only to help the patient be free of illusion and neurosis in making decisions. This requires great delicacy and objectivity on the part of the therapist. It may mean the therapist sometimes thinks that the client's decisions are not ethically good, objectively speaking. In such a case, the therapist may point out that the client's decisions are questionable or refer the client to an ethical counselor (clergyman, lawyer, friend), but the therapist should be careful not to take any responsibility for the client's decision. Thus the therapist ought to refer the client to ethical or spiritual advisers if it becomes apparent that the client's value system is inconsistent or inadequate.

A deeper problem, however, was raised by Philip Rieff (1968) in his book *The Triumph of the Therapeutic* and by others. Is it possible that the whole system of insight therapy as it originated with Freud has a built-in system of values or ideology that it inculcates? Thus many have accused psychoanalysis of being essentially a product of the middle class in opulent capitalist countries. They argue that it has taken on the political function of adjusting this middle class to a social system riddled with inherent contradictions. Freud (1930) himself, as we have already noted, saw all of civilization as the imposition of social controls on human beings' infinite and even contradictory drives. Consequently, every social system is a delicate balance between the repressive controls necessary for social life and work and the explosive drives of the id. In capitalist countries, as Rieff shows, the abundance of goods and the impersonal shape of social organization contribute to a much greater permissiveness, a society in which all types of behavior (between "consenting adults") is tolerable. Others, such as the proponents of radical sexual therapies, argue that as this permissiveness spreads, it will lead to social revolution.

Rieff predicts that we are embarking on a "therapeutic society" in which the "therapeutic man" will become typical. Such a person, whom Rieff pictures as the type successful psychoanalysis actually produces, is one who lives for a constant succession of intensely satisfying experiences, without any drive to realize some plan of life or some ultimate goal. This person is highly autonomous in the sense that he or she feels no guilt about seeking personal satisfaction in every situation, leaving the others involved to take care of themselves. This person is capable of satisfying intimate relationships but does not depend on any particular person for achieving these; thus he or she can move from one relationship to another without any sense of loss or guilt for infidelity.

If Rieff is correct—and certainly very different interpretations of the goals of psychoanalysis are given by Erik Erikson (1968), Erich Fromm (1975), Rollo May (1983), and such leaders in the field—the inherent ethic of psychoanalytical theory is to produce autonomous, hedonistic, goalless, conscienceless persons, the very sort ethicists have always condemned as selfish, loveless, and empty. Such persons are individualistic in the extreme, uncommitted to any social goals except the achievement of freedom to do what they please. Rieff's interpretation of psychoanalysis emphasizes Freud's belief that civilization—that is, social life—is always repression, not fulfillment, of fundamental human needs—a necessary evil. If this is the whole picture, it is difficult to see how a Freudian ethics could ever be compatible with either a Christian value system or a Marxist one. It is essentially an ideological defense of the style of life of those who profit from capitalism and who use their analysts to quiet their guilt.

Alan Bloom, in *The Closing of the American Mind* (1987), described the present generation of college students in terms similar to those employed by Rieff. Dominated by relativism, Bloom finds his subjects highly self-centered and devoid of commitment to family, religion, or country. Although Bloom attributes the causes of this malaise to many different factors, he does maintain: "Once Americans had become convinced that there was a basement to which psychiatrists have the key, their orientation became that of the *self*, the mysterious, true, unlimited center of our being. All our beliefs issue from it and have no other validation."

These accusations offered by Rieff and Bloom are very serious ones. They demand that:

1. The community of therapists must make a serious examination of social conscience and a purification of the theory, training, and practice of therapists, who must become conscious that the goals of therapy must be related to higher social and spiritual goals.
2. Clients should trust their therapists not as omnipotent fathers, but only for their limited skills. Clients also should receive guidance at the ethical (political and social) and spiritual levels from others as soon as they become sufficiently free emotionally to do so (Van Kaam, 1986).

Thus persons undergoing therapy should not change their system of values, divorce their partners, give up their religious vocation, or change their religion or their professional vocation merely under the influence of psychotherapy. The tendency to erect one of the many forms of therapy (including the various mystical cults now so popular) into a religion is a violation of the lines between the psychological level of personality and the ethical and spiritual levels and is doomed to end in disillusionment (Vitz, 1994).

In recent years, some of the Protestant and Catholic clergy and members of religious orders have discovered the value of psychotherapy and have come to place an excessive faith in it to meet all the needs of people for counseling, to the detriment of their confidence in the value of their own special roles as ethical and spiritual guides (Murnion, 1984). They have become preoccupied with getting in touch with their feelings, getting freed up, or developing a capacity for intimacy, and some have deserted the celibate life, the priesthood, or the ministry to become psychotherapists themselves so that they might "really" help people. A similar phenomenon has been experienced by the U.S. Jewish community, where psychotherapy has become a widespread substitute for the religious discipline of the Torah, the therapist has taken the place of the rabbi, and Freud the place of Moses.

Undoubtedly, religious people and the clergy in particular have sometimes been in real need of therapeutic experiences to correct an excessively repressive religiosity that disregarded their human emotional needs. Too often such persons have been discouraged from obtaining needed psychotherapy by the false notion that although morally good people may be physically ill, they cannot be mentally ill. Nevertheless, profound self-understanding and choice of one's life vocation require an exploration of the self that goes even deeper than psychology can penetrate and where ethical and spiritual guidance is of great value. What is needed are ethical and spiritual guides who genuinely appreciate the contributions of psychotherapy to human wholeness, but who pursue their own roles with a sense of their own mission. There is an important analogy between psychotherapy and spiritual purification, but it is an analogy, not an identity (Van Kaam, 1985).

12.5 ADDICTION OR CHEMICAL DEPENDENCY

Generally speaking, addiction is habituation to some practice harmful to the subject. Although the term *addiction* usually refers to habituation to drugs, one can also be addicted to other detrimental substances or activities, such as alcohol, tobacco, coffee, and excessive food, as well as too much sleep, too much work, and pursuit of sexual pleasure (Francis and Franklin, 1988). Many people use all these things in ways that do not destroy human equilibrium but some persons, for a variety of reasons not fully understood, become addicted to them. Their whole life is more and more absorbed by a single activity that distorts the personality, consumes physical and psychic energy, and often results in an intense self-centeredness, personality deterioration, and inability to communicate with others. Addiction or dependency on drugs and alcohol are more likely to result in such extreme symptoms. Thus this section addresses those addictions that are often referred to as *chemical dependency*.

One component of chemical dependency, and the most obvious, is its *hedonistic* character, although persons who are in other respects very ascetic may fall victim to it, precisely because they lack healthy pleasures in their lives. In the face of every difficulty of life, every tension or frustration, the chemically dependent person runs away from the loss of normal satisfaction and achievement by indulgence in the physical pleasure, relaxation, and euphoria of the addicting experience (Silvers, 1993). This search for pleasure, however, does not of itself constitute addiction; it also involves the increasing sense of guilt and helplessness that begin to accompany each overindulgence. The result is that the incipient addict begins to indulge not for the sake of pleasure itself, but to blot out the guilt and remorse for the consequences of previous indulgences. Furthermore, this vicious circle is reinforced by the use of psychological coping mechanisms of rationalization and denial that victims need to suppress guilt and pain, so that they become increasingly unable to perceive the real consequences of their behavior. Alcoholic persons, for example, frequently suffer from blackouts, repression, and delusional euphoric recall that so distort their memory that they actually have a very incomplete picture of what is happening to them.

Persons of very different personality types can become addicted, but a common feature is excessive *dependency* needs, sometimes masked by outward aggressiveness and competitiveness. Moreover, as addiction progresses, it tends to produce a pattern of behavior that overrides all temperamental differences. At one time addicts were thought to come mainly from the poorer classes, and undoubtedly addiction is common among some socially depressed groups. Recent research demonstrates, however, that chemical dependency can affect people of all backgrounds. Often gifted, talented, wealthy, and successful persons succumb to this severe personality problem (Smart and Murray, 1985).

Chemical dependency or addiction may be broadly classified as physiological or psychological. *Physiological addiction*, which causes a modification or need in the addict's physiological system, usually requires increasing doses of the addicting substance to obtain the same physiological effect. Moreover, in physiological dependence, withdrawal from the object of dependency—for example, heroin—results in severe physiological disturbance, even death, because the body has become so adapted to the presence of the substance in the system (Kosten, 1985a). In physiological addiction, however, the psychological component predominates; thus persons who lack this component can sometimes use even so highly addictive a drug as heroin without exhibiting the typical features of addiction. *Psychological dependency* itself results from a learned conditioned behavior pattern that leads the victim to anticipate the pleasure and release of tension, even when the substance does not notably modify the physiological system (Delbanco and Delbanco, 1995).

Chemical dependency, especially drug addiction, is one of the most highly publicized and most morally condemned social problems in the United States. Some of its most important facts and questions are, however, sometimes overlooked because of the widespread moral condemnation of such abuses. First, is chemical dependency more a personal or a cultural problem? Studies have shown that chemical addiction is especially serious in the United States. Is this because chemical addiction is merely a symptom of some larger American problem such as poverty, anomie, or spiritual deprivation (Kosten, 1985b)? The fact that drug users are at high risk for HIV infection because of their use of unsterilized hypodermic needles has still further complicated the problem.

Second, does the strict government control of addictive substances, especially drugs; the special moral disapproval; and the severe penalties for sale and use foment rather than solve the problem? Would chemical addiction be less of a problem in the United States if it were considered a medical or social problem rather than a moral and legal one (Szasz, 1977)? Removing the moral stigma from addiction to alcohol has been helpful in assisting many people to overcome this addiction. Would a similar response to the use of drugs, plus legalization of narcotics for sustaining treatment of addicts, be beneficial over a long period? While avoiding a naive optimism about easy solutions for chemical dependency, we must seek to learn from the experience of other nations in this regard, and above all these problems must be considered in the total context of American culture and its socialization process (Bissell and Royce, 1987).

Is this to say that the sense of moral guilt felt by the addict is merely neurotic? On the one hand, therapists speak of addiction as a "disease" in order to reduce its moral opprobrium and to achieve a more sympathetic attitude on the part of nonaddicts. On the other hand, an important part of therapy is to get addicts to accept moral responsibility for the harm they have done themselves and others through addiction (Wiley, 1995). This ambiguity can be cleared up if two points are kept in mind. First, chemical dependency is always a psychological disease because it involves an abnormal behavior pattern accompanied by the neurotic coping mechanisms already described. It can also be a physiological disease because it sometimes produces physiological dependency and usually produces widespread organic changes that greatly aggravate the condition. Second, *voluntary* acts must be distinguished from *free* acts. Addictive behavior is voluntary in the sense that it proceeds from an inner compulsion, but it always involves a restriction of freedom, since the addict becomes less and less able to perceive alternatives of action or to choose among them. In times of addictive need, the practical conscience of the addict is concerned totally with the need for a drink or a fix. He or she acts voluntarily, compulsively, but without free choice.

Thus actual consumption of addictive substances by addicts is seldom in itself a morally culpable act, and the guilt felt afterward is unrealistic and neurotic. Even the acquisition of the addiction often proceeds so gradually and subtly that it is difficult to judge that the addict knowingly and deliberately chose addiction. Nevertheless, it would be a mistake to think that the *whole* guilt felt by addicts is illusory. If it were, it would be difficult to explain why admission of responsibility has proved so important a part of therapy (Longa, 1995). The truth seems to be that the real moral responsibility of the addicted person lies in the obligation to ask and receive help from others when this is offered, since therapy cannot be effective until the addict accepts help. Acceptance does not take place all at once but passes through stages of (1) *admission* into treatment, (2) *compliance* with treatment (with hidden defiance and resistance), (3) *acceptance* or recognition of real need for health (with unrealistic anticipations of cure), and (4) *surrender,* that is, realistic acknowledgment and acceptance of the responsibility for lifelong change. Thus it is a mistake to reduce this complex situation either to a purely moral question or to a purely sociological or medical one. To deny all moral responsibility or capacity to change is to degrade addicts as persons, yet to pass judgment on their degree of responsibility is to misjudge the many ways in which they are victims of forces beyond individual control.

Treatment outcome studies in alcoholism indicate that a variety of treatment programs yield benefit and may be cost-effective; however, few studies exist that differentiate which programs are best for which types of patients. "So far the outcome literature reflects that patient factors such as having a stable family, stable job, less sociopathy, less psychopathology, and a negative family history for alcoholism are more powerful predictors of positive prognosis than is type of treatment" (Francis and Franklin, 1988).

Perhaps an even more effective way for health care professionals to combat chemical addiction is through preventive measures (Felthous, 1993). They can play an important role in combating the mentality in the United States that seems to predispose people for substance abuse and addiction (NIDA, 1986). Americans seem to think that every pain, every sorrow or frustration, can be overcome with a pill, potion, or injection of some type. Pharmaceutical firms constantly push drugs through advertising, and health care professionals often are used by such agencies to promote unnecessary drug use. Christian professionals will not share in this promotion because they realize that human pain, frustration, and sorrow simply cannot be suppressed. Human beings grow as persons by facing the difficulties and struggles of life realistically, "bearing one another's burdens" (Ga 6:2) as free people, not as slaves to a pleasure ethic. In saying this, we are not proposing an exaggerated stoicism as the Christian ideal, but a realistic effort to overcome the real causes of suffering rather than an escape into unconsciousness. Alcoholics Anonymous, which has led the way to the most successful methods of therapy for chemical dependency, has always emphasized that the addict cannot recover without a reaching out for a Higher

Power and a willingness to repair damage done to the neighbor and to be of service to the neighbor (Prochaska et al., 1992).

12.6 SEX THERAPY AND RESEARCH

Sexual Dysfunction

Sexual dysfunction is the inability to engage in satisfactory sexual expression; this may or may not be the result of a mental disorder, but is conveniently treated here. It is to be distinguished from deviant sexuality, which seeks satisfaction in abnormal ways. Such dysfunction is not an uncommon human problem and often is a contributing factor to marital discord, although perhaps it is as often an effect as a cause. What should be not only an expression but also a source of deepening love and commitment, rich in tenderness and joy, can be a source of profound depression and alienation. Couples frustrated and puzzled by sexual dysfunction are sometimes exploited by marriage counselors or sex therapists who are unqualified or irresponsible, since these disciplines are relatively new, rapidly expanding, and lacking in well-established professional or legal controls (APA, 1986b). Health care professionals can be of great help in preserving and improving family life if they are well-informed about the goals and effectiveness of sex therapy and the availability of reliable practitioners to whom couples may be referred (McCarthy, 1995).

The most common forms of sexual dysfunction for men are premature ejaculation, impotency, and secondary potency difficulties; for women, the most common forms are vaginismus and orgastic dysfunction (Masters and Johnson (1970, 1976). Contrary to the beliefs of some psychoanalysts, sexual dysfunction need not be a sign of a deep or severe psychic pathology; it can be the result of various relatively superficial maladjustments that impede spontaneity.

As Kaplan (1974) states, sex therapy "differs from other forms of treatment for sexual dysfunction in two respects: first, its goals are essentially limited to the relief of the patient's sexual dysfunction and, second, it departs from traditional technique by employing a combination of prescribed sexual experiences and psychotherapy." Thus sex therapy has a more limited objective than psychoanalysis or marital therapy. These latter two forms of assistance seek to help people with sexual dysfunction, but they concentrate more on the underlying conflicts and destructive interpersonal behavior that may give rise to such dysfunction. In sex therapy, however, the dysfunction is treated directly, and the therapy is complete when the couple is able to achieve a satisfactory sexual response (Levin, 1995).

During the past 30 years, centers for sex therapy have been widely established in the United States, but the original and most renowned center was founded in 1959 at Washington University in St. Louis by William Masters and Virginia Johnson. In 1974 this center, which offers therapy and trains professional therapists, was named the Reproductive Biology Research Foundation; later the name was changed to the Masters and Johnson Foundation. Other centers for research and treatment of sexual dysfunction exist at Cornell University and other university hospitals, but few centers combine research and therapy. In addition, many health care professionals, psychiatrists, psychologists, and special therapists offer sex therapy in private practice, as do the practitioners of dubious competency already mentioned (Crowe, 1992).

At the larger centers, the common sexual dysfunctions of married people are treated through an integrated combination of instruction and actual sexual experiences in which the couple explore a more relaxed, personalized approach to sexual relations freed from anxieties about "performance." The instructions are usually given by a man–woman team, and the actual experiences are engaged in privately by the couple in their home or a hotel near the therapy center. At the beginning of therapy, a thorough history is taken and a complete physical examination given. After therapy, which typically consists of about 10 days of instruction, a follow-up is made to see if the couple has successfully integrated the new approach to sexual relations into their ordinary living. More than 80 percent success is usually reported by such centers, which is remarkable considering the relatively short period of therapy compared to that required to meet other types of marital problems in marriage counseling (deSilva, 1993).

As a general rule, most centers and private therapists accept only married couples for treatment. At one time Masters and Johnson made use of paid surrogate partners for single persons and in special cases for married persons, but they have discontinued this much-criticized practice.

Ethical Risks of Sex Therapy

The principle of human sexuality indicates the importance for married couples to be able to express and deepen their love by satisfying sexual relations. The clinical experience of sex therapists today seems to show that when couples have good interpersonal relations, effective communication of attitudes and feelings, and a positive and anxiety-free attitude toward bodily intimacy and sensual enjoyment, sexual dysfunction is rare and special training unnecessary. In today's culture, however, many men and women find interpersonal communication, even at nonsexual levels, difficult and are inhibited in the spontaneous expression of their feelings both by inhibiting fears and by exaggerated competitive attitudes. Thus much of the need for sex therapy could be obviated by adequate preparation for marriage. From a Christian point of view, this education ought to express the intimate relation between the various meanings of sexuality as sensual satisfaction, as love and completion between man and woman, and as the source of the continuing life of the family and society, and it should show how permanent self-giving is the heart of the matter (Simpson, 1992).

When couples learn to communicate with each other honestly and lovingly, sexual adjustment is usually easy because intercourse is itself essentially a form of intimate communication. Effective sex education cannot be merely abstract but must include an experiential growth that enables persons to understand their own sexuality and to learn to relate to others as sexual persons through encounters appropriate to their age and personal maturity. Persons also need help, however, so that these growth experiences do not lead them down the dead-end paths of autoeroticism or a depersonalized search for satisfactions unrelated to the deeper meaning of sexuality as marital commitment.

Therefore, sex therapy undoubtedly may be necessary and ethically acceptable for married couples who need to overcome difficulties of miseducation or personal sexual development, provided that the prescribed sexual actions are performed with the married partner, and in view of the expression of marital love through complete sexual union and not as a substitute for it. It is desirable that a sufficient number of Christian health care professionals prepare themselves to provide such therapy in the context of a truly personalized attitude toward sexuality, lest such technical knowledge should be abused so as to further weaken family life rather than to promote and strengthen it (Atwood, 1992).

At present, no definite set of ethical standards exists for professionals involved in sexual therapy, although a group of prominent practitioners sought to develop such guidelines (Masters et al., 1980). *The Principles of Medical Ethics* of the APA (1981; 1986b), however, would seem to apply to sexual dysfunction counselors. Given the importance of the human activity involved, the need for definite moral standards is obvious. First, the same confidentiality required of anyone offering therapeutic treatment must be observed. Second, the persons involved should not be asked to perform actions that are immoral or contrary to their conscience. Thus use of surrogate partners as well as activities that are intentionally and directly masturbatory or otherwise deviant must be rejected. Third, therapists must not engage in sexual activity with patients. Unfortunately, studies show that these moral standards are sometimes violated. Violations of these principles will not only harm the patients, but will also destroy respect for sexual therapy and those who pursue it as a profession.

Unfortunately, sex therapists also often seem to approach their task from a purely scientific–technological point of view. One noted psychiatrist (Kaplan, 1974) completes her study of some of the literature with the lament, "There is a conspicuous absence of the word *love*." We cannot help but wonder, therefore, whether this approach may still further the depersonalization of human sexuality from which our culture suffers. Christians working in this field should exert leadership in the opposite direction.

Sexual Deviance

Sexual deviances are to be distinguished from sexual dysfunctions in that the object or action in which sexual satisfaction is sought is abnormal (Friedman and Douney, 1994). In discussing the principle of sexuality, we have explained how the Christian tradition in this matter defines normality, and we have dealt briefly with masturbation and with unethical forms of genital satisfaction within marriage. Psychiatry at present generally ignores such behaviors. It does, however, deal with *paraphilias,* such as fetishism, transvestitism, voyeurism, sadomasochism, zoophilia, pedophilia, etc. In contrast to sexual dysfunctions, these *paraphilias* are defined as conditions which "involve arousal in response to sexual objects or situations that are not part of normative arousal-activity patterns" and which interefere "to varying degrees, with the capacity for reciprocal and affectionate sexual activity" (Williams, 1988, p. 220). Psychosexual development in human beings is a very complex process, hence it is not surprising that such deviances occur and take such a variety of bizarre forms (Pontifical Council for the Family, 1996). They have been treated by the whole range of therapies we have mentioned, and by such ethically and medically questionable procedures as castration. Psychoanalytic theory explains these disorders as produced by the neurotic fear of normal sexual attraction, resulting from traumatic childhood events, which causes a transference of erotic desires to symbolic objects. Learning theorists think they are due to deviant sexual experiences (usually in puberty) which have been reinforced by sexual fantasies and masturbation (Abel, 1995).

Today, psychotherapists deal with these conditions by a multicomponent therapy which includes drugs, reconditioning, cognitive therapy, and training in social skills in relating to normal sexual partners. The paraphilia receiving most public attention is pedophilia, because of the victimization of children by trusted teachers, priests, and others. The belief that pedophiliacs are untreatable and can never learn to control their impulses is exaggerated (Jenkins, 1995). It can usually be brought under control, but pedophiliacs, who themselves have often suffered abuse as children, must guard themselves all their lives, as do "recovering alcoholics," and be guarded against occasions of relapse.

People suffering from such deviances are understandably regarded with fear and repugnance. When criminal, they require restraint and deterrance. Nevertheless, they retain human rights and dignity and should be regarded as suffering from mental disease due perhaps to childhood abuse or trauma for which they were not responsible, and their behavior may be so compulsive as to remove moral culpability. Their potential victims, however, must also be protected and their actual victims cared for and compensated insofar as possible.

An issue much debated is whether homosexual orientation is to be regarded as an abnormal condition. Up to 1973 it was generally so classified, but then the American Psychiatric Association replaced it in its diagnostic manual with the term "sexual orientation disturbance," in 1978 retained only "ego-dystonic" [distressful to the patient], and in 1987 dropped all reference. "Although controversy remains, the psychiatric community in general does not consider consensual homosexuality to be a mental disturbance" (Becker and Karoussi, 1988) even though DMS IV does contain the example of "persistent and marked distress about sexual orientation" (n. 302.9). Rejecting homosexuality as a psychological pathology, however, does not so much reflect a scientific judgment on the cause or nature of homosexuality as the view that to label homosexuality as abnormal is to stigmatize persons who are content with this condition and to encourage homophobia and discrimination against them.

"The factors responsible for the development of a sexual orientation are still unknown," (Becker and Karoussi, 1988, p. 601). However, since it is known that heterosexual orientation, although genetically based, is in part learned, it is probable that homosexuality is also a condition learned through a variety of childhood or pubertal experiences to which some subjects are genetically sensitive (Walker, 1983; Baily et al., 1993). Since the general population exhibits all degrees of heterosexuality and only about 3 to 4 percent of males and half as many females are exclusively homosexual, stereotyping individuals as "gay," "lesbian," or "straight" is questionable (Michaels et al., 1994). While some psychiatrists are pessimistic about changing this orientation, especially after adolescence, some report 30 percent cure in patients motivated to change (Nicolosi, 1991).

For Catholic psychiatrists, however, a problem arises from the fact that the Catholic Church, on the basis of the principle of personalized sexuality which defines the ability to enter into heterosexual marriage as normal to human nature, has taken sides in this controversy with those psychiatrists who continue to regard homosexual orientation as a "disorder" and its acting out in sexual behavior as objectively immoral (CDF, 1986; Hume, 1995). It rejects the notion that God created anyone homosexual or that homosexuality is a natural variety of sexuality. Rather, it is a disability to enter into successful heterosexual and fruitful marriage, which society has a responsibility to find ways of preventing or overcoming. Yet the Church also recognizes that the homosexual probably is not responsible for this disability and may well have diminished subjective culpability in acting it out. It also recognizes that "homophobia" in the sense of an exaggerated fear or dislike of the victims of this condition is itself a neurosis, while denial of the human rights and dignity of homosexuals is seriously unjust (CDF, 1995a; Peddicord, 1996). On the contrary, the Catholic community in particular has the responsibility to give special compassionate and understanding care for those suffering from this condition. It should also support them in their efforts to live as chaste celibates, as all Christians not in heterosexual marriage are required to do. Consequently, Catholic psychiatrists should promote research to discover the causes, prevention, and therapy of homosexuality, and should encourage homosexuals to seek such therapy and counseling as is presently available. For neither heterosexuals nor homosexuals is promiscuous sexual behavior either moral or medically safe.

Research

What has just been said of sex therapy also applies to sexual research and experimentation, including diagnostic procedures that may be used to determine the normality of sexual response, for example, to diagnose homosexual tendencies. Such research is legitimate and necessary to understand better the nature of human sexuality and the physiological or psychological pathologies to which it is subject. Such research, however, must be in accord with the principles already laid down (p. 348ff) for psychological experimentation with human subjects, which means that the experimental experiences must be designed to be therapeutic or truly educational for the subject and not depersonalizing or reinforcing of patterns inconsistent with the total health—moral and spiritual, as well as biological and psychological—of the human person.

Such conditions exclude, as we have already indicated for sex therapy, sexual acts between unmarried partners, especially the use of prostitutes, and certainly between the therapist and patient, although Riskin (1979) attempted to defend this. These conditions would seem also to exclude the use of subjects who are immature or otherwise lacking in mature control of their sexual impulses and behavior, unless the experiment itself tends to strengthen this control. The type of experiment, often reported, that exposes subjects to viewing photographs to measure sexual arousal is highly questionable because it involves risk of consent to illicit acts. Since, however, there could be a proportionate reason for such a risk, this type of experiment is not absolutely excluded. For example, the use of pictures for diagnostic purposes or for some benefit to the patient in conditioning experiments and therapy (e.g., in some operant conditioning therapies for homosexual orientation or compulsive anxiety) may be justified if the temptation involved is moderate and the subjects are warned that the purpose is not pornographic but simply to test automatic initial reactions.

Thus sexual therapy and sexual research can be carried on in an ethical manner. Basically, both sexual research and sexual therapy aim at helping people to express their love for one another more fully. However, great care and sensitivity must be observed in the practice of sexual therapy and in the experiments prompted by sexual research. In either case, the fundamental integrity of the persons involved must be respected. Thus actions that are in themselves immoral are not justified. Moreover, the activities involved in either research or therapy should be carried on in view of the fact that human love is not accomplished or developed through technique or knowledge alone. A deeper awareness and mutual communion must be present to enhance human love. Not only are these admonitions derived from an integral view of human nature and human love, but they also take into account a long-range view of human dignity. What have we gained if we learn everything there is to know about sexual activity but in the pursuit of pleasure learn less and less about fulfilling human love?

CONCLUSION

For many years, psychiatry and religion were at odds with one another. Leaders in both fields criticized and cast doubt upon one another and the disciplines they represented. Although a few pioneers of psychology such as William James treated religion sympathetically, others such as Sigmund Freud treated religion at best as an illusion which society would some day outgrow. On the other hand, theologians and philosophers often expressed a distrust of psychology and psychiatry that bordered on outright hostility. In contemporary times, however, psychiatrists and representation of religious conviction work hand in hand. For example, in an effort to encourage mental health professionals to view a patient's religion experience more seriously, the DSM (APA, 1994) includes a new entry entitled "Religious or Spiritual Problems." By recognizing religious problems as a category of concern distinct from any mental disorder, the revision reflects a move away from earlier tendencies of psychiatrists to treat religion as a delusion or a neurosis.

On the side of religion, movements toward reconciliation has also been realized. In 1994, Joseph English, M.D., the president of the American Psychiatric Association, led a delegation of members to meet with Pope John Paul II. Dr. English asked the pope to help overcome the myth that the mentally ill, even the homeless, suffer because of moral failure (Steintels, 1994). On the part of the Church, it seems that Pope John Paul II takes more account of psychology and psychiatry when writing encyclicals and moral exhortations. His admission that women facing the decision concerning abortion may be influenced by psychological pressures was somewhat of a breakthrough (*Gospel of Life*, n. 18, n. 99).

13
Suffering and Death

OVERVIEW

This chapter considers suffering and death, two concomitant realities of health care and medicine, from a Christian perspective. We begin by considering the response of health care professionals to suffering and death, analyzing the phenomenon of fear of death from the viewpoint of Christian spirituality (13.1; 13.2). In our present era we use two different sets of clinical signs to determine that human death has occurred. Thus the ethical evaluation of brain death is considered (13.3). Christian care for the dying and dead person requires truth telling (13.4) and respecting the remains of the person after death has taken place (13.5); these responsibilities are discussed next. Finally, we consider the ethical implications of suicide and euthanasia (13.6), and point out how these activities differ from allowing the person to die when medical therapy does not offer any benefit (13.7).

13.1 MYSTERY OF DEATH

Death and Human History

From time immemorial, human beings have viewed suffering and death and asked why. Why would a loving God allow people to suffer? Why would God allow a child to be born with Down's syndrome, or allow the father of a large family to undergo a mental breakdown, or allow a mother to be taken from her growing family when others, aging or without children, are left untouched? People both wise and callow have questioned the meaning of suffering and death since the beginning of time. In the Jewish and Christian traditions, some insight has been gained over the centuries concerning these concomitants of human existence (C. Lewis, 1943; Nouwen, 1972). Some of the knowledge and understanding is found in the Scriptures; much of it is in the oral tradition of churches and families. However, suffering and death remain mysteries—mysteries that will never be unraveled clearly and completely in this life—because they are bound up in the intimate life and love of God. Admitting that suffering and death are mysteries that cannot be solved fully in this life may seem to be a denial or delimitation of the human desire and power to know the truth. Actually, it is not a denial of human potential and aspiration. Rather, it is an admission that human beings are incapable of knowing everything, and that God plays a very important part in the life of any individual person or any group of persons.

To say that suffering and death are mysteries does not take them out of the realm of human investigation, nor does it mean that we should stand in helpless awe of them. After all, some of the great moments in human history are the result of human beings' efforts and success in conquering illness and disease. There is, however, a point beyond which human beings cannot go. Suffering will never be eliminated as long as human history continues, and each person must die. These ultimate truths are testimony to the power of the Creator, with whom humankind cooperates in the genesis and continuation of the human race, but who in the last analysis is the only ruler of the world, the Lord of the universe (John Paul II, 1995, n. 55).

Are Suffering and Death Punishment from God?

"Death was not God's doing; he takes no pleasure in the extinction of the living. To be—for this he created all" (Ws 1:13–14). "God had not wished to include suffering and death in man's destiny" (Pius XII, 1944). From where, then, came suffering and death? St. Paul says, "Through one man sin entered the world, and with sin death, death thus coming to all men inasmuch as all sinned" (Rm 5:12).

This original sin was essentially a sin of pride, the will to be like God not by using God's gifts to come closer to God in community, but to use these gifts to set up the human individual in self-centered domination of the world apart from God. It is this misuse of God's gifts from the beginning of the human race to this day that has prevented humankind from overcoming the natural causes of suffering and death. This misuse also introduced into the world countless unnatural causes and transformed natural death, which might have been a joyful completion of this life and a serene passage into a greater life, into a blind, terrifying mystery.

Human injustice has produced a world where the environment is polluted, where poverty and war spread disease and death. Thus it is plain that in large measure human suffering is the result of human folly. God has not punished the human race by blasting the earth with suffering and death like a thunderbolt from heaven; he has simply left us as a community to suffer the consequences of our own folly in hopes that it will finally awaken us to accept our responsibility to restore and preserve the good world God created for us and which we have made a world of suffering.

"But does that mean that if I am sick, I must have sinned?" That is a question that many sick people ask in moments of depression, and their distress is increased by their fear of guilt. Of course, in some cases in fact our sickness is the consequence of our own misbehavior, and God permits us to suffer the consequences of our own misuse of his gifts. If we are sick because of drug abuse, gluttony, laziness, sexual promiscuity, or recklessness, then in all honesty we must admit we brought this on ourselves.

If we are personally responsible for our suffering, we must then admit our responsibility and turn to a merciful God to help us repair our lives. But, as the Bible dramatically pictures in the Book of Job, innocent people also suffer and die. The birth-injured or genetically defective child, the hemophiliac infected by HIV blood, hard-working men and women exhausted by caring for their families—certainly such suffering is not a punishment from God. Yet it is ultimately a consequence of human sin, not of any sin of the victim, but of our human community past and present which could have prevented these tragedies or remedied them. Human intelligence if properly used can insure that the innocent cease to suffer from the sins of others. The innocent child is not responsible for being abused, but society is responsible for not rescuing the child. It is this responsibility that inspires all our efforts at medical research. We have already found remedies for many of these evils and can make progress in overcoming more. As we have misused God's gifts and brought suffering to the innocent, so we can also use these gifts of intelligence to repair the harm we have done. Thus health care professionals play an important role in God's redeeming work, together with Jesus Christ, the Healer, the conqueror of sin and death.

Death, Where Is Your Sting?

Even when people have turned their backs on God, he has not turned from them but has offered them forgiveness and restoration. In his mercy, however, God cannot deny their human freedom but has called them to return to him, not simply by restoring them to their innocent beginnings, but by a long history of struggle and learning from experience, an experience in which suffering is inevitable. For the Christian and for all who travel by less clearly marked out paths, God has revealed in Christ the direction of their journey and the power of grace by which it can be traveled (O'Meara, 1973). In baptism, according to St. Paul (Rm 6:1–11), through the cross of Christ humanity has died and been reborn in a new creation that will be completed in the resurrection of the body in eternal life. Human beings live now in such unity with Christ that all the events of their lives take on meaning from his life and death. Consequently, both the joy and the suffering of this life have a Christian meaning: its joys are signs of the hope for everlasting life in his kingdom, which is already present here on earth in promise; and its sorrows are a sharing in his cross through which a victorious resurrection is to be achieved.

Jesus came to conquer suffering and death. In what sense has he succeeded? People still get sick and continue to suffer, and death is inevitable. He conquered sickness, suffering, and death in the sense that he inspired us to overcome the evils that spread suffering and death. Even when we cannot escape suffering, Jesus gave it a new meaning, a new power. By believing in Jesus as Savior, by joining our suffering and death to his, humankind overcomes their evil (Schillebeeckx, 1981b). Although the results of original and actual sin are still present in life, they no longer dominate it. Rather, suffering and death are transformed into the very actions that help humankind fulfill its destiny.

Death is defined as the separation of body and soul, but it can be more than that. In their attempts to specify more clearly what it means to die, modern theologians have concentrated on death as a personal act of a human being, an act that terminates earthly existence but also fulfills it (CDF, 1979). Thus the person is not merely passive in the face of death, and death is different for the just than for the sinner. In the view of Rahner (1965), a view accepted and developed by many theologians, death is an active consummation, a maturing self-realization that embodies what each person has made of himself or herself during life. Death becomes a ratification of life, not merely an inevitable process (Boros, 1965). It is an event beyond our control, yet also a personal act in which the freedom of the person is intimately involved.

Dying with Christ is an adventure; it is a consequence of, but it need not be a condemnation for, sin. This is a new approach to death, yet it is thoroughly in keeping with the Christian tradition. Indeed, this view of death seems to describe more clearly the experience of Christ, who offered his life rather than have it taken from him, who completed his love and generosity in the final act of obedience to the Father: "It is consummated" (Jn 19:30). Not only pastoral care personnel but also those in other fields of the healing profession will enrich their own lives and the lives of their patients if they are able to communicate this notion of death.

13.2 FEAR OF DEATH

Denying Death

Because health care professionals are human, they tend to retreat from any phenomenon that causes fear or wonder. Death is such a phenomenon; it involves awe, fear, and mystery. For this reason health care professionals, just like other people, are tempted to avoid facing the evil of death (Cranford, 1985). The result of this fear has been studied by perceptive physicians and philosophers (E. Becker, 1973; Cassell, 1976; Aries, 1981; Hilfaker, 1985). When health care professionals are controlled by fear, they often deceive patients as to their true condition and neglect their need for understanding or comfort. Moreover, the occasion for personal spiritual growth is lost for both the patient and the health care professional, and the opportunity to help another human being prepare for death and eternal life is lost as well. Studies show that too many health care professionals retreat and cut themselves off from the dying patient completely (Landau and Gustafson, 1984). To put it another way, dying is not only a biological process, but also a psychological process that involves the health care professional as well as the patient.

Learning to Face Suffering and Death

To overcome fear and to help people die well, the health care professional must learn to handle the emotional strain that accompanies suffering and death and to deal with the ethical dilemmas sometimes encountered (R. Mack, 1984).

Although many helpful books on these topics are available, some clinical training in this area is also necessary. Every hospital staff should include people who specialize in the care of the dying. Their purpose is not only to help the dying patient work through fear, anger, and depression, but also to help the members of the healing team participate in the event of death in a way that is helpful for themselves (Gadow, 1980; P. Maguire, 1985). Otherwise health care professionals, no matter how well-educated or technically expert, will suffer psychological harm from their constant involvement in death. Is the high rate of alcoholism, suicide, and divorce among health care professionals in some way connected with stress over their inability to express their grief and sadness at the constant sight of death (Bosk, 1979)?

Given the power and prestige of the health care profession, acknowledging the importance of God in human life, the mystery of his presence as evidenced through suffering and death, is an important step in humanizing that profession. To accept limitation is to accept one's humanity. Health care professionals who assume a position of unlimited power in the process of healing have an outlook that is unrealistic. They think of themselves as the persons who cure, rather than realizing that it is God who cures and health care professionals who cooperate in this work by using the forces of nature.

Those who must deal with the dying have three options: (1) they can ignore the dying patient and thus become hardened and jaded; (2) they can relate to the dying patient in a sincerely personal manner without knowing how to deal with their own feelings; or (3) they may relate to the dying patient in a healthy way, recognizing the psychological strain that patient and professional undergo together (Fleyner, 1977). Taking this last option can teach a professional to value the experience of helping another fellow human being suffer and die in Christ, either with explicit Christian faith or perhaps simply with an openness to the mysterious future, which is the effect of Christ's grace in those who do not know him except under some other name or symbol. Few health care professionals, however, will be able to achieve this healthy, healing attitude without special training in the art of working with the dying.

Transformation by Christian Hope

In learning this art of the care for the dying, three points should be kept in mind. First, because suffering and death are obstacles to the fullness of life that Christians affirm, we have not only the right but the duty to try to overcome or mitigate them. Thus Christians should strongly favor medical research to conquer disease and to preserve and prolong life, for example, the crusade to eliminate heart disease and cancer or to make the environment more healthful. Medicine as a profession, as a science, and as an art has a Christian birthright.

Second, efforts by medical science to overcome the evils of sickness and suffering have not eliminated the healing role of prayer, which is also a part of the Christian heritage. Jesus healed physical as well as spiritual ills and commanded his followers not only to preach but also to heal and drive out demons (Mk 3:14–15). The reference to demons indicates the forces of evil that must be overcome for complete human healing in all the dimensions of the human person, spiritual and ethical, as well as psychological and physical; these forces are greater than merely human intelligence, even with the aid of science, can ever hope to achieve. Thus, to complete human healing necessitates turning to Jesus Christ, who, having died himself and risen, has conquered sin and death and who is the source of all healing powers, even those provided by modern medicine. Therefore health care professionals striving to help the suffering and the dying need to pray for and with them.

Third, although sickness and suffering have entered the world through sin, they are not themselves sinful, nor is the one who is suffering always the same one who has sinned. Jesus suffered because of the sins of others, and this is also true of innocent persons today. Thus health care professionals should see the sick as victims rather than as responsible for their own condition, unless in fact this responsibility is obvious. Even if they are in fact responsible, sick persons must then be helped to understand the forgiving mercy of God by which the road of hope is always open. The real problem of caring for the suffering and dying, therefore, is to help them realize that they can bring good out of evil by making their painful and frightening experiences a means of personal growth and a witness of courage to others who someday will have to meet the same test. The current situation of patients with acquired immunodeficiency syndrome (AIDS) emphasizes the importance of helping patients to approach death with a sound theological outlook. Although the situation of AIDS patients may be hopeless in regard to their physiological condition, the mercy of God is always open for them (USCC, 1987). Caregivers should help AIDS patients realize that they have not lost their human dignity (Kubler-Ross, 1987).

The Meaning of the Cross

Christian health care professionals will best succeed in this difficult task if they themselves understand suffering and death in terms of the suffering, death, and resurrection of Jesus Christ, which provides the only help in living hopefully with this mystery. Many health care professionals feel utterly defeated by the death of patients whom they have cared for and by the helplessness of even their best efforts in many cases to restore normal health. Only Christian hope has an answer for that despair. The sign of the Cross in Catholic hospitals stands for this profound attitude of hope.

Clearly, it takes more than words to accomplish this transformation of suffering and death. One must be willing to surrender to God through the person of Jesus Christ every day if one wishes to give new meaning and power to suffering and death. The small deaths one dies every day prepare a person for the larger and more important deaths and finally for the ultimate moment of meaning and power.

The perfection of Christian suffering and death is to accept it with hope and joy. This is not possible unless one works at it faithfully, relying on the unfailing grace of God. To communicate to patients effectively the meaning and power of death, health care professionals must have some experience of its reality themselves. Thus health care is more than a job, more than knowledge and technique. Basically, in its fullness it is a way of life that sees beyond the hurt, the sickness, the anguish; a way of life that enables one to look beyond the drudgery of daily reality, beyond the suffering in the hospital ward and the emergency room; a way of life that centers in God's love for his children, his ability to bring good out of evil, the suffering of Christ for all human beings, and his victorious resurrection.

13.3 DEFINING DEATH

The Dying Process and the Event of Death

When biologists speak of the death of any living organism, they refer to that inevitable and critical moment when an organism ceases to function as a specific, unified, homeostatic system and becomes disorganized into a mere collection of heterogeneous chemical substances (PCEMR, 1981). Sometimes, however, even after this moment, some tissues or cells of the former organism may continue temporarily to carry on some independent minimal life functions. From a biological point of view, the death of a human organism is similar to any death and is determined in much the same way, by various signs that the unifying life functions have ceased.

Yet the death of a human person is not just a biological event. Human death has a mystery about it because at death we lose touch irrevocably with a person who previously was able to communicate and to share our human community of thought, of love, of freedom, and of creativity (Kung, 1984). Human death is not merely a decay of an organism; it is the departure of a member of the human community. People all over the world have interpreted this departure of someone known and loved as the separation of a spiritual principle of life from its body. Science cannot close the door on such an explanation. Christians believe that the departed will return in their bodily personhood in a transformed existence, as Jesus did (Lk 24:36–43).

In any case, people often have the painful responsibility of determining when the death of another has occurred, because the time of death influences many other human decisions, such as inheritance, legal and moral rights possessed by the dying person, spiritual care for the dying person, and possibility of organ transplantation.

Dying is a process, but death is an event (Capron, 1986; White, 1992). We can be certain this event has not yet occurred as long as a person can communicate through speech or gesture. When such communication ceases, we can only judge by signs that are no longer distinctly and specifically human. We do not dare conclude, however, that death has occurred merely because such specifically human signs are no longer evident, as becomes very clear when we observe someone wake from sleep or coma (Evans, 1994).

Consequently, we are morally obliged to treat anybody who is apparently human (even in the fetal state) as a human person with human rights until we are sure that this body has become so disorganized that it no longer retains its human unity. To know this, we must be reasonably sure of three facts: (1) that the body does not now exhibit specific human behavior; (2) that it will not be able to function humanly in the future; and (3) that it no longer has even a minimal capacity for human functions because it has lost the basic structures required for integration of human functions, bodily and spiritual.

That third condition is required because medical experience has shown that persons who have been in apparent coma nevertheless have sometimes recovered human consciousness. Such resuscitation is possible as long as the essential structures of the human organism remain and the causes that inhibit their normal function can be removed. This is why some speculate that in the future the human body may be frozen and thawed out several years later. At the same time, there is no reason to deny that after true human death some cells or even organs of the human body may for a time (perhaps indefinitely if artificially supported) continue to exhibit some life functions. These functions are not those of the human organism as a unified entity, but merely a residual life at a level of organization comparable to that of plants and lower animals. Thus the essential point about determining human death is not to decide whether *any* life is present, but whether human life in the sense of a unified human person is still present (Grunstrand, 1986).

In the past, some signs of human death were always easy to identify. If rigor mortis or putrefaction occurred, even nonprofessionals were able to recognize that the human organism was irreversibly destroyed. Other less conclusive signs of human death were the absence of breathing and heartbeat, although it was known that these might sometimes be revived by such methods of resuscitation as were then available. When such efforts failed, death was judged certain. Physicians were required to pronounce the patient dead on the basis of such evidence and certify the time of death for legal purposes such as inheritance. Thus irreversible cessation of spontaneous heart and lung function became known as the *clinical* signs of death.

Need for New Clinical Definition of Death

In recent years, two developments have led to the proposal of a new set of clinical signs for determining human death (Canada Law Reform Commission, 1981; Cassell et al., 1972). First, machines have been perfected that artificially aid the function of the heart and lungs or that enable a person to be resuscitated after the heart and lungs have ceased to function for a short time. Often people recover full and spontaneous heart and lung function as a result of being temporarily assisted by such machines, proving that the essential structures of the unified human organism had not been destroyed. On the other hand, it seems possible that such machines may be able to maintain heart and lung function at least temporarily, even after this unity of the organism has ceased to exist, since the heart completely separated from the body can continue to beat, just as tissues in a test tube can continue to exhibit some residual life if nourished by an appropriate solution.

Thus such artificially sustained heart and lung action is not proof that human life still remains, yet as long as heart and lungs are sustained, it is impossible to verify the traditional signs of human death. Therefore the question arises: Are there other clinical signs that can be used, not to constitute a new definition of death, but rather as alternative criteria to establish the same essential fact, namely, that human life is no longer present because unified human function is not present and cannot be restored (New York Task Force on Medical Ethics, 1986; Halvey and Brody, 1993)?

The second, and perhaps more important, reason for seeking new clinical signs of death has been the recent advancement of techniques of organ transplantation. Such transplants are more likely to be successful if the organs are retrieved from a body through which blood continues to circulate. Thus transplant surgeons prefer to keep the cadaver of a dead donor on a respirator.

Clinical Criteria of Death

How, then, is it possible to be sure that the donor is in fact dead?

First, the traditional cardiovascular clinical signs are basic and sufficient and should be utilized if possible when determining death. The brain-death criteria, assessing function of the whole brain, should be employed only when traditional signs cannot be used because the dying person is dependent on a respirator or other form of artificial maintenance. If brain death is permitted to become the exclusive criterion for human death, no one would be judged dead without elaborate tests in a hospital. Present moral dilemmas about how to determine death are caused largely by excessive reliance on technology, and that excess should be moderated rather than encouraged.

Second, the new brain-death criteria must be ascertained by well-trained professionals. Human error and even carelessness must be anticipated and avoided. How can such errors be prevented when human life is at stake? Most criteria for brain death require more than one clinical observation of the patient. In the first set of criteria used to certify brain death, the "Harvard criteria," the observations were separated by 24 hours. At present, 6 to 12 hours between observations is considered sufficient. Moreover, persons applying the clinical criteria for brain death must be trained to recognize such conditions as hypothermia and drug-induced coma, which may produce a condition from which the patient can recover (Canada Law Reform Commission, 1981). Other safeguards require that the physician who certifies death should not be a member of a transplantation team, that might be overanxious to pronounce the donor dead. In some cases, the opinion of more than one physician is required before brain death is determined. One way or another, fail-safe procedures must be built into the process of using brain functions as the clinical signs to ascertain human death.

Third, and most serious, is the question about the nature of brain death itself (White, 1992; Byrne, 1993). It is critical that the criteria used to certify brain death establish that the person is dead, not merely dying or in a deep coma. Although the medical profession has accepted the general idea of using the activity of the brain as the main criterion in some cases to establish human death, exactly which specific signs should be used to determine that the total brain no longer functions has not been agreed upon by all (Halvey and Brody, 1993). For the most part, the criteria center on clinical observation, such as response to pain, cerebral function, brain-stem reflexes, and testing for apnea. These clinical observations are confirmed by use of an electroencephalogram (EEG) or blood-flow studies (Daniel et al., 1992).

Controversy About Defining Death

The variance in opinion as to the validity of brain-death criteria primarily results from theoretical issues. Thus one group of physicians maintains that cessation of neuronal activity in the brain is not sufficient to signify human death unless the cessation is proved to be irreversible and indicates destruction of all cerebral function (Byrne et al., 1979; Byrne and Nilges, 1993). This argument seemingly has been obviated by studying the circulation of blood in the brain by means of an angiogram or isotopes rather than by using an EEG to study neuronal activity. If the angiogram establishes that blood no longer circulates into the brain, the brain is dead because no way exists to restore activity to the brain when circulation ceases. The lack of blood circulation in the brain may also be proven through newer methods of imaging (Levy et al., 1987). Hence, when the whole brain is dead, the person is dead, since the organ that is the source of unified activity no longer functions, even though there may still be signs of residual cellular activity in the brain and other parts of the body.

Although it is not our purpose to settle any differences of opinion in regard to medical matters, we conclude that when total and irreversible function of brain activity is clinically proved, the person in question is dead because the form (soul) is no longer able to inform the matter (body). To date, many states have approved this method of discerning human death in so-called Definition of Death Legislation, and the need for national legislation in this regard has been recommended. The legislation of the various states requires that the signs indicate that total, not merely partial, death of the brain has occurred.

Would it be possible to declare a person dead if only some part of the brain, that is, the higher or neocortical centers on which specifically human thought processes apparently depend, did not develop fully or ceased to function (Younger and Bartlett, 1983; Lizza, 1993)? This view is defended by some who wish to use anencephalic infants as organ donors before total brain death occurs or who maintain that such infants may be aborted in the third trimester (Chervenak et al., 1984; Holzgreve et al., 1987; Seratini, 1993). The philosophers Robert Rizzo and Paul Yonder studied this question and declared (1973):

> We must ask whether the death of the cerebral cortex or neocortex signals human death, even though other parts may be still functioning for a time. . . . We offer the hypothesis that human death should be related to the cessation of functions distinctly human since breathing, heartbeat, and circulation are vegetative processes shared by other animals. . . . From all

clinical evidence the death of the neocortex marks the end of the physiological basis for human consciousness, that is, a consciousness unique in
its powers of reflection. It signals the end of the brain as a dynamic
integrated whole and presages in most cases the imminent death of other
cerebral systems (p. 226).

Despite some support for this position that cortical death constitutes human death (Veatch, 1993), this position presents several difficulties. First, if
people who have spontaneously functioning hearts and lungs but no other vital
signs are declared dead, what about people who have weak signs of "human
life" (R. Veatch, 1975)? If those in a deep and irreversible coma are declared dead
insofar as human life is concerned, what about people who are mentally retarded or senile? Do they show sufficient signs of human life to be kept alive?
Or should only minimal care be given to those who no longer have the functioning signs of human life that are associated with activity in the cortex of the
brain? Persons who argue for the elimination of retarded, senile, infirm, and
debilitated persons in certain circumstances believe partial brain death should
be accepted as a proper clinical sign for human death (Harris, 1985). However,
society must go very slowly in accepting such a definition unless it is willing to
bury people when they are still breathing and their hearts are pulsating spontaneously.

If the criteria of *partial* brain death were to be used as sufficient evidence
of death, ethical responsibility would require certitude about two facts. *First,* the
essential structures necessary and sufficient to constitute the unified organism
of the human person would have to be found in the cortical function of the
human brain, separated from the rest of the body. This certainly is plausible
from what is now known. *Second,* most of the brain would have to be considered
unnecessary for the specifically human functions of thinking and willing, but
existing only to maintain and move the body and supply the higher brain
centers with nourishing materials. This also is plausible, but the present state of
knowledge on this is far from certain (PCEMR, 1981; White, 1992). It is generally
recognized today that the brain is a system of subsystems that are intimately
interdependent. Although it is possible to localize such functions as speech and
sight in particular parts of the brain, this is not proof that only one such part is
involved in the function or even that it is its primary center, since inhibition of
a merely secondary or auxiliary part of a system may impede its function
(Gaddes, 1985; Rayport, 1992). Thus, at present, such localization of human
functions is merely tentative.

Therefore, although we accept total brain death as a sufficient criterion for
human death, we do not believe that partial brain death is sufficient. We do not
believe that death should be certified as long as patients are able to maintain
spontaneous breathing and heartbeat, since this constitutes strong evidence that
the brain, as the seat of the essential unity of the human body, is still living, even
if it is not evidencing its higher functions. Although even then there may be
reasonable doubts, the benefit of the doubt should be given to the rights of the
person.

13.4 TRUTH TELLING TO THE DYING

Breaking the News

"What to tell the patient" has been considered one of the more difficult and delicate ethical questions for health care professionals. The principle of professional communication, formulated in Chapter 8, p. 204, is relevant here. Not long ago, some physicians and other health care professionals thought that the less patients knew about their condition, the better would be the chances of recovery (Annas, 1994). Moreover, some health care professionals would even withhold information of impending death, fearing that such knowledge might lead a person to despair (Cope, 1968). In some parts of the world, this is still the practice of many physicians (Ishiwata and Sakai, 1994).

Because of an awakened moral sense by health care professionals and a sharper realization that patients have legal and moral rights that must be respected, however, today there is a much greater tendency to be open and honest with patients concerning their condition (Darvaal, 1993). In general, patients have the right to the truth concerning their condition, the purpose of the treatment to be given, and the prognosis of the treatment. The "Patient's Bill of Rights" of the American Hospital Association (AHA, 1972) states:

> The patient has the right to obtain from the physicians complete current information concerning diagnosis, treatment, and prognosis in terms the patient can be reasonably expected to understand (n. 3).

The *Ethical and Religious Directives for Catholic Health Services* (NCCB, 1994) declare:

> Catholic health care institutions offering care to persons in danger of death from illness, accident, advanced age, or similar condition should provide them with appropriate opportunities to prepare for death. Persons in danger of death should be provided with whatever information is necessary to help them understand their condition and have the opportunity to discuss their condition with their family members and care providers. They should also be offered the appropriate medical information that would make it possible to address the morally legitimate choices available to them. They should be provided the spiritual support as well as the opportunity to receive the sacraments in order to prepare well for death (D. 55).

Clearly, information concerning serious sickness or impending death is to be furnished even if the individual does not ask for it. Legal precedent as well as moral concern prompts this realization. Thus physicians and other health care professionals may not defend their lack of communication on the grounds that the patient did not wish to know and did not ask questions. In some hospitals, a patients' representative helps patients understand their situation, especially when surgery is anticipated. Whenever possible, the leader of the health care team, the physician, should be involved in explaining the situation to the patient.

Sensitivity to the Individual

Although health care professionals usually respect the rights of patients insofar as providing the proper information is concerned, difficult situations often arise and health care professionals hesitate to tell patients their true condition. For example, if patients with serious cases of cancer know their true condition, they might become despondent and lack the desire to live, thus contributing to their illness. People who are dying might become despondent, morose, and even suicidal if they know their true situation. With this in mind, the "Patient's Bill of Rights" states:

> When it is not medically advisable to give such information to the patient, the information should be made available to an appropriate person on his behalf (n. 8).

This statement is well-intentioned but also unsatisfactory and incomplete. It indicates that when health care professionals think that knowing the truth might harm the patient, they can fulfill their obligation by telling some friend or member of the family about the patient's condition and the prognosis. The statement does not indicate, however, what the member of the family or the friend is supposed to do with the information. To ensure Christian treatment for the patient, another dimension of the situation must be explored.

Even though medical personnel might fear untoward results if patients are informed of their true condition, this does not mean that patients should not be informed of the true situation. Health care professionals should remember in these cases the words of Dr. Eric Cassell (1976): "The depression in patients that commonly occurs after the diagnosis of a fatal disease seems to stem in part from the conspiracy of silence. The physician can be a great help by simply making it clear to the patient that he is available for open and direct communication." Thus the medical team, along with a friend of the patient or a member of the family, should work together and dispose the patient so that he or she will be able to accept the truth. Interviews with seriously ill or dying patients reveal that they do not wish to be kept continually in doubt about their condition. On the other hand, they do not want it revealed to them in an abrupt or brutal manner, according to Dr. Elisabeth Kubler-Ross in her seminal work in regard to dying patients (1969):

> When we asked our patients how they had been told, we learned that all the patients know about their terminal illness anyway, whether they were explicitly told or not, but depended greatly on the physician to present the news in an acceptable manner (p. 183).

Howard Brody (1981) assesses the practical situation aptly when he states:

> ... telling a patient something takes place over a span of time and is not a one-shot affair. Thus, the shading of phrases used, whether the truth is delivered all at once or in small doses, and the kind of follow-up are all

important parts of the ethical decision, as well as "tell" or "don't tell." A decision to reveal a grave prognosis, which may be "ethical" in itself, may become "unethical" if the physician tells the patient bluntly and then withdraws, without offering any emotional support to help the patient resolve his feelings. In fact, the assurance that the physician plans to see it through along with the patient, and that he will always make himself available to offer any comfort possible, may be more important than the bad news itself. In many of the "sour cases" that are offered as justification for withholding the truth, it may well be the absence of this transmission of compassion, rather than the telling of the truth, that produced the unfortunate results (p. 40).

Need for Trained Counselors

Because physicians are not always able to convey information concerning serious illness or impending death in a fitting manner, every health care facility has the moral obligation to include on its staff a person who is trained in the dynamics of helping patients accept sickness, suffering, and death in a Christian manner. The value of these pastoral care persons working closely with health care professionals is evident. Crisis counseling is not an arcane art, but on the other hand, one must be adequately prepared to perform it well. Well-meaning but untrained people can do other than good when trying to help in crisis situations.

Kubler-Ross (1978) maintains that to help others face death, one must be at peace with death oneself. The normal training for religious ministry does not prepare a person in this specialty. Several hospitals in the United States, however, have training programs to meet this need. The need for this service in hospitals is clear and has been recognized, but help in facing sickness and death is also necessary for people in a noninstitutional setting, such as for the poor and elderly.

In summary, increased knowledge of psychology and greater regard for the subjective process that accompanies sickness and dying has changed the ethical question in regard to truth telling. As Kubler-Ross declares: "The question should not be 'Should we tell?' but rather, 'How do we share this with the patient?'"

13.5 CARE FOR THE CORPSE OR CADAVER

Dignity of the Human Body

When a human being dies, the body is no longer vivified by the life-giving principle or soul by which it was constituted a substantial element of the human person. The cadaver of a person, then, is not a *human* body in the proper sense of the word. Insofar as is possible, the remains of a person should not be referred to as though the human person existed *in* the human body or was, so to speak, limited by the human body. Language of this nature is misleading because it implies a duality in human existence; in a certain sense, the living human person *is* the living human body. When persons die, they exist in a new form, in a sense incomplete, because they no longer have a body (Rahner, 1965). While existing in this life, the human person is a substantial unity of spirit (form) and body (matter), not an accidental juxtaposition of two distinct entities. The remains of a human body may resemble the body of a living person, and this resemblance may be prolonged through embalming; however, the remains are not a *human* body, but a mass of organic matter, decomposing into constitutive, organic elements.

If the corpse of a human person is not a human body, why are people so concerned about proper care for the remains of the deceased person? Why treat it with the respect and reverence that it usually receives? Respect and reverence are due the remains of a human being because of the sacredness of the human soul, which once informed the now-inert mass still bearing the person's image. For the Christian, the Orthodox Jew, and the Muslim, this body will also be reunited with the human soul in the resurrection and is thus eternal. As St. Paul says, "For just as in Adam all die, so too in Christ shall be brought to life" (1 Cor 14:21).

Jewish piety is expressed in the Old Testament book of Tobit, in which Tobit relates how one evening he was eating supper when news came of a man murdered in the street.

> I sprang to my feet, leaving dinner untouched, and I carried the dead man from the street and put him in one of the rooms, so that I might bury him after sunset. Returning to my own quarters, I washed myself, and ate my food in sorrow . . . And I wept. Then at sunset I went out, dug a grave, and buried him." (Tobit 3:4–7).

And this concern is expressed in the New Testament by the account of the care of the holy women and Joseph of Arimathea for the body of the crucified Jesus (Lk 23:50–56).

But even for those who do not share this faith in bodily resurrection, to mourn the person who will no longer be present in the same human manner as before, certain reverential actions are performed which express the love of the people who remain. Respect for the dead body, then, signifies respect for human life, respect for the Author of life, respect for the person who once existed in human form and who will exist again in the transformed body. Thus the actions and ritual that people follow when caring for the body of a deceased person have a meaning beyond their mere utility.

Although the commercialization of wake, funeral, and burial consistently has been criticized for its excesses (Mitford, 1975), the ritual care of the dead retains its meaning and worth in accord with the Judeo-Christian tradition. Having friends share the burden through liturgical services is also a source of strength and support for bereaved people. Thus the legitimate customs of people at the time of death are not signs of superstition or blind fear; rather, they bespeak a noble belief about life, its purpose, and the enduring strength of human love.

Cremation and Christian Burial

In the Judeo-Christian tradition, respect for the dead was usually displayed through burial of the corpse in the ground or in a mausoleum. Cremation of the remains, although not a common part of this tradition, has never been considered as disrespectful treatment. For a long time, however, cremation was forbidden in the Catholic Church because anti-Christian groups in the eighteenth century advocated cremation as a means of denying symbolically the immortality of the human person and the Resurrection. Thus, not because it was immoral in itself, but rather because of what it might signify, cremation was not an acceptable form of caring for the remains of a person in the Catholic Church according to the old Code of Canon Law (1917).

Because cremation is no longer associated with a denial of immortality today, although burying the dead is encouraged as the usual procedure, the discipline has changed and according to the Revised Code of Canon Law (1983) the total remains of a person or an amputated member, may be cremated if there is a serious reason (CDF, 1963; c.1176, par. 3). For example, if the custom of the country favors cremation, if there is danger of spreading disease, or if suitable grave sites cannot be obtained at a reasonable cost, cremation is legitimate. If the request involves no certain sign of disrespect for Christian faith, cremation may be requested by a dying person or the next of kin. Those who direct that their bodies are to be cremated, then, may be given the sacraments of the Church, as well as liturgical rites of burial, provided that the latter are not performed in the actual place of cremation.

A recent TV drama, otherwise usually well-informed on legal and medical matters, turned on the supposed refusal of "Christian burial" to a suicide. While in former times there were Catholic customs concerning the right of burial in Catholic cemeteries which had been ritually blessed, today such exclusion is rarely invoked, especially in the case of suicides, since the Church passes no judgment on their responsibility (Coriden, 1985). While in the case of the death of notorious criminals the local bishop may require that the funeral rites be private, the Church respects and prays for all the dead.

Autopsy

Autopsy is the examination of a cadaver performed to provide greater medical knowledge concerning the cause of death. Occasionally, the benefit of an autopsy will be to provide knowledge about a rare or contagious disease. In such cases, the good of the community would overrule the rights of the next of kin, and if the next of kin were not willing, the court could order that an autopsy be performed. In cases of violent death or unattended death, an autopsy is required by law, no matter what wishes are expressed by the next of kin.

Usually, however, the purpose of an autopsy is not to trace the etiology of a rare disease nor to discover unknown or violent causes of death. More frequently, autopsies are performed to help health professionals achieve a higher level of efficiency in the care of the living. The autopsy rate of a hospital is usually a good sign of concern for excellence and offers a gauge of professional integrity and interest in scientific advancement (Altman, 1988). Through autopsies, the diagnosis and treatment a person received can be evaluated and staff members encouraged to observe a high level of proficiency. For this reason, autopsies should be encouraged and people should be encouraged to look on them as an ordinary part of the medical care process. Needless to say, the human remains of a person should always be treated with utmost respect during an autopsy.

Organ Donation

In accord with the respect due to the remains of a human person, no organs should be removed from a corpse, nor should the body be dismembered in any way, unless a sufficient reason justifies such an action. Usually the next of kin or the person to whom the corpse is committed for care has the legal right to determine if organs may be removed from the body and if an autopsy may be performed (*Pierce v. Swan Point,* 1872). The right of the next of kin in regard to caring for the human body is not absolute. It may be superseded by statements made by the person while still alive, for example, through the Uniform Anatomical Gift Act, or by the needs of society, for example, when an autopsy might help stave off a contagious disease. In the future, the need of organs for donation in society may change our assumptions in regard to family rights to donate organs of the deceased (Guttmann and Guttmann, 1993). In Europe, donation of organs meets less juridical opposition (Hors et al., 1993).

The Uniform Anatomical Gift Act is "designed to facilitate the donation and use of human tissues and organs for transplantation and other medical purposes and provide a favorable legal environment for such activities" (Lehrman, 1988). At present all 50 states have enacted the Gift Act, thus enabling persons who are of sound mind and 18 years of age or older to give all or part of their bodies to persons or institutions authorized to practice or perform research medicine or to engage in tissue banking, with the gift to take effect at death. This law also recognizes the right of the next of kin to donate the body or any part for the same purpose, but in most states the law declares that if there is a conflict between the donor and the next of kin, the wishes of the donor have precedence. The person or institution to whom the donation is made need not accept the gift. If the gift is accepted, following removal of the part named, the body is transferred to the next of kin or other persons under obligation to dispose of the body. If the whole body is retained for research at a medical school, it will often be cremated upon completion of the research. In such cases there may not be a wake but a funeral service; a memorial Mass, for example, is usually celebrated without the corpse being present if the person was Catholic.

Theoretically, protection from civil and criminal proceedings that might result from the removal of organs or experimentation on the corpse is granted by the Gift Act to all persons concerned, including physicians, next of kin, funeral directors, and medical examiners. However, in practice if the next of kin refuses the request for organ retrieval, even if the deceased person had signed an anatomical gift donation card, hospitals and physicians will usually follow the decision of the next of kin because they fear malpractice charges. Persons interested in donating a part or all of their body at death should inform their families of their desire so that if possible conflicts will be avoided.

From a Christian point of view, the practice of donating organs and one's body for scientific research is ethical and even to be encouraged if a true need exists. Pius XII (1956a) and John Paul II (1984d; 1995, N. 86) have both issued statements approving of donation of blood when offered for "the love of neighbor, which forms the inspiring motive of the gospel message and which has been defined as the *new commandment*."

Sale of Organs from the Dead

Another ethical question, however, does not admit such an easy solution: Is it immoral to accept or solicit payment for the gift of certain organs? Although some have defended such practices, other authors (Ramsey, 1970; Dorozynski, 1993) maintain that abuses could arise very quickly if cadaver organs were sold or contracted for money. Ramsey points out that blood replaces itself, whereas human organs do not. With this latter opinion we agree. If society is to live in a humane manner, generosity and charity, rather than monetary gain and greed, must serve as the basis for donation of functioning organs. The National Organ Transplant Act (McDonald, 1988) prohibits the sale of human organs, although reasonable payments for expenses incurred by the health facility or donor are allowed.

Because of what it represents, the remains of a human person should be treated with respect and reverence. Health care professionals should never allow their frequent experience of human death to inure them to the great mystery and sacredness of human life. The danger in the practice of medicine is that people become blase or insensitive about suffering, death, and human remains to cover their own feelings of fear, inadequacy, or lack of faith. Although such feelings are often unconsciously motivated, they are nonetheless destructive of humane Christian health care. Moreover, it bespeaks a personality defect on the part of the health care professional that requires a new orientation toward the act and experience of death.

13.6 ASSISTED SUICIDE AND EUTHANASIA

An Age-Old Question

Suicide is the choice to destroy one's own life, and "assisted" suicide is formal cooperation with the suicide of another. It should be obvious from our discussion of the principle of legitimate cooperation that it cannot be ethical for a health care professional to cooperate formally with suicide if suicide itself is unethical. *A fortiori* if assisting suicide is immoral, killing a person without their consent, even with the intention of relieving their suffering, cannot be ethical. Hence we will first discuss the morality of suicide, then of assisted suicide, then of euthanasia (mercy killing), and finally in the last section of this chapter the question of whether letting a patient die is ethically distinct from euthanasia.

It is important to be clear (Novak, 1971; John Paul II, 1995, N. 66) that the issue here is not whether all persons who commit suicide are to be morally condemned. No doubt most persons who take their own lives do so because they are so emotionally disturbed that they act compulsively, or at least their perception of objective reality is so distorted by their anguish and depression that their freedom of choice is greatly restricted.

Thus actions of suicides are not to be evaluated ethically at all, or at least it may be assumed that they act in good faith and are subjectively guiltless. Many experts in suicidology today seem to take it for granted that all suicides are compulsive and irrational (Durkheim, 1951; Menninger, 1938). Can this assumption really be made, or is there the possibility that the decision about whether to live or to take one's life may be a genuine ethical choice for some people who have the capacity to make a free and deliberate choice (Battin, 1994)? Only if suicide is a free and rational choice can we talk about the *morality* of suicide.

The Greeks and Romans both condemned and defended suicide (Choron, 1972; Noyes, 1973), as did Eastern cultures (Holck, 1974). The Epicureans, who considered pleasure and peace of mind the highest human goods, argued that it was better to kill oneself than to endure life if it had become more painful than pleasurable or peaceful. The Stoics, who believed that virtue or self-control was the highest good, argued that it was permissible to kill oneself if suffering or torture might force one to lose self-control or act ignobly, or where a choice had to be made to perish in a shameful way or "die with dignity." Dualists, such as some Platonists (but not Plato himself), agnostics, and Manicheans taught that the soul, which is the real person, is burdened by the body in this life or in many reincarnations; thus suicide might be justified as a laying down of this burden.

Even in Christian Europe, men and women have been regarded as heroic if they committed suicide for the sake of honor. Recently, some Catholic Irishmen and Buddhist Vietnamese have used suicide by self-starvation or self-immolation as a protest against perceived injustice. In the notorious Johnstown, Guyana, and Waco, Texas, mass suicides and more recently in other suicides by cult groups in Europe and Japan, millenialist religious delusions have motivated groups of people to self-destruction.

The monotheistic religions of Judaism, Christianity, and Islam have always opposed suicide, however, because they regard life as God's gift, which his children are to use as faithful stewards (John Paul II, 1995, n. 66). Moreover, these monotheistic religions, unlike others, hold that eternal life is not the survival of a disembodied soul, nor endless reincarnation, but resurrected life with God. Consequently, Christians cannot escape accounting to God for stewardship of the life given them in their worldly existence, nor can they reject the body that will always be part of them. This view was already anticipated by the great Greek philosopher Plato, who argued that suicide is a rejection of duty to one's body, to the community of which the person is a part, and to God who gave the person life. In a very different way, another great philosopher, Kant, argued that suicide is the greatest of crimes because it is a person's rejection of morality itself, since a person must be his or her own moral lawgiver (see section 7.2, p. 153). To kill oneself is to treat oneself as a thing (a means) rather than as a person.

The Christian churches, especially the Catholic Church, have always firmly opposed suicide, as the document of the Congregation of the Doctrine of the Faith *Declaration on Euthanasia* (CDF, 1980a) stated:

> Intentionally causing one's own death, or suicide, is equally as wrong as murder; such an action on the part of a person is to be considered as a rejection of God's sovereignty and loving plan. Furthermore, suicide is also often a refusal of love for self, the denial of the natural instinct to live, a flight from the duties of justice and charity owed to one's neighbor, to various communities or to the whole of society.

Is There a Right to Control One's Own Death?

Today, however, the Christian stand against suicide is again being questioned (Quill et al., 1992b; Brody, 1992b; Beauchamp, 1994). The Protestant moralist Joseph Fletcher (1960) has said, "The real issue is whether we can morally justify taking it into our own hands to hasten death for ourselves (suicide) or for others (mercy killing) out of reasons of compassion." Fletcher answers this in terms of his own situationism, according to which the only command of God is to "act lovingly." This leads Fletcher to a form of situation ethics that justifies any means if it is effective for achieving loving ends because, "If we will the end, we will the means." Consequently, it appears to him that there are many situations in which persons can will their own death for the good of others (as a war prisoner fearing torture that may cause him to reveal the hiding place of others) or in which others may be put to death out of compassion for their sufferings, assuming that they would want this to be done for them.

Such views have been promulgated in the United States by the Hemlock Society and other societies. Recently the case of Dr. Jack Kevorkian, who in Michigan has publicized that he has many times assisted patients in committing suicide with fatal devices he has invented, and legislative acts and court decisions have brought the issue of suicide and physician-assisted suicide sharply into focus. "Dr. Death," as he is known in the press, has claimed that his intention is not to kill but to relieve suffering and that he hopes to promote the legalization of euthanasia. Andrew Greely reported recently (Greely, 1996) that 75 percent of Americans think doctors should be able to end a terminal patient's life if the family requests it.

Although even Catholic moralists who are proportionalists have generally rejected suicide, some have argued that the natural law against suicide and euthanasia admits exceptions. Thus Daniel Maguire, in *Death by Choice* (1974, 1984), maintains:

> What he [the proportionalist Peter Knauer, SJ] means is that the taking of innocent life is wrong if there is no commensurate reason for taking it. . . . At the theoretical level, then, Knauer's ethical theory allows for euthanasia, suicide, or abortion under his dominant rubric of "commensurate reason." He slips out from under the old rule against intentionally taking innocent human life and comes up under the position that commensurate reason is what counts (p. 69).

Maguire admits that Knauer and McCormick "are not willing to go as far as their theories"; that is, they consider mercy killing and suicide to be wrong because no proportionate good could come from allowing exceptions. However, Maguire is willing to follow the theory to its ultimate conclusions, and he states, "The morality of terminating life, innocent or not, is an open question, although it is widely treated as a closed one (p. 112)." Maguire believes termination of life can be moral or immoral according to the circumstances that give it moral meaning. He also claims that the traditional argument that suicide violates God's dominion over human life is not persuasive, since if God gives us a share in his dominion over our life in most matters, as he clearly does, why not over our death as well?

In general, these proportionalists believe that to make an absolute rule against suicide is, under some circumstances, to fail to respond compassionately to useless human suffering or to draw subtle distinctions that indicate the Pharisaic legalistic mentality repudiated by Christ. Humanists, emphasizing the autonomy of the individual, tend to favor the right of all persons to determine when their own life shall cease (Engelhardt, 1986c; Miller et al., 1994). If, for the sake of discussion, we accept this position, what values and countervalues, then, need to be balanced to decide in particular circumstances whether suicide is permissible? The usual advantages often mentioned can be summarized as follows:

1. Suicide gives the human person full autonomy since he or she can choose to live or die, to be part of society or reject it.
2. Suicide enables a person to leave life with dignity, instead of enduring useless suffering, being a burden to others, and so forth, or suffering mental disease or unjustified disgrace and dishonor.
3. Suicide may enable one to avoid temptation to treacherous or ignoble acts that destroy one's personal integrity or that may be harmful to others, such as the revelation of secrets under torture.
4. Suicide relieves one's family, and also society, of burdens, so that their resources can be used for something better.
5. Suicide can be an act of heroic sacrifice for others, such as the kamikaze pilots in World War II.
6. Suicide can be a protest against social injustice, such as the Buddhist

monks who burned themselves in protest against tyranny in Vietnam or the Irish Catholic hunger strikers.

The following reasons against suicide are also frequently mentioned:

1. Suicide is an intrinsic evil for a person to reject living out life to its full, since there is opportunity for personal growth as long as conscious suffering or conscious endurance is possible.
2. Suicide is contradictory to the very basis of morality, since by this act the person gives up all other moral responsibilities.
3. Suicide is not a road to immortal life, since that life is mysterious, and whether this is the proper way to enter it is not known.
4. By suicide the individual withdraws himself or herself from the community that has given him or her life and deprives it of a unique member.
5. Suicide is a rejection of God because it is a rejection of God's gift of life.
6. Suicide deeply hurts a person's loved ones and discourages them in their own task of living.

Suicide Is Intrinsically Immoral

Even in a proportionalist methodology, when these various values are weighed one against another in concrete cases, the reasons given to justify suicide are either social or personal. As regards the social reasons that persons might believe they have a duty in justice or charity to kill themselves for the good of others, society has no right to require some of its members to directly sacrifice their life for others, although it can require that they perform some positive action for the common good, which may involve the risk or even the certainty that they may incur death. Thus those who kill themselves because they believe this will benefit others are following an exaggerated sense of moral obligation, while at the same time they are failing to fulfill their social obligation to continue to participate in the life of the community.

It is probable that the personal reasons for suicide often underlie the social arguments. Basically, persons kill themselves because "there is no other way out" (Siegl and Tuchel, 1985). The question, therefore, is whether this can ever be reasonably said to be true. There is no doubt that one can *feel* this way easily enough, but can one conscientiously judge that it is really the case? Essentially, human persons are historical beings oriented to the future. As Albert Camus wrote (1956):

> There is but one truly serious philosophical problem and that is suicide . . . Even if one does not belive in God, suicide is not legitimate . . . From the moment life is accepted as a good, it is a good for all . . . in a man's attachment to life, there is something stronger than all the ills in the world.

As long as there is hope for a future, suicide is clearly unreasonable. When hope in the future is closed off, suicide may appear a rational thing to do. In a

Christian scheme of values, however, hope in God grounds the future. By God's providence even the most painful situations not only can be endured, but also may be extremely important events in the completion of earthly life. In a secular humanist system in which ultimately no one cares for us except ourselves, this may not be true, but Christians ought to wait on the God who gave them life, since he knows best how to prepare them for the mystery of eternal life with him (John Paul II, 1995, n. 66).

As for Maguire's argument that, "If God shares with us a stewardship over life, why not over death?" it should be noted that our stewardship over life presupposes that we *preserve* our life, not destroy it. Suicide is a rejection of God's gift of life and therefore of God the giver, not a use of that life in the service of the purposes for which God gave it.

Thus attempts to balance the various values of suicide lead back to the conclusion that suicide is intrinsically and always wrong, since in all circumstances it constitutes an abdication of one's responsibility to live out life in community with other persons and with God (Grisez, 1977). Actually underlying all the modern arguments for suicide is the error of the absolute autonomy of the individual, that is, the notion that each of us ought to have total control of our own lives and therefore of our own deaths. In fact we do not create ourselves, but are part of a human society and of a universe which has its origin in God. According to the principle of stewardship and creativity, the Creator has made us partners in his wise governance of the world and we must work in cooperation with him, not contradictory to his guidance. To reject his gift of life is to reject our relation to God and to humanity.

The old saying holds, "While there is life, there is hope." Moreover, even beyond this life there is hope in God, if we have not rejected God here and now.

Physician-Assisted Suicide

When persons freely choose to die and ask to be killed, they are not only committing the crime of suicide but also compounding it by making another a partner in the crime. To yield to such a request is false compassion (J. Sullivan, 1952), although no doubt some persons like Dr. Kevorkian rationalize their actions. To have true compassion for the person who has made such a decision is to realize that the person feels hopeless, alienated from community, and doubtful of God's love. Mercy entails staying by such a person's side and through friendship helping him or her to recover hope. The mercy killer in such a case is really adding a final rejection to the many rejections that have already driven the person to that point of despair (Iglesias, 1984). True compassion is to do everything possible to alleviate pain—and modern medicine, if properly used, can always reduce pain to the level of the endurable—and to be with the sufferer in this trial.

On the other hand, if the sufferer is no longer really free to make a truly human decision but is pleading to be put out of the pain or depression that has taken away his or her capacity to think straight, the mercy killer is simply a murderer putting to death someone no longer able to protect himself or herself

(Barry, 1994). Health care professionals have the responsibility to do all they can to relieve suffering by legitimate means but, as we have seen, assisting in a suicide is not a legitimate means.

Euthanasia

The word *euthanasia* is derived from two Greek words that mean "good death" or "happy death." For centuries the term referred to an action by which a person was put to death painlessly, usually to avoid further suffering from an incurable disease or to end an irreversible comatose condition. *Webster's New International Dictionary* (5th ed.), for example, defines *euthanasia* as "a mode or act of inducing death painlessly as a relief from pain." Euthanasia in this sense is often called "mercy killing" or even "death with dignity."

The public discussion of this issue, however, is often confused by authors who speak of "passive" and "active" euthanasia (Greek for "good death"); by "passive euthanasia" they mean the withdrawal of life supports from patients when such supports are no longer beneficial but harmful. It is better to avoid this language and to follow the definition used by Congregation for the Doctrine of the Faith in the *Declaration on Euthanasia* just cited: "By euthanasia is understood an action or omission of an action which of itself or by intention causes death in order that all suffering may be eliminated" (CDF, 1980a).

It is essential to note that according to this definition, although euthanasia can be performed either by commission or omission, it is performed by omission only if "the intention" of the omission is to "cause death in order that all suffering may be eliminated." When the omission does not have this purpose, but is the result of a decision that treatment to sustain life is no longer beneficial to the patient and therefore no longer obligatory, the action is not euthanasia, and its moral justification will be discussed in the last section of this chapter. Confusion is also caused by the use of the term "death with dignity," since this can beg the question "What is 'dignity' in death?" Certainly, if mercy killing is murder, to be murdered is not to die with dignity, but to have one's dignity as a human being denied in the most flagrant way.

In the traditional meaning of the term, euthanasia could be performed with or without the consent of the person to be put to death. In the Judeo-Christian tradition, euthanasia without the consent of the patient is equated with murder and with consent of the patient is both suicide and murder. Today the proponents of euthanasia generally defend it in this latter form, where the patient's consent is given or at least presumed, so that it amounts to assisted suicide (Dworkin, 1993).

Yet deciding to help with suicide in order to relieve suffering very often becomes a decision to relieve that suffering even when the patient does not or cannot consent. Evidence for this is supplied by the history of the medical profession in The Netherlands, a country otherwise known for its respect for human rights. In that country the government announced that while its laws forbade euthanasia, the mercy killing of patients with their consent would not be prosecuted, provided physicians reported what they were doing (Keown,

1992). The result was that about 3 percent of deaths were reported as euthanasia, and about half of these as performed *without the consent* of the patients (Van Delden et al., 1993). This government has now legalized euthanasia under certain restrictions, but it is not at all clear how this limitation will be enforced.

If the motives of mercy killers are examined, their claim that they did it for the sake of the victim cannot be accepted easily. The real motive may well be that a relative or the health care professional did not want to accept the responsibility of helping the dying person to the end. Often the killer says, "I loved my mother, I couldn't bear to see her suffer!" It is true in such a case that the killer could not bear to see her suffer, but the quality of that love is not so certain. No doubt, however, sometimes mercy killers are themselves not free enough from tortured feelings to make a sane decision. Medical personnel hardly have such excuses. By consenting to help their patients die, they may simply be evading the painful and threatening task of adequate spiritual care for the dying, which is discussed in Chapter 14. As for the type of euthanasia used by the Nazis, in which patients were put to death without their consent because they were senile, insane, or defective, or as genocide, few in the United States today would defend such a practice, but some are beginning to discuss the morality of euthanasia for infants with serious birth defects or for people in a comatose condition (Finkel et al., 1993; Harris, 1994).

Generally, the medical profession has rejected euthanasia (AMA, 1988b, 1994a), as is evidenced by the Hippocratic Oath as well as by more recent codes of medical ethics, such as The Geneva Declaration (WHO, 1957) and the Helsinki Statement of the World Health Organization (WHO, 1964). However, the tendency of the medical profession in the United States to prolong the act of dying even after the patient does not benefit from life-prolonging therapy has caused many people to opt for euthanasia as a certain manner of ending life when medical therapy is no longer beneficial (Nowell-Smith, 1994). The fear of prolonged dying has also led to creation of the living will (Marzen, 1986), and when the living will proved to be unsatisfactory, to creation of the durable power of attorney for incompetent people (Peters, 1987). Although the living will and durable power of attorney are not unethical and may even be helpful in some cases, they do not of themselves eliminate the decision-making problems that arise at the time of death (Emmanuel and Emmanuel, 1992).

As we discuss next, ethical treatment of patients at the time of death depends on a clear understanding of the ethical norms for withholding and withdrawing life support from persons with fatal pathology. Generally, the Christian churches have rejected euthanasia (Park Ridge Center, 1991). The teaching of the Catholic Church in the *Declaration On Euthanasia* (CDF, 1980a) states:

> It is necessary to state firmly once more that nothing and no one can in any way permit the killing of an innocent human being, whether a fetus or an embryo, an infant or an old person, or one suffering from an incurable disease, or a person who is dying. Furthermore, no one is permitted to ask for this act of killing for himself or herself or for another person entrusted

to his or her care, nor can he or she consent to it either explicitly or implicitly. Nor can any authority legitimately recommend or permit such an action. For it is a question of the violation of the divine law, an offense against the dignity of the human person, a crime against life, and an attack on humanity (p. 512).

Even more definitively, Pope John Paul II in the encyclical *The Gospel of Life* (*Evangelium Vitae*, 1995, n. 65), says:

> In communion with the bishops of the Catholic Church I confirm that euthanasia is a grave violation of the law of God, since it is the deliberate and morally unacceptable killing of a human person. This doctrine is based upon the natural law and upon the written word of God, as transmitted by the church's tradition and taught by the ordinary and universal magisterium.

This means that this teaching is for the Catholic conscience infallible and unchangeable moral truth.

13.7 LETTING DIE

Prolonging Life or Prolonging Dying?

If euthanasia by commission is always wrong, is it always wrong to withhold or withdraw life supports such as a respirator or artificial nutrition and hydration from a patient? Is that not euthanasia by omission? Probably nothing has promoted the movement for the legalization of euthanasia more than the dramatization by the press of the horrors of modern dying hooked up to machines in a tangle of tubes. No wonder so many seem to think that the only alternative to being kept alive with a respirator and intubation is legalized euthanasia! Since most people dread the thought of dying in such a condition, they are beginning to accept mercy killing and assisted suicide, which they believe is now the only way "to die with dignity." This, like many other dilemmas with which our technological culture confronts us, is false. The moral tradition of the Catholic Church has always denied that physical life need be prolonged at all costs (NCCB, 1986; Gula, 1991). Most recently, in the encyclical *The Gospel of Life* (*Evangelium Vitae*, 1995), John Paul II writes:

> Euthanasia must be distinguished from the decision to forgo so-called "aggressive medical treatment," in other words, medical procedures which no longer correspond to the real situation of the patient, either because they are by now disproportionate to any expected results or because they impose an excessive burden on the patient and the patient's family. In such situations, when death is clearly imminent and inevitable, one can in conscience "refuse forms of treatment that would only secure a precarious and burdensome prolongation of life, so long as the normal care due to the sick person in similar cases is not interrupted" [quote from CDF

document *Declaration on Euthanasia*, 1980a]. Certainly there is a moral obligation to care for oneself and to allow oneself to be cared for, but this duty must take account of concrete circumstances. It needs to be determined whether the means of treatment available are objectively proportionate to the prospects for improvement. To forego extraordinary or disproportionate means is not the equivalent of suicide or euthanasia; it rather expresses acceptance of the human condition in the face of death.

Ordinary and Extraordinary Means

To understand this traditional teaching of the Catholic Church, a number of misunderstandings must be cleared up. First, it should be noted that the pope uses the terms "extraordinary or disproportionate means" as equivalents. It was traditional in Catholic moral theology to say that "ordinary means" of medical treatment are obligatory, but "extraordinary means" are not, until the Congregation for the Doctrine of the Faith in its Declaration on Euthanasia (CDF, 1980a) supplemented this terminology with the concept of "the proportion of benefit to burden" (O'Rourke, 1988a).

The older terminology had led to misunderstanding between ethicists and health care professionals. Physicians use "ordinary" to describe an accepted or standard medical procedure. A procedure or medicine that is new or untested or is still in the experimental stage is called "extraordinary." Thus, from the physician's point of view, something that was once extraordinary, such as cardiac angioplasty, may become ordinary because its therapeutic worth is proven. From an ethical perspective, on the other hand, a morally obligatory means to prolong life is "ordinary," while a means which is optional (not obligatory) is "extraordinary."

In an ethical perspective, ordinary means to prolong life are "all medicines, treatments, and operations which offer a reasonable hope of benefit for the patient and which can be obtained or used without excessive expense, pain, or burden; extraordinary means are all medicines, treatments, and operations which cannot be used or obtained without expense, pain, or other burden" (Pius XII, 1957; Connery, 1980). When determining whether a particular medicine, procedure, or mechanical device is an ordinary or extraordinary means of medical care, one must consider the condition of the patient as well as all the social and familial circumstances. Hence, an *a priori* list of ordinary and extraordinary means of life support from the ethical perspective cannot be constructed. Before evaluating the means to prolong life as ordinary or extraordinary in the ethical sense, one must consider the condition of the patient.

Several ethicists (McCormick, 1984a; Showalter and Andrew, 1984) prefer not to use the terms *ordinary* and *extraordinary* at all, and replace them by the terms *proportionate* and *disproportionate*. This has the risk of succumbing to the proportionalist methodology on which these moralists rely, but which in the encyclical *The Splendor of Truth* (John Paul II, 1993) has been rejected by the Church (cf. 8.1). Instead, we prefer to retain the older terms but to define them as does the *Declaration on Euthanasia* by the proportion of benefit to burden, while at the same time maintaining, contrary to proportionalism, the principle that *direct* killing is intrinsically and always unethical, although "letting die" when therapy will not benefit the patient (indirect killing in accord with the principle of double effect) is ethically justifiable.

Benefit and Burden of What?

Besides the confusion of the notion of the "proportion of benefit to burden" with proportionalism, other problems about how to apply the principle of benefit versus burden in initiating or continuing life supports have arisen. If we are to weigh the proportion between benefit and burden, we must ask three questions: The benefit and burden of what? To whose benefit or burden? How are benefit and burden to be measured?

As to the first of these questions, some hold that the benefit and burden estimation applies only to "medical procedures" which can sometimes be withheld and not to "normal" or "comfort care" which must always be given (Pontifical Academy of Sciences, 1985, p. 959). Therefore, they argue that since feeding and giving drink to patients who cannot feed themselves is "normal" or "comfort care" which must always be given; artificial nutrition and hydration must also be "care" and not a "medical procedure," and hence must always be supplied. But "medical procedures" can also be a form of "normal care," and feeding and hydrating by intubation is obviously a form of medical intervention (Meisel, 1994). Therefore, the ethical issue is whether a particular form of "care" is of real benefit, no matter whether it be "medical" or not. Moreover, classical moral theology held that taking food and drink even in a normal manner ceases to be obligatory for a patient if its benefit no longer exceeds its burden.

Persons who are in a state of persistent cognitive–affective deprivation give no indication that they experience pain, so it is difficult to know what "comfort care" could mean in their case. In hospices and nursing homes for religious, artificial nutrition and hydration are seldom used when there is little hope of restoring cognitive–affective function, yet such institutions are considered the epitome of comfort care for the dying.

Others argue that the only kind of "burden" which can be weighed against the benefit of prolonging life is the burden of the procedures to be withheld or withdrawn, and not any of the other burdens that may result from the need to care for the patient whose life will be sustained. Thus, they argue that since the procedure of nutrition and hydration by IVF is relatively inexpensive, causes only minor pain, and can often be administered by nonprofessionals at home, it is only a minor burden.

But in fact such procedures, when they have to be undergone day after day, can become quite painful to conscious patients and very burdensome to the caregiver, especially when the patient is unconscious. When one decides to provide life support in such cases, one is also creating a situation in which one is responsible for the total care of the patient. One must, therefore, take into account not only the burdens of such a procedure as starting an IVF but the burdens of total care, which may lead to the neglect of one's other responsibilities. Furthermore, one must take account of the fact that the indignity of existing in a state of persistent cognitive–affective deprivation can be counted as a serious burden to the patient, even if the patient is unconscious, along with the burdens the family may endure in caring for a person in such a condition.

Again, to some people it seems more justification is needed to remove life supports once they have been used than never to begin their use, because, they think, in the former instance one is killing the patient. But to withhold life supports if they are required is just as serious a sin of omission as to withdraw them when they are needed. Conversely, if it is not obligatory to begin their use, it is not obligatory to continue their use.

Finally, some grant that it is permissible to withhold or withdraw a respirator but not to withhold or withdraw the artificial supplying of nutrition and hydration. They say that to omit nutrition is to "starve" the patient. They also argue that to give food and drink, unlike supplying a respirator, is a fundamental Christian duty, that it is associated with the sacrament of the Eucharist, and that it is natural, while the respirator is not. Also, they point out that it is not certain the patient will die when the respirator is removed, since sometimes patients, like Karen Quinlan, begin to breathe on their own, while to stop nutrition and hydration will certainly kill.

No doubt these arguments have some basis in our intuitive feelings about the fundamental need for nourishment, but they do not stand up under critical examination. When the respirator is removed there is still a grave risk of death, and one much quicker than from lack of food and water. Nor are food and drink any more necessary or more basic to us than the oxygen supplied by the respirator. We have just as much a duty to give people air as food and drink when they cannot supply these for themselves.

Whose Benefit and Whose Burden?

Although some admit that some burdens can exceed the value of physical life, they will admit this is so only in situations where prolonging life simply prolongs the suffering of actual dying. Otherwise, they maintain, the benefit of life at any level is so great that it exceeds any burden. They point out the danger of encouraging euthanasia, if one admits arguments based on the "quality of life" rather than the essential, incommensurable preciousness of life itself. Hence, they restrict the withdrawal of life supports to situations when the disease is "terminal" and "death is imminent" (May, 1987; Grisez, 1996).

Even the encyclical *The Gospel of Life* (John Paul II, 1995), in the passage already quoted, only mentions withdrawal of life supports "when death is clearly imminent and inevitable." Since, however, this encyclical also continues to cite the CDF Declaration on Euthanasia, which gives a wider scope to the benefit versus burden criterion, we believe that *The Gospel of Life* intends only to illustrate the criterion of benefit versus burden with the most obvious and uncontroverted case, and cannot be read to change the traditional teaching nor to restrict the criterion to that situation alone.

This problem arose in the Karen Quinlan and Paul Brophy cases, when the lower courts refused permission to remove life-support mechanisms because they said "death was not imminent." The lower courts, and some other interested parties used the terms "imminent death" or "terminal condition" to show that because the life supports had already been applied the person could not be said to be dying. Nevertheless, the Supreme Courts of New Jersey and Massachusetts, when reversing the lower courts in the Quinlan and Brophy cases realized that "imminent death" was not the ethical issue (Meisel, 1995). Rather, they considered whether or not the therapy was truly beneficial and whether or not it imposed a grave burden on the patients. This method of evaluating the moral obligation of using or foregoing medical therapy is followed consistently by Catholic ethicists.

We would observe that it can reasonably be argued that even when persons whose life is supported in an irreversible unconscious state may technically be physiologically "stable" and may remain in that state for very long periods, they are in fact "terminally ill" and really "dying" (although of course their death is not "imminent"). In the normal course of nature their pathology is actually causing their death, although that dying process has been slowed to a snail's pace by the life-support technology. When these procedures cease, the person dies directly from the existing pathology and only indirectly from the withdrawal of life support.

Nor can our reply to this argument about the dying process be refuted by saying, "But we are *all* dying." In the normal course of adult life the body is aging but has the capacity to recover from trauma, and thus is not dying. Experienced physicians, however, can sometimes detect that a patient's condition is such that he or she will from that point on go steadily downhill to death because the body no longer has the power of recovery. It is at this critical point that it becomes reasonable to say that the patient is "dying," though the unpredictable time of death is still remote, not "imminent."

Again, some will not admit that patients can so deteriorate as to be beyond the possibility of benefit. Present medical knowledge distinguishes between patients in "the locked-in state," in "coma," and in the "persistent vegetative state" (PVS). Those in the rare "locked-in state" have at least some periods of conscious awareness and can respond to others at least by eye movements, but are otherwise paralyzed and unable to speak. Those in *coma* are totally unconscious as if asleep, while those in PVS show signs of arousal and may grimace or make other reflex movements, but show no signs of awareness or response to communication (Plum and Posner, 1982). While in rare cases persons have returned to consciousness after long periods in the two former states, it is medically probable that PVS patients have suffered severe, irreversible brain damage and never recover awareness.

Though PVS patients can be physiologically stabilized for long periods, even years, they can have no psychic functions since these depend on higher brain centers (American Society of Neurosurgeons, 1986). In some cases this severe brain damage has been verified by brain imaging or autopsies. If such PVS patients were not kept alive at least by artificial hydration and nutrition and sometimes by respirators, they would soon die. Yet some will still argue that sustaining life benefits them because: (1) recovery of awareness is remotely possible, perhaps by a miracle (Childs and Mercer, 1996); (2) they are better off alive than dead; (3) at least the caregivers are benefitted by their exercise of charity in behalf of so totally helpless a person. We will evaluate this opinion only after we have answered our third question about the measurement of benefit.

It should be noted, however, that although the PVS patients can have no burden of pain (Ashwal and Cranford, 1995), they may be said to have the burden of indignity. Most people, its seems, regard the possibility that they might be sustained in this dreadful condition as an indignity which they would never permit if they had the choice.

Some also hold that the only person whose burden should be considered is the patient. Hence for the unconscious patient, and particularly the patient in PVS who will never regain awareness, no procedure can be any burden at all, since they are unconscious. It is clear, however, in the documents of the Church, that the burden both to the patient and to those who have the responsibility of the patient's care must be taken into account. As Directive 57 of the ERD (NCCB, 1994) states: "Disproportionate means are those that in the patient's judgment do not offer a reasonable hope of benefit or impose excessive expense on the family or the community." We have already shown that, in deciding to continue life support, caregivers undertake the responsibility to supply not only special procedures but the total care of the patient. In the case of PVS patients, this may last for many years and require around-the-clock attention.

Therefore, it is necessary to consider the burdens that arise from social, psychological, and spiritual circumstances, as well as those that arise from physical circumstances. A father who contracts cancer may determine that, rather than spend his life savings on surgery and hospitalization, he will devote his savings to the education of his children, allowing the cancer to take its natural course. A person undergoing dialysis may determine that the therapy is too burdensome from a social point of view. A person who might survive if on a ventilator 24 hours a day may decide that living in that condition would put too much strain on his or her family and may ask to have the respirator removed (CHA, 1993).

If a patient can judge that some form of care is excessively burdensome, so can the patient's proxy when the patient becomes incompetent to make such a decision. Today one must also consider the burden to society of medical practices that lead to the irreversibly unconscious survival of a large number of persons whose care may occupy professional and other resources needed to care for those who will certainly benefit far more (Callahan, D 1993).

How Are Benefits and Burdens to Be Measured?

The question, "How are benefits and burdens to be measured?" has produced the most controversy in determining whether a means is extraordinary and therefore not obligatory. Pro-life activists, in their laudable concern to oppose anything that might favor the trend toward euthanasia, sometimes treat physical life as an absolute good. They argue that since without life we cannot achieve any other good, life is the greatest of goods, or that it is incomparable to and incommensurate with any other good. Hence it is difficult for them to concede that the burden of sustaining life could ever exceed the value of physical life (Pro-Life Committee, 1992).

Certainly, God gave us the gift of human life to show forth his goodness and love (Gn 1). We in turn show our love for God by respecting and fostering the gift of human life. As Jesus taught, love for God leads us not only to love ourselves, but to love others as well (Mt 22:37). One way to show our love for God, for ourselves, and for others is to prolong human life. Nevertheless, although earthly human life is a great good which makes possible our striving for other goods, Sacred Scripture indicates that it is not the absolute and ultimate good (Senay, 1981), since it is only a way to eternal life, from which it takes its full meaning.

Therefore, by the principle of double effect, the choice of another good may justify the *indirect* surrender of human life either for oneself or for another (Mangan, 1949). In these circumstances, one does not choose death. Rather, one chooses another good, foreseeing that death will result as an unwanted and indirect effect of that choice. Jesus on the cross, for example, in order to carry out the mission given him by his Father, freely permitted himself to be crucified rather than to be silent, escape, or use force against his killers whom he had come to save. Martyrs surrender their lives rather than deny God in their hour of crisis. They choose the good of professing their faith. Soldiers die for the freedom of their country. Many health care professionals have died caring for the sick in times of plague or war. Thus Christians have always maintained that life surrendered indirectly for a greater good than one's own physical life is not suicide. Thus physical life is not an absolute good which outweighs all burdens required to preserve it.

Thus we return to the question of how to evaluate the benefit of any form of health care whether a patient is actually dying or not, but especially in cases where the dying process has begun. Moral theology has always held that "benefit" for the human being cannot be measured in merely physical terms, but rather in terms of the life goal of the total person, soul and body. Physical life is a great human value, but it is subordinated to the eternal destiny of the whole person.

Pope Pius XII (1957) in a classic address cited in *The Gospel of Life* (John Paul II, 1995, n. 65), answered our question by stressing that the spiritual purpose of life should be the goal to which medical care is ultimately directed and by which its benefit is to be evaluated. He declared:

> Normally one is held to use only ordinary means [to sustain life]—according to the circumstances of persons, places, times, and cultures—that is to say, means that do not involve any grave burdens for oneself or for another. A more strict obligation would be too burdensome for most people and would render the attainment of higher, more important good too difficult. *Life, health, all temporal activities are in fact subordinated to spiritual ends.*

In other words, the means to prolong life may be withheld or withdrawn if these means do not help a person strive for the spiritual purpose of life, or if they impose a grave burden on the person or the person's caregivers in regard to striving for that purpose (Schindler, 1988). This places the ethical question squarely in the context of the traditional Christian view that all our free decisions must be measured by our ultimate goal, eternal life with God. As Jesus said, "Seek first the kingdom of God and his righteousness, and all these things will be given you besides" (Mt 6:33). It is also in accord with the commonsense observation that we are not morally obliged to do what does nobody any good.

To prolong life, therefore, is of benefit only when it gives the person opportunity to continue to strive to achieve the spiritual purpose of life (O'Rourke and deBlois, 1992). In order to strive for the spiritual purpose of life, one needs some degree of cognitive–affective function. Hence some writers (Barry, 1986) are mistaken when they claim that a means is beneficial as long as it prolongs human life, even at the minimal level of physiological function without reasonable hope of restoring the capacity necessary for spiritual function. Others (May, 1987) mistakenly maintain that as long as there is no physical pain for the patient there is a moral obligation to prolong life, even if the medical diagnosis states that the person is in an irreversible coma or persistent vegetative state and will not regain cognitive–affective function.

Hence to judge the "benefit" of earthly life, especially mere physical survival, we must ask what possibility of spiritual advance it offers. As long as any consciousness is possible to us, even in a state of suffering, we can perform acts of faith, of love, and of hope that will bring us closer to God and our neighbor, but when this becomes no longer possible because consciousness and freedom have been irrevocably lost by deterioration of the brain, the artificial prolongation of life by medical techniques used merely to demonstrate human ingenuity ceases to be of any real benefit to the subject.

Continuing Controversies

The differences of opinion about the meaning of "benefit" and "burden" have become especially evident in regard to the use of artificial nutrition and hydration for patients in persistent vegatative state (PVS) (Lynn, 1986). As we have seen in the foregoing discussion, even among moralists who are not proportionalists and who base their views squarely on magisterial teachings, some insist that hydration and nutrition can be withheld or withdrawn from patients only if death is imminent, or if the burden of the procedure itself is excessively painful; while others maintain that artificial nutrition and hydration should be evaluated as one would evaluate any other medical treatment, such as a respirator (AAN, 1989; AMA, 1994a). Thus, if cognitive–affective function cannot be restored, the artificial nutrition and hydration may be withheld or withdrawn because there is no moral obligation to continue using ineffective medical means (Annas, 1985c; Cranford, 1984; O'Rourke, 1986; Weir and Gostin, 1990). Yet others would maintain that artificial nutrition and hydration may be withheld or removed only if the therapy constitutes a grave physical burden (May, 1987;

New Jersey Catholic Conference, 1987; Louisiana Catholic Bishops, 1995). We have already stated the arguments which are offered by both sides of the question. The *Ethical and Religious Directives* say:

> *Directive 58.* There should be a presumption in favor of providing nutrition and hydration to all patients, including patients who require medically assisted nutrition and hydration, as long as this is of sufficient benefit to outweigh the burdens involved to the patient.

All can agree that in this matter serious abuses are possible. Hence decisions not to sustain human life ought always to be conservative. It is in this sense that we understand that there is a "presumption in favor of providing hydration and nutrition to all patients." But presumptions yield to facts, and consequently the real issue remains the estimation of benefits and burdens involved. When those who have responsibility for the care of an irreversibly unconscious person act on the basis of a careful and conservative diagnosis of PVS or some other condition in which present medical science has no ability to enable the person to continue human acts, further life support can only be judged "aggressive" and "extraordinary," and thus ceases to be obligatory. Such care by its very nature is highly burdensome to the caregivers and is an indignity to the patient. "Normal" or "comfort care" that avoids any pain or indignity to the dying patient always remains obligatory, but it need not include the continuation of nutrition and hydration by intubation.

While *The Gospel of Life* and other magisterial documents, including that issued by the U.S. National Conference of Bishops and embodied in the *Ethical and Religious Directives*, do not explicitly adopt this position, they carefully leave the way open to it, since it is essentially a prudential matter to be decided in the circumstances of each case rather than by a routine rule. We have, however, tried in the foregoing to make clear the sound principles which must be prudentially employed.

The Declaration on Euthanasia (CDF, 1980a) sums up the problem and its answer:

> It is also permissible to make do with the normal means that medicine can offer. Therefore one cannot impose on anyone the obligation to have recourse to a technique which is already in use but which carries a risk or is burdensome. Such a refusal is not the equivalent of suicide; on the contrary, it should be considered as an acceptance of the human condition or a wish to avoid the application of a medical procedure disproportionate to the results that can be expected or a desire not to impose excessive expense on the family or the community.

The difficulty of decision making is especially acute when treatment for newborn infants with birth defects is in question. Without forgetting that direct killing of the innocent is always wrong, parents and health care professionals must recognize that in some cases continuing life support of the newborn cannot really be judged beneficial to the child and may be greatly burdensome to the parents (cf. McCormick, 1974b; Kolata, 1993). Aggressive care of handicapped and genetically deprived infants should be instituted, in accord with the ethical questions: Is the care effective? Will it impose a grave burden if the treatment is continued? The attitude that the life of every infant must be prolonged as much as possible, no matter what impairment, is ethically unacceptable on the principles we have enunciated and was also recognized in the original Baby Doe regulations of the Federal Government (Federal Register, 1983).

Finally, we want to emphasize that the fears of pro-life activists that anything less than a policy of supporting life at all costs will give support to euthanasia is not only inconsistent with the traditional wisdom of Catholic moral theology, but is also unwise in the present political scene. As we noted at the beginning of this section, the fear is widespread among elderly people that they will be forced to spend their last days hooked up to complicated medical apparatus, and that their desire to die in a natural and dignified manner will be ignored by hospitals concerned only to protect themselves from litigation. Therefore, if the only alternative to such a fate is euthanasia, the elderly will vote for its legalization.

Who Decides

Who makes the difficult and delicate ethical decision that life should or should not be prolonged and that a certain means is ordinary or extraordinary? Some place the burden primarily on the physician (M. Smith, 1993); some believe it should be the duty of the courts to protect the rights of incompetent patients (Horan and Grant, 1984); others propose that ethics committees become involved in the discussion (Fletcher and Hoffman, 1994). Clearly the physician is involved in the decision in an integral manner and has the responsibility of considering the condition of the patient and determining the medical prognosis; that is, whether the means in question will cure, help appreciably, or have no effect on the dying patient (Pellegrino and Thomasma, 1993). There are, however, other circumstances to be considered, in addition to the medical effectiveness of the means. What about expense, pain, spiritual and social burden? Only the patient or the family can decide concerning these circumstances. Thus the essential right to make a decision as to what would be an ordinary means and what would be an extraordinary means from an ethical point of view belongs to the patient (Merz, 1993). With the guidance of the physician, often in consultation with family members, the patient decides what actions should be performed and which should be omitted. The physician-patient relationship is expressed aptly in this manner (Pius XII, 1957):

> The rights and duties of the doctor are correlative to those of the patient. The doctor, in fact, has no separate or independent right where the patient is concerned. In general, he can take action only if the patient explicitly or implicitly, directly or indirectly, gives him permission.

The statement of the AMA (1994) corresponds with this thinking:

> The principle of patient autonomy requires that physicians respect the decisions to forego life sustaining treatment of a patient who possesses decision making capacity . . . if a patient is incompetent, a surrogate decision maker should be identified.

The most difficult problems arise when the patient is incompetent to decide concerning proper medical treatment (Hubbard, 1993). Special care must be taken to defend the right to life of such persons. Some physicians are tempted, for example, to judge too easily that newborn children who suffer from a serious handicap are not to be treated (Bopp, 1993). On the other hand, parents who have just been informed that a newborn is handicapped may too quickly decide to allow such children to die. Patients who are severely depressed may also refuse treatment that they would have accepted in a better frame of mind. There is evidence also of serious neglect of patients in long-term care facilities who are allowed to go untreated (Lidz, 1992). Consequently, great caution is always necessary in "letting die" decisions for incompetent persons.

This has led some to argue that the rights of incompetent patients are best defended by an appeal to the courts, where the adversary process ensures greater protection (Hoefler, 1992). It is also debated whether the courts should accept "substituted judgment" or "best interest of the patient" as the criteria for its own decisions (deBlois, 1994). To date, in a whole series of cases, *Quinlan, Saikewicz, Perlmutter, Spring, Eichner Conroy, Jobes, Brophy, Greenspan, Lawrence,* and many others, the courts have approved the withholding of treatment which is ineffective or imposes an excessive burden, even if death might result (Meisel, 1996).

In our opinion, only in cases of conflict where one of the parties believes that the rights of the patient are imperiled should there be recourse to the courts. Ordinarily, however, the physician should counsel the guardians by giving a medical opinion as to risks and benefits, and the guardians should make the decision on the basis of the patient's best interest, that is, to decide what is beneficial for the patient, given the circumstances that prevail. Best interest of the patient should respect the patient's reasonable wishes, if these wishes are known. However, the prior wishes of the incompetent patient should not be considered as the sole criterion for determining treatment because in the face of prevailing circumstances, the patient's prior wishes may be unreasonable. "Where the proper and independent duty of the family is concerned, they are usually bound only to the use of ordinary means" (Pope Pius XII, 1957).

Recently the federal government, through the Patient Self Determination Act, 1990 (HCFA, 1992), encouraged the use of advance directives, a document to be signed by patients stating who is to make medical decisions in their interest if they become incompetent. Every state now has either a living will statute or a health care power of attorney statute. "Advance directive statutes do not create the right to make an advance directive, rather their primary purpose is to confer immunity for individual and institutional health care providers who rely on advance directives and they prescribe procedures which must be followed if statuatory immunity is to be available" (Meise, 1995, p. 356). Certainly such documents may make it easier for relatives of the person to know the person's wishes and to feel comfortable with exercising proxy consent. They may also protect health care professionals in case of malpractice suits.

Although it is ethically permissible to sign such documents, we should be aware that they do not solve all problems (SUPPORT Study, 1995). Changes in medical practices and in our own wishes may result in such directives becoming irrelevant or counterproductive, nor can we foresee all the circumstances in which these directives may have to be applied. Probably the better provision for the future is to make as sure as we can that those who will have responsibility for our care if we become incompetent, both our family and our physician, *understand our moral convictions and attitude toward death.* Then they will have the information necessary to make a good decision for us even in changing circumstances.

Pain

Dying patients are often, but not always, in pain, and questions arise about the proper medical treatment. The following considerations are offered to help make ethical decisions concerning pain control (O'Rourke, 1992).

First, pain is not an absolute human evil. Although suffering is to be alleviated whenever possible, it is not of itself a moral evil nor without supernatural and human benefits when rightly used (see also chapter 13.1). Some will scoff at this view of life, but the Christian tradition holds that great spiritual good can come out of suffering when this is joined to the suffering of Jesus. Christian teaching in this regard is often misrepresented, but it does not imply a masochistic desire for pain, nor does it stand in the way of medical progress. As one group of Christians who have investigated the situation (Amulree et al., 1975) maintain, "A terminal illness can be transformed into a time for which everyone concerned is grateful."

Second, alleviating pain by means of medicine or even by surgery does not constitute euthanasia, even if the suffering person's life might be shortened as a result of the medical or surgical procedure (CDF, 1980a; John Paul II, 1995, n. 65). In this case, the direct object of the act is to relieve pain; if life is shortened, it is an accidental, even though foreseen, result. This view is expressed succinctly in the *Ethical and Religious Directives* (NCCB, 1994):

> *Directive 61.* Patients should be kept as free of pain as possible so that they may die comfortably and with dignity, and in the place where they wish to die. Since a person has the right to prepare for his or her death while fully conscious, he or she should not be deprived of consciousness without compelling reason. Medicines capable of alleviating or suppressing pain may be given to a dying person, even if this therapy may indirectly shorten the person's life, so long as the intent is not to hasten death. Patients

experiencing suffering that cannot be alleviated should be helped to appreciate the Christian understanding of redemptive suffering.

It should be noted that: (1) the "compelling reason" for rendering a patient unconscious (provided of course that the person has already had the opportunity to receive the sacraments) could be that no other way of relieving extreme pain can be found. Thus the argument that euthanasia is necessary to relieve unbearable pain is false, since it is always possible as a last resort short of death to render the patient unconscious. (2) The argument used by some advocates of euthanasia that their intent is not to kill but to relieve suffering is an evasion, since in fact their intention is to kill as a means to relieve suffering. It thus fails to meet the condition of the principle of double effect, which requires that the means used not be intrinsically evil.

The opportunity to use suffering as a means of spiritual growth is not destroyed if pain-killing drugs are used. Rather, the individual and those who care for him or her have the right to use such drugs in a way that will permit the best use of the patient's remaining energies and time of consciousness, so that the patient can complete life with maximal composure.

Third, in recent years medical and psychological breakthroughs have occurred in regard to severe pain (Foley, 1991; Cleeland et al., 1994; American Pain Society, 1992). Medically speaking, pharmaceutical and surgical procedures make it possible to control and alleviate severe pain in the hospital and at home. Severe and excruciating pain, then, is hardly a realistic excuse for direct euthanasia or suicide. Moreover, an even more startling discovery in the control of pain has been made by people in the hospice movement (Saunders, 1994). Case studies demonstrate that pain is alleviated and controlled when human concern and care are given to the elderly. The ultimate human pain seems to be loneliness and the feeling of dying alone. If these feelings are overcome, it seems that pain is not such a prominent factor, even for those who are dying of debilitating disease (Kubler-Ross, 1969, 1978; Torrens, 1985).

Pastoral Norms

In summary, the following pastoral norms for decision making in regard to allowing a patient to die can be formulated:

1. A physician may admit that a patient is incurable and cease trying to effect a cure; however, physicians should not cease trying to find a remedy for disease itself.
2. As long as there is a slight hope for curing patients or checking the progress of their illness, the physician should use the available remedies at hand, if this is the desire of the patient or proxy. However, the patient or proxy may refuse treatment if it is ineffective or constitutes a serious burden to the patient, the family, or even society (NCCB, 1994, D. 57). The burden may be psychic, social, or spiritual, as well as physiological.

3. The patient, considering his or her medical prognosis as well as other spiritual and temporal circumstances of life, should determine in consultation with the physician whether a particular means is ordinary or extraordinary from an ethical point of view.

4. If the means are ordinary, they must be used; if the means are extraordinary, they may be used but need not be. Minimal means of maintaining the patient's comfort and well-being are always considered ordinary means.

5. If the patient is unable to make the pertinent decisions, family members, in consultation with the physician, should have the right and obligation to determine whether the means in question are ordinary or extraordinary and whether extraordinary means will be used. In making this decision, the family should decide as the patient would and for the benefit of the patient, not solely for the benefit of the family.

6. Such documents as the *Advanced Directive: A Christian Perspective* may be used by patients as a means of informing family and physician and as a help in preparing for death (deBlois, McGrath, O'Rourke, 1991). We do not, however, favor that such documents be given legal status. Although legal documents are not in themselves wrong, they do not solve the problems of decision making, and potentially they may led to disrespect for human life and inhumane care for the dying.

CONCLUSION

Many of the acute ethical issues in health care are concerned in one way or another with suffering and death. We have indicated that we believe it is essential for health care professionals to be able to face death in a spiritual and psychologically balanced manner. Otherwise, they will be unable to care for patients in a beneficial and personally fulfilling manner. Moreover, we call attention to the social developments in regard to suffering and death. Inflicting death is a new method of solving human problems. A unique responsibility belongs to health care professionals in circumventing and opposing the incipient "culture of death." "The deepest inspiration and strongest support of a health care professional lies in the intrinsic and undeniable ethical dimension of the health care profession, something already recognized by the still relevant Hippocratic Oath, which requires all doctors to commit themselves to absolute respect for human life and its sacredness" (John Paul II, 1995, n. 89).

PART 5

Pastoral Ministry in Health Care

This book deals with persons seeking health, with the health care professionals who serve them in this search, and finally with some of the many difficult ethical decisions professionals and health seekers have to make together. This concluding Part 5, which consists of a single chapter, deals with members of the health care team whose professional status is often not recognized, yet who have a very special, integrative role to perform on that team and its ethical decision making, namely the pastoral care ministers and chaplains. The men and women who carry on this work are, for the most part, highly qualified and able to minister to patients at their deepest level of need. Since a Catholic health care institution is a community of healing and compassion, the care offered is not limited to the treatment of a disease or bodily ailment but embraces the physical, psychological, social and spiritual dimensions of the human person" (ERD 1994, p. 9).

Much of the material in this section may seem to be liturgical rather than ethical. It sums up the ethical purpose of this book, however, because medical ethics is concerned not with rules about forbidden procedures, but with a healing process that respects the individual sanctity of the individual person and seeks to restore the person to full participation in the community. We first show that pastoral care is needed on the health team not as an adjunct to psychotherapy or social work, but precisely in its service to human persons in their search for spiritual health (14.1), which we argued in Chapter 2 is essential for total health, and also in service to the hospital staff itself (14.2). We then discuss the ways in which the pastoral ministry can make this contribution to health care through spiritual counseling (14.3) and the celebration of the Word and the Sacrament (14.4). In this way, a truly caring and sympathetic community can be formed in which the crisis of ethical decisions can best be met. Finally, in 14.5 we conclude by discussing the ways in which the pastoral minister can assist professionals, patients, and their families in the actual process of ethical decision making.

14
Pastoral Care and
Ethical Decisions

OVERVIEW

Much of the material in this section may seem to be liturgical rather than ethical. It sums up the ethical purpose of this book, however, because medical ethics is concerned not with rules about forbidden procedures, but with a healing process that respects the sanctity of the individual person and seeks to restore the person to full participation in community. We first show that pastoral care is needed on the health team not as an adjunct to psychotherapy or social work, but precisely in its service to human persons in their search for spiritual health (14.1), which we argued in Chapter 2 is essential for total health, and also in service to the hospital staff itself (14.2). We then discuss the ways in which pastoral ministry can make this contribution to health care through spiritual counseling (14.3) and the celebration of Word and Sacrament (14.4). In this way, a truly caring and therapeutic community can be formed in which the crises of ethical decisions can best be met. Finally, in 14.5 we conclude by discussing the ways in which the pastoral minister can assist professionals, patients, and their families in the actual process of ethical decision making.

14.1 PASTORAL MINISTRY AND THE HEALTH CARE TEAM

Need for Pastoral Health care

If Christian ministry is to be Christ-like, care for the sick undoubtedly is an essential part of it. At least a third of the Gospel according to St. Mark, aside from the passion narrative devoted to Jesus' own suffering and death, is devoted to accounts of how Jesus healed the physically and mentally sick. His care for the sick seems to have been the clearest evidence to others of his mission from the Father and of the life-giving truth of his preaching.

Studies devoted to the history of pastoral care (Clebsch and Jaekle, 1964; Holifield, 1983) conclude that, traditionally, religious ministry has four functions: (1) to heal, (2) to sustain, (3) to guide, and (4) to reconcile. Whereas by healing and sustaining they have in mind something broader than physical and psychological healing and encouragement in times of sickness, it is obvious that ministers cannot heal and sustain if they are not intimately concerned with problems of physical and psychological health. Furthermore, we show in later sections that guidance and reconciliation are in some respects especially effective when they occur in times of health crisis. The *Ethical and Religious Directives for Catholic Health Care Services* (ERD, 1994) says:

> Directed to spiritual needs that are often appreciated more deeply during times of illness, pastoral care is an integral part of Catholic health care. Pastoral care encompasses the full range of spiritual services, including a listening presence; help dealing with powerlessness, pain, and alienation; and assistance in recognizing and responding to God's will with greater joy and peace (Part Two: Introduction).

The hospital in Western culture (6.3) originated in the religious care of the sick and only with the rise of humanism in the eighteenth century began to subordinate that concern to purely medical care. Even in the nineteenth century, however, the nursing profession in its modern form was the creation of Florence Nightingale, herself inspired by the Christian ideals of the Anglican Church and her work inspired by the tradition of the Catholic nursing sisters.

Today, however, in many hospitals, pastoral care is left to occasional visiting ministers who are treated much as any other visitor. In others a chaplain is provided, but he or she is regarded by the medical staff simply as a convenience to the patients such as the hospital barber or proprietor of the gift shop. It is becoming much more common, however, even for public hospitals to include a department of pastoral care as a recognized part of their therapeutic work. The men and women of such a department are still often regarded as somewhat less than professional colleagues of the medical staff, who think of them according to outmoded stereotypes (Vande Creek and Shopland, 1991).

The first reason for this situation is the secularization of the medical profession, which believes itself neutral to religious concerns. This is the case even in many, perhaps most, Catholic and other church-related hospitals, where a large part of the medical staff may not be members of the sponsoring church. Even when a Catholic hospital has a largely Catholic medical staff, these health care professionals may still conceive their own tasks as rigidly separated from the concerns of pastoral care. Our interpretation of this secularization, on which we insist throughout this book, is that it is neither neutral, nor genuinely pluralistic, but sincere fidelity to humanism as an equivalent religion.

Thus the question arises as to whether a purely secular hospital serving principally humanist patients (who make up probably at least 40 percent of the American public) should have a pastoral care department and, if so, what its character should be. We believe that such a health care facility would still need a pastoral care department. The purpose of such a department would be to help patients deal with the existential (spiritual) problems that arise so acutely in times of illness or dying. The recent spate of books and articles on death and dying, many written from a purely humanist point of view, are evidence of this concern (Kubler-Ross, 1969; Rachels, 1983; Battin, 1994). Also, this need cannot be met adequately by psychotherapists or social workers. Some psychotherapists have developed an existential psychology to deal with human problems at this deeper level. For reasons already given in Chapter 12, however, this exceeds the professional competence of therapists, who are not ordinarily prepared to deal with philosophical issues concerning the meaning of life and with questions of ethical evaluation.

Since today most hospitals are pluralistic, a counselor working from the viewpoint of humanism must also be prepared to assist patients of other faiths. To do so, the humanist counselor must be able to take an honestly ecumenical approach, not scorning the value systems of Catholics, Protestants, Jews, Muslims, Hindus, Buddhists, Native Americans, or Afro-Americans. To do this adequately, a humanist spiritual care department would probably have to include some professionals committed to the major faiths.

The same standards, on the other hand, should hold also for church-sponsored health care facilities. In a Catholic hospital, pastoral care should be thoroughly Catholic, but as the Second Vatican Council has taught, being truly Catholic requires accepting pluralism and ecumenism. Thus Catholic hospitals should provide pastoral care for the large number of humanist patients who say they "have no religion," are "not interested in religion," and so forth (Directive 22, NCCB, 1994). Such care should respect the system of values by which humanist patients live and should avoid denominational pressures. At the same time, it should not neglect the need of such patients to deal with the problems of suffering, death, alienation, and loneliness on their own terms.

A second reason for the ambiguous situation of pastoral care in many hospitals is that in fact the chaplain or others occupied in pastoral care lack specialized professional training to work with the sick. Although all ministerial education includes general skill in pastoral health care, assignments to a chaplaincy or pastoral care department in a modern hospital require specialization. Catholic hospitals only recently have begun to move away from the period when the local bishop supplied the hospitals of his diocese with a chaplain priest, often one unable to accept a regular pastoral assignment because of age or illness, but who could reside at the hospital and administer the sacraments. Catholic hospitals are now hiring only those chaplains certified for special training and competency in health care.

Appointment to the Pastoral Care Staff

In Catholic hospitals, the pastoral care staff usually includes at least one priest, deacon, whether temporary or permanent, several religious or lay people, and in some facilities pastoral representatives of churches other than Catholic. All members of the pastoral staff are denominated as chaplains, even though at one time this term was reserved for ordained clergy (NACC, 1995).

The *Ethical and Religious Directives* require that priests and deacons be appointed to the pastoral care staff of Catholic health care facilities by the local bishop in collaboration with the local institution (NCCB, 1994, D. 21). Religious and laity, it seems, are appointed by the administration of the facility, as is the director of the pastoral care team. If the director is not a Catholic however, then his or her appointment must also be approved by the local bishop. While the appointment of pastoral care personnel from other churches is recommended in Directive 22, the process of appointment is left to "diocesan policy." Since few dioceses have policies in this regard, the freedom of the administration to appoint persons to this task seems reasonable. Finally, it seems that an appointment to the pastoral care staff, whether by bishop or administration, carries with it the special designation needed to constitute one as a minister of the Church (O'Meara, 1983). For this reason, we use the words chaplain and minister interchangeably in this section.

Preparation of Pastoral Care Professionals

The development of *clinical pastoral education* (CPE) as the result of the pioneering work of Anton Boisen (1936, 1945) and its accreditation through a national association involved a shift to a more psychotherapeutic approach to the sick (Hiltner, 1969; Cobb, 1977; Derrickson and Ebersolo, 1986). This shift agreed in some respects with the traditional Protestant emphasis on pastoral counseling, but it produced a certain tension in ministerial identity for those who found it hard to reconcile the moralistic and evangelistic emphasis of their tradition with modern psychotherapy's stress on guiltless self-expression.

Because of their emphasis on sacramental ministry, in which counseling was often largely restricted to hearing confessions, Catholics were slower to accept the new psychotherapeutic approach. After the Second Vatican Council, however, CPE began to be a regular part of priestly formation in many seminaries, and the National Association of Catholic Chaplains (NACC) began to develop its own programs and certification in specialized pastoral ministry. Here again the tension between traditional types of ministry and psychotherapeutic emphasis has not yet been completely resolved (Duffy, 1983).

Although CPE or its equivalent has served to make ministers of pastoral health care more professional and has thus somewhat improved their status with medical staffs, it has also raised the question as to whether pastoral care is simply another form of psychotherapy and social work. Until pastoral care people themselves have a clearer theology of pastoral care and a surer sense of their specific identity, they will have difficulty being accepted as professionals by hospital administrators and medical staffs. To sum up, the *Ethical and Religious Directives* state:

> A Catholic health care organization should provide pastoral care to minister to the religious and spiritual needs of all those it serves. Pastoral care personnel—clergy, religious, and lay alike—should have appropriate professional preparation, including an understanding of these Directives (D. 10).

Pastoral Care and Other Health Care Services

In seeking their proper role in health care, pastoral care personnel often claim that they deal with the whole person or the patient as a person, whereas other health care professionals are more concerned with special parts of the person.

On the contrary, some physicians believe that it is the medical doctor who is the only complete health care professional, who must therefore head the health care team and make the final decision in all matters. Thus the physician deals with health care as a whole, while other members of the team, including pastoral care persons, deal only with special or incidental aspects of the patient's health problem (6.4). Thus such a physician sometimes consider the ministry of the pastoral care as merely partial, auxiliary, or incidental and resents as presumptuous and intrusive any claim on the part of pastoral care to deal with the whole person.

This controversy about whole and part can be clarified by realizing that different wholes are in question. In viewing the patient under the aspect of *physical* health, the physician is the chief of any health care team and *de jure* has the ultimate decision in presenting to the patient an evaluation of a possible course of treatment, although *de facto* a nurse, dietician, physical therapist, or pharmacist may actually know more about the patient. The ultimate decision, however, remains with the patient or those responsible for the incompetent patient (Katz, 1994).

As whole persons in making their decisions about how to use the services of the health care team, patients must take into consideration other aspects of personality than physical health. Consequently, patients need the help and counsel of the psychotherapist, the ethical counselor, and the spiritual guide. In taking such counsel, it is clear that to the patients, physical health is only a *part* of the problem; in this problem the ethical and spiritual aspects are more inclusive than the psychotherapeutic or physical aspects of the person's health (see Chapters 1 and 2). From this point of view, patients, after receiving the physician's advice, may need to take ultimate counsel with their minister, priest, or some other equivalent spiritual guide. Sensitive physicians are quick to realize this and are happy not to stretch their responsibility beyond their professional competence for physical or, perhaps, mental health.

Nevertheless, chaplains, insofar as they stand for the personhood of the patient in its totality and its ultimately spiritual character, have the obligation to defend the patient as a person in conflict situations, against both unjust actions of the staff and imprudence or negligence of the family or other guardians.

On behalf of the whole person, the first task of the health care ministry is to help patients understand the several dimensions of any health decision. Thus in a hospital it is reasonable that the pastoral care department play a significant role in receiving and dismissing patients. Entering patients need to look forward to their experience in the hospital as one over which they have genuine control, and they should leave it feeling they are prepared to go on with normal life. Chaplains can help patients achieve this sense of self-control at a time when patients often feel they are helpless.

The foregoing tasks of the health care ministry, however, important as they are, remain secondary to its specific and central task of helping patients grow through their experience of sickness and convalescence or of death. But before discussing this principal work of health care ministry, we must discuss the responsibility of the pastoral care people for the other members of the health care team.

14.2 MINISTRY TO THE HOSPITAL STAFF

Not only the patients are persons, but so also are the members of the administrative and medical staffs and all the auxiliary personnel. Today it is well recognized in hospitals that the mental health of the staff is an important factor in the therapy of the patients (Fath, 1985). In fact, in any health care facility the effectiveness of health care depends in large part on the type of interpersonal relations that exist among its staff. Ultimately, this is a spiritual problem, since physicians, nurses, and others engaged in the very difficult vocation of caring for the suffering and confronting the crises of life and death are engaged in their own spiritual struggle.

Staff members need help to maintain their sense of dedication, their courage, and their human compassion against all temptations of routine, cynicism, callousness, and ambition. If the Christian Church from a long and often bitter historical experience has accepted the motto *ecclesia semper reformanda* ("the Church needs constant renewal"), this must be equally true of hospitals and the health care profession. Only on the basis of this constant effort to renew Christian humanism within the staff is there any real hope of sound ethical judgment in the care of patients.

Intrastaff Problems

The pastoral care department as a whole will be concerned with bringing to the hospital's attention administration issues of interpersonal relationships within the staff that affect the workings of the institution and the good of the patients. Most pastoral care ministers soon learn of many of these interpersonal issues informally through members of the administrative and medical staffs who come to them for counsel and encouragement.

Although pastoral care people usually attempt to help those who come to them with such intrastaff difficulties with as much tact as they can muster, accusations of interference in medical or administrative matters can easily result. For pastoral care people to react to such criticism by confining their concern to private counseling often seems like neglect of responsibility to the institution and the patients it serves.

First, we would suggest that the chaplain or director of the pastoral care department or some representative of that department who is especially competent should be included on the ethics committee of the hospital. This will provide a channel for raising ethical issues.

Second, the staff should be thoroughly informed of the religious and counseling services that the pastoral care department is ready to provide to them. It is important here, for example, that a Catholic hospital let the personnel know they are welcome at the Eucharist and for personal confession or counseling. It is also important (and often neglected) to let non-Catholics know that the department has considered their needs, studied them, and made some provision for them in a way that is convenient and free of embarrassment.

Third, the director should have a recognized procedure by which discussion can be facilitated with the administration, with the medical staff, with whatever group represents the nurses, and with the union or other representative body of the hospital employees, concerning issues of interpersonal relationships that the members of the pastoral care department may have observed are affecting patient or institutional welfare. Naturally, administrators may be reluctant to give the director this formal access to groups in the hospital with which the administration may be at odds. Unless such recognized access exists, however, the director or chaplain will not be able to play that role of arbitrator and peacemaker which must be a primary and spiritual ethical concern of any truly human institution. Ethics is always concerned about the tension between justice and social harmony. It is absurd to speak of an institution's concern for medical ethics if it does not recognize the need for this type of peacemaking as a truly ministerial function.

Coministry

If the pastoral care department is to fulfill this role, its members must have a profound respect for those who dedicate their lives to the healing profession and should acknowledge that Christian ministry to the sick is not a monopoly of the pastoral care department (Lawler, 1994). For Catholics, the Second Vatican Council (1965c) reemphasized the ancient concept of "the universal priesthood of the believers," according to which Christ's ministry is not confined to ordained clergy. In its three-fold function of teaching, shepherding, and worshiping, this ministry is shared in a variety of ways by every member of the Christian community so that all Christians are ministers along with Christ, who himself is the Servant of the Father (O'Meara, 1983). Consequently, all Christians also share in pastoral ministry to the sick. Jesus made this one of the responsibilities for love of neighbor on which all persons are to be judged (Mt 25:31, n. 46).

In a very special way, therefore, the physicians, nurses, administrators, and all the members of a hospital staff are carrying out not merely a secular service but a genuine Christian ministry of healing, deriving its authority from Christ's own healing work and witnessing to his continuing presence in the world. Thus the pastoral care department not only should refrain from monopolizing the religious aspect of health care, but should also carry on an educational effort to help the hospital staff appreciate the spiritual and ethical values of their own professional work (CHA, 1994).

With this respect for their coministers should also come an increased sensitivity by pastoral care people to how some medical professionals are warped or destroyed as persons by the tensions under which they work. From such insight should come a creative effort to suggest and develop ways in which justice, charity, and peace can heal the "wounded healers" (Nouwen, 1972). Finally, it is important that the pastoral care department itself provide a model of true humanity and good interpersonal relations.

14.3 SPIRITUAL COUNSELING IN HEALTH CARE

Trust

We have discussed some of the functions which the religious minister can perform as an integrator of health care in the interest of the total health of the human person, but we have not yet discussed the specifically spiritual role of the minister. The reason that some have confused pastoral care with psychotherapy is because they are uncertain about what "spiritual ministry" really means or how it can contribute significantly to the patient's healing. To discuss this problem, we first begin with the question as to how spiritual counseling differs from psychological counseling as these occur during a person's stay in a hospital or longterm care facility. By counseling, we mean the effort to offer spiritual help through conversation or direction. We do not intend to intimate that every chaplain is *ipso facto* a professional counselor realizing that this title is often subject to state licensing.

Persons who are ill are faced with potentially serious problems:

1. They may fear suffering and death.
2. They may face the uncertainties of diagnosis and prognosis and fear about the pain or embarrassment of various testing or treatment procedures either unfamiliar to them or all too painfully familiar.
3. They may face the tedium of a long stay in the health care facility under circumstances they find either boring or excruciating.
4. They suffer separation from their regular work, friends, and family and are not comfortable in the new situation.
5. They may be worried and perhaps feel guilty about the various responsibilities at home that they cannot handle.
6. They suffer from a sense of deprivation of privacy and of freedom, almost as if they were imprisoned.
7. They may feel puzzled about *Why has this happened to me?* and may interpret their sickness as punishment for moral guilt or experience the "silence of God." They may also anticipate further guilt through failure in courage and hope.
8. They may feel alone and deserted in meeting all the foregoing, and their sense of dignity, worth, and membership in the human community may be diminished by real moral guilt for which God's forgiveness is truly needed. Their prayer is that of Psalm 41:

> Once I said, Lord, have pity on me;
>> heal me, though I have sinned against you.
> My enemies say the worst of me:
>> "When will he die and his name be perish?" . . .
> Against me they imagine the worst:
>> "A malignant disease fills his fame";
>>> and "Now he lies ill, he will not rise again."

Spiritual ministers in their own proper role are called on to help patients in these struggles and may also be called on to help members of the health team who are faced with similar problems both in their personal lives and in their professional involvement with patients. The first task of the spiritual guide is to establish *trust*, but this trust differs from that on which most professional relations are based because it has a type of ultimacy. People often seek out a spiritual minister to confide in when they can no longer trust their lawyer, physician, or even their psychiatrist.

Yet many patients do not even trust a minister, and when the chaplain visits them they are thinking, What is his or her game? Is she trying "to save my soul," to make a convert out of me? Is he looking for an offering? Or for a confession? Thus chaplains must build up trust on the foundation not of words but of behavior. A chaplain must keep promises, maintain contact, and be available to help in whatever difficulty is bothering the patient or to look for someone who can help. A chaplain must also be nonjudgmental, empathetic, and very careful about confidentiality. Finally, a chaplain's care is expected to extend beyond the patient to the patient's family.

Nevertheless, as in other counseling, this trust has its limits, and ministers must make clear to those they serve that a spiritual counselor has limited powers (Nouwen, 1990). Otherwise, the trust between chaplain and patient will soon appear to be violated. Thus chaplains should explain that (1) they cannot work miracles at will, or change structures, or get the patient out; (2) they cannot be continuously present and can give only limited time to any one patient; and (3) their role is primarily that of a listener, counselor. All this should become clear in the implicit or explicit counseling contract. It is up to counselors to set these limits tactfully and to remember that they are dealing with patients who in their weakened condition have undergone considerable psychological regression, which makes them as dependent and demanding as a child in relation to its parents. The chaplain should give the patient permission for this dependency, but a limited permission. If such limits are not set, the minister will soon find that the patient interprets much that the minister does as a betrayal of trust.

Caring in the Name of the Christian Community

This trust between a spiritual guide and the spiritual pilgrim, between a shepherd and the straying sheep, takes its special character first from the charism of the minister as a person *ordained* sent by the Church. The spiritual guide is an "apostle," that is, one sent by the Church in the name of God on whom the Spirit of God has been invoked by the prayers of the Christian community. Even when guides are not ordained, their ministry must somehow be authorized by the Christian community if it is to be given that special trust that should characterize it (McBrien, 1987). We believe as mentioned above (p. 439 this chapter), that "being sent" is accomplished for persons in Catholic health care facilities through their appointments, either by the bishop or the administration of the facility, to the pastoral care staff. Physicians and psychotherapists in their white coats are often invested with an analogous charisma, as explained in Chapter 4, in speaking of the priestly character of the whole healing profession, but this is only an analogy to the charism of the spiritual guide.

A minister, particularly if young and humble, may find the reverence shown him by a client because of this charism very embarrassing and even unreal. The young chaplain might prefer simply to be on friendly terms with a patient, not to be invested with a halo of mysterious power. Timothy seems to have had the same problem, judging from the advice Paul gave him, "Do not let people disregard you because you are young, but be an example to all the believers in the way you speak and behave, and in your love, your faith, and your purity" (1 Tm 4:12). If ministers have set appropriate limits to their role, however, this charismatic function will not expand absurdly. Yet within these limits, they should accept honestly the task of speaking for God and in his name, however awesome that claim may be.

This requires spiritual counselors to reflect constantly on two realities: first, that God is acting through them to accomplish what is quite beyond their own abilities and, second, that unless they acknowledge their own human limits, they will be placing obstacles in the way of God's work. Ministers who have this correct perception of their own role will not attempt too much, put themselves under impossible strains, or feel guilty at an inability to solve all problems of all patients. On the other hand, they will feel and communicate to patients unlimited hope in the loving power of God and a sense of each patient's dignity in God's eyes and their own (McBrien, 1987). They should make a special effort to make sure if possible that when patients leave a facility they will retain a connection to the Christian community or know how to form such a connection if it has not existed before.

Some ministers are so secularized that they feel more comfortable in a psychotherapeutic role than in a spiritual one and thus fail their patients by refusal to speak in God's name. They avoid talking with patients about spiritual issues, praying with them, or inquiring about their need for the sacraments as if these were forbidden or offensive topics. Patients may very well read this as a lack of faith on a minister's part and thus as a threat to the patient's own faith, which is already sorely tried by doubts and anxieties raised by the patient's condition. Ministers who find themselves in a quandary about their own pastoral identity should attempt to resolve this ambiguity through spiritual guidance and perhaps psychotherapy if they are going to fulfill their responsibility of helping patients in *their* quandaries (Thayer, 1985).

Discernment

The minister, like a psychotherapist, is a listener and a reflector through whom the realities of the patient's situation become clearer to the patient and more manageable. Furthermore, like the psychotherapist, the minister listens not just to what the patient seems to be saying superficially, but to what the patient, perhaps unconsciously, is trying to say nonverbally and symbolically (Wicks et al., 1985).

The psychotherapist, however, is listening for the message that rises from the patient's subconscious emotional drives, whereas the minister as a spiritual therapist is listening for a message that comes from a still deeper level, from that place the Scripture calls the "heart," that is, from the spiritual interior of the person's being where the person is committed to some sort of ultimate values and to some fundamental insight into reality (Nouwen, 1990). In most patients, as in most everyone, this commitment and vision is dim and confused indeed; yet it is the source of all personal life, where people really live and where they really die. "Out of the depths I call to you O Lord, O Lord hear my voice" (Psalm 130). It is this voice *de profundis* to which the minister must listen. Moreover, a spiritual guide is not looking, as is the psychotherapist, for the psychic energies and motivations that flow from human instinctual needs, but for the work of the Holy Spirit in the patient, the signs of faith, hope, and love, and the spiritual forces of sin and alienation that oppose these. This is the spiritual level of human functioning discussed in Chapter 2 (Fichter, 1981; Kelsey, 1982).

The patient may raise these questions directly by saying, "Why has this happened to me, Father? Have I sinned? Am I going to be punished? What will happen to me if I die?" or "I don't seem to be able to pray now that I am sick," and so forth. Today in a secularized society, however, such questions are seldom asked *directly*. Even if they are, the chaplain may very well suspect that they do not really come from the spiritual level of personality but are merely the pious language that some people (especially those who are from a fundamentalist religious background) use in speaking of purely physical or psychological problems (Browning, 1987). Also, the patient may think that this is the way you are supposed to converse with a minister, who is supposed only to talk that type of religious language. Therefore the counselor has to listen to religious questions inherent in pseudoreligious language (Hoff, 1984). In both cases counselors must go deeper to find the really spiritual level in the patient.

This requires patience, and it is usually a mistake to begin asking spiritual questions of a patient with whom the needed level of trust has not yet been established. On the other hand, experienced spiritual counselors learn how to cut through other levels of small talk and psychological talk to the issues with which they have to deal. Simple directness is ordinarily not resented by patients. Catholics are usually not alarmed and even expect "Father" to ask them if they want to go to confession or receive communion and to make some further tactful inquiry if they refuse. *Directness* is not bluntness or insensitivity. It is rather a form of respect for a patient, a refusal simply to play games.

This respect for the person demands that the minister not take advantage of the patient's weak condition (D. McNeill et al., 1982). It is unethical to try to force conversion of patients, accuse them of supposed sin, make demands for prayer or faith, and so forth. It may seem incredible that some ministers carry on such a preaching attack on patients, but many patients will report unpleasant experiences of being confronted by zealous ministers in a hospital and being embarrassed or pressured. Reports of such experiences have done much to prejudice physicians and nurses against the ministerial profession.

The minister who exerts this pressure fails to trust in God's providence, by which God is using the patient's experience of illness as an occasion of possible spiritual growth. The Spirit of God is already at work in the sufferer in ways that are not labeled religious. The minister must recognize this growth process and cultivate it, helping patients to understand what is going on in their own terms (Egan, 1986).

A specific responsibility for ministers is not only to deal with the patient's spiritual problems, but also to help him or her become vividly aware of the real presence of God and of the Church as the People of God in the patient's life in this very event of sickness, where the patient may feel abandoned and isolated. Ministers are themselves a visible sign or sacrament of this presence, incarnating God, as it were, in a tangible, human, imperfect, but real form.

Also, it is not enough that ministers provide this witness of God's presence only to members of their own church. Too many ministers assume that they have responsibility only to their own parishioners or to those of their own denomination and that others will resent their presence. Usually, however, this is not the case. Most laity are less ecclesiastically defined than we think. For them any minister, even a rabbi, is still a "man of God" and as such ought to have some interest in them as "children of God." Even the humanist is seldom content with the silence of humanism in the face of the ultimate questions and is resentful if the religious minister writes him off as a nonbeliever.

Objectives of Pastoral Care

As a spiritual adviser, the minister's primary task is really a very simple but not easy one. It is to say, as much or more by presence, attitude, and nonverbal symbols as by the exhortatory Word, that God is present to sick persons in their fear or suffering, that God as loving, caring Father, as cosuffering Lord Jesus, as Healing Spirit is present and acting, but this presence is in *mystery*. That is, it exceeds human rational empirical comprehension because it leads to an open future. This implies a spiritual awe before the *mysterium tremendum*. The sick person, as did Job, feels guilty and yet is not clear how he or she is guilty. There is a sense of *judgment*. The minister should not deny this. Indeed, a minister symbolizes this judgment. The minister also overcomes judgment, however, by being a sign of mercy and reconciliation (Holst, 1985).

Sickness may be the time of genuine conversion in which persons truly find God for the first time in their lives or after a long time of forgetfulness and separation. The minister must affirm the reality of this invitation of divine mercy, but that is not the whole of the minister's responsibility. Conversion is the beginning of a new life, but that life has to be lived authentically or it will be lost again. Consequently, one of the chief aims of spiritual counseling is to assist converts to begin to grow daily in the Christian life and to plan practically to continue that growth once they have returned to the routine situations of everyday life.

It is important also that the minister, in helping sick persons realize God's presence, also make vivid to them that the minister is a sign of the concern of God's people, of the Christian community or church, for a suffering brother or sister. Sickness is in Old Testament terms a type of "uncleanness," and the patient may experience a "leprosy" of loneliness, alienation, and "excommunication" as an outcast from life and the human community. This is especially true of patients with acquired immunodeficiency syndrome (AIDS). The minister removes this excommunication and reunites the lonely one with the community that is praying for him or her. Recall how Jesus, healing a leper, sent him to a priest to be readmitted to the Jewish community (Mk 1:44). Recall as well, how Jesus might indicate that the cured person should "sin no more," but he never asked people how they became sick or how they contracted their pathologies.

Hospitals today, for various reasons, do not encourage long stays unless really necessary. This means that for most patients the contact with pastoral care is brief. Hence it must be focused on assuring the patient that God through the Christian community is at their side in a difficult moment and that when they leave the hospital it will still be concerned and available to help.

14.4 CELEBRATING THE HEALING PROCESS

Word and Sacrament

The specific spiritual task of pastoral care, however, is not exhausted simply by the counseling situation. It must not be confined to talking about the presence of God, but it must deepen into *experiencing* that presence in prayer, worship, celebration, and communion (Catechism, n. 1135 ff.).

Today, when most chaplains and other ministers as well are training in clinical pastoral education (CPE) programs, they sometimes feel a tension between the model of the chaplain as a pastoral counselor, whose main task is to engage in a therapeutic psychological process with the patient, and the former model of the pastor as the one who reads the Scriptures, prays with and exhorts the patient, and administers the sacraments (Holst, 1985). These two models seem opposed to each other. In particular, one seems aimed at removing feelings of guilt and giving feelings of interpersonal warmth and confidence and getting clients "in touch with their feelings," whereas the other tends to generate guilt and to impose a formalized religious response that covers up a patient's real experience.

Actually the two models, when they are well understood, are complementary and can reinforce each other. We have already shown how pastoral counselors by their own presence are already a *sacrament*, that is, a sign of the presence of God. The Word of God first came to human beings not in the text of the Bible that records his coming, but in the incarnation of Jesus Christ, who came to the sick and suffering, shared their suffering, and healed them by his touch (Schillebeeckx, 1981b). Ministers, because they are sent by Jesus, are the living witnesses, "other Christs," and a sign of Christ's care for the patient. Therefore, everything that the minister does to witness this tender concern, this ability to empathize, to listen, and not to judge, is a sacrament of Jesus' presence. Even humor and light banter, if their purpose is precisely to establish real communication, resemble the wit that Jesus constantly displayed in his preaching and parables. Above all, the down-to-earthiness—the freedom from stuffiness, self-righteousness, and elitism that can be the curse of the clerical state—is in imitation of Jesus, who did not hesitate to eat with sinners in simple fellowship.

Thus, when ministers read the Scripture with patients, they should already have placed the Scripture in a human relational context in which the Word of God can be truly understood. Prayer also must grow out of this living context; that is, it should be natural for two people who have come to share a common concern to give it prayerful expression. A minister should not be praying in front of an embarrassed patient who feels as if something is "being laid on him" in which he has no part. An opening for prayer will come, however, only if the patient senses that the minister's concern for him or her goes *deep,* deeper than the mere professional interest. The Scriptures used should be chosen just because they help to make real the presence of Jesus, especially in his power to forgive, heal, and lead one into the fullness of life (John Paul II, 1984a).

The Catholic priest is more likely than the Protestant minister or the rabbi to be concerned about the administration of the sacraments in the hospital setting. These, too, must be understood not as some ritual intruding into a real situation, but as a ritualization of a process of healing that is already occurring. The primordial sacrament is the touching Jesus used when he healed the leper. "Moved with pity, he said to him, 'I do will it. Be made clean.' The leprosy left him immediately, and he was made clean" (Mk 1:41–42). It indicates the intimate presence, the care, the community, the power of life between Jesus and the sick and outcast. When a chaplain does what is so natural, namely, to hold the hand of sick persons to give them reassurance that the minister is there, that they are not alone, that is the primordial sacramental rite on which all the other sacraments are based—*human bodily contact* as a sign of *spiritual presence.*

Anointing the Sick

In administering the sacraments, using the new rites that the Catholic Church and other liturgical churches have recently improved precisely for this purpose, ministers must try to enhance this character of human contact already present in the counseling situation. What ministers have done as good pastoral counselors, they now deepen and intensify by a sign that combines the verbal word of Scripture with the nonverbal sacramental act.

The new rite of Anointing of the Sick brings this out clearly (see Paul VI, *Apostolic Constitution on the Sacrament of Anointing the Sick,* 1972; Catechism, n. 1500 ff.). It is not merely for the dying, as formerly, but for any person seriously ill. *Serious* should be judged here not merely in physical terms, but also in psychological terms. Thus, when anyone is sick enough that the minister suspects that the thought of possible death with its deep anxiety has entered his or her mind and produced fear and the threat of despair, then the spiritual and perhaps physical healing of the sacrament is needed and should be given. Whenever there is question of major surgery or of any disease that patients know sometimes leads to death and thus raises this fear in their own minds, ministers can anoint. They should not anoint when the illness is one in which recovery is assured and that consequently does not appear to contain any serious threat.

What is the meaning of this rite? First, it is not merely something done by a priest to a patient. Even when ministers are alone, they are there to represent not only God, but also the Christian community (Rahner, 1963). In fact, God is the center of the Christian community, so the priest as minister is there to represent the Trinitarian community into which all Christians are incorporated in the Second Person Incarnate by their baptism. The anxiety of sick persons is that by their illness they are outcasts, aliens to this community. Patients experience this by their isolation from usual daily life and by the threat of death that might take them away forever. What such patients need is the reassurance that their people and their God are still with them. The priest supplies the sign of this by *touching* a patient. This touch means "presence," "acceptance," and as such is common to all the sacraments. It is a special type of touch in this case, however, a *healing* touch because it is the "anointing with oil," a common form of healing remedy that has the sense of soothing pain and infusing life and movement. Its significance as a spiritual healing is given by the words spoken.

This actual form of the sacrament is also preceded by brief scriptural passages that can be expanded. This is in keeping with the general principle of the new rites that each sacrament should begin with a proclamation of the Word of faith, since it is faith that opens the person to God's work and is the beginning of God's gifts.

Communal Nature of the Anointing of the Sick

Although the sacrament is valid with only the priest and the recipient present, this is not the ideal way to perform it. A study made in several public hospitals shows that the physicians and nurses frequently resent the visit of the priest to perform "the Last Rites" (Nolin, 1972). There are several reasons for this. One is the notion, now out of date, that these rites seal the fate of the patient and therefore mark the failure of the medical profession, something that health care professionals hate to face. Again, professionals think the rites may frighten and depress the patient. Another reason, however, is that the priest seems to be a "medicine man" who has been brought in as competition to the medical profession because the family has given up on the physician's efforts. An additional reason is the exclusive character of the rite. Even in Catholic hospitals when the priest arrives, the physicians, nurses, and family often leave the room as if what was going on was merely private and not an act communal prayer. Finally, there is sometimes a simple objection to an outsider coming in to do something for the person, as if the hospital were not all-sufficient.

These misunderstandings can be traced to what is really poor pastoral theology and practice. If the purpose of the sacrament is to help patients escape their sense of isolation, it is best if family and friends can be present, which would include when possible the nurse and physician. Furthermore, if the sacrament is not to mark the end of life, but to help in the healing process, both physical and spiritual, it is certainly not separated from or in competition with the medical work of the hospital. Rather, it is part of that healing process. In fact, it is a celebration of God's healing work, which God performs not only through the ritual, but also through the *ministry* of the physicians, nurses, and administration. Priests are not the only ministers of health; they are part of a psychosomatic healing *team*, every member of which is called by God to a healing work and empowered by him through their natural gifts and education. The priest's special role on this team is to make explicit and eucharistic (thankful) the work of all.

It is essential to realize that the sacraments are not performed merely in the ritual moment. Rather, they are the celebration of a culminating moment (not necessarily the last) of the saving work of God that has gone on for some time through what are apparently merely secular events. Therefore, it is fitting not only that physicians and nurses be present at the anointing, but also that they participate in it by reading the Scriptures or saying some of the prayers and by imposing hands on the patient or making the sign of the cross. Priests, in their instruction and commentary and by additions to some of the prayers, if necessary, should thank God for the healing gifts and work of the medical staff. It would be very appropriate for patients also at this time to express their thanks to the physicians and nurses.

This expansion of the ritual can best be done when the sacrament takes place at the Eucharist in the hospital chapel, but it can also be done in the hospital room or ward when the physician can be present. The patient's confession when this is necessary would, of course, be done privately before the ceremony begins. The proper rite for the dying patient is not the Anointing of the Sick but the reception of *Viaticum,* or final communion (NCCB, 1994, D. 16.). This is the expression of the sick person's communion and unity with the Church on earth, which prays for his or her swift passage to the eternal banquet. Thus this communion should be shared with others present if possible.

Special Problems About the Sacrament of the Sick

When an emergency arises and someone must be anointed who has not yet received the sacrament in an illness, it is necessary to perform it quickly; but if the patient recovers consciousness, it is possible to hold a healing service of prayer so that the patient can more fully participate in the fruits of the sacrament. In the case of a person who is doubtfully alive, the Sacrament of Anointing should be administered, but the new ritual forbids it to be given to someone who has already died.

Previously priests were advised to administer the sacrament to someone who had recently died—up to two or three hours—if the death had been sudden. The ritual no longer prescribes this. In the present liturgical transition, however, when many people are still poorly instructed with regard to the Sacrament of Anointing, a Catholic family may be very disconsolate to hear that the sacrament was not received. Priests, therefore, may prudently judge in given circumstances whether they might better administer the anointing conditionally, where there is still some doubt (even minimal) that life still remains, for the sake of the family. Perhaps a better procedure is to assure the family that the patient received the proper rites of the Church, meaning by this that the priest has prayed for the departed and blessed the body, since in such circumstances these are the proper rites according to the present discipline. It is important to instruct people that the Church prays daily for all its members and that no one departs this life without the powerful intercession of the Church. In these ecumenical times, chaplains should not hesitate to administer anointing to non-Catholics who might present themselves at a general anointing service, since they probably are baptized and of good faith. If not, the sacrament still constitutes a prayer for their healing.

The Sacrament of Reconciliation

Unfortunately in recent years many Catholics do not make frequent use of the Sacrament of Reconciliation, i.e., "confession." Conversion is not easy for anybody, since it means deep change of heart and life. Unless we are reminded of its urgency, we put it off. Moreover, not a few Catholics today have not been well instructed on why confession is important or even how to go about its proper performance. Sickness is sometimes the reminder that we need and it is important that pastoral care facilitate conversion. Jesus' message was, "This is the time of fulfillment. The kingdom of God is at hand. Repent and believe in the good news!" (Mk 1:15). The good news is that God through his ministers helps us to repent and believe and thus opens up to us the joy of belonging to his kingdom. Those who have deeply experienced this joy of forgiveness and new hope now can make sickness into a blessing.

In his encyclical "On Reconciliation and Penance" (1984a), Pope John Paul II has given a full explanation of this sacrament and has said of "contrition," or the sorrow for sin which it requires, the following:

> *Conversion* and *contrition* are often considered under the aspect of the undeniable demands which they involve and under the aspect of the mortification which they impose for the purpose of bringing about a radical change of life. But we do well to recall and emphasize the fact that *contrition* and *conversion* are even more a drawing near to the holiness of God, a rediscovery of one's true identity which has been upset and disturbed by sin, a liberation in the very depth of self and thus a regaining of lost joy, the joy of being saved, which the majority of people in our time are no longer capable of experiencing. . . . It is the act of the Prodigal Son who returns to his Father and is welcomed by him with the kiss of peace. It is an act of honesty and courage. It is an act of entrusting oneself, beyond sin, to the mercy that forgives. Thus we understand why the confession of sins must ordinarily be individual and not collective, just as sin is a deeply personal matter. But at the same this confession in a way forces sin out of the secret of the heart and thus out of the area of pure individuality, emphasizing its social character as well, for through the minister of pen-

ance it is the ecclesial community, which has been wounded by sin, that welcomes anew the repentant and forgiven sinner.

Because sin is an injury to oneself and one's neighbor as well as a rejection of God's guidance and love, conversion is not just an act between God and the sinner, but between them and Christian community as well. While we can ask God's forgiveness alone, this is not complete until we have also asked the forgiveness of the community, which can be pronounced only by an ordained priest who represents the Christian community and has been sent by God to announce his mercy.

This Sacrament of Reconciliation or *Rite of Penance* (Catechism, N.1449, 1482) for the sick can be celebrated in the form of a penance service in the hospital chapel or even in the ward, with the invitation to all who wish to make individual confession and receive absolution. Such a service is an opportunity for the priest to deal with the question of sin and guilt and the meaning of suffering and of mercy and hope. When confession is made in a ward, it should be remembered that if it is difficult to achieve sufficient privacy, the penitent can be instructed simply to make a general acknowledgment of sins and to speak of them in detail in a future confession.

Baptism and Eucharist

If the patient is unbaptized and wishes to become a Catholic Christian, the new ritual should be followed (RCIA, 1993). When patients have been baptized as Protestants but wish to be Catholic, they should be received as members of the Catholic community and confirmed (Kiesling, 1974). What about the infant in danger of death or the unconscious dying person?

Today even some Catholics are raising questions about infant baptism. This, however, seems to have Pelagian overtones because it implies that the grace of God can only be received on one's initiative. In truth, baptism is a sign of the pure gift of God, the gift of faith and justification that comes to people without any merit on their part merely because they do not reject it. Before the infant is born, he or she is already subject to the grace of God through the prayers of the Church. Infant baptism is the public ratification of accepting infants, alienated from God through no fault of their own by the sins of society (original sin), into union with the Three Persons of the Trinity. This act of incorporating the infant into the life of the human community begins biologically and sociologically with conception and birth. Why, then, should not the infant also be incorporated into the redeemed community of the Church? Jesus said, "Let the children come to me; do not prevent them, for the kingdom of God belongs to such as these" (Mk 10:14), meaning not that children because of their innocence are in no need of grace, but that they do not reject this gift as adults often do. Consequently, it is certain that baptism can be validly conferred on the child from the moment of conception and probable that it can be conferred on any unconscious adult (although not certain, since the person may have positively rejected the grace of God).

From this some theologians in the past concluded that it is essential that all children in danger of death, even in utero, should be baptized and encouraged the baptism of all doubtfully baptized adults who had not actually refused baptism. This was based on the idea that salvation without baptism (at least *in voto,* i.e., "baptism of desire") was impossible, since it is a matter of faith that persons can only be saved through Christ and thus through his Church. Augustinian theologians came to the inescapable but embarrassing conclusion (to a Christian believing in God's mercy, as Augustine strongly did) that unbaptized children are damned. St. Thomas found a way out of this embarrassment by pointing out that it is possible (1) for unbaptized children to enjoy a natural happiness (Limbo) even if they are not admitted to the inner mystery of God, the existence of which they have never been aware, and (2) for unbaptized adults to be saved by an implicit desire for baptism if they have conscientiously followed what light God has given them.

The *Catechism of the Catholic Church* (#1257) teaches:

The Lord himself affirms that Baptism is necessary for salvation [Jn 3:5]. He also commands his disciples to proclaim the Gospel to all nations and to baptize them [Mt 28:9, n. 20]. Baptism is necessary for salvation for those to whom the Gospel has been proclaimed and who have the possibility of asking for this sacrament. The Church does not know of any means other than Baptism that assures entry into eternal beatitude; this is why she takes care not to neglect the mission she has received from the Lord to see that all who can be baptized are "reborn of water and the Spirit." *God has bound salvation to the sacrament of Baptism, but he himself is not bound by his sacraments.*

Thus the Catholic Church does not deny that the grace of Christ in ways known only to God can be given to anyone in the world without baptism, but it strives to fulfill its commission from Christ to preach the Gospel to all and to offer baptism to those who accept it and to their children. Moreover, the *prayer* of the Church for all persons is often efficacious even when it cannot be ritually expressed in the sacraments (see 1 Co 7:14). Thus theologians today generally are of the view that infants dying before baptism can already be graced through the prayer of the Church (especially of the child's family) and by that grace of Christ will enter into the intimate mystery of God. The Sacred Congregation for the Doctrine of the Faith (CDF, 1980b) says in its Instruction on Infant Baptism, "As for infants who have died without baptism, the Church can do nothing but commend them to the mercy of God, as in fact she does in the funeral rite designed for them" (USCC, 1969, n. 82).

Nevertheless, it still is obligatory to administer baptism to manifest the concern of the Church and thus to keep alive the consciousness of the dignity of the human person from the first moments of existence (CDF, 1980b; USCC, 1971b). Consequently, nurses and physicians should baptize infants who are in danger of death and even miscarried fetuses who exhibit human form and some sign of life. They should pour water on the child (on the head, if possible) so as actually to touch its skin and should say, "I baptize you in the name of the

Father, the Son, and the Holy Spirit." In this way they express Christian reverence and fellowship with this little person who will forever be part of the Trinitarian community. If the infant is surely dead, baptism should not be administered, but the family of the infant may be assured that God's mercy has been implored through the prayers of the Church.

For the dying unconscious adult, it is permissible also to perform such a baptism with the condition, "If you are not baptized, I baptize you." Clearly this is not a grave obligation unless the person has asked to be baptized before lapsing into unconsciousness. This should not be done in a merely mechanical manner (trying to baptize everyone in the hospital, etc.) but only when there is some sign or probability that the person if conscious would be receptive of the sacrament. In our U.S. culture, secularized as it is, surveys have shown that the great majority of people have at least some belief in God and reverence for Jesus and thus would be open to whatever help the Church has to offer in prayer and sacrament. As part of the physician and nurse's care for particular persons in their charge whom they believe have given some indication that they might wish such baptism, they may confer it on dying infants or conditionally on unconscious persons, provided this can be done without offense to their families. Again, this shows the Church's concern for a person who has providentially come under the care of the Catholic community.

The Eucharist

The Eucharist is the supreme sacrament and sign of the Christian community, indicating that such patients remain a part of that community, even when absent from the public worship assembly, and that they are destined for eternal life with the community (Catechism, N. 1211, 1374). It is a life-giving, health-giving sacrament, since the eating of bread and drinking of wine are the basic symbols of the power to live and under these signs Jesus, the Lord of Life, is himself present to give us eternal life. After Jesus raised the daughter of Jairus, "He told them to give her something to eat" (Lk 8:55). Again, St. Paul believed (1 Co 11:27–31) the unworthy reception of the Eucharist leads to sickness and death because this hypocrisy cuts a person off from the God of the living.

Today the Eucharist is often distributed by auxiliary ministers, as well as by the priest. This is appropriate, since in the earliest days communion was taken from the public assembly to the homes of the sick. In a hospital it would be appropriate when possible (and the current practice with regard to the fast before communion makes this easy) to have the patients who wish to listen to the Mass in the chapel on closed-circuit radio or television then to be brought communion immediately after the Mass. In this way the union between Mass and communion would be emphasized. It is essential in any case that communion in the health care facility should not be reduced to a routine in which someone pops in and out of a room to place a wafer in a sleepy patient's mouth. We would suggest at least a card containing Scripture reading and prayers that a patient can use while preparing for communion.

Lay Ministers

What can ministers who are not priests do? Today religious sisters and brothers and laypeople share in the sacramental ministry. We have already mentioned that anyone can administer baptism who intends to do what the Church does in this most necessary of all sacraments. It has been theologically disputed whether it might be possible for the Church to delegate to a deacon or even to nonordained persons the Anointing of the Sick, as Confirmation has been delegated by bishops to priests, but according to the *Catechism of the Catholic Church* (#1461–1467 and 1516), this is not valid. It is permitted, however, for deacons and nonordained persons, men or women, to hold a service of healing (U.S. Catholic Conference, 1979). This can consist of Scripture readings, prayers, and the laying on of hands for the sick. They can also make use of blessed oil as a sacramental. It would seem, however, that in such services it should be made clear to all that what is taking place is not a sacrament in the strict sense. This does not mean, however, that the prayer is inefficacious. Jesus said, "Where two or three are gathered together in my name, there am I in the midst of them" (18:20). Rather, it is *preparatory* to the full public visit of the priest to the sick as a representative of the whole Christian community. Just as the physician's arrival completes the care given to patients by nurses, even if the physician does nothing additional except to approve and confirm what has already been done, so the priest approves, confirms, and completes the healing prayer of a local group and of auxiliary ministry. This is not a mere formality but an expression of the unity and public witness of the Church.

It should be remembered, too, that deacons, sisters, brothers, and other visitors, although they cannot give sacramental absolution, can truly help a sick person to conversion and reconciliation with God and neighbor in an efficacious way. We are not proposing revival of the "confession to a layman," which was common in the Middle Ages when a priest was not available, but are emphasizing that today in pastoral counseling such confession often takes place spontaneously. When it does, the ministers who are not priests should help such patients make an act of contrition and then encourage them to have a priest hear their confession when it becomes possible. They should also assure patients that here and now the mercy of God is truly present in prayer and that with this trust in God's mercy they should be at peace. The reason for confession later is to ratify and complete by the public acknowledgment of the priest as a representative of the Church a conversion that has already taken place. There is no reason for nonordained ministers to believe that because they are not ordained, they cannot help patients achieve this reconciliation here and now.

The Sacraments and Bioethics

The foregoing discussion of sacramental ministry may sound liturgical rather than ethical, but it sums up the ethical message of this book. That is, medical ethics has to do not with certain rules about forbidden procedures, but with a healing process by which the dignity of every human person in all its dimensions is respected by the community and the sick person is restored to full life in community. Unethical behavior tends to exclude persons from the deepest sharing of communal life centered in the Trinity. Ethical behavior fosters this communion. This ethical vision with its perception of the true scale of values is summed up and expressed in the sacraments, especially in the Eucharist. A Catholic health facility that really understands the healing character of the sacraments will have a perfect model for an ethical treatment of the patients. The sacraments represent for us how Jesus in love went about treating sick people.

What makes a Catholic hospital different from all other hospitals? Its vision of the sick is a eucharistic vision, carried out in all details of the treatment of the patient and the mission of the healing team.

14.5 ETHICAL COUNSELING AND PASTORAL CARE

Respecting the Patient's Value System

Don Browning, in *The Moral Context of Pastoral Care* (1976), ably argues for renewed stress on the ethical dimension of pastoral care. He believes that the Christian emphasis on spiritual relation to God by grace must never be allowed to eradicate the memory of its Jewish origins in the Torah, in the law understood not as a death-dealing formalism but as a true discipline of life through which the seeds of grace can be cultivated. A Christian spirituality that neglects moral obligation, or that speaks of love but forgets justice, is foreign to the teaching of Jesus, who came not to destroy the law but to fulfill it (Mt 5:17–19). Systematic theologians have the task of relating and balancing law and grace, but pastoral care counselors have to live with the tension, neglecting neither grace nor discipline.

We have been arguing in this chapter that the primary task of pastoral care is *spiritual* guidance and celebration, yet the purpose of this book has been to deal with *ethical* questions confronted by health care professionals and their patients. Certainly, ministers frequently have to be of help to professionals and patients in their struggles to make such ethical decisions. What is the relation between *spiritual* and *ethical* guidance? Section 2.3 shows that the spiritual and ethical dimensions of the human person, although interrelated, are not identical. Spiritual counseling deals with the ultimate, existential questions, the problems of commitment to certain fundamental values or life goals. Ethical counseling in the strict sense, on the other hand, deals with the decisions that must be made about actions that have to be taken to achieve these goals. In brief, the former deals with *ends;* the latter, with the *means.*

Some theologians, especially of the Lutheran tradition (Thielicke, 1969), question whether ethics in this sense is relevant for a Christian. Are Christians not in danger of self-righteousness and legalism the moment they begin to measure their actions by some ethical system? For such theologians, Christian life is a spontaneous grateful response to God's gracious forgiveness, a loving response that can only be distorted by any ethical calculation of ends and means.

Nevertheless, other Protestant theologians such as Gustafson (1983) recognize that although our ethical decisions must be motivated by faith and love, they also require a rational decision-making process. Thus, although the main task of pastoral care is spiritual, it must also extend to assisting professionals and patients to live out their spiritual commitments by prudent decisions about concrete actions.

This book has been devoted to providing ethical guidance for health care decisions, but in concluding we still have to ask: What is the responsibility of a minister or a pastoral care department in medical-moral decisions?

In answering this question, the first difficulty to consider is how a minister can be an ethical counselor to persons who, in a pluralistic culture, are committed to such different value systems. As spiritual counselor, a minister may have to deal with someone who is struggling with a strictly spiritual problem that involves commitment to a value system, but as ethical counselor, the client's value system is not in question. The problem is its application. How are counselors to help if they do not share the client's value system?

Chapter 7 argues that different value systems cannot be simply reduced to some common denominator, but rather are *analogous* to each other, that is, fundamentally different yet having much in common. Consequently, we believe that in pastoral care it is possible to proceed ecumenically to find a common ground for ethical decisions between different value systems, whether these differences separate pastor and patient or members of the health team. Such an ecumenical method depends on (1) clarity about one's own values and fidelity to them, (2) respect for the values of others and their fidelity to these, and (3) a common effort to find a basis for mutual dialogue and action. Since at a time of sickness patients are seldom in any condition to rethink their whole outlook on life, an ethical counselor should in general not disturb the patient's basic commitment unless it becomes apparent that such issues at the spiritual level have to be faced because the patient is already struggling with them. Consequently, the counselor must deal with a Jew within the Jewish ethical tradition, a Baptist within the Baptist tradition, a humanist within a humanistic set of values. Pressure to proselytize patients to one's own faith are an unfair exploitation of the sick (Browning, 1983).

Next we must ask: What is the goal of ethical counseling? How can patients be helped within the context of their value system to achieve a free and informed conscience and to arrive at prudent ethical decisions? Human decisions to be ethical first must be free. The sick suffer from various limitations of their psychological freedom (Clair, 1993). When their illness is mental, this freedom is severely restricted or even eliminated by neurosis or psychosis. When it is physical, however, the sick still suffer some degree of unfreedom because of the weakness, mental confusion, depression, and so forth, consequent on their physical condition, and also because they are confined to a narrow and unfamiliar social situation. Thus the sick patient is often not able to think clearly and realistically.

Ethical counseling, therefore, must first aim at creating an atmosphere in which the patient's freedom is maximized. Until some area of genuine freedom opens up for the patient, ethical discussion is useless. When such an opening is achieved, the counselor must strive to keep ethical discussion confined to just that area of freedom and not waste time with what seem to be ethical arguments but are in fact only the expression of emotional conflict. The means to achieving this increased freedom are essentially the techniques of psychotherapy, which the minister needs to understand and use in a modest way, referring more difficult problems to members of the health team who are professionally skilled in such therapy. Religious ministers have something special to contribute to this freeing process, however, because they can help to lift the burden of existential fear or hopelessness that may be one of the chief obstacles to freedom. Patients who are confident of God's loving and forgiving care have a peace of mind even in the face of suffering and death that makes it possible for them to face difficult decisions with serenity and sanity.

Subjective and Objective Morality

Once the counselor is assured that the patient is sufficiently free to deal with an ethical decision, the counselor's next objective should be to help the patient arrive at a decision that is prudent and thus at least *subjectively* good, that is, according to the patient's honest conscience, even when the counselor is not convinced that this decision is *objectively* good (*Osservatore Romano*, 1989). There are three reasons why such a gap between subjective and objective morality may occur or may seem to the counselor to exist (see p. 99, 3.4): (1) the patient may have a different value system than the counselor; (2) the patient's decision may appear inconsistent with the patient's own value system; and (3) the patient's decision may be inconsistent with the facts of the situation as the counselor perceives these facts.

In the first case, as already said, the counselor generally should not attempt to convert the patient to the counselor's own value system but should help the patient to make decisions consistent with the patient's own values. In the second case, the counselor should do what is possible to help the patient to make a self-consistent decision, since only then will the decision be conscientious and subjectively right. In the third case, the counselor should try to help the patient perceive the facts of the situation correctly. Nevertheless, in this last case the counselor should remember that one's perception and interpretation of facts is influenced by one's value system and personal experience, so that it may not be possible for patient and counselor to come to an agreement on the facts.

The reason that the counselor first should be concerned to help the patient come to a subjectively honest decision is two-fold: (1) because the patient always retains primary responsibility for health decisions (3.1), and (2) because the proximate norm of all moral decisions is the conscience of the agent (3.4, 8.1). Ethically it is more important that persons do what they sincerely believe to be right at a given stage of their moral development than that they do what is objectively right. Because we live in a sinful world, and each of us suffers from the darkness of mind and hardness of heart resulting from our own sins, the Word of God is received by us in obscurity. Only little by little do we move forward into the light, as is so eloquently witnessed in the Old Testament by the history of the Chosen People. What is most essential is that we keep moving forward, even if our steps are frequently missteps. For those who make mistakes in good faith, experience is self-corrective. The New Testament shows how Jesus (unlike the Pharisees) is more concerned with the faith and goodwill of sinners than he is with their conformity with a law of which they are often ignorant and to which they do not know how to comply. St. Paul (1 Co 8) also urges respect for the conscience of others, even when they are mistaken and immature in their moral understanding.

The task of the counselor, however, does not stop with helping a patient arrive at a subjectively prudent and conscientious decision. The fact that a decision is honest does not prevent it from being harmful to others or even to the one who makes the decision when actually it is an *objectively* wrong decision. Honest mistakes do not injure moral integrity, destroy spiritual relations to God and neighbor, or prevent some spiritual growth, but they do have consequences from which we and others suffer. Moreover, Christian morality is creative; it is a response to God's call to move forward toward him and to share in his redemptive work. This divine call is often present in the crisis of sickness and dying. Consequently, the counselor cannot be content simply to ratify, as it were, decisions made by a patient within the narrow limits of the patient's routine morality.

On the one hand, if the counselor sees that the patient's decision may in fact be clearly injurious to the patient or to others (e.g., if the patient is thinking of suicide or abortion), the counselor has to do what is possible to prevent this harm, even when the counselor is convinced of the subjective honesty of the decision (5.2) (Kemp, 1993). On the other hand, the counselor may judge that it is necessary in particular cases to confront the patient with the challenge inherent in the decision that has to be made. Thus the counselor must raise disturbing questions that ultimately go beyond the ethical level to the spiritual level of the patient's value system. Obviously, counselors must be very cautious about disturbing sick people in this manner, yet they should have the courage to do so when the patient's own behavior signals that such probing and confrontation are necessary. The wonderful scene of Jesus and the Samaritan woman (Jn 4:4–30) shows how the Spirit of God can be at work in the human conscience, revealing itself by the uneasiness, the denial, the defiance, and the disguised cries for help that a spiritually sensitive and experienced counselor can recognize. In these cases the apparent subjective honesty of the client masks a hidden conflict of conscience that cannot be resolved without probing that goes beyond the subjective to a new and deeper perception of reality.

It is no simple matter for a counselor to balance these two counseling aims of subjective and objective conscience. Formerly, it would seem that the clergy were too quick to impose objective moral standards on the people, with little sensitivity to the moral development or experience of different individuals. Today, with the growth in psychological understanding of individual differences and of the developmental aspects of morality, it would seem that the opposite temptation prevails. The axiom *people must make their own conscientious decisions* has often been pushed so far that ministers have lost interest in objective morality.

A disturbing example of this was provided by the way in which many clergymen who had been active as draft counselors during the Vietnam War then went on to become "abortion counselors" (Moody, 1971; Nathanson and Ostling, 1979). In both cases they believed they were serving the cause of human rights, and they probably contributed significantly by reason of their clerical prestige both to ending the war and to liberalizing the antiabortion laws. Yet the accounts of some of them concerning their experience as counselors in the latter cause show that they seemed to have thought that compassion for the woman was the only ethical issue involved in abortion. They saw no inconsistency in their concern for the napalmed children of Vietnam and their lack of concern for the salined fetuses of the United States.

The reason this apparent inconsistency was discussed so little was because these counselors saw their task purely in terms of the individual subjective conscience of the client. When the client was a conscientious objector, the counselors supported his decision to refuse service in the war. When the client was a pregnant woman who honestly believed it would be wrong for her to bear her child, they supported her decision and were ready to help her find a safe clinic and to help her overcome any sense of guilt (Nathanson, 1979). The concern for the subjective conscience of the client in both cases was certainly proper, but we have to ask whether it was enough. Does not the counselor also have to face the question of the objective justice or injustice of the war and also the question of the rights of the unborn child? Although counselors cannot impose their personal judgment about the objective justice in either instance, they cannot simply avoid the issue. Rather, the minister must do what is possible to prevent objective harm and to challenge the judgment of the patient when signs indicate that such challenge may be an opportunity for successful moral growth. Another example of the same problem is the present campaign to legalize "assisted suicide." Some counselors and some physicians seem to think that if people want to kill themselves and are sincere in their decision, they should be assisted to carry it out.

Christian Discernment

An important aspect of this moral growth for the Christian is the deepening of the vital relation between the conscience of the individual and the conscience of the Christian community. The Holy Spirit guides us not merely privately, but also through dialogue within the historical Christian Church. Ethical counselors frequently find great immaturity in Catholic clients with regard to the relation between personal conscience and what they understand to be the official teaching of their Church. What is a counselor to do when confronted by patients who express such dilemmas as the following? (1) I know the Church condemns this, but I don't think God will condemn me. (2) I think I have to do this, but I am afraid I will have to go to hell for doing it. (3) I know the Vatican has condemned this, but why can't you as a priest give me permission to do it? (4) I have made up my mind, but I want to know what you think. (5) I am not going to confess this because I know the confessor will argue with me. (6) I guess I will just have to go ahead and do this and then go to confession afterward. (7) I am going to do what I think is right, but I guess this means I will have to leave the Church. (8) I did what I thought was right, but I still feel guilty about it.

Moreover, counselors find such difficulties not only in patients, but also in dealing with the professional staff who:

1. May separate their professional opinions and their obedience to Church teachings into mental compartments, making no effort to reconcile their professional and their Christian lives;
2. Complain that the bishops and priests are ignorant of medical problems and always behind the times in the ethical regulations they impose on the medical profession;
3. Complain that there is too much variation in the guidance given by different priests or different dioceses and there is a lack of clear enforcement of Church teachings; and
4. Object to taking time from their work to discuss moral issues because such discussions come to no clear conclusions.

Finally, such difficulties are compounded by the fact that the members of the pastoral care department itself may have widely different ethical views and may themselves be struggling with the tension between official Church teaching, the diverse views of theologians, and their own pastoral experience.

We have argued previously (3.4) that such difficulties are not unusual in the Christian community, since it is a historical, catholic, pilgrim people in which the pastors must struggle to keep the flock unified and continuously on its march; yet the diversity of experiences and talents must play their complementary and sometimes conflictual roles. The pastoral role in the situation of a health care facility is not to deny tension and conflict, but to help the persons involved make a contribution to the growth of all. Jesus welcomes into his following a great variety of people at various levels of moral growth, providing for the weak and challenging the strong. St. Paul followed this pattern, with special emphasis on helping the Christians of each community mature in conscience.

In carrying out this educative task, ministers should first emphasize, as we have attempted to do in this book, the primary values and principles of Christian living as they apply to the healing process. These principles should not be presented as rules, but as goals to be creatively achieved in a loving and generous response to the grace of God, after the pattern of the Good Samaritan (Lk 10:25–37), who saw in the injured man in the ditch the call of God. The professional or the patient who has these goals at heart and uses the knowledge and imagination available to reach them will act in a truly humane and Christian way, enlightened by the Holy Spirit.

Christians open to the Spirit in this way are not negligent of or ungrateful for the guidance given by the pastors of the Church, whether that guidance has the certitude of the Gospel or simply the authority of pastors doing what they can to apply the Gospel in a given time or place according to the lights they possess. On the other hand, mature Christians know that God requires of them personal decisions based not only on pastoral guidance, but also on their own gifts and experience.

The final task of ethical counselors, therefore, is to help those they counsel mature in conscience and live in peace with the responsibility for their own decisions, content with the assurance that God calls us to share in his own task of healing a wounded world. Indeed all those engaged in health care can be confident that the words addressed by Jesus to the apostles applies also in a very real way to them, "Proclaim the kingdom of God and heal the sick!" (Lk 9:2) and also in other words, "Amen, I say to you, whatever you did for one of these least brethren of mine, you did for me" (Mt 25:40).

CONCLUSION

The hospitals in Western culture originated because of a desire to give spiritual care to dying people. At the time of origination spiritual care was often the only help that could be given to people with fatal pathologies. As time progressed and medical science achieved the power to heal people with serious illnesses, the tendency to weaken the efforts at spiritual ministry. Indeed the SUPPORT Study (cf. Chapter 13) and anecdotal experience seem to indicate that physicians have a very difficult time meeting the needs of dying patients. Dying and death become experiences outside the pale of medical competence. While pastoral care personnel are competent to help dying patients, the solution to the problem of caring for dying patients in a compassionate manner does not lie in separating pastoral care from medical care. Rather, physicians must be convinced of the need to minister to dying patients, even though pastoral care persons may have skills better suited for the care of the dying.

In contemporary times, inducing death is often looked upon as a solution to human problems. In the care of people suffering from fatal pathologies, because of pain, depression, or a feeling of absurdity, some recommend suicide or assisted suicide as reasonable choices. But human problems are not solved through killing innocent people. Hence, the added emphasis needed upon excellent pastoral care ministers in all health care facilities.

Bibliography

AAMC: Association of American Medical Colleges, Panel on the General Professional Education of the Physician and College Preparation for Medicine, *GPEP Report,* Washington DC, 1984.

ABA: American Bar Association, "Lawyers Reject AMA Solution to Crisis," *Medical World News* 27 (5), March 10, 1986, 24.

Abel, G., "Sexual Abuses," *Psychiatric Clinics of North America,* 18 (1), March, 1995, 139–53.

Abramowitz, Stephen, "Psychosocial Outcomes of Sex Reassignment Surgery," *Journal of Consulting and Clinical Psychology* 54 (2), 1986, 183–189.

ACGME: Accreditation Council for Graduate Medical Education, "Regulations in regard to abortion training," February, 1995, revised June, 1995.

Ackerman, Terrence F., "Fooling Ourselves with Child Autonomy and Assent in Non-Therapeutic Clinical Research," *Clinical Research,* 1979, 345–348.

Aday, Luann, *At Risk in America: The Health and Health Care Needs of Vulnerable Populations in the United States,* San Francisco, CA: Jossey-Bass, 1993.

Aday, Luann; Fleming, Gretchen; and Andersen, Ronald, *Access to Medical Care in the U.S.: Who Has It, Who Doesn't,* Chicago: Pluribus Press, 1984.

Adcock, David F.; Sear, Alan M.; and Yates, Eugene W. "Ownership of the Medical Radiograph," *Southern Medical Journal,* 1991, April 84(4), 447–450.

Adler, Mortimer J., *The Time of Our Lives: The Ethics of Common Sense,* New York: Holt, Rinehart and Winston, 1970, ch. 17, 185 ff.

Aertnys, Joseph; Damen, Charles. *Theologia Moralis,* Rome, Marietti, 1947, cooperation; vol. 1, n. 398.

Agras, W. Stewart; and Berkowitz, Robert, "Behavior Therapy," in *Textbook of Psychiatry,* John Talbott; Robert Hales; and Stuart Yudofsky, eds. Washington, DC, American Psychiatric Press, 1988, 891–905.

AHA: American Hospital Association
    1972 "Patient's Bill of Rights," Chicago: American Hospital Association Press.
    1986a "Cost and Compassion," Chicago: American Hospital Association.
    1986b "Hospital Responsibility Is in Requesting Organ Donations," *Technical Advisor Bulletin,* Sept. 15.

Aiken, Linda; Mechanic, David, *Applications of Social Science to Clinical Medicine and Health Policy,* Newark: Rutgers University Press, 1986.

Alexander, Leo, "Medical Science Under Dictatorship," *New England Journal of Medicine* 241, 1949, 39–47. Reprinted in *Child and Family* 10, 1971, 40–57.

Allport, Gordon W.
    1937 *Personality: A Psychological Interpretation,* New York: Henry Holt, 24–50.
    1961 *Pattern and Growth in Personality,* New York: Holt, Reinhart, and Winston.

Alpern, Kenneth D., ed. *The Ethics of Reproductive Technology,* New York: Oxford University Press, 1992.

Alpert, Joseph S., *A Clinician's Companion: A Study Guide for Effective and Humane Patient Care,* Boston: Little Brown, 1986.

Altman, Lawrence
    1987 *Who Goes First: The Story of Self-Experimentation in Medicine,* New York: Random House.
    1988 "Sharp Drop in Autopsies Stirs Fear that Quality of Care May Also Fall," *New York Times,* July 21, 1988.
AMA: American Medical Association
    1986 *Health Plan for America,* Chicago: AMA.
    1987a AMA Special Task Force on Professional Liability and Insurance, *Journal of the American Medical Association* 257 (6), Feb. 13, 810–812.
    1987b *Health Policy Agenda for the American People,* Chicago: AMA.
    1988a Report of the Council on Ethical and Judicial Affairs, "Ethical Issues Involved in Growing AIDS Crisis," *Journal of the American Medical Association* 259, 1360.
    1988b "AMA House Delegates Reject Euthanasia," *New York Times,* June 28, 1988.
    1988b "Euthanasia and Physician-Assisted Suicide: Lessons in the Dutch Experience," *Issues in Law and Medicine,* 10 (1), Summer, 1994, 81–90.
    1988c "News at Deadline: AMA Accepts Registered Care Technologist," *Hospitals* 14, July 10.
    1988d *Director of Graduate Medical Education Programs, 1988–89,* Chicago: AMA.
    1994a Council on Ethical and Judicial Affairs, Code of Medical Ethics, "HIV Infected Patients and Physicians" (9:131); "Withholding and Withdrawing Life Sustaining Medical Treatment," n. 2:20.
    1994b Council on Ethical and Judicial Affairs, Code of Medical Ethics, "Anencephalic Infants as Organ Donors," *Journal of the American Medical Association* 2:23; 2: June, p. 161; 9:131.
    1995a "Ethical Issues in Managed Care," *Journal of the American Medical Association* 273 (4), 330–335.
    1995b Council on Ethical and Judicial Affairs. "The Use of Anencephalic Neonates as Organ Donors," *Journal of the American Medical Association,* 273, 1995, 1614–18.
    1996 *Physician Characteristics and Distribution in the United States 1995–1996,* Chicago, IL: AMA Publications.
AMA News June 1996 "New Bioethics Panel to study genetics research subjects," p. 10.
American Fertility Society, Ethics Committee of the, "Ethical Considerations of the New Reproductive Technologies," *Fertility and Sterility,* 46 (Supplement 1), 1986.
American Neurological Association, "On Certain Aspects of Care and Management of PVS Patient," *Neurology,* January, 1989, p. 125.
American Pain Society, *Principles of Analgesic Use in the Treatment of Acute Pain and Cancer Pain,* Skokie, IL: American Pain Society, 1992.
American Society of Neurosurgeons, in *Patricia Brophy v. New England Sinai Hospital,* (Mass. Sup. Court, Jud. Ct. Sept. 11, 1986), cited p. 12.
Amulree, Lord, et al., *On Dying Well: An Anglican Contribution to the Debate on Euthanasia,* London: Church Information Service, 1975.
Anderson, W. French
    1985 "Human Gene Therapy: Scientific and Ethical Considerations," *Journal of Medicine and Philosophy* 3, Aug 10, 275–291.
    1994 "Genetic engineering and our humanness," *Human Gene Therapy,* 5 (6) June, 755–759.
Andrews, Lori
    1985 *State Laws and Regulations Governing Newborn Screening,* Chicago: American Bar Foundation.
    1994 *Assessing Genetic Risks: Implications for Health and Social Policy,* Washington: National Academy Press.
Andrusko, Dave; and Bond, Leslie, "Harvesting the Living," *Call to Conscience,* ch. 9, Washington: National Right to Life Conference, 1988.

Angoff, Nancy Rockmore. "Do Physicians Have an Ethical Obligation to Care for Patients with AIDS?" Yale *Journal of Biology and Medicine*, May–June, 1991, 201–224.

Annas, George
1973 "The Patients Have Rights: How Can We Protect Them?" *Hastings Center Report* 9, 8–9.
1979 "Denying the Rights of the Retarded: The Phillip Becker Case," *Hastings Center Report* 9, 18–20.
1985a "Is Genetic Screening Test Ready When the Lawyers Say It Is?" *Hastings Center Report* 6, Dec. 15.
1985b "The Phoenix Heart, What We Have to Lose," *Hastings Center Report* 3, June 15, 1985, 15–16.
1985c "Fashion and Freedom: When Artificial Feeding Should be Withdrawn," *American Journal of Public Health*, 175 (6) 685–688.
1994 "Informed Consent, Cancer and the Truth in Prognosis," *New England Journal of Medicine*, 330 (3) January 20, 1994, 223–225.
1995 "Reframing the debate on health care reform by replacing our metaphors," *New England Journal of Medicine*, 332 (11), March 16, 744–746.

APA: American Psychiatric Association
1978 *Task Force on ECT*, Washington, DC: American Psychiatric Association.
1981 *The Principles of Medical Ethics with Annotations Especially Applicable to Psychiatry*, Washington: APA.
1985 Task Force, *Seclusion and Restraint: The Psychiatric Uses*, Washington, DC, APA.
1986a "Unethical Behavior, Incompetency, and Impairment in the Ethical Decision Process," *Ethics Newsletter*, APA 2(1), Jan.–Feb.
1986b "Sexual Involvement Between Psychiatrists, Their Students, Supervisors, Colleagues, and Employees," *Ethics Newsletter*, APA 2(2), Apr.–May.
1993 Commission on AIDS, "AIDS Policy Position Statement on Confidentiality Disclosure and Protection of Others," *American Journal of Psychiatry*, May, p. 852.
1994 *Diagnostic and Statistical Manual of Mental Disorders* DSM IV, 4th edition, Washington, DC: APA.

Applebaum, Paul, et al., "False Hopes and Best Data: Consent to Research and Therapeutic Misconceptions," *Hastings Center Report* 17(2), April 1987, 16–30.

Appleton, William S., "The Importance of Psychiatrists' Telling Patients the Truth," *American Journal of Psychiatry* 129, 1972, 742–745.

Aquinas, Saint Thomas, *Summa Theologiae*. Gilby, Thomas, OP, ed., New York: McGraw-Hill, 1976; On the body: vol. 11, I, 75, 4, ad. 2, 76, 1 ad. 6; On the principle of totality: vol. 38, II-II, q. 65, 1 c., q. 94, a2.; I-II, q. 100 a1, a3.

Aries, Philippe, *The Hour of Our Death*, New York: Alfred A. Knopf, 1981.

Arieti, Silvano, *The Intra-Psychic Self: Creativity and its Cultivation*, New York: Basic Books, 1967.

Aristotle
Politics, Richard McKeon, ed, Chicago: University of Chicago Press, 1950.
Nicomachean Ethics, Richard McKeon, ed, Chicago: University of Chicago Press, 1950.

Arizona Medical Examiners, "Care for AIDS Patients," *Journal of Arizona Medical Association*, 3:1987.

Arkes, Hadley
1992 "On 'Delayed Hominization': Some Thoughts on the Blending of New Science and Ancient Fallacies," in Russell E. Smith ed., *The Interaction of Catholic Bioethics and Secular Society*, Braintree, MA: The Pope John Center, 1992, 143–162.
1994 "Abortion Facts and Feelings," *First Things*, 42 April, 1994, 34–38.

Ashley, Benedict
1972 "A Psychological Model with a Spiritual Dimension," *Pastoral Psychology* 23, 31–40.

1976   "A Critique of the Theory of Delayed Hominization," in *An Ethical Evaluation of Fetal Experimentation: An Interdisciplinary Study,* Donald G. McCarthy and Albert S. Moraczewski, OP, eds., St. Louis: Pope John XXIII Medical-Moral Research and Education Center, 113–133.

1985   *Theologies of the Body,* Braintree, MA: Pope John XXIII Medical-Moral Research and Education Center.

1987   "How the Roman Catholic Position on Euthanasia Developed," Report to the Catholic-Methodist Dialogue.

1990   "The Chill Factor in Moral Theology: An In-depth Review of *The Critical Calling: Reflections on Moral Dilemmas Since Vatican II*" by Richard McCormick, The *Linacre Quarterly,* November 1990, p. 66–77.

1995   *Spiritual Direction in the Dominican Tradition,* NY: Paulist Press.

1996   *Theologies of the Body,* 2nd edition, Braintree, MA: Pope John XXIII Center.

Ashley, Benedict M.; and Albert S. Moraczewski, "Is the Biological Subject of Human Rights Present from Conception?" Peter J. Cataldo and Albert S. Moraczewski, eds., *The Fetal Tissue Issue: Medical and Ethical Aspects,* Braintree, MA: Pope John Center, 1994.

Ashley, Joann, *Hospitals, Paternalism and the Role of the Nurse,* New York: Teacher's College Press, 1976.

Ashwal, S.; and Cranford, R., "Medical Aspects of the Persistent Vegetative State—A Correction," *New England Journal of Medicine,* 333(2), July 13, 1995, p. 130.

Atkinson, Gary M., "Persons in the Whole Sense," *American Journal of Jurisprudence,* 22, 1977, 86–117.

Atkinson, Gary M.; and Moraczewski, Albert S., OP, *Genetic Counseling: The Church and the Law,* St. Louis: Pope John XXIII Medical-Moral Research and Education Center, 1980.

Atwood, J. "Constructing a Sex and Marital Therapy Frame: Ways to Help Couples Deconstruct Sexual Problems," *Journal of Sex and Marital Therapy,* 18(3), Fall, 1992, 196–218.

Austin, C.R., *Human Embryos: The Debate on Assisted Reproduction,* Oxford: Oxford University Press, 1989.

Australian Research Commission, *Human Embryo Experimentation in Australia,* Senate Select Committee on Human Experimentation Bill, Australian Government Printing Office, 1985, p. 25.

Auxter, Thomas, *Kant's Moral Theology,* Macon, GA: Mercer University Press, 1982.

Aviram, Uri; and Shnit, Dan, "Psychiatric Treatment and Civil Liberties in Israel: The Need for Reform" *Israel Journal of Psychiatry and Related Sciences* 21(1), 1984, 3–18.

Axelrod, David; et al., "Physician Competence: Whose Responsibility?" *Medical Staff News* 3 May 1988.

Ayer, A.J., *Language, Truth and Logic,* London: Gollancz, 1936.

Baily, James; Pillard, Richard; Neale, Michael; and Agyel, Yvonne, "Heritable Factors Influence Sexual Orientation in Women," *Archives of General Psychiatry* 50(3) 1993, 217–223.

Bakken, Kenneth. *The Call to Wholeness: Health as a Spiritual Journey,* New York: Crossroad Publishing Co., 1985.

Baldessarini, R., *Chemotherapy in Psychiatry*, Cambridge, MA: Harvard University Press, 1985.

Baldwin, D; et al. "Changes in Moral Reasoning During Medical School," *Academic Medicine,* September, 1991.

Ball, John; and Rubin, Elaine, "Academic health centers: structures and strategies for coping with the managed care environment," Washington, DC: Association of Academic Health Centers, 1995.

Bandura, A., *Social Foundation of Thought and Action,* Englewood Cliffs, NJ: Prentice-Hall, 1986.

Barber, Bernard "Some Problems of the Sociology of Professions," in *The Professions in America,* Kenneth S. Lynn, ed., Boston: Houghton Mifflin, Daedalus, 647–865, 1965.

Barden, Howard; et al., "The Costs and Benefits of Screening P.K.U. in Wisconsin," *Social Biology* 31(1), Spring 1984, 1–17.

Barkow, John, *Darwin, Sex and Status, Biological Approaches to Mind and Culture,* Toronto: University of Toronto Press, 1989.

Barlow George; and Silverberg, James, eds., *Sociobiology: Beyond Nature/Nurture? Reports, Definitions, Debates,* Boulder, CO: Westview Press, Inc., 1980.

Barnett, H. A.; and Kaserman, D. "The shortage of organs for transplantation: exploring the alternatives," *Issues in Law and Medicine,* 9(2) Fall, 1993, 117–137.

Barnlund, Dean C., "The Mystification of Meaning: Doctor-Patient Encounters," *Journal of Medical Education* 51, 1976, 716–725.

Baron, Charles H., "Fetal Research: The Question in the States," *Hastings Center Report* 15(2), Apr. 15, 1985, 12–16.

Baron, Richard J., "Bridging Clinical Distance: An Empathic Rediscovery of the Known," *Journal of Medicine and Philosophy* 16, 1981, 5–24.

Barron, James, "Group Requiring Abortion Study," *NY Times,* February, 1995.

Barry, Robert
  1986 "Withholding and Withdrawing Treatment," *Journal of the American Medical Association* 256(4), July 25, 1986, 469–71.
  1994 *Breaking the Thread of Life: On Rationale Suicide,* New Brunswick, NJ: Transaction Publishers.

Bashim, Yvonne, "Doctoring The Genes," *Science* 84(10), Dec. 5, 1984, 52–60.

Battin, Margaret, *The Least Worst Death: Essays in Bioethics on the End of Life,* New York: Oxford University Press, 1994.

Bauer, Arthur, *Legal and Ethical Aspects of Fetal Tissue Transplantation,* Austin, TX: R.G. Landes, 1994.

Baulieu, Etienne-Emile
  1989 "Contragestin and Other Clinical Applications of RU 486, an Antiprogesterone at the Receptor," *Science,* 245 September 22, 1351–1357.
  1991 "Improvements seen for RU 486 abortions," *Science,* 254, October 11, 198 ff.

Bayer, Edward
  1982 *Oppression Within Marriage and Prevention of Pregnancy by Artificial Means,* Rome: St. Thomas University.
  1985 *Rape within Marriage: A Moral Analysis Delayed,* Lanham, MD: University Press of America.

Bayer, Ronald, *Homosexuality and American Psychiatry: The Politics of Diagnosis,* Princeton, NJ: Princeton University Press, 1987.

Bayer, Ronald; Levine, Carol; and Wolt, Susan, "HIV Antibody Screening: An Ethical Framework for Evaluation," *Journal of the American Medical Association* 256 (13), Oct. 3, 1986.

Bayley, Corrine; and McCormick, Richard A., SJ, "Sterilization: The Dilemma of Catholic Hospitals," *America* 143, Oct. 18, 1980, 222–225.

Beauchamp, Thomas, "Suicide" in *Matters of Life and Death: New Introductory Essays in Moral Philosophy,* Tom Regan, ed., New York: McGraw-Hill, 1994, 69–120.

Beauchamp, Tom L.; and Childress, James, *Principles of Biomedical Ethics,* New York: Oxford University Press, 1979; 2nd edition, 1983; 3rd edition, 1994.

Beauchamp, Tom L.; and McCullough, Lawrence B., *Medical Ethics: The Moral Responsibilities of Physicians,* Englewood Cliffs, NJ: Prentice-Hall, 1984.

Beauchamp, Thomas; and Walters, Leroy, "The Management of Medical Information," In their *Contemporary Issues in Bioethics,* 4th edition, Belmont, CA: Wadsworth, 1994.

Beck, Aaron; et al., *The Prediction of Suicide,* Philadelphia: Charles Press, 1986.

Becker, Ernest, *The Denial of Death.* New York: Free Press, 1973.

Becker, Howard S., "The Nature of a Profession," in *Education for the Professions,* Nelson B. Henry, ed., 61st Yearbook of the National Society for the Study of Education, 2nd ed., Chicago: University of Chicago Press, 1960, 27–46.

Becker, Judith; and Kavoussi, Richard, "Sexual Disorders," in *Textbook of Psychiatry*, John Talbott; Robert Hales; and Stuart Yudofsky, eds., Washington, DC: American Psychiatric Press, 1988, 587–604.

Bedate, C.A.; and Cefalo, R.C., "The Zygote: To be or not to be a person," *Journal of Medicine and Philosophy*, 14, 1989, 641–645.

Beitman, Bernard D.; and Klerman, Gerald L., *Integrating Pharmacotherapy and Psychotherapy*, Washington, DC: American Psychiatric Press, 1991.

Bellah, Robert
    1986 et al., *Habits of the Heart: Individualism and Commitment in American Life*, New York: Harper & Row.
    1991 et al., *The Good Society*, NY: Random House.
    1992 *Autonomy and Responsibility: The Social Basis of Ethical Individualism in Revisioning Philosophy*, Albany, NY: Sung Press.

The Belmont Report: Ethical Principles and Guidelines for the Protection of Human Subjects of Research, 2 vols., U.S. National Commission for the Protection of Human Subjects of Biomedical and Behavioral Research. Washington, DC: U.S. Government Printing Office, 1978.

Benjamin, Martin
    1985 "Lay Obligation in Professional Relations," *Journal of Medicine and Philosophy* 1, Feb. 10, 1985, 85–103.
    1988 "Medical Ethics and Economics of Organ Transplantation," *Health Progress*, March, 47.

Berger, L. Peter; and Luckmann, Thomas, *The Social Construction of Reality: A Treatise in the Sociology of Knowledge*, Garden City, NJ: Doubleday, 1966.

Bergin, A.E.; and Payne, I.R., "Religiosity of Psychotherapists: A National Survey," *Psychotherapy*, 27, 1991 3–7.

Beriman, Daniel; and Navarro, Vincente, *Health and Work Under Capitalism: An Alternative Perspective*, Amityville, NY: Baywood Publishing, 1983.

Berk, Marc; Schur, Claudia; and Cantor, Joel, "Ability to obtain health care: recent estimates from the Robert Wood Johnson foundation national access to care survey," *Health Affairs*, Fall 1995, 4:139–146.

Berlant, Jeffrey Lionel, *Profession and Monopoly: A Study of Medicine in the United States and Great Britain*, Berkeley: University of California Press, 1975.

Berlin, Fred, "Ethical Use of Psychiatric Diagnosis," *Psychiatric Annals* 13(4), Apr. 1983, 321–331.

Bernardin, Joseph
    1986 "The Consistent Ethic of Life," *Health Progress* 67(6), July 1986, 48–51.
    1995 "Making the Case for Not-for-Profit Health Care," *Health Progress*, February 1995.

Bertalanffy, Ludwig von, *General System Theory; Foundations, Development, Applications*, New York: Dover Publications, 1968.

Billings, Evelyn; and Westmore, Ann, *The Billings Method; Controlling Fertility without Drugs or Devices*, 5th ed., Victoria, Australia: Gorbon and Gotch, 1985.

Billings, John
    1983 *The Ovulation Method*, 7th ed., Melbourne: Advocate Press, 1983.
    1989 *Nota Critica:* " 'When Did I Begin?' by Norman M. Ford," *Anthropotes*, (1)119–127.

Birch, Charles, *The Liberation of Life: From the Cell to the Community*, New York: Cambridge University Press, 1981.

Birmingham, William, *What Modern Catholics Think About Birth Control*, New York: New American Library, Signet Books, 1964.

Bishop, Anne; and Scudder, John. *Nursing Ethics, Therapeutic Caring Presence*, Lynchburg, VA: College of Virginia, 1996.

Bissell, LeClair; and Royce, James, *Ethics for Addiction Professionals*, Center City, MN: Hazelden Foundation, 1987.

Black, Peter. "Declarations of Brain Death in Neurosurgical and Neurological Practice," *Neurosurgery* 15(2), Aug. 1984, 170–174.

Black, Peter; and Szasz, Thomas, "The Ethics of Psychosurgery: Pro and Con," *The Humanist* 37, 1977, 6–11.

Blackeslee, Sandra, "Behind the Veil of Thought," *New York Times* (March 21, 1995) p. B7 & 10.

Blank, Robert; and Bonnicksen, Andres, L., eds., *Emerging Issues in Biomedical Policy*, Vol. 11, Debates over authority in medical decision making: new challenges in biomedical experimentations. NY: Columbia University Press, 1993.

Blaskiewicz, Robert, private correspondence, March 26, 1996.

Blendon, Robert; Brodie, Mollyann; and Benson, John, "What happened to Americans' support of the Clinton plan," *Health Affairs* 14:2 Summer 1995:7–24.

Blendon, Robert J.; and Donelan, Karen, "Discrimination Against People with AIDS," *New England Journal of Medicine* 319(15), Oct. 13, 1988, 1022.

Block, Sidney; and Chodoff, Paul, eds. *Psychiatric Ethics*, New York: Oxford University Press, 1981.

Bloom, Alan
1987 *The Closing of the American Mind: Education and the Crisis of Reason*, New York: Simon and Schuster.
1990 ed. *Confronting the Constitution*, Washington, DC: American Enterprise Institute.

Blum, Henrick L.
1983 *Expanding Health Care Horizons: From General Systems Concept of Health Care to a National Policy*, Oakland: Third Party Publications.

Blum, Richard H., *A Common Sense Guide to Doctors, Hospitals and Medical Care*, New York: Macmillan, 1964.

Blumstein, J. "The use of financial incentives in medical care: the case of commerce in transplanting organs," *Health Matrix*, 3(1), Spring, 1993, 1–30.

BMA, British Medical Association, *Our Genetic Future: The Science and Ethics of Genetic Technology*, New York: Oxford University Press, 1992.

Bodlund, O., et al., "Personality traits and disorders among transsexuals," *Acta Psychiatrica Scandinavia*, 88:5, November, 1993, 322–27.

Boff, Leonardo
1986 *Liberation Theology: From Dialogue to Confrontation*, San Francisco: Harper and Row.
1992 *Faith on the Edge: Religion and Marginalized Existence*, Trans. Barr, Maryknoll, NY: Orbis Books.

Boisen, Anton T.
1936 *Exploration of the Inner World*, New York: Harper & Row, Torchbooks.
1945 *Religion in Crisis and Custom*, New York: Harper.

Bok, Derek, "Needed: A New Way to Train Doctors", *Connecticut Medicine* 48(11), Nov. 1984, 741–48.

Bole, Thomas
1989 "Metaphysical accounts of the zygote as a person," *Journal of Medicine and Philosophy*, 14, 647–653.
1992 "The Licitness of Inducing the Non-viable Anencephalic Fetus," *HCE Forum* 4(2), 121–133.

Boorse, C., "On the Distinction Between Disease and Illness," in *Concepts of Health and Disease Interdisciplinary Perspectives*, Reading, MA: Addison-Wesley, 1981.

Bopp, James, "Petition for a Writ of *Certiorari* to the United States Court of Appeals for the Tenth Circuit." *Issues in Law and Medicine*, 9(1), Summer, 1993, 81–95.

Boros, SJ, Ladislaus, *The Mystery of Death*, New York: Herder & Herder, 1965.

Bosk, Charles
1979 *Forgive and Remember, Managing Medical Failures*, Chicago: University of Chicago Press.

1986 "The Health Care System: Overview," in James Childress, et al., *Biolaw* vol. 1, Frederick, MD: University Publications of America, 9–27.

Bourgeois, P.; and Schalow, F., "The Integrity and Falleness of Human Existence," *Southern Journal of Philosophy* 25, 1987, 123–132.

Bourke, Vernon, *History of Ethics* 2 vol, NY: Doubleday Image Books, vol. 1, On Voluntarism, 1970, 147 ff.

Bowker, John, *Problems of Suffering in the Religions of the World*, NY: Cambridge University Press, 1970.

Boyle, Joseph, "Toward Understanding the Principle of Double Effect," *Ethics* 90, 1980, 527–538.

Boyle, P.; and Callahan, D., "Managed Care in Mental Health: The Ethical Issues," *Health Affairs*, Fall 1995, 7–22.

Boyle, Philip; and O'Rourke, Kevin, "Presumed Consent for Organ Donation," *America* 155(15), Nov. 22, 1986, 326–332.

Bradford, Roberta. "Obstacles to Collaborative Practice," *Nursing Management*, 20:4, 1989, p. 72.

Brahms, Diana, "Doctor's Duty to Answer Patients' Inquiries," *The Lancet* 1 (8538), Apr. 18, 1987, 932.

Braude, Peter; Bolton, Virginia; and Moore, Stephen, "Human gene expression first occurs between the four and eight-cell stages of preimplantation development," *Nature*, 332, March 31, 1988, 459–461.

Breggin, Peter R.
1972 "New Information in the Debate Over Psychosurgery," *Congressional Record*, March 30, E3380–86.
1979 *Electroshock: Its Brain-Disabling Effects*, New York: Springer Publishing Co., 1979.

Brennan, Carl H, "Restoring Intimacy to the Physician-Patient Relationship," *Health Progress*, March 75(2), 1994, 80, 79.

Brenner, Brooks, "The Showing of Psychiatry," *Academic Psychiatry*, 18(2), Summer, 1994, 11–81.

Brint, Steven, *In an Age of Exgens: The Changing Role of the Professional in Politics and Public Life*, Princeton, NJ: Princeton University Press, 1994.

Brodeur, Dennis. "Toward a Clear Definition of Ethics Committees," *Linacre Quarterly* 51(3) August 1984:233–247.

Brodie, Janet, *Contraception and Abortion in Nineteenth Century America*, Ithiaca, NY: Cornell University Press, 1994.

Brody, Baruch A.
1975 *Abortion and the Sanctity of Human Life: A Philosophical View*, Cambridge, MA: MIT Press.
1983 "Autonomy and Paternalism: Some Value Problems; A Utilitarian Perspective, A Deontological Perspective," ch. 12–14 in his *Ethics and its Applications*, New York: Harcourt Brace Jovanovich, 159–198.

Brody, Baruch, A., et al., "Morality and Sex Change," *Hastings Center Report* 11, 1981, 8–13.

Brody, Howard
1981 *Ethical Decisions in Medicine*, 2nd ed., Boston: Little, Brown, 37–72.
1992a *The Healer's Power*, New Haven: Yale University Press.
1992b "Assisted Death—A Compassionate Response to a Medical Failure," *New England Journal of Medicine*, 327(19), November 5, 1384–88.

Bromley, Dorothy Dunbar, *Catholics and Birth Control: Contemporary Views on Doctrine*, Old Greenwich, CT: Devin-Adair Publications, Inc., 1965.

Brower, Leslie A., "The Health Care Team: Who Calls the Plays?" in *Biomedical Ethics: A Community Forum*, Henry M. Sondheimer, ed., Syracuse: SUNY Medical Center, 1985, 135–142.

Brown, J. B.; et al., "Natural Family Planning," *American Journal of Obstetrics and Gynecology* 157, Oct. 1987, 1082.

Browning, Don
1976   *The Moral Context of Pastoral Care,* Philadelphia: Westminster Press.
1983   *Religious Ethics & Pastoral Care,* Philadelphia: Fortress Press.
1987   *Religious Thought and the Modern Psychologies: Critical Conversation in the Theology of Culture,* Philadelphia: Fortress Press.

Bruce, Jo Anne Czecoswki, "Access of Patient to Health Records," In her *Privacy and Confidentiality of Health Care Information,* second edition. Chicago, IL: American Hospital Publishing, 1988, 161–182.

Bultmann, Rudolf, *Jesus and the Word,* New York: Charles Scribner's Sons, 1958.

Burling, T. "A Cognitive Behavioral Therapeutic Community Treatment Outcomes," *Addictive Behaviors,* 19(6), November–December, 1994, 621–629.

Burtchaell, James T., ed., *Abortion Parley,* Kansas City: Andrews and McMeel, 1980.

Byers, David, "Global Population and the Dialogue between Religion and Science," *Proceeding: ITEST,* St. Louis: ITEST Foundation, 1996.

Byrne Paul; et al., "Brain Death, An Opposing Viewpoint," *Journal of the American Medical Association* 242, 1979, 1985–1990.

Byrne, Paul; and Nilges, Richard, "The Brainstem in Brain Death: A Critical Review," *Issues in Law and Medicine,* 9(1), Summer, 1993, 3–21.

Caffara, Carlo, "The Ecclesial Identity and Mission of the Family," in *The Family Today and Tomorrow,* St. Louis: Pope John XXIII Medical-Moral Research and Education Center, 1985.

Cahill, Lisa Sowle, "The Embryo and the Fetus: New Moral Contexts, *Theological Studies,* 54, 1993, 124–42.

Cahn, Steven, *Saints and Scamps: Ethics in Academia,* Totowa: NJ: Rowman & Littlefield, 1986.

Califano, Joseph, *America's Health Care Revolution,* NY: Random House, 1985.

Callahan, Daniel
1970   *Abortion Law, Choice, Morality,* New York: Macmillan.
1973a   *The Tyranny of Survival and Other Pathologies of Civilized Life,* New York: Macmillan.
1973b   "The WHO Definition of Health," *Hastings Center Studies* 1(3), 77–87.
1981   "Arguing the Morality of Genetic Engineering," in *Medical Ethics and the Law: Implications for Public Policy,* Marc Hiller, ed., Cambridge, MA: Ballinger, 441–449.
1987a   "Surrogate Motherhood: A Bad Idea," *New York Times,* Jan. 20.
1988   *Setting Limits: Medical Goals in an Aging Society,* New York: Simon and Schuster.
1993   *The Troubled Dream of Life: Living with Mortality,* New York: Simon and Schuster.

Callahan, Joan, ed. *Ethical Issues in Professional Life,* NY: Oxford University Press, 1988.

Callahan, Sidney, "Ethical Issues of Unconventional Therapies," *Health Progress,* 74:7, September 1993, 42–43.

Campbell, Courtney S. "Gifts and Caring Duties in Medicine," In: Campbell, Courtney S., Lusting, B. Andrew, eds. *Duties to Others,* Boston, MA: Kluwer Academic, 1994, 181–197.

Campion, Edward W. "Why Unconventional Medicine?" *New England Journal of Medicine,* 328(4), January 28, 1993, 282–283.

Camus, Albert
1956   *The Rebel,* preface, p. 3, p. 8, New York: Vintage Books, p. 6.
1972   *The Myth of Sisyphus and Other Essays,* trans., Justin O'Brien, New York: Alfred Knopf, 1955.

Canada Law Reform Commission. *Criteria for the Determination of Death,* Ottawa: The Commission, 1981.

Canadian Medical Association Journal, "Confidentiality, Ownership, and Transfer of Medical Records," 133(10), Nov. 15, 1985.

Candilis, Philip; Wesley; and Robert; Wichman, Allison, "A survey of researchers using a consent policy for cognitively impaired human research subjects," *IRB A Review for Human Research Subjects,* 15 (6), November–December, 1993, 1–4.

Capps, Walter H., ed., *The Future of Hope: Essays by Block, Fackenheim, Motlmann, Metz, and Capps,* Philadelphia: Fortress Press, 1970.

Capron, Alexander M.
1984 "Current Issues in Genetic Screening," in Humber, James; et al., ed., *Biomedical Ethics Review 1984,* Clifton, NJ: Humana Press, 121–149.
1986 "Determination of Death," in Katherine Benesch, et al., eds., *Medicolegal Aspects of Critical Care,* Rockville, MD: Aspen Publishers, 109–132.
1993a "Duty, Truth and Whole Human Beings," *Hastings Center Report,* 23:4, July–August, 13–14.
1993b "Ethical implications of studies in molecular genetics: an emerging issue," in Bankowiski and Levine, eds. *Ethics and Research on Human Subjects,* Geneva: Council for International Organizations of Medical Science.

Carmi, Ammon, "Genetic Engineering," *Medicine and Law* 3, Aug. 2, 1983, 181–192.

Carnes, Patrick, *Sexual Addiction,* Minneapolis: Comp-Care Publications, 1983.

Carrick, Paul, *Medical Ethics in Antiquity: Philosophical Respectives on Abortion and Euthanasia,* Boston: D. Riedl, 1985.

Carson, Sandra A.; and Buster, John E., "Ectopic Pregnancy," *The New England Journal of Medicine,* 329, October 14, 1993, 1174–1180.

Carton, Sharon, "The Poet, the Biographer and the Shrink: Psychiatrist-Patient Confidentiality and the Anne Sexton Biography," *Entertainment and Sports Law Review,* 10:2, 1993, 117–164.

Cassel, Christine, "Ethical Issues in Mental Health Care of the Elderly," in *Geriatric Mental Health,* J.P. Abrahams, ed., New York: Grune and Stratton, 1984, 229–241.

Cassell, Eric. *The Healer's Art,* New York: Lippincott, 1976.

Cassell, Eric, et al., "Refinements in Criteria for the Determination of Death: An Appraisal," *Journal of the American Medical Association* 221, 1972, 48–53.

Cassens, Brett, "Social Consequences of the Acquired Immune Deficiency Syndrome," *Annals of Internal Medicine* 103(5), Nov. 1985, 768–771.

Cassirer, Ernst, *The Philosophy of Symbolic Forms,* vol. 1, New Haven: Yale University Press, 1953, 86–93.

Cataldo, Peter J., "Reproductive Technologies," *Ethics and Medics,* 21, January, 1996, 1–3.

Cataldo, Peter; and Moraczewski, Albert. *The Fetal Tissue Issue: Medical and Ethical Aspects,* Braintree, MA: Pope John Center, 1994.

Catechism of the Catholic Church, Collegeville: Liturgical Press, 1994.

Cavanaugh, John R., *The Popes, The Pill and The People,* Milwaukee: Bruce Books, 1964.

CCHCM: Commission for Catholic Health Care Ministry, "A New Vision for a New Century," Livonia, MI: Commission Control Office, 1988, 62.

CDC: Centers for Disease Control, "Update: Human Immunodeficiency Virus Infection in Health Care Workers Exposed to Blood of Infected Patients," *Morbidity and Morality Weekly Report* 36, 1987, 285–289.

CDF: Congregation for the Doctrine of the Faith
1963 "Cremation," in *Canon Law Digest* 6, Milwaukee, WI: Bruce Books p. 666 ff.
1974 *Declaration on Procured Abortion,* May, translated in *Osservatore Romano,* Dec. 5.
1975a "Declaration on Certain Problems of Sexual Ethics," *Vatican Council II: More Postconciliar Documents,* vol. 2, Austin Flannery, OP, ed., Northport, NY: Costello Publishing, 1982:486–499.
1975b "Doctrinal Congregational Statement on Sterilization," (March 13), in *Commentary of National Conference of Catholic Bishops,* Washington, DC: United States Catholic Conference, 1978.

1979 "The Reality of Life After Death," (March 11), in *Vatican Council II: More Postconciliar Documents*, vol. 2, Austin Flannery, OP, ed., Northport, NY: Costello Publishing Co., 1982, 500–504.

1980a "Declaration on Euthanasia," (May 5) in *Vatican Council II: More Postconciliar Documents*, vol. 2, Austin Flannery, OP, ed., Northport, NY: Costello Publishing Co., 1982, 510–517.

1980b "Instruction on Infant Baptism," (Oct. 20) in *Vatican Council II: More Postconciliar Documents*, vol. 2, Austin Flannery, OP, ed., Northport, NY: Costello Publishing Co., 1982, 510–517.

1984 "Instruction on Certain Aspects of the Liberation Theology,' " Boston: St. Paul Editions.

1986 "The Pastoral Care of Homosexual Persons," *Origins*, 377(16), November 13, p. 377 ff.

1987 "On Respect for Human Life," *Origins* 16(40) March 19:697–709.

1989 "The Moral Norms of Humanae Vitae," *Origins* 18(38) March 2.

1990 "Instruction on the Ecclesial Vocation of the Theologian," *Origins*, 20:8, July 5, 117–125.

1994 *Catechism of the Catholic Church*, Collegeville: Liturgical Press, 1994.

Cessario, R. *The Moral Virtues and Theological Virtues*, Notre Dame, IN: Notre Dame University Press, 1991.

de Chardin, Pierre Teilhard. *The Phenomenon of Man*, New York: Harper and Row, 1964.

CHA: The Catholic Health Association of the United States

1987 "Responses to the Vatican Document on Reproductive Technologies," *Hospital Progress* Jul–Aug:45–65.

1993a *Care of the Dying: A Catholic Perspective*, Part III, St. Louis, MO.

1993b *Integrated Delivery Systems*

1994 "Leaders for the new reality" *Ministry Perspectives*, 3.

Charlesworth, Max, *Bioethics in a Liberal Society*, NY: Cambridge University Press, 1993.

Charman, Robert C. *At Risk: Can the Doctor-Patient Relationship Survive in a High-Tech World?* Dublin, NH: W.L. Bauhan, 1992.

Charon, Rita; and Williams, Peter, "Medical Education," *Academic Medicine*, 70(9), September, 1995.

Charter of the Rights of the Family, Vatican City: Vatican Polyglot Press, 1983.

Chayet, Neil L., "Confidentiality and Privileged Communication," *New England Journal of Medicine* 275, 1966, 1009–1010.

Chervenak, F.A.; Farley, Margaret, Walters, Leroy; et al., "When is Termination of Pregnancy During the Third Trimester Justifiable," *New England Journal of Medicine* 310, 1984, 501–504.

Childress, James. *Who Should Decide: Paternalism in Health Care*, New York: Oxford University Press, 1982.

Childs, N.; and Mercer, W., "Late Improvement in Consciousness After Post-Traumatic Vegetative State," *New England Journal of Medicine* 334 (1), January 4, 1996, 24–25.

Chiles, John A.; Carlin, Albert S.; Benjamin, Andrew H.; and Beitman, Bernard D. "A physician, a non-medical psychotherapist, and a patient: The Pharmacotherapy-Psychotherapy Triangle," Bernard D. and Gerald L. Klerman, *Integrating Pharmacotherapy and Psychotherapy*, Washington, DC: American Psychiatric Press, 1991, 105–120.

Choron, Jacques, *Suicide*, New York: Charles Scribner Sons, 1972.

CIC: *Code of Canon Law*, 1983, Canon 1176; Canon 1203; Canon 1917.

Clair, Jeffery; and Allman, Richard, eds., *Sociomedical Perspectives on Patient Care*, Lexington, KY: University Press of Kentucky, 1993.

Clark, Angus, ed., *Genetic Counseling: Practice and Principles*, New York, NY: Routledge, 1994.

Clark, D.M., et al., "A Comparison of Cognitive Therapy, Relaxation, and Imipramine in the Treatment of Panic Disorder," *British Journal of Psychiatry*, 164(6), June, 1994, 759–769.

Clayton, Ellen. "What the Law says about Reproductive Genetic Testing and What it Doesn't," In Rothenberg, Karen; and Thompson, Elizabeth, eds., *Women and Prenatal Testing: Facing the Challenges of Genetic Technology*, Columbus, OH: Ohio State University Press, 1994.

Clebsch, William A.; and Jaekle, Charles R., *Pastoral Care in Historical Perspective*, New York: Jason Aronson, 1964.

Cleeland, Charles, et al., "Pain and Its Treatment in Out-Patients with Metastatic Cancer," *New England Journal of Medicine*, 330(9), March 3, 1994, 592–596.

Clements, Colleen, "Common Psychiatric Problems and Uncommon Ethical Solutions," *Psychiatric Annals* 13(4), April 1983, 289–301.

Clouser, K. Danner, *Teaching Bioethics: Strategies, Problems, and Resources*, New York: The Hastings Center Monograph: Plenum Press, 1980, 77.

Clouser, K. Danner; Culver, Charles M.; and Gert, Bernard, "Malady: A New Treatment of Disease," *Hastings Center Report* 11, 1981, 29–37.

Cobb, John B., *Theology and Pastoral Care*, Philadelphia: Fortress Press, 1977.

Code of Canon Law, A Test and Commentary, NY: Paulist Press, 1985.

Cohen, Jacques; and Tombin, Giles. "The science fiction and reality of embryo cloning," *Kennedy Institute of Ethics Journal*, 4(3), September, 1994, 187–192.

Cohen, S.K., "Psychoanalysis and Psychotropic Medication," *Journal of the American Psychoanalytic Association*, 43(1) 1995, 15–17.

Cole, C. et al., "Treatment of Gender Dysphoria," *Texas Medicine*, 90(5), May, 1994, 68–72.

College of Healthcare Executives, *The Future of Healthcare: Changes and Choices*, Chicago: Arthur Andersen Co., 1987.

College of Physicians Health and Public Policy Committee, "Acquired Immunodeficiency Syndrome," *Annals of Internal Medicine* 104(4), Apr. 1986, 575–581.

Collins, Francis. "Evolution of a vision: genome project origins, present, future, challenges, and far reaching benefits," *Human Genome News*, 7(3), September, 1995, p. 3.

Colombotos, John; and Kirchner, Corrine, *Physicians and Social Change*, New York: Oxford University Press, 1986.

Congar, Yves. *Le foi et la théologie*, Paris, du Cert c.4, p.1, 1962; 1977.

Connell, R.J., "A Defense of 'HV'," *Laval Theologique et Philosophique* 26, 1970 57–88. Criticism by W.R. Albury, and reply by L. Connell, *Laval Theologique et Philosophique* 27, 1971, 135–149.

Connery, John, SJ
1977 *Abortion: The Development of the Roman Catholic Perspective*, Chicago: Loyola University Press.
1980 "Prolonging Life: The Duty and Its Limits," *Catholic Mind*, Oct. 11, 43–57.
1981 "Catholic Ethics: Has the Norm for Rule Making Changed?" *Theological Studies* 42, 1981, 232–250.

Conrad, Peter; and Kern, Rochelle, eds., *The Sociology of Health and Illness*, New York: St. Martin's Press, 1981.

Cook, Elizabeth; and Jeleng, Ted, Wilcox, Clyde, *Between Two Absolutes: Public Opinion and the Politics of Abortion*, Boulder, CO: Westview Press, 1992.

Cope, Oliver, *Man, Mind and Medicine*, Philadelphia: Lippincott, 1968.

Coriden, James; Green, Thomas; and Heintschel, Donald, *The Code of Canon Law Text and Commentary*, New York: Paulist Press, 1985.

Couch, Nathen, et al., "The High Cost of Low Frequency Events: The Anatomy of Surgical Mishaps," *New England Journal of Medicine* 304, 1981, 634–637.

Council of Europe. "Opinions on the Use of Dead Human Embryos for Industrial and Commercial Purposes," in *Council of Europe*, 37th Session, Strasbourg: The Council, 1985: 1–9.

Council of Trent, Decrees and Documents, 1563.

Cournos, Francine; Faulkner, Larry; and Fitzgerald, Larry; et al., "Report of the Task Force on Consent to Voluntary Hospitalization," *Bulletin of the American Academy of Psychiatry and Law,* 215(3), 1993, 293–307.

Cousins, Norman. "How Patients Appraise Physicians," *New England Journal of Medicine* 313(22) Nov. 28, 1985, 1422–1424.

Cox, Harvey, ed., *The Situation Ethics Debate,* Philadelphia: Westminster Press, 1968.

Cramer, D.W., et al., Tubal Infertility and the Interuterine Device, *New England Journal of Medicine* 312, 1985, 941–947.

Cranford, Ronald
    1984 "Termination of Treatment in the Persistent Vegetative State," *Seminars in Neurology* 4(1), March 1984, 36–44.
    1985 "Life, Death, Awareness, and Suffering," in *Social Responsibility: Business, Journalism, Law, Medicine,* Louis Hodges, ed., Lexington, VA: Washington & Lee University, 41–50.
    1988 "The Persistent Vegetative State: The Medical Reality," *Hastings Center Report* (Feb/March), 25–32.

Crashaw, R. et al., "Patient-Physician Covenant," *Journal of the American Medical Association,* 273, (1996), p.1553.

Crauford, D.; and Harris, R., "Ethics of Predictive Testing for Huntington's Chorea: The Need for More Information," *British Medical Journal* 293(6541), July 26, 1986, 249–251.

Creighton Group on HIV Confidentiality, "Confidentiality and its Limits: Ethical Guidelines for HIV Infection," *Creighton Law Review,* 25(4), June, 1992, 1439–1460.

Crespi, R., "Ethical aspects of patenting in biotechnology," *Cancer Detection and Prevention,* 17(2), 1993, 323–327.

Crews, Frederick, "The Myth of Repressed Memory," Parts I and II, *The New York Review of Books,* 41(19), November 17, 54–59; 42(20), December 1, 49–58, 1994.

Crissman, Susan, and Betz, Linda, "Education and Image: Critical Issues Confronting the Nursing Profession," *Journal of Contemporary Health Law & Policy* 3, Spring 1987, 174–184.

Cronin, John, *Catholic Social Principles,* Milwaukee: Bruce Books, 1950.

Crooij, Marinus, et al., "Termination of Early Pregnancy by the 3Beta-Hydroxysteriod Inhibitor Epostane," *The New England Journal of Medicine,* 219, September 29, 1988, 813–817.

Crowe, M., "Sex Therapy: The Successes, the Failures, the Future," *British Journal of Hospital Medicine,* 48(8), October, 1992, 474–479.

Cubb, E., et al., "A pilot study on teaching natural family planning in general practice," in *Natural Family Planning Current Knowledge and New Strategies for the 90's,* Washington, DC: Georgetown University Press, 1990.

Culver, Kenneth, "Splices of Life: Genetic Therapy Comes of Age," *Science* (1), January, 18–24, 1993.

Cunningham, Bert, *The Morality of Organic Transplantation,* Washington, DC: Catholic University of America Press, 1944.

Cuomo, Mario, "Religious Belief and Public Morality," *The Human Life Review* 11(1–2), Spring 1985, 26–40.

Cupples, Brian; and Cochnauer, Myron, "The Investigator's Duty Not to Deceive," *I.R.B.: A Review of Human Subjects Research* 7(5), Oct. 1985.

Curran, Charles E.
    1968 *A New Look at Catholic Morality,* Notre Dame: Fides Publishers.
    1973 "Sterilization, Roman Catholic Theory and Practice," *Linacre Quarterly,* May, 103.
    1975 *Ongoing Revision; Studies in Moral Theology,* Notre Dame: Fides Publishers, "On specificity of Christian ethics," pp. 1–37; "Theology of compromise," pp. 187–190; "Principle of double effect," pp. 173–209; "Cooperation," pp. 210–228.

1977a *Themes in Fundamental Moral Theology,* Notre Dame: University of Notre Dame Press.

1977b *Issues in Sexual and Medical Ethics,* Notre Dame: University of Notre Dame Press.

1978 "Ten Years Later: Reflections on the Anniversary of Humanae Vitae," *Commonweal,* July 7, 1978, 425–230.

1979 *Transition and Tradition in Moral Theology,* Notre Dame: University of Notre Dame Press.

1982 *American Catholic Social Ethics: Twentieth Century Approaches,* Notre Dame: University of Notre Dame Press.

1984 *Critical Concerns in Moral Theology,* Notre Dame: University of Notre Dame Press.

1985 *Directions in a Fundamental Moral Theology,* Notre Dame: University of Notre Dame Press.

1988 *Tensions in Moral Theology,* Notre Dame: Notre Dame Press.

Curran, Charles E.; and Hunt, Robert E., *Dissent in and for the Church; Theologians and Humanae Vitae,* New York: Sheed & Ward, 1969.

Curran, Charles E.; and McCormick, Richard A., SJ,

1979 "Moral Norms and Catholic Tradition," *Readings in Moral Theology* No. 1, New York: Paulist Press.

1980 "The Distinctiveness of Christian Ethics," *Readings in Moral Theology* No. 2., New York: Paulist Press.

1986 *Official Catholic Social Teaching,* Mahwek, NJ: Paulist Press.

1988 *Dissent in the Church,* New York: Paulist Press.

Curran, William J., "Medical Peer Review of Physician Competence and Performance: Legal Immunity and the Anti-Trust Laws," *New England Journal of Medicine* 316 (10), March 5, 1987, 597–598.

Curran, William J.; and Cassells, W., "The Ethics of Medical Participation in Capital Punishment with Intravenous Drug Injection," *New England Journal of Medicine* 302, 1980, 226–230.

Curzer, Howard, "Is Care a Virtue for Health Care Professionals?" *Journal of Medicine and Philosophy,* (1) February 18, 1993.

Daling, et al., "Primary Tubal Infertility in Relation to the Use of an Intrauterine Device," *New England Journal of Medicine* 312, 1985, 937–91.

Daly, T.V.

1987 "Identifying the Origin of Life: The Search for a Marker Event for the Origin of Human Life," *St. Vincent's Bioethics Center Newsletter,* 5, March, 4–6,

1988 "Individuals, Syngamy and the Origin of Life," 6, December, 1–7.

Daniel, David, et al., "Brain Imaging in Neuropsychiatry" in *Textbook of Neuropsychiatry,* Washington, DC: American Psychiatric Press, 1992.

Darvall, Leanna, *Medicine, Law and Social Change: The Impact of Bioethics, Feminism and Rights Movement on Medical Decision Making,* Brookfield, VT: Dartmouth Publishing Company, 1993.

Davis, John Jefferson

1984 *Abortion and the Christian,* Phillipsburg, NJ: Presbyterian Reformed Publishing.

1985 *Evangelical Ethics Issues Facing the Church Today,* Phillipsburg, NJ: Reformed Publishing Co.

Davis, Nancy, "Morality and Biotechnology," *Southern California Law Review,* 65 (1) November, 1991, 27–40.

deBlois, Jean

1991 with McGrath, Mary; and O'Rourke, Kevin, 3 "Advance Directives," *Health Progress,* July–Aug, p. 27–31.

1994 with Norris, Patrick; and O'Rourke, Kevin, *A Primer for Health Care Ethics,* DC: Georgetown University Press., consent, p.72–73; ectopic pregnancy, 208–210.

1995 "The American health care system and the pursuit of health," in Magill, G., ed. *Values and Public Life*, University Press of America, 199–224.

Dedek, John F.
1972 *Human Life: Some Moral Issues*, New York: Sheed & Ward.
1979 "Intrinsically Evil Acts: An Historical Study of the Mind of St. Thomas," *The Thomist* 43, 385–413.

Deeken, Alfons, *Process and Permanence in Ethics*, New York: Paulist Press, 1974.

Delbanco, Andrew; and Delbanco, Thomas, "A.A. at the Crossroads," *The New Yorker*, March 20, 1995.

Delhaye, Phillipe; et al., "Déclarations épiscopales du monde entier," Jan Grootaers and Gustave Thils, eds., *Pour Relire Humanae Vitae*, with commentaries by eds., Paris: Duculot.

Dellapenna, Joseph W., "Abortion and the Law: Blackman's Distortion of the Historical Record," in *Abortion and The Constitution*, Dennis Horan; Edward Grant; and Paige C. Cunningham, eds., Georgetown: Georgetown University Press, 1987.

DeMarco, Donald T.
1988 "Catholic Moral Teaching and TOT/GIFT," with a "Response" by Donald J. McCarthy, *Reproductive Technologies, Marriage and the Church*, Braintree, MA: Pope John Center, 122–144.
1991 "Zygotes, Persons, and Genetics," *Ethics and Medics*, 16 (1), 3–4.

Denes, Magda, *Necessity and Sorrow: Life and Death in an Abortion Hospital*, New York: Basic Books, 1976.

Denham, M. J., "The Ethics of Research With the Elderly," *Age and Aging* (6), Nov. 13, 1984, 321–327.

Dennett, Daniel C., *Consciousness Explained*, Back Bay/Little Brown, 1995.

Dent, June, "Obtaining Informed Consent for HIV Antibody Testing, the Decision Making Process," *Counseling Psychology Quarterly*, 2(1), 1989, 73–77.

Derrickson, Paul; and Ebersolo, Myron, "Lasting Effects of CPE, A Five Year Review," *Pastoral Care* 30, March 1986, 5.

deSilva, P., "Management of Female Sexual Difficulties," *British Journal of Clinical Psychology*, 11(2), June, 1993, 125–134.

Devereux, George, *A Study of Abortion in Primitive Societies*, New York: International Universities Press, 1976 [1955].

Dewey, John, *Reconstruction in Philosophy*, Boston: Beacon Press, 1948 [1920], ch. 7.

DHEW: Department of Health, Education, and Welfare
1975 The National Commission for the Protection of Human Subjects of Biomedical and Behavioral Research, *Research on the Fetus*, Washington, DC: U.S. Government Printing Office.
1978 National Commission for Protection of Human Subjects of Biomedical and Behavioral Research, *Report and Recommendations, Institutional Review Boards*, DHEW (o.s.) 78–0008, 1978.

DHHS: Department of Health and Human Services
1986 Task Force on Organ Transplantation, *Organ Transplantation: Issues and Recommendations*, Rockville, MD; DHHS, April.
1995 *Integrity and Misconduct in Research*, Public Health Service.

Diamond, Eugene F., "Games People Play with Abortion Data," *Linacre Quarterly*, November, 1991, 35–38.

Diamond, James, J., "Abortion Animation, and Biological Hominization," *Theological Studies*, 36, 1975, 305–324.

Dickens, Bernard, "Abortion, Amniocentesis and the Law," *American Journal of Comparative Law* 34(2), Spring 1986, 249–270.

Dickson, David, "Europe Split on Embryo Research," *Science* 242, Nov. 25, 1988, 1117.

Dickstein, Morris. "Columbia Recovered," *New York Times Magazine*, May 15, 1988, 32 ff.

DiNoia, J. *The Diversity of Religions: A Christian Perspective,* Washington, DC: Catholic University of America, 1992.

Doms, Herbert, *The Meaning of Marriage,* NY: Sheed & Ward, 1939.

Donabedian, Avedis, "Quality in Health Care: Whose Responsibility is it?" *CME Seminar,* Clearwater, FL: American Board of Quality Assurance, 1994.

Donceel, Joseph
    1970 "Immediate Animation and Delayed Hominization," *Theological Studies* 31(1), 76–105.
    1985 "Catholic Politicians and Abortion," *America,* Feb. 2, 81–83.

Doran, Kevin, *What is a Person? The Concept and the Implications for Ethics.* Lewiston, NY: Edwin Mellen Press, 1989.

Dorman, J., "The History of Psychosurgery," *Texas Medicine,* 91(7), July, 1995, 54–61.

Dorozynski, Alexander, "Europe Condemns Sale of Organs," *British Medical Journal,* 307, September, 1993, 6907–756.

Dougherty, Charles
    1985 *Ideal, Fact, and Medicine,* Lanham, MD: University Press.
    1995 "Institutional Ethics Committees," in Reich, Warren, ed. *Encyclopedia of Bioethics Revised edition,* NY: Simon & Schuster Macmillan, 402–412.

Downie, R.S. "The Doctor-Patient Relationship," In: Gillon Ranaan, *Principles of Health Care Ethics,* NY: Wiley Publishing, 1994, 343–352.

Drane, James, "Anencephaly and the interruption of pregnancy: policy proposals for HECs," *HEC Forum,* 4, February, 1992, 103–119.

Dresser, Rebecca; and Whitehouse, Peter, "The incompetent patient on the slippery slope," *Hastings Center Report,* 24(4), July–August, 1994, 6–12.

Drucker, Peter F., "Freudian Myths and Freudian Realities," in *Adventures of a Bystander,* New York: Harper and Row, 1978, 83–99.

Duff, Raymond; and Hollinshead, August, *Sickness and Society,* NY: Harper and Row, 1968.

Duffy, Regis, *A Roman Catholic Theology of Pastoral Care,* Philadelphia: Fortress Press, 1983.

Duke, Kathryn Swenz, "Hospitals in a changing health care system," *Health Affairs* 15:2, Summer 1996, 49–62.

Duke, Leela, "Amniocentesis Debate Continued," *Economic and Political Weekly* 18(38) September 17, 1983, 1633–35.

Dulles, Avery
    1988 "What is the Role of a Bishops' Conference," *Origins* 17 (46), Apr. 28, 1988, 789–796.
    1991 "The Magisterium, theology & dissent," *Origins* 20:42 (March 128, 1991): 692–696.

Durkheim, *Suicide,* Glenco, IL: Free Press, 1951.

Duska, Ronald; and Whaelen, M. *Moral Development a Guide to Piaget and Kohlberg,* New York: Paulist Press, 1975.

Dworkin, R. *Life's Dominion: An Argument about Abortion, Euthanasia and Individual Freedom,* NY: Knopf, 1993.

Easthope, Gary, *Healers and Alternative Medicine: A Sociological Explanation,* Brookfield, VT: Gower Publishing, 1986.

Ebert, Robert; and Ginzberg, Eli; et al., "The Case for Medical Education Reform," in *Health Affairs Supplement,* 1988.

Edelman, D.A., "IUD Complications in Perspective," *Contraception* 36(1), 1987, 159–67.

Edelman, D.A.; McIntyre, S.; and Harper, J., "A Comparative Trial of the Contraceptive Sponge and Diaphragm," *American Journal of Obstetrics and Gynecology* 150, 1984, 869.

Edelman, Gerald, *Neural Darwinism: The Theory of Neuronal Group Selection,* New York: Basic Books, 1987.

Edelstein, Ludwig, *Ancient Medicine: Selected Papers*, O. and C. Tembia, eds., Baltimore: Johns Hopkins Press, 1967.

Edleman, Gerald, *The Remembered Present: A Biological Theory of Consciousness*, New York: Basic Books, 1995.

Edwards, Lilian, "The right to consent and the right to refuse: more problems with minors and medical consent," *Juridical Review*, 1, January, 1993, 52–73.

Egan, Gerard, *The Skilled Helper*, 3rd ed., Monterrey, CA: Brooks-Cole, 1986.

Ehrman, Lee; et al., "The Supreme Court and Patenting Life," *Hastings Center Report* 10, 1980, 1–15.

Eichna, Ludwig, "Medical Education 1975–1979: A Student's Perspective," *New England Journal of Medicine* 303, 1980, 727–732.

Eige, Francis, ed. *The Professions in Ethical Context: Vocations to Justice and Love*, Villa Nova, PA: Villa Nova University Press, 1986.

Eisenberg, John, *Doctors, Decisions and the Cost of Medical Care*, Ann Arbor: Health Administration Press, 1986.

Eisenberg, Leon, "Health Care for Patients or For Profit?" *American Journal of Psychiatry* 143 (8), Aug. 1986, 1015–1019.

Elliott, Carl, "The Risks of Insanity: Commentary on Psychopathic Disorders, A Category Mistake," *Journal of Medical Ethics*, 17, 1991, 89–90.

Ellul, Jacques
1965 *The Technological Society*, New York: Alfred A. Knopf.
1980 *The Technological System*, New York: Continuum Publishing Co.

Ellwood, Paul; Enthoup, Alain; and Etheridge, Lynn, "The Jackson Hole Initiatives for the 21st Century American Health Care System," *Health Economics*, Vol. 1, 1992, 149–168.

Ely, John, "The Wages of Crying Wolf," *The Yale Law Journal*, Apr. 1973, 935.

Emanuel, Ezekial
1988 "Do Physicians Have an Obligation to Treat Patients with AIDS?" *New England Journal of Medicine* 318(25), June 23, 1686–1690.
1991 *The Ends of Human Life*, Cambridge, MA: Harvard University Press, Chapter 1.
1994 "Euthanasia, Historical, Ethical and Empiric Perspectives," *Archives of Internal Medicine*, 154(17):1890–901, 1994 Sep 12.
1995 "The Beginning of the End of Principalism," *Hasting Center Report*, July–Aug 1995, 25:4:37–38.

Emanuel, E.; and Emanuel, L., "Proxy Decision Making for Incompetent Patients: An Ethical and Empirical Analysis," *Journal of the American Medical Association*, 267(15), April 15, 1992, 2067–71.

Enarson; et al., "An Overview of Reform Initiatives in Medical Education 1906 through 1992," *Journal of the American Medical Association*, 268(9), 1992, 1141–1143.

Engel, G.L., "The Clinical Application of the Biopsychosocial Model," *Journal of Medicine and Philosophy* 6(2), 1981.

Engelhardt, H. Tristram, Jr.
1977 "Some Persons Are Humans, Some Humans Are Persons, and the World Is What We Persons Make It," in *Philosophical Medical Ethics*, Stuart C. Spicker and H. Tristram Engelhardt, Jr., eds., Boston: Reidel, 183–194.
1986a "Endings and Beginnings of Persons' Death, Abortion and Infanticide," in *The Foundations of Bioethics*, New York: Oxford University Press, 202–249.
1986b *The Foundation of Bioethics*, New York: Oxford University Press, 107–110.
1986c "Suicide and the Cancer Patient," *CA Cancer Journal for Clinicians* 36(2), Mar.–Apr., 105–109.
1992 "The Search for Universal System of Ethics: Post Modernist Disappointment," in *Ethical Problems in Dialysis and Transplantation*, Boston: Kluwer.
1995 *The Foundations of Bioethics*, 2nd edition, NY: Oxford Press.

England, M. J.; and Goff, V. *New Directions for Mental Health Services,* San Francisco, CA: Jossey-Bass, 1993.

Engler, R. L.; et al., "Misrepresentation and Responsibility in Medical Research," *New England Journal of Medicine* 317, 1987, 1383–389.

Erde, Edmund, "Defining Health, Disease and Their Bearing on Medical Practice," *Ethics in Science and Medicine* 6, 1979, 31–48.

Erikson, Erik, *Identity: Youth and Crisis,* New York: W.W. Norton and Co., 1968.

Evans, Martyn, "Against Brainstem Death," in *Principles of Health Care Ethics,* Raanan Gillon, ed., New York: Wiley, 1994.

Ewan, Christine, "Teaching Ethics in Medical Schools," *Medical Teacher,* 8(2), 1986.

Fackleman, K. A., "Researchers 'clone' human embryos," *Science News,* October, 1994:22–25.

Faden, Ruth; and Beauchamp, Thomas, *A History and Theory of Informed Consent,* New York: Oxford Press, 1986, 161.

Farrell, Dave, "The WD Report: The Impossible Choice," *Woman's Day,* 6, June 1995, 87–90.

Fath, Gerald, OP, "Pastoral Counseling in the Hospital Setting," in *Clinical Handbook of Pastoral Counseling,* ed., Robert Wicks; Donald Parsons; and Donald Capps, eds., NY: Paulist Press, 349–360.

Federal Register, July 5, 1983, Vol. 48, 129, 30846, "Nondiscrimination on the Basis of Handicap Relating to Health Care for Handicapped Infants."

Feldman, David
    1986a *Health and Medicine in the Jewish Tradition,* New York: Crossroad Publishing Co., 1986.
    1986b "The Matter of Abortion," in his *Health and Medicine in the Jewish Tradition,* New York: Crossroad Publishing Co., 1986.

Felthouse, A.R., "Substance Abuse and the Duty to Protect," *Bulletin of the Academy of Psychiatry and the Law,* 21(4), 1993, 419–26.

Fetsch, Susan; and Minturn, Mary. "Strengthening the Nurse's Role as Patient Advocate," *Bioethics Forum,* Winter 1994 (10):15–19.

Fichter, Joseph H., *Religion and Poor: The Spiritual Dimensions of Health Care,* New York: Crossroad Publishing Co., 1981.

Fingarette, Herbert; and Hasse, Ann Fingarette, *Mental Disabilities and Criminal Responsibility,* Berkeley: University of California Press, 1979.

Finkel, Norman, et al., "Right to Die, Euthanasia and Community Sentiment: Crossing the Public/Private Boundary," *Law and Human Behavior,* 17(5), October, 1993, 487–506.

Finnis, John
    1983 *Fundamentals of Ethics,* Washington, DC: Georgetown University Press.
    1991 *Moral Absolutes: Tradition, Revision, and Truth,* Washington, DC: Catholic University of America Press.

Fisher, Anthony, "'When Did I Begin' Revisited," *Linacre Quarterly,* 58(3), 1991, 59–68.

Fisher, R. A.
    1989 et al., "Frequency of heterozygous complete hydatidiform moles, estimated by locus-specific minisatellite and Y chromosome-specific probes," *Human Genetics,* 82, 259–63.
    1991 "Frequency of Heterozygous Complete Hydatiformmoles," *Human Genetics,* 82(1989):259–63.

Flaman, "When Did I Begin? Another Critical Response to Norman Ford," *Linacre Quarterly,* 58(4), 1991, 39,55.

Flannery, Austin, "Hierarchies Give Pastoral Advice on *Humanae Vitae,*" *Doctrine and Life* 19(2), Feb. 1969.

Fletcher, John
    1982 *Coping with Genetic Disorders: A Guide for Clergy and Parents,* San Francisco: Harper and Row.

1983   "The Evolution of the Ethics of Informed Consent," in Kare Berg and Erik Knat, eds., *Research Ethics,* New York: Alan R. Liss.

1985   "Ethical Issues in and Beyond Prospective Clinical Trials of Human Gene Therapy," *Journal of Medicine & Philosophy* 3, Aug. 10, 293–309.

Fletcher, John; and Hoffman, Diane," Ethics Committees: Time to Experiment with Standards," *Annals of Internal Medicine,* 120(4) February 14, 1994, 335–338.

Fletcher, Joseph

1954   *Morals and Medicine,* Boston: Beacon Press.

1960   "The Patient's Right to Die," *Harpers,* Oct., 138–143.

1974   "Four Indicators of Humanhood: The Enquiry Matures," *Hastings Center Report* 4, 4–7. With replies in Correspondence I 5(4), 43–45.

1979   *Humanhood: Essays in Biomedical Ethics,* Buffalo: Prometheus Press.

1982   "Situation Ethics Revisited," *Religious Humanism* 16, Winter, 9–13.

1988   *The Ethics of Genetic Control: Ending Reproductive Roulette,* Buffalo: Prometheus Books.

Flexner, Abraham, *Medical Education in The United States and Canada,* Carnegie Foundation for the Advancement of Teaching, Bulletin 4, Boston: Marymount Press, 1910. Reprinted Washington, DC: Science and Health Publications, 1960.

Fleyner, John, "Dying, Death, and the Front Line Physician," in *Dying and Death,* ed., David Burton, New York: Williams, 1977.

Flynn, A., "Natural methods of contraception," *Maternal and Child Health,* 16, 1991, 148–53.

Foley, K.M., "The Relationship of Pain and Symptom Management to Patient Requests for Physician-Assisted Suicide," *Journal of Pain and Symptom Management,* 6, 1991, 289–297.

Ford, Amasa *et al. The Doctor's Perspective: Physicians View Their Patients and Their Practice,* Cleveland: Case Western Reserve University, 1967, 139 ff.

Ford, John C.; and Grisez, Germain, "Contraception and the Infallibility of the Ordinary Magisterium," *Theological Studies* 39(2), June 1978, 258–312.

Ford, John C., and Kelly, Gerald, SJ, *Contemporary Moral Theology,* 2 vols., Westminster, MD: Newman Press, 1964 (on contraception, vol. 2, 245–275).

Ford, Norman, *When Did I Begin?: Conception of the Human Individual in History, Philosophy and Science,* Cambridge, MA: Cambridge University Press, 1988.

Fordney-Settlage, Diane S.; Motoshima, Masanabu; and Tredway, Donald S., "Sperm Transport From the External Cervical Os to the Fallopian Tubes in Woman: A Time and Quantitation Study," *Fertility and Sterility* 24, Sept. 1973, 655–661.

Forer, Lois G., "Medical Services in Prisons: Rights and Remedies," *American Bar Association Journal* 68, May 1982, 562–565.

Foster, John, "A Defense of Dualism," in *The Case for Dualism,* John Smythies, ed., Charlottesville, VA: University Press of Virginia, 1989.

Foucault, Michael, *The Birth of the Clinic: An Archaeology of Medical Perception,* New York: Pantheon, 1973.

Fox, Ellen; Arnold, Robert; and Bordy, Baruch. "Medical Ethics Education: Past, Present and Future," *Academic Medicine,* 70(9), September 1995.

Fox, Renee, *Essays in Medical Sociology,* Philadelphia: University of Pennsylvania, 1988.

Fox, Renee; and Swazy, Judith P.

1978   *The Courage to Fail: A Social View of Organ Transplant and Dialysis,* 2nd ed., Chicago: University of Chicago Press, 1978.

1992   "Leaving the field," *Hastings Center Report,* 22(5) September-October, 1992, 9–15.

Francis, Richard; and Franklin, John, "Alcohol and Other Psychoactive Substance Use Disorders," in *Textbook of Psychiatry,* John Talbott, et al., eds., Washington DC, American Psychiatric Press, 1988, 313–356.

Francke, Linda Bird, *The Ambivalence of Abortion,* New York: Random House, 1978.

Francoeur, Robert. "We Can—We Must: Reflections on the Technological Imperative," *Theological Studies* 33, 428–439, 1972.

Frankena, William
    1980 *Thinking About Morality*, Ann Arbor: University of Michigan Press.
    1985 "The Potential of Theology for Ethics," in *Theology and Bioethics: Exploring the Foundations and Frontiers*, E. Shelp, ed., Boston: D. Reidel, 49–64.

Freedman, D., "The Search: Body, Mind and Human Purpose," *American Journal of Psychiatry*, 149, 1991, 858–866.

Freeman, Harrop A., *Counseling in the United States*, San Francisco: Jossey-Bass, 1967.

Freidson, Eliot, *Profession of Medicine: A Study of the Sociology of Applied Knowledge*, New York: Dodd, Mead, and Co., 1971.

Frenkiel, Nora, "Family planning: baby boy or girl," *New York Times*, November 11, 1993, C-1.

Freud, Sigmund
    1920 *Beyond the Pleasure Principle*, in *Complete Works*, vol. 18, London: Hogarth and Institute of Psychoanalysis, 1958.
    1930 *Civilization and its Discontents*, in *Complete Works*, Vol. 20, London: Hogarth and Institute of Psychanalysis, 1958.

Freymann, JohnGordon, *The American Health Care System: Its Genesis and Trajectory*, New York: Medcom, 1974.

Friedman, Emily, "The 'Dumping' Dilemma: Finding What's Fair," *Hospitals* 56 (18), Sept. 16, 1982, 75–84.

Friedman, Richard; and Douney, Jennifer, "Homosexuality," *NEJM* 331(4) October 6, 1994, 923–929.

Fromm, Erich, *Crisis of Psychoanalysis*, New York: Fawcett World Library, 1975.

Fuchs, Josef, SJ
    1971 "The Absoluteness of Moral Terms," *Gregorianum* 52, 415–458.
    1980 "Sin of the World and Normative Morality," *Gregorianum* 61, 67.
    1984 *Christian Ethics In A Secular Arena*, Washington, DC: Georgetown University Press.

Fulford, K.W.M.; and Hope, Tony, "Psychiatric Ethics: A Bioethical Ugly Duckling," In Gillon, Raana, ed., *Principles of Health Care Ethics*, NY: Wiley, 1994, 681–695.

Fumento, Michael, "Fetal attraction," *The American Spectator*, 3, July, 1992, p. 36.

Gabriel, Trip, "High Tech Pregnancies: Test, Hopes, Limits," *New York Times*, January 7, 1996.

Gaddes, William, *Learning Disabilities and Brain Function*, New York: Springer-Verlag, 1985.

Gadow, Sally, "Caring for the Dying: Advocacy or Paternalism," *Health Education* 3, 1980, 387–398.

Galdston, Iago, *Social and Historical Foundations of Modern Medicine*, New York: Brunner-Mazel, 1981.

Gallagher, John
    1981 "Magisterial Teaching from 1918 to the Present," in *Human Sexuality and Personhood*, St. Louis: Pope John XXIII Medical-Moral Research and Education Center.
    1985 *Is the Human Embryo a Person: A Philosophical Investigation*, Toronto: Human Life Research Institute.

GAO: General Accounting Office
    1987 *Medical Malpractice: Characteristics of Claims Closed in 1984*, Washington, DC: GAO.
    1993 *Organ Transplants: Increased Effort Needed to Boost Supply and Ensure Equitable Distribution of Organs*, Washington, DC, April.

Garfield, Jay L.; and Hennessey, Patricia, eds., *Abortion, Moral and Legal Perspectives*, Amherst: University of Massachusetts Press, 1984.

Garrison, Fielding H., *An Introduction to the History of Medicine*, 4th ed., Philadelphia: W.D. Saunders Co., 1960 [1929].

Garry, D. J., "Are there really alternatives to the use of fetal tissue from elective abortions in transplantation research?" *New England Journal of Medicine* 327(22) November 26, 1992, 1592–1595.

Gatch, Milton M., *Death: Meaning and Morality in Christian Thought and Contemporary Culture*, New York: Seabury Press, 1969.

Gaylin, Willard, "Skinner Redux," *Harpers*, Oct. 1973, 48–56.

Gazzaniga, Michael. *Nature's Mind: The Biological Roots of Human Nature*, NY: Basic Books, 1992.

GBI: Committee on Bioethical Issues of the Bishops of Great Britain and Ireland
    1986a "Use of the Morning After Pill in Cases of Rape," *Origins* 15(39) March 13:633–638.
    1986b "A Reply: Use of the Morning After Pill in Cases of Rape," *Origins* 16(13), September 11:237–238.

Gelbard, Alene, "Population Growth, Development, and Women: A Consensus?" in *Proceeding ITEST* ed, Robert Brungs, St. Louis, MO: ITEST Foundation, 1995.

Gemuth, Saul, "The Reproductive Glands," in *Physiology*, Robert Berne and Matthew Levy, eds., St. Louis: C.V. Mosby Co., 1988.

Gerbert, Barbara; Bleecker, Thomas; Maguire, Bryan T.; et al. "Physicians and AIDS: Sexual Risk Assessment of Patients and Willingness to Treat HIV-infected Patients," *Journal of General Internal Medicine*, 7(6) Nov-Dec, 1992, 657–664.

Gerhardt, Uta, *Ideas About Illness*, NY: University Press, 1989.

Gervais, Karen; and Miles, Steven, "RU-486: New Issues in the American Abortion Debate," report for the Center for Biomedical Ethics, Minneapolis, MN, 1990.

Gianelli, Diane. "Embryo research approved with a catch," *AMA Medical News*, December 10, 1994.

Gilbert, Scott F. "Cleavage: Creating multicellularity," In: *Developmental Biology*, 3rd ed., Sunderland, MA: Sinauer Associates, 1991, Chapter 3, 75–98. 1991.

Gilder, George, *Wealth & Poverty*, New York: Bantam, 1982.

Gilleman, Gerard, *The Primacy of Charity in Moral Theology*, Westminster, MD: Newman Press, 1961.

Gillick, Muriel R. "From Confrontation to Cooperation in the Doctor-Patient Relationship," *Journal of General Internal Medicine*, 1992, Jan–Feb, 7(1), 83–86.

Gilligan, Carol
    1993 *In a Different Voice*, Cambridge, MA: Harvard University Press.
    1995 *Moral Voices, Moral Selves*, co-author, J. Hekman, University Park, PA: Pennsylvania State University Press.

Gillon, Raanan
    1986a "The Principle of Double Effect and Medical Ethics," *British Medical Journal* 292(6514), Jan. 18, 193–194.
    1986b "Doctors and Patients," *British Medical Journal* 292(6518), Feb. 15, 466–469.
    1986c "Doctors and Patients," *British Medical Journal* 292(6518) Feb. 15, 466–469.
    1987 "Aids and Medical Confidentiality," *British Medical Journal* 294(6588) June 27, 1675–1677.
    1994 ed., *Principles of Health Care Ethics*, New York: Wiley.

Ginsberg, Eli, et al., *The Coming Physician Surplus*, Totowa, NJ: Rowman and Allanheld, 1984.

Glaser, William A., *Social Settings and Medical Organization: A Cross-National Study of the Hospital*, New York: Atherton, 1970.

Glass, Bentley
    1975 *Human Heredity and Ethical Problems*, Philadelphia: Philadelphia Society for Health and Human Values.

Glover, Jonathan, *What Sort of People Should There Be? Genetic Engineering, Brain Control and Their Impact on Our Future World*, New York: Free Press, 1985.

Goffman, Erving, *Asylums: Essays on the Social Situation of Mental Patients and Other Inmates*, Chicago: Aldine, 1962.

Goldberg, Abbot, "The Peer Review Privilege: A Law in Search of A Valid Policy," *American Journal of Law* 10(2), Summer 1984, 151–167.

Goldenring, John M.
1984   "Denial of antipregnancy prophylaxis in rape victims," *New England Medical Journal*, 3, December 20, 1984, 1637.
1985   "The brain-life theory: Towards a consistent biological definition of humanness," *Journal of Medical Ethics*, 11, 1985, 198–204.

Goldner, Jesse, "An overview of legal control and the regulator implications of taking Professor Katz seriously," *Saint Louis University Law Journal*, 38(1), Fall, 1993, 63–134.

Goldschmidt, Timothy, *The Human Career, The Self in the Symbolic World*, Cambridge, MA: Blackwell, 1991.

Goldstein, Robert, "Tarasoff and the Practice of Psychotherapy," *American Journal of Psychiatry*, 150, August, 1993, p. 1278.

Goleman, Daniel, "Psychologists Dispute Value of Antidepressants," *New York Times*, November 30, 1995.

Golub, Edward, *The Limits of Medicine: How Science Shapes Our Hope for a Cure*, NY: Random House, 1994.

Goode, William J., "The Theoretical Limits of Professionalization," in *The Semi-Professions and Their Organization*, Amitai Etzioni, ed., New York: Free Press, 1969, 266–313.

Goodman, Lenn E.; and Goodman, Madeleine J., "Prevention: How Misuse of a Concept Undercuts its Worth," *Hasting Center Report* 2, Apr. 16, 1986, 26–38.

Goodwin, Candice. "Personal Property vs. Public Health," *New Scientist*, 140:1903, 1993, p. 25.

Granfield, Patrick, *The Limits of the Papacy*, New York: Crossroad Publishing Co., 1987.

Greeley, Andrew
1976   "Council or Encyclical," *Review of Religious Research* 18, Fall, 3–24.
1991   "Live and Let Die: Changing Attitudes" *Christian Century*, vol. 108, Dec. 4:1124–25.
1996   *General Social Survey Trends 1972–1994*, Chicago: National Opinion Research Council (NORC), 1996.

Green, S. A., "The Ethical Limits of Confidentiality in the Therapeutic Relationship," *General Hospital Psychiatry*, 17(2), March, 1995, 80–84.

Green, Ronald M., "Conferred Rights and the Fetus," *Journal of Religious Ethics* 2, Spring 1974, 55–76. Reply by James Childress, "A Response," *Journal of Religious Ethics* 2, Spring 1974, 77–84.

Greene, Majorie. *Dimensions of Darwinism: Themes & Counter Themes in Twentieth Century Evolutionary Theory*, New York: Cambridge University Press, 1983.

Greenfield, S. et al., "Variations in Resource Utilization Among Medical Specialties," *Journal of the American Medical Association*, 267 (2), 1992, 1624–1630.

Greer, Germaine, *Sex and Destiny, The Politics of Fertility*, New York: Harper and Row, 1984.

Gregorek, Joseph, "Guide for Treating Rape Victims Emphasizes Compassion, Respect," *Health Progress* 69 (7), Sept. 1988, 71–72.

Griese, Orville, *Catholic Identity in Health Care*, Braintree, MA: Pope John Center, 1987, n. 46, Ogino-Knaus, p. 37–38.

Grimes, David A. "Technology Follies: The Uncritical Acceptance of Medical Innovation." *Journal of the American Medical Association*, 269 (23) June 16, 1993, 3030–3033.

Grimes, David A.; and Cook, Rebecca J. "Mifepristone (RU-486)—An Abortifacient to Prevent Abortion?" *The New England Journal of Medicine*, 327, October 8, 1992, 1088–89.

Grisez, Germain G.
1964   *Contraception and the Natural Law*. Milwaukee: Bruce Books.

1970a *Abortion: The Myths, the Realities, the Arguments,* Washington, DC: Corpus Books. 282–287.

1970b "Toward a Consistent Natural-Laws Ethics of Killing," *American Journal of Jurisprudence* 15, 65–96.

1977 "Suicide and Euthanasia," in *Death, Dying and Euthanasia,* Dennis J. Horan and David Mall, eds., Washington, DC: University Publications, 742–818.

1983 *The Way of the Lord Jesus,* Chicago: Franciscan Press, "probabalism," p. 293.

1988 *Beyond the New Morality,* 3rd edition, co-author, Russell Shaw, Notre Dame, IN: University of Notre Dame Press.

1990 "When Do People Begin?" in *The Ethics of Having Children, Proceedings of the American Catholic Philosophical Association,* 63, 27–47.

1992 "When Do People Begin," in *Abortion: A New Generation of Catholic Responses,* Heaney, Stephen, ed. Braintree, MA: Pope John XXIII Center, 1992, p.1–27.

1993 *Living a Christian Life,* Vol. 2, Quincy, IL: Franciscan Herald Press.

1996 "Difficult Moral Questions," *Linacre Quarterly* 63(2) Spring 1996, p. 44.

Grisez, Germain; and Boyle, Joseph M. Jr., *Life and Death with Liberty and Justice,* Notre Dame: University of Notre Dame, 1979, 229–236 against Tooley.

Grisez, Germain and Sullivan, Francis. "The Ordinary Magisterium's Infallibility," *Theological Studies* 55(4) December 1994:720–738.

Grobstein, Clifford

1983 "A Biological Perspective on the Origin of Human Life and Personhood," in Shaw and Doudera eds., *Defining Human Life,* Ann Arbor, MI: Alpha Press.

1988 *Science and the Unborn,* New York, NY: Basic Books.

Gross, B.A., "Natural Family Planning Indicators of Ovulation," *Clinics in Reproductive Fertility* 3, Jan. 1987, 91–117.

Grudstrand, Karen, *Redefining Death,* New Haven: Yale University Press, 1986.

Grudzinskas, J.G.; and Nysenbaum, A.M., "Failure of Human Pregnancy after Implantation," Seppälä, Markku and R.G. Edwards, eds. *In Vitro Fertilization and Embryo Transfer,* Annals of the New York Academy of Science, 442, 1985, 38–44.

Guerrero, Rodrigo, "Possible Effects of the Periodic Abstinence Method," in *Proceedings of a Research Conference on Natural Family Planning,* W.A. Uricchio, ed., Washington, DC: Human Life Foundation, 1973, 84–96.

Gula, Richard

1991 "Moral Perspectives on Euthanasia," *Studies in Christian Ethics,* 4(1), 1991, 22–39.

1994 "Euthanasia and Assisted Suicide," St. Louis, MO: Catholic Health Association.

Gurdon, J.B., "The Generation of Diversity and Pattern in Animal Development," *Cell,* 68, January 24, 1992, 185–199.

Gustafson, James M.

1975 *Can Ethics be Christian?* Chicago: University of Chicago Press.

1978 *Protestant and Roman Catholic Ethics: Prospects for Rapprochement,* Chicago: University of Chicago Press.

1983 *Ethics from a Theocentric Perspective,* vol. 1 (1983), vol. 2 (1984), Chicago: University of Chicago Press.

1994 "A Christian perspective on genetic engineering," *Human Gene Therapy,* 5(6), June, 747–754.

Gutierrez, Gustavo

1977 *Liberation and Change,* Atlanta: John Knox Press.

1990 *The Truth Shall Make You Free,* Trans. O'Connell, Maryknoll, NY: Orbis Books.

Guttmann, Astrid; and Guttmann, Ronald, "Attitudes of Healthcare Professionals and Public Toward the Sale of Kidneys for Transplantation," *Journal of Medical Ethics,* 19(3), September, 1993, 148–153.

Haan, Norma, *On Moral Grounds,* New York: New York University Press, 1985.

Haas-Wilson, Deborah, "The economic impact of state restrictions, parental consent and notification laws," *Journal of Policy Analysis and Management*, 12(3), Summer, 1993, 498–511.

Hage, J. "Medical requirements and consequences of sex reassignment therapy," *Medical Science and the Law*, 35(1), January, 1995, 17–24.

Hagland, Mark, "An Interview with Richard Doyle: The Milliman and Robertson Guidelines," *Hospitals*, 23(9), December 3, 1995, p. 47.

Halley, Martin; et al. *Medical Malpractice Solutions: Systems and Proposals for Injury Compensation*, Springfield, IL: Charles Thomas Company, 1989.

Halvey, Amir; and Brody, Baruch, "Brain Death: Reconciling Definitions, Criteria and Tests," *Annals of Internal Medicine*, 19(6), September 15, 1993, 519–525.

Hammet, Theodore, *AIDS in Correctional Facilities: Issues and Options*, Washington, DC: U.S. Department of Justice, 1986.

Hampton, Harriette, "Care of the woman who has been raped." *New England Journal of Medicine*, 332(4), January 26, 1995, 234–37.

Hanley, Robert, "Surrogate Deals for Mothers Held Illegal in New Jersey," *New York Times* February 3, 1988, 1A.

Hannink, James G., *Persons, Rights, and the Problem of Abortion*, (Ph.D. diss.) Michigan State University, 1975, 42–172. Against Tooley's argument.

Harbison, Jean, "Gilligan, A Voice for Nursing," *Journal of Medical Ethics* December, 1992, 18, 64, 202–205.

Hardin, Garret
     1974   "Living on a Lifeboat," *Biosciences* 24; 561–568.
     1993   *Living within Limits: Ecology, Economics, and Population Taboos*, NY: Oxford University Press, 1993.

Hare, R.M. "Moral Reasoning About the Environment," *Journal of Applied Philosophy* 4 (1), 1987:3–14.

Häring, Bernard, CSSR
     1966   *The Law of Christ*, 3 vols., Philadelphia: Westminster Press.
     1973   *Medical Ethics*, Notre Dame: Fides Publishers.
     1976   "New Dimensions of Responsible Parenthood," *Theological Studies*, 37, 1976, p. 120.
     1992   *My Witness for the Church*, New York: Paulist Press, 1992.

Harper, Robert A., *Psychoanalysis and Psychotherapy: 36 Systems* Englewood Cliffs, NJ: Prentice–Hall, 1959, 152–155.

Harrington, Anne, ec., *So Human a Brain: Knowledge and Values in the Neurosciences*, Boston, MA: Birdhauser, 1992.

Harris, John
     1985   *The Value of Human Life*, London: Routledge, and Kegan Publications.
     1994   "Not all Babies Should Be Kept Alive As Long As Possible," in *Principles of Health Care Ethics*, Raanan Gillon, ed., New York: Wiley.

Harrison, Beverly Wildung, *Our Right to Choose Toward A New Ethic of Abortion*, Boston: Beacon Press, 1984.

Hartman, Rhonda, "The privacy implications of Professor Andrews' proposed mandatory registering of bone marrow donations," *University of Pittsburgh Law Review*, 54(2), Winter, 1993, 531–558.

Hastings Center Institute of Society, Ethics, and the Life Sciences: Research Group on Ethical, Social, and Legal Issues in Genetic Counseling and Genetic Engineering, "Ethical and Social Issues in Screening for Genetic Disease," *New England Journal of Medicine* 286, 1972, 1129–1132.

Hatcher, Robert A., et al., *Contraceptive Technology, 1986–1987*, 13th ed., New York: Irvington Publications, 1987.

Hatfield, Agnes; and Lefley, Harriet, *Surviving Mental Illness: Stress, Coping, Adaptation*, NY: Guildford Press, 1993.

Hauerwas, Stanley. *A Community of Character: Toward a Constructive Christian Social Ethic*, Notre Dame: University of Notre Dame Press, 1981.

Hay, P.; Sachdev, P.; Cumming, S.; Smith, J. S.; Lee, T.; Kitchener, P.; and Matheson, J., "Treatment of obsessive-compulsive disorder by psychosurgery," *Acta Psychiatrica Scandinavia* 87(3), March 1993, 197–207.

HCFA: Health Care Financing Administration.
  1992 "Advance Directives," *Federal Register* 57, Reg. 8194.
  1993 "National health expenditures," *Health Care Financing Review* 16:1 Fall, 1994.

Healy, Edwin, SJ, *Medical Ethics*, Chicago: Loyola University Press, 1956, "On cooperation," 102–108.

Heaney, Robert, et al. *The Fullness of Life: Catholic Medical Education for the 21st Century*, Omaha, NY: Creighton University Press, 1991.

Heaney, Stephen J., "Aquinas and the Presence of the Human Rational Soul in the Early Embryo," *The Thomist* 56 (1992): 19–48.

Helmchen, H. "Ethical Problems in Psychiatric Everyday Practice," *Japanese Journal of Psychiatry & Neurology* 48 (1994) Supplement p. 53–61.

Hendren, Hardy; and Lillehi, Craig, "Pediatric Surgery," *New England Journal of Medicine* 319(2), Jul. 14, 1988, 89–96.

Henry, William E.; Sims, John; and Spray, Lee, *The Fifth Profession: Becoming a Psychotherapist*, San Francisco: Josey-Bass, 1971.

Herranz, Gonzalo, "RU 486: The "Abortion Pill," *Origins* 23, May 23, 1991, 21, 2, 28–33.

Hesburgh, Theodore, ed. *the Challenge and Promise of a Catholic University*, Notre Dame, IN: University of Notre Dame Press, 1994.

Highwater, Jamake. *Myth and Sexuality*, NY: NAL Books, 1990.

Hilfaker, David, *Healing the Wounded*, New York: Parthenon Books, 1985.

Hilgers, Thomas W., MD
  1977 "Human Reproduction: Three Issues," *Theological Studies* 38, 136–152.
  1980 "The New Technologies of Birth," in *The New Technologies of Birth and Death*, St. Louis: Pope John XXIII Medical-Moral Research and Education Center, 29–55.
  1993 "Norplant," *Linacre Quarterly* 60 (1993): 64
  1994 *The Scientific Foundations of The Ovulation Method*, Omaha, NE: Pope Paul VI Institute Press, 1980.
  1995 "The Natural Methods for the Regulation of Fertility: The Authentic Alternative, *Linacre Quarterly* 62 (1995):52–59.

Hiltner, Seward, *Pastoral Counseling*, Nashville, TN: Abingdon Press, 1969.

Hilts, Philip. "HMOs are turning to spiritual healing," *New York Times* (December 12, 1995):B10.

Hitchcock, James
  1982 *What is Secular Humanism*, Ann Arbor: Servant Books.
  1984 "The Seamless Garment Unfolds," *The Human Life Review* 4, 15–30.

Hite, Shere
  1976 *Hite Report on Female Sexuality*, New York: Macmillan.
  1981 *Hite Report on Male Sexuality*, New York: Alfred A. Knopf.

Hittinger, Russell. "Resolving conflicting normative claims in public policy," in Gerard Magill, ed. *Abortion and Public Policy*, Omaha, NE, Creighton University Press, 1996.

Hoefler, James, Kamoic, P., "The Right to Die: State Courts Lead Where Legislatures Fear to Tread," *Law and Policy*, 14(4) October 1992, p. 337–380.

Hoff, Lee Ann, *People in Crisis: Understanding and Helping*, Menlo Park, CA: Addison-Wesley Publications, 1984, ch. 2.

Hogan, John; and Flannery, Austin, *Humanae Vitae and the Bishops: The Encyclical and Statements of National Hierarchies*, Shannon: Irish University Press, 1972.

Holbrook, David, "Medicare Ethics and the Potentialities of the Living Being," *British Medical Journal* 291(6493), Aug. 17, 1985, 459–462.

Holck, Frederick H., ed., *Death and Eastern Thought,* Nashville: Abingdon Press, 1974.

Holder, Angela Roddy, "Amniocentesis, Genetics, Counseling, and Genetic Screening," in her *Legal Issues: Pediatrics and Adolescent Medicine,* New Haven, CT: Yale University Press, 1985.

Holifield, E. Brooks, *A History of Pastoral Care in America from Salvation to Self-Realization,* Nashville: Abingdon Press, 1983.

Holleman, Warren; Edwards, David; and Matson, Christine. "Obligations of physicians to patients and third party payors," *Journal of Clinical Ethics,* 5 Summer 1994:113–120.

Holmes, "Psychopathic Disorders: A Category Mistake?" *Journal of Medical Ethics,* 17 (1991) p.77–85.

Holmes, Helen, "Sex Preselection: Eugenics for Everyone?" in *Biomedical Ethics Review,* James Humber, ed., Clifton, NJ: Humana Press, 1985, 39–71.

Holst, Lawrence, ed., *Hospital Ministry; The Role of the Chaplain Today,* New York: Crossroad Publishing Co., 1985.

Holzgreve, H., et al., "Kidney Transplantation from Anencephalic Donors," *New England Journal of Medicine* 316 (17), Apr. 23, 1987, 1069–1070.

Hook, Sidney, *Towards an Understanding of Karl Marx,* New York: John Day, 1953; *Manifesto of the Communist Party,* p. 72.

Hoose, Bernard, *Proportionalism: The American Debate and its European Roots,* Washington, DC: Georgetown University Press, 1987.

Horan, Dennis, J., et al, *Abortion and the Constitution, Reversing Roe vs. Wade Through the Courts,* Washington, DC: Georgetown University Press, 1987.

Horan, D.J.; and Grant, E.P., "The Legal Aspects of Withdrawing Nourishment," *Journal of Legal Medicine* 5 (4), 1984, 595–632.

Horowitz, L.C., *Taking Charge of Your Medical Fate,* New York: Random House, 1988.

Hors, et al, "Toward a European Charter for Transplantation Ethics," *Transplantation Proceedings* 25 (1 pt 2) February 1993, 1697–8.

Howsepian, A.A. "Who and What are We," *Review of Metaphysics* 45(3) March, 1992, p. 483–502.

Hoyninger-Huene, Paul. *Reductionism and Systems Theology in the Life Sciences,* Boston, MA: Kluwer Publications, 1989.

Hoyt, Robert, ed., *The Birth Control Debate: Interim History from the Pages of the National Catholic Reporter,* Kansas City: National Catholic Reporter, 1969.

Hsiao, William, *Cost-Based Relative Social Values,* Washington, DC: DHHW, 1988.

Huang, T.T., "Twenty Years of Experience in Managing Gender Dysphoric Patients," *Plastic and Reconstructive Surgery* 96(4), September 1995, p. 921–930.

Hubbard, Bishop Howard, "What Role For Surrogate Decision Makers?" *Origins* 22 (34) February 4, 1993, p. 576–579.

HUGO: Human Genome Organization, "Statement on the Principled Conduct of Genetics Research," Bethesda, MD: HUGO, Americas, Inc., March 21, 1996.

Hugo, John, *St. Augustine on Nature, Sex and Marriage,* Chicago: Scepter Press, 1968.

"Humanist Manifesto," *The New Humanist* 6, May-June 1933. Reprinted in *The Humanist* 33, Jan.–Feb. 1973, 13–14.

"Humanist Manifesto II," *The Humanist* 33, Sept.–Oct. 1973, 4–9.

Hume, Basil Cardinal. "Note on Church Teaching Concerning Homosexual People," *Origins* 24:45 (April 27, 1995) p. 765–769.

Hume, Kevin, "Latest Research Findings: The Pill and IUD," *Proceedings of First International Congress for the Family,* Madras Congress, 1983.

Hursthouse, Rosalind, *Beginning Lives* (Oxford: Basil Blackwell/Open University). Criticizes Tooley, pp.107–117.

Hussey, Edmund, "Needed: A Theology of Priesthood," *Origins* 17(34), Feb 4, 1988, 517–583.

Idziak, Jeanine, *Divine Command Morality,* Lewiston, NY: Edwin Mellen Press, 1980.

Iglesias, Teresa. *Euthanasia and Clinical Trends, Principles and Alternatives,* London: Linacre Center, 1984.

Illich, Ivan D.
 1972 "Technology and Conviviality," in *To Create a Different Future: Religious Hope and Technology,* Kenneth Vaux, ed., New York: Friendship Press, 40–66.
 1976 *Medical Nemesis: The Expropriation of Health,* New York: Pantheon Books.

Illich, Ivan D., et al., *Disabling Professions,* Boston: Marion Boyars Publications, Ltd., 1978.

International Congress of Moral Theology, *Humane Vitae: Twentieth Anniversary Dopo,* Milan, Italy: Edizioni Press, 1988.

Institute of Medicine, *The Nation's Physician Workforce,* Washington, DC: National Academy Press, 1996.

Irving, Dianne Nutwell
 1992 "Scientific and Philosophical Expertise: An Evaluation of the Argument on 'Personhood'," *Linacre Quarterly* Feb. 3, 1992.
 1993a "The Impact of 'Scientific Misinformation' on Other Fields: Philosophy, Theology, Biomedical Ethics, Public Policy," *Accountability in Research* (Feb. 1993):1–24.
 1993b *Begging Lives,* Oxford, Blackwell.

Ishiwata, Ryuji; and Sakai, Akio, "The Physician-Patient Relationship and Medical Ethics in Japan," *Cambridge Quarterly of Healthcare Ethics* 3(1) Winter 1994, 60–6.

ITEST, 1975, Institute for Theological Encounter with Science and Technology, *Brain Research: Human Consciousness,* St. Louis: ITEST Publications, 1976.

Jackson, Jesse, "Political Campaign Speech," *Des Moines Register,* Jan. 16, 1988.

Jacobs, Seth, "Determination of Medical Necessity: Medicaid Funding for Sex Reassignment Surgery," *Case Western Reserve Law Review,* vol. 31, 1980, 179.

Janssens, Louis, "Ontic Evil and Moral Evil," *Louvain Studies* 4, 1972, 115–156.

Janus, Samuel; and Janus, Cynthia, *The Janus Report on Sexual Behavior,* NY: Wiley, 1993.

JCAHO: Joint Commission for Accreditation of Health Care Organizations "Manual for Hospitals," Chicago, IL: American Hospital Assoc., 1993

Jecker, Nancy. "Managed competition and managed care," *Clinical Ethics* 10:3 (August 1994):527–540.

Jecker, Nancy; and Selt, Donnie. "Separating care and cure; an analysis of historical and contemporary images of nursing and medicine," *Journal of Medicine and Philosophy* 16, 1991:285–306.

Jenkins, Philip, *Pedophiles and Priests* (New York: Oxford, 1995).

John XXIII, "Christianity and Social Progress (Mater et Magistra)," in *Social Justice: The Catholic Position,* Washington, DC: Consortium Press, 1975.

John Paul II
 1980a Encyclical Letter: *"Dives in Misericordia,"* Origins 10(26), Dec. 11.
 1980b "The Patient is a Person," (Oct. 23, 1980) *The Pope Speaks* 26(1).
 1980c "Lust and Personal Dignity," *Origins* 10(19), Oct. 23, 303.
 1981a Encyclical Letter: "On Human Work," *Origins* 11(15), Sept. 24, 255.
 1981b *Familiaris Consortio,* "On the Human Family," *Origins* 11 (28–29), Dec. 24.
 1984a "On Reconciliation and Penance," *Origins* 74(27), Dec. 20, 442.
 1984b *Reflections on Humanae Vitae,* Boston: St. Paul Editions.
 1984c "The Priest in an Indifferent World," *Origins* 14(8), July 12, 1984, 122–130.
 1984d "Blood and Organ Donors," (1985) *The Pope Speaks* 30:1 (1984): 1–2.
 1986 "Medicines at the Service of Man," (Oct. 24, 1986) *Health Progress,* Apr. 1087.
 1987a "Sollicitudo Rei Socialis," *Origins* 17(33) March 3.
 1987b "The Catholic Schools in the 80s," *Origins* 17(17), Oct. 8, 279–282.
 1988 On U.N. Bill of Rights, "Serving the Cause of Human Rights," *Origins* Jan. 26, 1989, 18, 33, 541–544.
 1991a "To the Participants at the 1st International Congress on the Transplant of Organs," Insegamenti, 1481: 1711.

1991b   *"Centesimus Annus"* (The 100th Year), *Origins* 6:23 (November 14):363–367.

1993   Splendor of Truth (*Veritatis Splendor*) *Origins* 23(18) Oct. 14.

1995   Gospel of Life (*Evangelium Vitae*) *Origins* 24:42 (April 6, 1995) n. 30, 35, 48.

Johnson, Gale D., *Population Growth and Economic Development Policy Questions*, Washington, DC: National Academy Press, 1986.

Johnson, Mark vs. Jean Porter, "Delayed Hominization," *Theological Studies*, 56 (Dec., 1995):743–771.

Jonas, Hans

1979   "Toward a Philosophy of Technology," *Hastings Center Report* 9, 34–43.

1984   *The Importance of Responsibility: In Search of an Ethics for the Technological Age*, Chicago: Chicago University Press, 1984.

Jones, D. Gareth. "Medicine's future: technology or a person-centered profession?" *Humane Medicine* 8:1 January 1992:50–55.

Jones, James, *Bad Blood: The Tuskegee Syphilis Experiment*, New York: Free Press, 1982.

Jonsen, Albert R.

1968   *Responsibility in Modern Religious Ethics*, Washington, DC: Corpus Books.

1985   "Organ Transplants and the Principle of Fairness," *Law, Medical and Health Care* 1, Feb. 13, 37.

1990   "The duty to treat patients with AIDS and HIV infection," in Gostin, Lawrence, ed. *AIDS and the Health Care System*, New Haven, CT: Yale University Press, p. 155–168.

Joseph, D.H. "Cognitive Therapy: A Well Thought Out Strategy," *Nursing Forum* 30:2 (1995) p. 13–21.

Jung, Carl, et al., *Man and His Symbols*, London: Aldus Books, 1964, rev. ed. 1984.

Kahn, Eva, *Clinical Genetics Handbook*, Orabell, NJ: National Genetics Foundation, 1987.

Kaiser, Irwin, "Fertilization and the Physiology and Development of Fetus and Placenta," in *Obstetrics and Gynecology*, David Danforth and James Scott, eds., Philadelphia: J.B. Lippincott, 1986.

Kaiser, Robert Blair, *The Politics of Sex and Religion*, Kansas City: Leaven Press, 1985.

Kambic, R. "Roman Catholic Church–sponsored natural family planning services in the United States," *Advances in Contraception* 10 (June 1994): 85–92.

Kanigel, Robert, "Uncertain of Our Gods," *Notre Dame Magazine* 17(2), Summer 1988, 34–42.

Kaplan, Helen Singer, *The New Sex Therapy*, New York: Brunner/Mazel, 1974, 86.

Kaplan, Robert. "Health related quality of life in patient decision making," *Journal of Social Issues* 47:4 (Winter 1991):69–90.

Karp, David A. *Speaking of Sadness: Depression, Disconnection, and Meaning of Illness* (New York: Oxford University Press, 1995).

Kass, Leon

1985   *Toward A More Natural Science, Biology and Human Affairs*, New York: Free Press, 65 ff.

1987   "The Limits of Genetic Inquiry," *Hastings Center Report* 17(4), August 1987, 5–11.

Kassirer, Jerome. "Managed care and the morality of the marketplace," *New England Journal of Medicine* 353:1 July 6, 1995:50–54.

Katz, Fred. "An SS physician," in his *Ordinary People and Extraordinary Evil, a Report on the Beguilings of Evil*, Albany, NY: State University of New York Press, 1993.

Katz, Jay

1984   *The Silent World of Doctor and Patient*, New York: Macmillan, 1984.

1992   "Duty and Caring in the Age of Informed Consent and Medical Science," *Human Medicine*, July 8, 1992:187–197.

1993   "Ethical and clinical research revisited," *Hastings Center Report*, 23:5 (Sep-Oct, 1993):31–39

1994   "Reflections on unethical experiments and the beginnings of bioethics in the United States," *Kennedy Institute of Ethics Journal* 4:2 June 1994:85–92.

Katz, Jay; Capron, Alexander M.; and Swift-Glass, Elenor, *Experimentation with Human Beings*, New York: Russell Sage Foundation, 1972.

Kauffmann, Christopher
1976 *Tamers of Death*, New York: Crossroad Publishing Co.
1978 *The Ministry of Healing*, New York: Crossroad Publishing Co.

Keane, Philip
1977 *Sexual Morality: A Catholic Perspective*, New York: Paulist Press.
1984 *Christian Ethics and Imagination*, Ramsey, NJ: Paulist Press.

Keenan, James; Kaveny, Kathy, "Ethical Issues in Health Care Restructuring," *Theological Studies* 5(6), March 1995. 136–150.

Keenan, James; and Kopesteiner, Thomas, "The Principle of Cooperation," *Hospital Progress*, April 1995, p. 26.

Kelagham, et al., "Barrier-Method Contraceptives and Pelvic Inflammatory Disease," *Journal of American Medical Association* 248, 1982, 185.

Kelly, David F., *The Emergence of Roman Catholic Medical Ethics in North America*, New York: Edwin Mellen Press, 1979.

Kelly, Gerald, SJ, "The Morality of Mutilation: Toward a Revision of the Treatise," *Theological Studies* 17, 322–344, 1956.

Kelly, James, "Residual or Prophetic: The Cultural Fate of Roman Catholic Sexual Ethics of Abortion and Contraception," *Social Thought* 12, Spring 1986, 3–18.

Kelsey, Morton, *Prophetic Ministry: The Psychology and Spirit of Pastoral Care*, New York: Crossroad Publishing Co., 1982.

Kemp, Evan, "Paternalism, disability and the right to die," *Issues in Law and Medicine*, 9:1 (Summer 1993):73–79.

Keown, John, "The Law and the Practice of Euthanasia in the Netherlands." *The Law Quarterly Review*, 108 January 1992, p. 51–78.

Kevles, Daniel and Hood, Leroy, *The Code of Codes: Scientific and Social Issues in the Human Genome Project*, Cambridge, MA: Harvard University Press, 1992.

Kiesling, Christopher, OP
1970 *The Future of the Christian Sunday*, NY: Sheed and Ward.
1974 *Confirmation and Full Life in the Spirit*, Cincinnati: St. Anthony's Messenger Press.
1986 "On Relating to the Persons of the Trinity," *Theological Studies* 47, 1986, 599–612.

Kindred, Michael, "The Legal Rights of Retarded Persons in 20th Century America," in *Ethics and Mental Retardation*, Loretta Koppleman and John Moshop, eds., Boston: Riedel, 1984.

King, J. Charles, "The Inadequacy of Situation Ethics," *Thomist* 34, 1970, 423–427.

King, Patricia. "Rights within the therapeutic relationship," *Journal of Law and Health* 6:1 (1991–92):31–60.

Kinsey, A. C., et al,
1948 *Sexual Behavior in the Human Male*, Philadelphia: William Saunders.
1953 *Sexual Behavior in the Human Female*, Philadelphia, William Saunders.

Kippley, John F., "Catholic Sexual Ethics: The Continuing Debate on Birth Control," *Linacre Quarterly* 41, 1974, 8–25.

Klaus, Hanna, MD; and Brennan, J., MD, "Terminology and Care Curricula in Natural Family Planning," Los Angeles: Natural Family Planning Physicians' Conference, 1981.

Klerman, Gerald L., "Ideological Conflicts in Integrating Pharmacotherapy and Psychotherapy," in Klerman, G.; and Beitman, B., eds., *Integrating Pharmacotherapy and Psychotherapy* (Washington, DC: American Psychiatric Press, 1991), pp. 2–20.

Kluge, Eibe-Henner
1993a "The Physician as Entrepreneur," *Canadian Medical Association Journal*, 149:2, 1993, p. 204–205.

1993b   "Advanced Patient Records: Some Ethical and Legal Considerations Touching Medical Information Space," *Methods of Information in Medicine* 32, (April 1993), p. 95–103.

Knauer, Peter, "The Hermeneutic Function of the Principle of Double Effect," *National Law Forum* 12, 1967, 132–162.

Knight, R.P., "The Comparative Clinical Status of Conditioning Theories and Psychoanalysis," in *The Conditioning Theories*, Joseph Wolpe, Andrew Slater, and L.J. Reyna, eds., New York: Holt, Rinehart and Winston, 1966, 3–20.

Knox, Ronald, *Enthusiasm*, New York: Sheed & Ward, 1950, 231–318.

Koester, Helmut, "*Nomos Physeos*: The Concept of Natural Law in Greek Thought," in *Religions in Antiquity: Essays in Memory of Erwin Ramsdell Goodenough*, Jacob Neusner, ed., Leiden: E. J. Brill, 1968, 521–541.

Kohlberg, Lawrence
1973   "Indoctrination Versus Relativity in Value Education," *Theology Digest* 21, Summer, 113–119. Reprinted from *Zygon* 6, 1971, 285–310.
1981   *Essays on Moral Development*, San Francisco: Harper & Row.

Kolata, Gina.
1993   "Baby's sad life highlights cost of futile care," *New York Times*, October 6.
1995   "Gene therapy fails to yield benefits, two studies find," *New York Times*, September 28, 1995.

Koop, C. Everett
1986   "Surgeon General's Report on Acquired Immune Deficiency Syndrome," *Journal of the American Medical Association* 20, Nov. 28, 1986, 256.
1987   "Doctors Who Shun AIDS Patients are Assailed by Surgeon General," Phillip Boffey, *New York Times*, Sept. 9, 1987, A1.

Koppleman, Loretta, "Consent and Randomized Clinical Trials: Are They Moral or Design Problems?" *Journal of Medicine and Philosophy* 4, Nov. 22, 1986, 317–345.

Kosnick, Anthony R., et al., *Human Sexuality: New Directions in American Catholic Thought*, New York: Paulist Press, 1977.

Kosten, T.R.; Rounsaville, B.J.; and Kleber, H.D.
1985a   "Comparison of Clinician Ratings to Self-Reports of Curing Detoxification of Opiate Addicts," *American Journal of Alcohol Abuse* 11, 1–10.
1985b   "Ethnic and Gender Differences Among Opiate Addicts," *International Journal of Addiction* 20, 1143–1162.

Krason, Stephen
1983   *The Supreme Court's Abortion Decision: A Critical Study of the Shaping of a Major American Public Policy and a Basis for Change*, Ann Arbor: University Microfilms International, 1983.
1991   *Liberalism, Conservatism and Catholicism: An Evaluation of Contemporary Political Ideologies in Light of Catholic Social Teaching*, New Rochel, NY: CUF, 1991.

Krieger, Lloyd, "Price and Service," *Barron's Weekly*, August 14, 1995, p. 47.

Kristof, Nicolas, "More Insurers Screen Applicants for AIDS," *New York Times*, Dec. 26, 1985, D1, D4.

Krugman, Saul, "The Willow Brook Hepatitis Studies Revisited: Ethical Aspects," *Review of Infectious Diseases*, Jan. 1986, 157–162.

Kubler-Ross, Elisabeth
1969   *On Death and Dying*, New York: Macmillan.
1978   *To Live Until We Say Good-By*, Englewood Cliffs, NJ: Prentice-Hall.
1987   *AIDS: The Ultimate Challenge*, New York: Macmillan.

Kung, Hans, *Eternal Life: Life After Death as a Medical, Philosophical, and Theological Program*, Garden City, NY: Doubleday, 1984.

Kurtz, Paul, 1969
1983   *In Defense of Secular Humanism*, Buffalo: Prometheus Books.
1988   *Forbidden Fruit: The Ethics of Humanism*, Buffalo: Prometheus Books.

Lamm, Richard *et al. Critical Challenges: Revitalizing the Health Professions for the Twenty-first Century,* San Francisco, CA: Pew Health Professions Commission, 1995, p. 28.

Laine, D.; and Davidoff, F. "Patient-centered medicine," *JAMA* 275:2 January 10, 1996:152–156.

Lain-Entralgo, P., *The Therapy of the World in Classical Antiquity,* Rather & Sharp, trans., New Haven: Yale University Press, 1970.

Lain-Entralgo, P., *La Medicina Hypocrite,* Madrid: Revista de Occidente, 1970.

Landau, Richard; and Gustafson, James, "Death is Not the Enemy," *Journal of the American Medical Association* 252(17), Nov. 2, 1984, 2458.

Landis, David A. "Physician distinguish thyself: conflict and covenant in a physician's moral development," *Perspectives in Biology and Medicine* 36:4 summer 1993:628–641.

Langan, John, "The Christian Difference in Ethics," *Theological Studies* 49 (1), Mar. 1988, 131.

Lappé, Marc
 1972 "Moral Obligations and the Fallacies of 'Genetic Control,'" *Theological Studies* 33, 411–427.
 1987 "The Limits of Genetic Inquiry," *Hastings Center Report* 17(4) August p. 5–10.

Lauritzen, Paul, "What Price Parenthood?" *Hastings Center Report,* March/April, 1990, pp. 38–46.

Lavin, Michael, "Mutilation, Deception, and Sex Changes," *Journal of Medical Ethics* 13, 1987, 86–91.

Lawler, Michael. *A Theology of Ministry,* Kansas City, Sheed and Ward, 1994.

Lawler, Ronald; Boyle, Joseph; and May, William E., *Catholic Sexual Ethics,* Huntington, in: *Our Sunday Visitor,* 1985, Revised edition, 1996, "On Sterilization," p. 170–172.

Lazurus, Jeremy. "Sex with Former Patients Almost Always Unethical," *American Journal of Psychiatry* 149:7 (July 1992) p. 855–860.

Leahey, Richard; and Levin, Roger. *Origins Reconsidered in Search of What Makes Us Human,* NY: Doubleday, 1992.

Lederberg, Joshua, "A Geneticist Looks at Contraception and Abortion," *Annals of Internal Medicine* 67, 1967, 26–27.

Lee, Phillip, et al., "Physicians's Competence: Whose Responsibility," *Medical Staff News,* May 1988.

Lee, Robert, "Confidentiality and medical records," in Dyer, Charles (ed) *Doctors, Patients and the Law,* Boston, MA: Blackwell Scientific, 1992, p. 29–43.

Lehmann, H. E., "Problems with Ethical Aspects of Psychotropic Drug Use," *Progress Inc.,* 1979.

Lehrman, Dorothy, ed., *Fetal Research and Fetal Tissue Research,* Washington, DC: Association of American Medical Colleges, June 1988.

Leiden, Jeffrey. "Gene therapy: promises, pitfalls, and prognosis," *NEJM* 333:13 (September 28, 1995):871.

Lejeune, Jerome, Testimony in Maryville, Tenn. case, 1989. *Child and Family,* 21, 1, pp. 7–52.

Lejeune, Jerome; Ramsey, Paul; and Wright, Gerard, "The Question of *In Vitro* Fertilization," *Studies in Law, Ethics and Medicine,* London: Society for Protection of Unborn Children, 1984.

Leo XIII, *Rights and Duties of Capital and Labor* (Rerum Novarum), see Misner, Paul, *Social Catholicism in Europe,* NY: Crossroads Publishing, 1991, Chapter 11.

Levin, Arthur, *Talk Back to Your Doctor: How to Demand (and Recognize) High Quality Health Care,* Garden City, NY: Doubleday, 1975.

Levin, J. S.
 1994 "Religion and Health: Is There an Association, Is it Valid, and Is it Causal?" *Social Science & Medicine,* 38 (1994) p.1475–1482.
 1995 "What is Clinical Sexuality," *Psychiatric Clinics of North America* 18:1 (March 1995) p.1–6.

Levine, Robert

    1981 *Ethics and Regulations of Clinical Research,* Baltimore: Orban and Schwartzenberg, 2nd ed. 1986.

    1983 "Informed Consent in Research and Practice: Similarities and Differences," *Archives of Internal Medicine* 143(6), June, 1229–1231.

    1985 "Institutional Review Boards and Collaborations Between Academia and Industry: Some Counterproductive Policies and Practices," *Circulation* 72 (2), Aug., 148–150.

Levine, S. "Gender disturbed males," *Journal of Sex and Marital Therapy,* 19;2 (Summer 1993):131–141.

Levy, Charlotte, *The Human Body and the Law: Legal and Ethical Considerations,* NY: Oceana Publications, 1983, 90.

Lewis, C. S., *The Problem of Pain,* NY: Macmillan, 1943.

Lewontia, R.C.; Rose, Steven; and Kamin, Leon, *Not in Our Genes,* New York: Pantheon Books, 1984.

Lidz, Charles, et al, *The Erosion of Autonomy in Long-Term Care,* New York: Oxford University Press, 1992.

Lifshitz, Samuel, "Rape," in *Principles and Practice of Emergency Medicine,* George Schwartz, et al., eds., Philadelphia: Saunders, 1986.

Lifton, Robert Jay

    1986 *The Nazi Doctors,* New York: Free Press.

    1982 "Medicalized Killing in Auschwitz," *Psychiatry* 45(4), Nov., 283–297.

Light, Donald, *Becoming Psychiatrists,* New York: W.W. Norton and Co., 1980.

Lindenberg, Svend; and Poul, Hytel, "In vitro studies of the peri-implantation phase of human embryos," Van Blerkom, Jonathan and Pietro M. Motta, *Ultrastructure of Human Gametogenesis and Early Embryogenesis* (Boston: Kluwer Academic Publishers, 1989), pp. 209–211.

Linzer, N., "Ethical Issues in Professional Behavior," *Forum* 22, Spring 1986.

Lipp, Martin. *The Bitter Pill: Doctors, Patients and Failed Expectations,* New York: Harper & Row, 1980.

Lippman, A. "Led (Astray) by Genetic Maps: The Cartography of the Human Genome and Health Care," *Social Science and Medicine,* 35:12, (December 1992):1469.

Lizza, John, "Persons and Death: What's Metaphysically Wrong with our Current Statutory Definition of Death?" *Journal of Medicine and Philosophy* 18(4) August 1993, 351–74.

Llewellyn-Thomas, H., "The Measurement of Patients' Values in Medicine," *Medical Decision Making* 2(4), Winter 1982, 449–462.

Lock, Stephen; and Wells, Frank, eds. *Fraud and Misconduct in Medical Research,* London: BMJ Publishing Group, 1993.

Loewy, Erich, "Physicians and Patients: Moral Agency in a Pluralistic World," *Journal of Medical Humanities and Bioethics* 1(1), 1986, 57–68.

London, Perry

    1964 *The Modes and Morals of Psychotherapy,* New York: Holt, Rinehart and Winston.

    1969 *Behavior Control,* NY: Harper and Row.

Longabaugh, R. "Matching Treatment Focus to Patient Investment and Support," *Journal of Consulting and Clinical Psychology* 63:2 (April 1995) p. 296–307.

Lopata, A., Kohlman, D. J.; and Kellow, G. N., "The Fine Structure of Human Blastocysts Developed in Culture," in *Embryonic Development* ed. by M. C. Burger and R. Weber, Part B: Cellular Aspects, (New York: Alan R. Liss, 1982): 69–85.

Lothstein, L. M., "Sex Reassignment Surgery: Historical, Bioethical, and Theoretical Issues," *American Journal of Psychiatry* 139, 1982, 417–426.

Lotstra, Hans, *Abortion: The Catholic Debate in America,* New York: Irvington Publishers, 1985.

Louisiana Catholic Bishops, *Approaching Death, The Moral Choices*, Louisiana Catholic Conference, New Orleans, 1995.

Ludmerer, Kenneth M., *Learning to Heal: The Development of American Medical Education*, New York: Basic Books, 1985.

Lumsdon, Kevin. "Faded glory: is this nursing's last stand?" *Hospitals* 69:23 December 5, 1995:30–38.

Lurie, Nicole, et al., "Termination of Medi-Cal Benefits, A Follow-Up Study One Year Later," *New England Journal of Medicine* 314 (19), May 8, 1986, 1266–1268.

Lynn, Joanne, ed., *By No Extraordinary Means: The Choice to Forego Life-Sustaining Food and Water*, Bloomington, IN: Indiana University Press, 1986.

Lynoe, Niels; Mattson, Bengt; Sandlund, Mikael. "The Attitudes of Patients and Physicians Toward Placebo Treatment," *Social Science and Medicine* 36:6, 1993, p. 767–774.

Lyons, Joseph P. "The American medical doctor in the current milieu: a matter of trust," *Perspectives in Biology and Medicine*, 37:3 Spring 1994:442–459.

Machan, Tibor R., *The Pseudo-Science of B.F. Skinner*, New York: Arlington House, 1974.

MacGillivray, Doris; Campbell, M.; and Thompson, Barbara, eds. *Twinning and Twins* (New York: John Wiley and Sons, 1988).

MacIntyre, Alisdair
    1979 "Seven Traits for Designing our Descendants," *Hastings Center Report* 9, 5–17.
    1981 *After Virtue*, Notre Dame, IN: Notre Dame University Press, 1981.

Mack, Arien, *Death in American Experience*, New York: Schocken Books, 1973.

Mack, J. E. "Power, Powerlessness, and Empowerment in Psychotherapy," *Psychiatry* 57:2 (May 1994) p. 178–198.

Mack, Robert, "Lessons From Living With Cancer," *New England Journal of Medicine* 311 (25), Dec. 20, 1984, 30–35.

Macklin, Ruth
    1982 *Man, Mind and Morality: The Ethics of Behavior Control*, Englewood Cliffs, NJ: Prenctice Hall.
    1985 "Mapping the Human Genome: Problems of Privacy and Free Choice," in *Genetics and the Law*, Aubrey Milunsky and George Annas, eds., New York: Plenum University Press, 107–114.
    1994 *Enemies of Patients*, NY: Oxford University Press, 1994.

MacNamara, Vincent, *Faith & Ethics*, Washington, DC: Georgetown University Press, 1986.

Macquarrie, John, *Three Ethical Issues*, New York: Harper & Row, 1970, Ch. 4, "Rethinking the Natural Law," 82–110.

Maguire, Daniel
    1974 *Death by Choice*, Garden City: Image Books, rev. 1984.
    1986 *The Moral Revolution: A Christian Humanist Vision*, New York: Harper & Row.

Maguire, P., "Barriers to Psychological Care for the Dying," *British Medical Journal* 291 (6510), Dec. 14, 1985, 1711–1713.

Mahoney, John, *Bioethics and Belief* (London: Sheed and Ward, 1984).

Mahkorn, S.; and Dolan, W., "Sexual Assault and Pregnancy," in *New Perspectives in Human Abortion*, Hilgers, T; Horan, D.; Mall, D., eds., Frederick, MD: University Publications of America, 1981.

Mahowald, Mary; Silver, Jerry; and Racheson, Robert, "The Ethical Options in Transplanting Fetal Tissue," *Hastings Center Report* 7(1), Feb. 1987, 9–15.

Malaspina, Delores; Zuithin, Mathew; and Kaufman, Charles. "Epidemiology and Genetics of Neuropsychiatric Disorders," in Yudofsky, Stuart, and Hors, Robert, *Textbook of Neuropsychiatry*, Washington, DC: American Psychiatric Press, 1992.

Malone, Patrick, "Death Row and the Medical Model," *Hastings Center Report* 9, 1979, 5–7.

Mangan, J., "An Historical Analysis of the Principle of Double Effect," *Theological Studies* 10, 1949, 40–61.

Mann, J. I.; Vessey, M. P.; Thorogood, M.; and Doll, S. R., "Moycardial Infarction in Young

Women with Special Reference to Oral Contraceptive Practice," *British Medical Journal* 2, 1975, 241–245.

Manning, Willard, et al. *The Cost of Poor Health: A Rand Study,* Cambridge, MA: Harvard University Press, 1991.

Many, Seth, "Psychiatrists, State Hospitals, and Civil Rights," *New York State Journal of Medicine* 80 (12), Nov. 1980.

Marco, G. J.; Hollingworth, R. M.; and Durkam, W. F., *Silent Spring Revisited,* Washington, DC: American Chemical Society, 1987.

Marcus, Ruthanne, and CDC Surveillance Group, "Surveillance of Health Care Workers Exposed to Blood from Patients Infected with the Human Immunodeficiency Virus," *New England Journal of Medicine* 319(17), Oct. 27, 1988, 1119.

Marcuse, Herbert
1964 *One-Dimensional Man: Studies in the Ideology of Advanced Industrial Society,* Boston: Beacon Press.
1972 *Counter Revolution and Revolution,* Boston: Beacon Press.

Margo, Curtis, "Selling Surgery," *New England Journal of Medicine* 314(24), June 12, 1986, 1575–76.

Margolis, Joseph, "Thoughts on Definitions of Disease," *The Journal of Medicine and Philosophy* 11(3) 1986, p. 233–236.

Maritain, Jacques
1929 *Three Reformers: Luther, Descartes, Rousseau,* rev. ed., London: Sheed & Ward, 54 ff.
1947 *The Person and the Common Good,* NY: Charles Scribner & Sons, 1947.

Marmer, Stephen. "Theories of Mind and Psychopathology," in *Textbook of Psychiatry* J. Tabot, ed., Washington, DC: American Psychiatric Press, 1988, p. 129–141.

Marmoc, Judd, ed., *Homosexual Behavior: A Modern Reappraisal,* New York: Basic Books, 1980.

Marquis, Don, "An Argument that All Prerandomized Clinical Trials Are Unethical," *Journal of Medicine and Philosophy* 11(4), Nov. 1986, 367–383.

Martelet, Gustave, SJ
1969 *L'Existence Humaine et L'Amour, Pour Mieux Comprendre L' Encyclicque Humanae Vitae,* Paris: Desclee, 1969.
1981 "A Prophetic Text Under Challenge: The Message of *Humanae Vitae,*" in *Natural Family Planning: Nature's Way/God's Way,* Anthony Zimmerman, SVD, ed., Collegeville, MN: DeRance Inc. and Human Life Center, 1981, 153–167.

Martin, Douglas; and Meslin, Eric. "The Give and Take of Organ Procurement," *Journal of Medicine and Philosophy,* 1994 February 19(11) 61–78.

Martin, Barry; and Bean, Grahm. "Competence to consent to ECT," *Convulsive Therapy* 8:2 (June 1992):92–102.

Marzen, Thomas, "The Uniform Rights of the Terminally Ill Act: A Critical Analysis," *Issues in Law and Medicine* 1(6), May 1986, 441–475.

Maslow, Abraham J., *Motivation and Personality,* 2nd ed., New York: Harper & Row, 1970.

Masters, William H.; and Johnson, Virginia
1966 *Human Sexual Response,* Boston: Little, Brown.
1970 *Human Sexual Inadequacy,* Boston: Little, Brown.
1976 *The Pleasure Bond,* New York: Bantam Books, paperback edition.

Masters, William H.; et al., *Ethical Issues in Sex Research and Therapy,* Boston: Little, Brown, vol. 1 1977, vol. 2 1980.

Masters, William H.; Johnson, Virginia E.; and Kolodny, Robert, *Masters and Johnson on Sex and Human Loving,* Boston: Little, Brown, 1986.

Mathieu, Deborah. "Ending the experiment: dilemmas of the experimental/therapeutic distinction." in Blank, Robert; and Bonnicksen, Andrea eds. *Emerging Issues in Biomedical Policy: An Annual Review* V.11 NY: Columbia University Press, 1993, p. 1247–263.

May, Rollo, *Freedom and Destiny,* New York: Dell Books, 1983.

May, Thomas. "The nurse under physician authority," *Journal of Medical Ethics* 4 December 19, 1993:223–227.

May, William E.

1976 "Proxy Consent to Human Experimentation," *Linacre Quarterly* 43, 73–84.

1977 "Sterilization: Catholic Teaching and Catholic Practice," *Homiletic and Pastoral Review* 77, Aug,–Sept., 9–22.

1983 *Contraception and Catholicism,* Front Royal, VA: Christendom Publishing.

1984 "Aquinas and Janssens: On the Moral Meaning of Human Acts," *The Thomist* 48, 566–606.

1987 "Sexual Ethics and Human Dignity," in *Persona Verita e Morale,* Rome: Citta Nuova Edditrice, 477–494.

1991 "Zygotes, Embryos and Persons," *Ethics and Medics,* 16:10 October, 2–4.

1994 "The Management of Ectopic Pregnancies: A Moral Analysis," Cataldo, Peter, and Albert Moraczewski eds. *The Fetal Tissue Issue: Medical and Ethical Aspects,* Braintree, MA: Pope John Center, 1994, pp. 121–147.

May, William F., *The Physician's Covenant: Images of the Healer in Medical Ethics,* Philadelphia: Westminster Press, 1983.

McBrien, Richard, *Ministry: A Theological, Pastoral Handbook,* New York: Harper & Row, 1987.

McCabe, Herbert, OP, *What Is Ethics All About?* Washington, DC: Corpus Books, 1969.

McCartney, James

1986 "Catholic Positions on Withholding Sustenance for the Terminally Ill," *Health Progress* Oct. 67(8):38–40.

1987 *Unborn Persons, Pope John Paul II, and the Abortion Debate,* NY: Peter Ang.

McCarthy, B. "Learning from Unsuccessful Sex Therapy Patients," *Journal of Sex and Marital Therapy,* 21:1 (Spring 1995) p. 31–8.

McCarthy, Donald G.

1983 "Infertility Bypass," *Ethics and Medics* 8(10), Oct.

1988 "TOTS is for Kids," *Ethics and Medics* 13(12), Dec.

McClendon, James. *Ethics,* Nashville: Abingdon Press, 1986.

McCloskey, Elizabeth. "The patient self determination act" *Kennedy Institute of Ethics Journal* 1:2 (June 1991): 163–169.

McCombie, S.C., "The Cultural Impact of the AIDS Test: The American Experience," *Social Science and Medicine I* 23(5), 1986.

McCormick, Richard A.

1973 *Ambiguity in Moral Choice,* 1973 Pere Marquette Theology Lecture, Milwaukee: Marquette University.

1974a "Proxy Consent in the Experimentation Situation," *Perspectives in Biology and Medicine* 118, Autumn, 2–20.

1974b "To Save or Let Die: The Dilemma of Modern Medicine," *Journal of the American Medical Association* 229, 172–176.

1976 "Experimentation in Children: Sharing in Sociality," *Hastings Center Report* 6, 41–46.

1977 "Man's Moral Responsibility for Health," *Catholic Hospital* 5, 609.

1981 *Notes on Moral Theology,* Washington, DC: University Press.

1984a *Health and Medicine in the Catholic Tradition,* New York: Crossroad Publishing Co., 140.

1984b *Notes on Moral Theology,* Lanham, MD: University Press of America.

1987 "Begotten, Not Made," *Notre Dame Magazine* 15 (3), Autumn, 22–26.

1990 "The Embryo Debate 3: The First 14 Days." *The Tablet,* (March 10, 1990):301 ff.

1991a "The Preembryo as Potential: A Reply to John A. Robertson," *Kennedy Institute of Ethics Journal,* 1, 4:303–305.

1991b "Who or What is the Preembryo?" *Kennedy Institute of Ethics Journal* 1:1–15.

1993 "Veritatis Splendor and Moral Theology," *America* 169, Oct. 30, 8–11.

1994 "Some Early Reactions to Veritatis Splendor," *Theological Studies* S(55), 481–506.

1995a "The Catholic hospital today: mission impossible?" *Origins* 24:39 (March 16, 1995): 648–652.

1995b "Does Christianity Make a Difference," *Christian Bioethics*, 1995:7:97–102.

McCormick, Richard A. and Ramsey, Paul, eds., *Doing Evil to Achieve Good*, Chicago: Loyola University Press, 1978.

McCullough, Lawrence, "Methodological Concerns in Bioethics," *Journal of Medicine and Philosophy* 11(1), Feb. 1986, 17–37.

McDonagh, Enda, *Doing the Truth: The Quest for Moral Theology*, Notre Dame, IN: University of Notre Dame Press, 1979.

McDonald, J. C., "The National Organ Procurement and Transplantation Network," *Journal of the American Medical Association* 259, 1988, 725–726.

McDonald, Margaret, "ECT: Lothar Kalinowsky Remembers," *Psychiatric News*, May 5, 1978.

McDowell, Jan; and Newell, Claire, *Measuring Health: A Guide to Rating Scales and Questionnaires*, New York: Oxford University Press, 1987.

McElhinney, Thomas. "Medical ethics in medical education: finding and keeping a place at the table," *Journal of Clinical Ethics* 4:3 (Fall 1993):273–275.

McFadden, Charles J.

1967 *Medical Ethics*, 6th ed., Philadelphia: F.A. Davis Co., "On cooperation," 357–372, "On truthfulness and professional secrecy," 389–414.

1976 *Dignity of Life: Moral Values in a Changing Society*, Huntington, IN: *Our Sunday Visitor*, 186ff.

McGrath, Patrick J. "On Not Re-interpreting *Humanae Vitae*," *Irish Theological Quarterly* 38, 1976, 130–143.

McGrath, J.; and D. Solter, "Completion of mouse embryogenesis requires both the maternal and paternal genomes," *Cell* (1984): 179–183.

McHugh, James. "What is the Difference Between a 'Person' and a 'Human Being' with the Law," *Review of Politics* 54(3) Summer 1992, p. 445–461.

McInerny, Ralph, "Fundamental Option," in *Persona Verita Morale*, Rome: Citta Nuova Edditrice, 1987, 427–434.

McNeill, D. R.; Morrison, P. A.; and Nouwen, H. J., *Compassion*, Garden City: Doubleday, 1982.

McNeill, John J., *The Church and the Homosexual*, Mission, KS: Sheed, Andrews & McMeel, 1976.

Mechanic, David, "Physicians and Patients in Transition," *Hastings Center Report* 15(6), Dec. 1985, 9–12.

Mehl, Roger, *Catholic Ethics and Protestant Ethics*, Philadelphia: Westminster Press, 1971.

Meier, Levi, ed., *Jewish Values in Bioethics*, New York: Human Services Press, 1986.

Meisel, Alan

1982 "The Rights of the Mentally Ill Under State Constitutions," *Law and Contemporary Problems* 45(3), 7–40.

1995 "Barriers to Forgoing Nutrition and Hydration in Nursing Homes," *American Journal of Law and Medicine* 21(4) p. 335.

Menninger, Karl

1938 *Man Against Himself*, New York: Harcourt Brace.

1958 *Theory of Psychoanalytic Technique*, New York: Basic Books, "On transference," 77–98.

1968 *Crime of Punishment*, New York: Viking Penguin.

Merkelbach, Benedictus, OP, *Summa Theologiae Moralis*, 10th ed., 3 vols., Burge, Belgium: Desclee de Brouwer, 1949, vol. 1, "On cooperation," 487–492.

Mershey, Harold, "Variable Meanings for the Definition of Disease," *The Journal of Medicine and Philosophy*, 1986, 215–232.

Merton, Robert, K., "Some Thoughts on the Professions in American Society," (Presidential Address), Brown University, 1960.

Merz, Jon, "On a Decision Making Paradigm of Medical Informed Consent," *Journal of Legal Medicine* 14(2), June 1993, p. 231–264.

Meyer, J. K., "Psychiatric Considerations in the Sexual Reassignment of Non-Intersex Individuals," *Clinics in Plastic Surgery* 1, 1974, 275–283.

Meyer, J. K., et al, "Sex Reassignment: Follow Up," *Archives of General Psychiatry* 36(9), Aug. 1979, 1010–1015.

Michaels, Stuart, et al. *The Social Organization of Sexuality*, Chicago: University of Chicago Press, 1994.

Michels, Robert; and Marzak, Peter, "Progress in Psychiatry," *New England Journal of Medicine*, 329(8), August 19, 1995, 552–557.

Michjeda, Maria. "Fetal Tissue Transplantation; Miscarriages and Tissue Banks," in *The Fetal Tissue Issues*, Cataldo and Moraczewski, eds., Braintree, MA: Pope John Center, 1994:1–14.

Milhaven, John Giles, "Thomas Aquinas on Sexual Pleasure," *Journal of Religious Ethics* 5, 1977, 1576–181.

Miller, Franklin, et al., "Regulating Physician-Assisted Death," *New England Journal of Medicine* 33(2) July 14, 1994, 119–123.

Mills, Michael; Wofsy, Constana; and Mills, John, "The Acquired Immune Deficiency Syndrome: Infection Control and Public Law," *New England Journal of Medicine* 314(14), Apr. 3, 1986, 931–926.

Minogue, Brendon, *Bioethics: A Committee Approach*, Sudbury, MA: Jones & Bartlett, 1996.

Minow, Martha. "The Role of Families in Medical Decisions." *Utah Law Review* (1) 1991, p. 1–24.

Mitford, Jessica, *The American Way of Death*, 2nd ed., New York: Simon & Schuster, 1975.

Mizratti, Terry, *Getting Rid of Patients*, New Brunswick: Rutgers University Press, 1981.

Modde, Margaret, "The Christian Faithful and the Health Care Ministry," *Health Progress* 66(7), Sept. 1985, 75–82.

Modell, Bernadette
> 1982 "Social Aspects of Prenatal Monitoring for Genetic Disease," *The Future of Prenatal Diagnosis*, Edinburgh: Churchill Livingston, 1982.
> 1992 "Ethical aspects of genetic screening," *Annals of Medicine* 24:6 (December 1992); 549–555.

Moffic, Steven; Coverdale, John; and Bayer, Timothy. "Ethics Education for Psychiatry," *The Journal of Clinical Ethics* 2:3 (Fall 1991) p.161–166.

Mohr, James, *Abortion in America: The Origins and Evolution of National Policy 1800–1900*, New York: Oxford University Press, 1978.

Moline, Jon, "Professionals and Professions: A Philosophical Examination of an Ideal," *Social Science and Medicine* 22 (5), 1986, 501–508.

Monod, Jacques, *Chance and Necessity An Essay on the Natural Philosophy of Modern Biology*, NY: Alfred Knopf, 1971.

Monteleone, James A., MD, "The Physiological Aspects of Sex," in *Human Sexuality and Personhood*, St. Louis: Pope John XXIII Medical-Moral Research and Education Center, 1981, 71–85.

Moody, Howard, "Abortion: Woman's Right and Legal Problem," *Christianity and Crisis* 31, 1971, 27–32.

Moore, G. E., *Ethics*, New York: Oxford Press, 1965 (original 1903).

Moore, Keith L.
> 1988 *The Developing Human: Clinically Oriented Embryology*, 4th ed., Philadelphia: Saunders, 1988.
> 1989 *Before We Are Born: Basic Embryology and Birth Defects*, 3rd ed., Philadelphia: Saunders, 1989.

Moore, Lorna, *The Bicultural Basis of Health: Expanding Views of Medical Anthropology*, Prospect Heights, IL: Waveland Press, 1987.

Moore, Robert; and Mockel, Daniel, eds. *Jung and Christianity in Dialogue* NY: Paulist Press, 1990.

Moore, Wilbert E.; and Rosenblum, Gerald W., *The Professions: Roles and Rules*, New York: Russell Sage Foundation, 1970, 51–65, 174–186.

Moraczewski, Albert
    1990 "Personhood: Entry and Exit," in *The Twenty-Fifth Anniversary of Vatican II: A Look Back and a Look Ahead*, ed. Russell E. Smith. Braintree, MA: The Pope John Center.
    1996 "Managing Tubal Pregnancy Part II," *Ethics and Medics*, 21(8) August 1996.

Morreim, E. Haavi
    1993 "Impairment and Impediments in Patient Decision Making: Reframing the Competency Question," *Journal of Clinical Ethics* 4:4, 1993, p.294–307.
    1995 "Moral justice and legal justice in managed care: the ascent of contributive justice," *The Journal of Law, Medicine, and Ethics* 23:3 (Fall, 1995): 236–247.

Mossman, Douglas; and Hart, Kathleen. "How Bad is Civil Commitment? A Study of Attitudes Toward Violence and Involuntary Hospitalization," *Bulletin of the American Academy of Psychiatry and the Law*, 21:2 (1993) p.181–194.

Moyers, Bill. *Healing and the Mind*, NY: Doubleday, 1993, *passim*.

Mullady, Brian. *The Meaning of the Term "Moral" in St. Thomas Aquinas*, Rome, Liberea Editrice Vaticana, 1986.

Mulvanney, Kieran, "The Other Side of Animal Rights," *New Scientist* 109(1502), April 3, 1986, 52–53.

Munetz, Mark R.; Lidz, Charles; and Meisel, Alan, "Informed Consent and Incompetent Patients," *Journal of Family Practice* 20(3), Mar. 1985, 273–279.

Murnion, "A Sacramental Church in a Sacramental World," *Origins* 14(6), June 21, 1984, 81–90, especially p. 88.

Murphy, Francis X., *Catholic Perspectives on Population Issues II*, vol. 35, Washington, DC: Population Reference Bureau, Feb. 1981.

Murray, J.; et al, "Informed Consent for Research Publication of Patient Related Data," *Clinical Research* 32(4), Oct. 1984, 404–408.

Murray, Joseph, E., "Decisions on the Frontlines of Surgery," *Harvard Medical*, 1986, 18–24.

NACC: National Association of Catholic Chaplains, "Formal Statement of Definition for Standards," *Newsletter*, August 31, 1995.

NAS: National Academy of Science, "Confronting AIDS, Update 1988," Washington, DC: 1988.

Nash, George. *The Conservative Intellectual Movement in America Since 1945*, New York: Basic Books, 1976

Nathanson, Bernard
    1983 *The Abortion Mentality*, New York: Fall, 1983
    1992a "The Science of Chemical Abortifacients", Pope John Center, *The Interaction of Catholic Bioethics and Secular Society*, Russell E. Smith, ed. Braintree, MA: The Pope John Center, 1992, pp. 133–143.
    1992b "Licensed to kill," *National Review* 44 (February 3, 1992): 44–47.

Nathanson, Bernard, and Ostling, Richard, *Aborting America*, New York: Doubleday, 1979.

National Academy of Science: see NAS

National Coalition: National Coalition on Catholic Health Care Ministry, Silver Spring, MD, Resource 10, (1995):5.

National Institute of Drug Abuse: see NIDA

Navarro, Vincente, *Crisis in Health and Medicine: A Social Critique*, New York: Tavistock Publications, 1986.

NCCB: National Conference of Catholic Bishops

1973 *Statement on Population,* Washington, DC: United States Catholic Conference.

1974 *Documentation on the Right to Life and Abortion,* Washington, DC: United States Catholic Conference.

1977 *Commentary on Reply of Sacred Congregation for the Doctrine of the Faith on Sterilization in Catholic Hospitals,* Sept. 15.

1980 "Statement on Tubal Ligation," *Origins* 10(11) May 28.

1985 "Pastoral Plan for Prolife Activities: A Reaffirmation," *Origins* 15 (24), Nov. 28.

1986 Committee for Prolife Activities, "Statement on Uniform Rights of the Terminally Ill Act" (June 26, 1986) *Origins* 16 (12), Sept. 4, 1986, 222–224.

1994 "Ethical and Religious Directives for Catholic Health Services" *Origins* 24(27), December 15, 1994, 449–464.

NCR: National Catholic Reporter, "Rome Document Sparks Firestorm Reaction: Even Critics Admit it Should not be Ignored," April 3, 1987.

Nelson, D. M., *The Priority of Prudence.* University Park, PA: University of Pennsylvania, 1992.

Nelson, James. "Duties of Patients to their Caregivers," in Courtney, Lustig, eds, *Duties of Others,* Boston, MA: Kluwer Academic, 1994, p. 199–214.

Neppe, Vernon; and Tucker, Gary. "Neuro Psychiatric Aspects of Seizure Disorders," in *Textbook of Neuropsychiatry,* Yudofsky, Stuart; and Hales, Robert, eds., 1992.

New Jersey Catholic Conference, "Providing Food and Fluids to Severely Brain-Damaged Patients," *Origins* 16(32) Jan. 22, 1987, 584.

New York Task Force on Medical Ethics, *The Determination of Death,* New York: The Task Force, 1986.

New York Times

1988 "Pressure to Regulate *in vitro* Fertilization Groups as Demand Rises," July 27.

1996 "AMA Opposes Taking Organs from Brain Abnormal Babies," January 7, p. 11A.

Ngyan, William, and Sahat, Nadia, *Diagnostic Recognition of Genetic Disease,* Philadelphia: Lea and Debiger, 1987.

Nicolosi, J., *Reparative Therapy of Male Homosexuality,* Northvale, NJ: J. Aronson.

NIDA: National Institute of Drug Abuse, *Drug Use Among American High School Students and other Young Adults,* Washington, DC: U.S. Department of Health and Human Services, 1986.

Niebuhr, H. Richard, *The Responsible Self,* New York: Harper & Row, 1963.

NIH: National Institutes of Health

1985 "Consensus Conference: Electroconvulsive Therapy," *Journal of the American Medical Association* 254 (15), Oct. 18, 1985, 2105–08.

1987 *Human Somatic Cell Gene Therapy Prospects for Treating Inherited Diseases,* Washington, DC: NIH.

1994 *Report on the Human Embryo Research Panel,* Washington, DC: National Institutes of Health, September 27.

1996 *The Nation's Physician Workforce* National Academy Press, 1996.

Nilstan, Tore. "Theory and methods for research on ethical issues in dementia care," *Scandinavian Journal of Caring Sciences,* 6:3 (1992):173–177.

Nolan, Martin, "The Principle of Totality in Moral Theology," in *Absolutes in Moral Theology,* Charles E. Curran, ed., Washington, DC: Corpus Books, 1968.

Nolin, Kieran, OSB, "Attitudes of Medical Staff to Sacramental Ministry in Public Hospitals," paper read at Institute of Religious and Human Development, Texas Medical Center, Houston, 1972.

Noonan, John T.

1965 *Contraception: A History of Its Treatment by the Catholic Theologians and Canonists,* New York: Harvard University Press, "On zero population growth," 18–25, "On Church's middle course in sex ethics," 56–106, rev., 1987.

1967 "Abortion and the Catholic Church: A Summary History," *Natural Law Forum* 12, 85–131.

1970a "An Almost Absolute Value in History," in *The Morality of Abortion: Legal and Historical Perspectives*, John T. Noonan, Jr., ed., Cambridge, MA: Harvard University Press, 1–59.

1970b ed., *The Morality of Abortion: Legal and Historical Perspectives*, Cambridge, MA: Harvard University Press.

1979 *A Private Choice: Abortion in America in the Seventies*, New York: Free Press.

1985 "An Almost Absolute Value in History," *Human Life Review* 11(1–2), Winter-Spring 1985, 125–178.

1993 "Development in Moral Doctrine," *Theological Studies* 54, 662–677.

Nouwen, Henri J.

1972 *The Wounded Healer: Ministry in Contemporary Society*, Garden City, NY: Doubleday.

1990 *In the Name of Jesus*, NY: Crossroads.

Novak, David

1971 *Suicide and Morality*, NY: Scholars Press.

1985 *Halakah in a Theological Dimension*, Chico, CA: Scholars Press.

Nowell-Smith, Patrick, "In Favor of Voluntary Euthanasia," in *Principles of Health Care Ethics*, Raanan Gillon, ed., New York: Wiley, 1994.

Noyes, R., Jr., "Seneca on Death," *Journal of Religion and Health* 12, 1973, 223–240.

Nozick, Robert, *Philosophical Explanations*, Cambridge: Belknap Press, 1981.

Nugent, J. Kevin (ed.) *The Cultural Context of Infancy*, Norwood, NJ: Ablex Publishing, 1989.

O'Callaghan, D. F., "Humanae Vitae in Perspective: Survey of Recent French Writing," *Irish Theological Quarterly* 37, 1970, 309–321.

O'Connell, Timothy, *Changing Catholic Moral Theology: A Study of Josef Fuchs*, doctoral dissertation, Ann Arbor: University Microfilms, 1974.

O'Donnell, Thomas

1976 *Medicine and Christian Morality*, Boston: St. Paul Press, 66 ff., (original ed. 1957).

1994 "Modern 'Treatment' of Ectopic Pregnancy," *The Medical-Moral Newsletter*, 31 (March, 1994), p. 1–1.

O'Donovan, Oliver, *Begotten or Made*, New York: Oxford University Press, 1984.

Olshansky, Ellen Francis; and Sammons, Lucy, "Artificial Insemination: An Overview," *Journal of Obstetric Gynecological and Neonatal Nursing* 14(6), Nov. 1985, 49–54.

O'Meara, Thomas

1973 *Loose in the World*, New York: Paulist Press.

1983 *Theology of Ministry*, New York: Paulist Press.

Ong, Walter J. "Yeast: a parable for Catholic higher education," *America* April 7, 1990:347–63.

O'Neil, E. H. *Health Professions: Education for the Future*, San Francisco, CA: Pew Health Care Commission, 1994.

Oppenheimer, Gerald; and Padgug, Robert, "AIDS: The Risk to Insurers, The Threat to Equity," *Hastings Center Report* 16 (5), Oct. 1986, 18–22.

O'Rourke, Kevin

1975 "Fetal Experimentation: An Evaluation of the New Federal Norms," *Hospital Progress* 56, Sept., 60–69.

1986 "The A.M.A. Statement on Tube Feeding: An Ethical Analysis," *America* 155(15), Nov. 22, 321–28.

1987 "Institutional ownership as an ethical issue," in *Health Care Ethics*, Anderson, Gary, ed, Rockville, MD: Aspen Press, 1987, 235–250.

1988a "Responsibility for Physician's Competence," *Ethical Essays*, St. Louis: St. Louis University Medical Center, June.

1988b "Two Ethical Approaches to Research on Human Beings," *Health Progress,* October.

1992 "Pain Relief: The Perspective of Catholic Tradition," *Journal of Pain and Symptom Management,* November 1992, p. 485–91.

1996a "Ethical opinions in regard to the questions of early delivery of anencephalic infants," *Linacre Quarterly,* Summer 1996.

1996b "Health Care Models: New and Old," op. ed. *St. Louis Post Dispatch,* February 16, 1996, p. 6C.

1996c "An Open Letter to Germain Grisez," *Health Progress,* November–December, 1996.

O'Rourke, Kevin; and Boyle, Philip, *Medical Ethics: The Sources of Catholic Teachings,* Washington, DC: Georgetown University Press, 1993, 2nd ed.

O'Rourke, Kevin; and deBlois, Jean, "Removing Life Support: Motivations, Obligations," *Health Progress,* July/August 1992, p. 20–28.

Ory, H. W., "Association between Oral Contraceptives and Myocardial Infarction, A Review," *JAMA* 237, 1977, 2619–1622.

Ory, H.W.; Forrest, J.D.; and Lincoln, R., *Making Choices: Evaluating the Health Risks and Benefits of Birth Control Methods,* New York: Guttmacher Institute, 1983.

Osmond, Daniel. "A physiologist looks at purpose and meaning in life," in *Evidence of Purpose: Scientists Discover the Creator,* John Templeton, ed., NY: Continuum, 1994 p.133–167.

Osmundsen, John A., "We Are All Mutants—Preventive Genetic Medicine: A Growing Clinical Field Troubled by a Confusion of Ethicists," *Medical Dimensions* 2, 1973, 5–7, 26–28.

Osservatore Romano, "The Moral Norms of 'Humanae Vitae'" *Origins* 18:38 (March 2, 1989).

Ossi, Robert, "Mildred, is it Fun to be a Cripple? The Culture of Suffering in Mid-Twentieth Century American Catholicism," *The South Atlantic Quarterly,* 93(3) Summer 1994, 547–590.

OTA: Office of Technology Assessment
1984 "Human Gene Therapy: Background Paper," Washington, DC: OTA, Dec.

1988 *Infertility, Medical and Social Choices,* Washington, DC: OTA, n. 307.

1993 *Biomedical Ethics in US Policy,* US Government Printing Office, OTA-BP-BBS-105.

Outka, Gene
1968 *Norm and Context in Christian Ethics,* New York: Charles Scribners Sons.

1972 *Agape: An Ethical Analysis,* New Haven: Yale University Press.

Palca, Joseph, "The Pill of Choice?" *Science* 245 (Sept. 22, 1989): 1319–1323.

Palmour, Jody, *On Moral Character: A Practical Guide to Aristotle's Virtues and Vices,* Washington, DC: Archon Institute, 1988.

Paris, John, "When Burdens of Feeding Outweigh Benefits," *Hasting Center Report* 16(1), Feb. 1986, 30–32.

Paris Statement of 1966, in *A Catholic/Humanist Dialogue,* Paul Kurtz and Albert Dondeyne, eds., Buffalo: Prometheus Books, 1972, 3 ff.

Parisi, P.; M. Gatti, G. Prinzi; and G. Capterna, "Familial incidence of twinning," *Nature,* 304 (Aug. 18, 1983): 626–9.

Park Ridge Center, *Active Euthanasia, Religion, and The Public Debate,* Chicago, IL: Park Ridge Center, 1991.

Parker, Lisa. "Bioethics for human geneticists, models for reasoning and methods for teaching," *American Journal of Human Genetics* 54:1 (January 1994): 137–147.

Parsons, Talcott, *The Social Systems,* Glencoe, IL: Free Press, 1951.

Pastrana, Gabriel. "Personhood and the Beginning of Human Life," *The Thomist* 41 (1977): 247–294.

Paul VI

   1967   *The Development of Peoples* (Popolorum Progressio), March 26, Washington, DC: United States Catholic Conference.

   1968   *Humanae Vitae: Encyclical Letter on the Regulation of Births,* Washington, DC: United States Catholic Conference.

   1971a   *A Call to Action: Apostolic Letter on Eightieth Anniversary of "Rerum Novarum,"* May 14, Washington, DC: United States Catholic Conference.

   1971b   "Justice in the World," issued by Synod of Bishops, *The Pope Speaks* 16, 377–384.

   1972   *Apostolic Constitution on the Sacrament of Anointing the Sick,* Washington, DC: United States Catholic Conference.

   1974   Message to President of United Nations General Assembly, Dec. 10, 1973, *The Pope Speaks* 18, 304–307.

Payer, Lynn. *Medicine and Culture: Varieties of treatment in the US, England, W. Germany and France,* NY: H. Holt, 1988.

PBC: Pontifical Biblical Commission. "The Interpretation of the Bible in the Church," *Origins* 23:29 (January 6, 1994):497–524.

PCJP: See Pontifical Council on Justice and Peace

PCEMR: See President's Commission for the Study of Ethical Problems in Medicine and Biomedical and Behavioral Research.

Peddicord, Richard, *A Question: Sexual Ethics or Social Justice,* Kansas City, MO: Sheed and Ward, 1996.

Pellegrino, Edmund

   1981   "The Moral Foundations for Valid Consent," in *Proceedings of the Third National Conference on Human Values and Cancer,* Washington, DC: American Cancer Society.

   1985a   "Relevance and Utility of Courses in Medical Ethics: A Survey of Physicians' Perceptions," *Journal of the American Medical Association* 253(1), Jan. 4, 49–53.

   1985b   "The Virtuous Physician, and the Ethics of Medicine" in *Virtue and Medicine Explorations in the Character of Medicine,* E. Shelp, ed., Boston: D. Reidel, 237–255.

   1987   "Altruism, Self-Interest and Medical Ethics," *Journal of the American Medical Association* 258(14), Oct. 9, 1139–40.

Pellegrino, Edmund D.; and Thomasma, David C.

   1981   *What is Medicine?: A Philosophical Basis of Medical Practice,* New York: Oxford University Press, 58–81.

   1988   *For the Patient's Good: The Restoration of Beneficence in Health Care,* New York: Oxford University Press.

   1993   *The Virtues in Medical Practice,* New York: Oxford University Press, 1993.

   1996   *The Christian Virtues in Medical Practice,* NY: Oxford University Press, 1996.

Penrose, Roger, *Shadows of the Mind: A Search for the Missing Science of Consciousness,* New York: Oxford, 1995.

Pennsylvania Catholic Conference, "Guidelines for Catholic Hospitals Treating Victims of Sexual Assault," *Origins* 22 (May 6, 1993):810.

Pereda, J.; and H. B. Croxato, "Ultrastructure of a seven-cell human embryo," *Biology of Reproduction* 18 (1978):481.

Peredo, Jaime; and Mario Coppo, "Ultrastructure of Two-Cell Human Embryo Fertilized in Vivo," Seppälä, Markku, and R. G. Edwards, *In Vitro Fertilization and Embryo Transfer,* ed., (New York: Annals of the New York Academy of Science, vol. 442, 1985), pp. 416–419.

Perico, Giacoma. "Response and moral questions," *La Civilta Cattolica* (June 1993) Rome.

Perlin, Michael. "Tarasoff and the Dilemma of the Dangerous Patient: New Directions for the 1990's," *Law and Psychology Review,* 16, (Spring 1992), p. 29–63.

Perry, Ralph, *General Theory of Value,* Cambridge: Harvard University Press, 1980.

Peschle, Henry, *Christian Ethics* Volume II, Dublin: Goodly & Neal, 1978, 479.

Peters, David, "Advance Medical Directions: The Case for the Durable Power of Attorney for Health Care," *The Journal of Legal Medicine* 8(3), 1987, 437–464.

Petersdorf, Robert G., "Medical Education for the Future: A Mandate for Change," *Internist* 27(5), May 1986, 17–20.

Peterson, Herbert, et al., for the U.S. Collaborative Review of Sterilization Working Group, "The Risk of Pregnancy After Tubal Sterilization," *American Journal of Obstetrics and Gynecology*, 174(4), April 1996, 1161–1171.

Peterson, Michael R., "Psychological Aspects of Human Sexual Behavior," in *Human Sexuality and Personhood*. St. Louis: Pope John XXIII Medical-Moral Research and Education Center, 1981.

Petitti, Diana; Sidney, Stephen; Berstein, Allan; Wolf, Sheldon; Quesen, Berry, and Ziel, Charles, "Stroke in Users of Low Dose Contraceptives," *NEJM* 335(1), July 4, 1996, 8–15.

Petrila, John, "Mental Health Therapies," in *Bio-Law Vol. 1*, Frederick, MD: University Publications of America, 1986, 177–215.

Pew Commission (Pew Health Professions Commission)
1993   *Contemporary Issues In Health Professions Education and Workforce Reform*, Center for Health Professions, University of California, San Francisco.
1995   *Critical Challenges: Revitalizing the Health Professions for the 21st Century*, Center for Health Profession, University of California, San Francisco, p. 26 ff.

Philibert, Paul, "Lawrence Kohlberg's Use of Virtue in His Theory of Moral Development," *International Philosophical Quarterly* 15, 1975, 455–479.

Phillipe, P., "Genetic Epidemiology of Twinning," *American Journal of Medical Genetics*, 20 (1985):97–105.

Physicians' Desk Reference, Oradell, NJ: Medical Economics Co., 1986.

Piaget, Jean, *The Moral Judgment of the Child*, New York: Free Press, 1965 [1929].

Piccione, Joseph. Private letter, (October 6, 1995).

Pieper, Josef, *Leisure, the Basis of Culture*, New York: New American Library, 1964.

Pierce vs. Swan Point Cemetery, 10 Rhode Island, 227, (1872).

Pietroferg, John, *Counseling: An Introduction*, New York: Houghton Mifflin, 1983.

Pilote, Louise, et al., "Regional Variation Across the United States in the Management of Acute Care Myocardial Infarction," *NEJM* 333:9 (August 31, 1995) p. 565–572.

Pinckaers, Servais, *The Sources of Christian Ethics*, Washington, DC: Catholic University Press, 1995.

Pincus, Jonathan, "Ethical Issues in Forensic Neurology," *Seminars in Neurology* 4(1), 1984, 87–91.

Pius XI, "Casti Connubii," Dec. 31, 1930, *The Human Body: Papal Teachings*, Boston: St. Paul Editions, 1979 [1960], n. 4–12.

Pius XII
1944   "Allocution to the Italian Medical-Biological Union of St. Luke" (Nov. 12), *The Human Body: Papal Teachings*, Boston: St. Paul Editions, 1979 [1960], n. 165–179.
1951   "Allocution to Italian Midwives" (Oct. 29) *The Human Body: Papal Teachings*, Boston: St. Paul Editions, 1979 [1960], n. 243–315.
1952   "Allocution to the First International Congress of Histopathology" (Sept. 14), *The Human Body: Papal Teachings*, Boston: St. Paul Editions, 1979 [1960], n. 349–381.
1956a   "Allocution to a Group of Eye Specialists" (May 14), *The Human Body: Papal Teachings*, Boston: St. Paul Editions, 1979 [1960], n. 637–649.
1956b   "Allocution to Second World Congress on Fertility and Sterility," The Human Body: Papal Teachings, Boston: St. Paul Editions, 1979 [1960], n. 650–666.
1957   "Prolongation of Life," (Nov. 24) Issues in Ethical Decision Making, Gary Atkinson, ed., St. Louis: Pope John XXIII Medical-Moral Research and Education Center, 1976.

Plato, *Republic* (III, 405A) London, Penguin Books, 1970.

Plum, Fred; and Posner, Jerome, *The Diagnosis of Stupor and Coma,* Philadelphia: F.A. Davis Co., 1982, 315.

Poddimatam, Feliz, *Fundamental Option and Mortal Sin,* Bangalore, Asian Trading Corporation, 1986.

Polkinghorne, JC. *Reason and Reality: The Relationship Between Science and Theology,* Philadelphia, PA: Trinity Press, 1991.

Pontifical Academy of Science, *The Artificial Prolongation of Life, and the Exact Determination of the Moment of Death,* Oct. 31, 1985.

Pontifical Council for the Family
  1996a "The Truth and Meaning of Human Sexuality," *Origins* 25:32, February 1, 1996, 529–552.
  1996b "The Holy See and Population," Diarmuid Martin, in *Proceeding of ITEST,* Robert Brungs, ed., St. Louis: ITEST Foundation, 1996.

Pontifical Council on Justice and Peace, "Church and Human Right," *Osservatore Romano* (Eng. ed.) 6, 1973; Oct. 23, 6–10; Oct. 30, 8–9; Nov. 6, 6–8; Nov. 13, 9–10.

Population Crisis Committee, "Issues in Contraceptive Development," *Population,* May 1985, 153.

Powsner, Rhoda, and Hemmersaith, Frances, "Medical Malpractice Crisis: The Second Time Around," *Journal of Legal Medicine* 8(2), 1987, 283–304.

PCEMR: President's Commission for the Study of Ethical Problems in Medicine and Biomedical and Behavioral Research
  1981 "Report on the Definition of Death Legislation," Washington, DC: U.S. Government Printing Office.
  1982a *Making Health Care Decisions: The Ethical and Legal Implications of Informed Consent in the Patient-Practitioner Relationship,* 3 vol., Oct.
  1982b *Splicing Life: The Social and Ethical Issues of Genetic Engineering with Human Beings,* Nov.
  1982c "Substantive and Procedural Principles of Decision Making for Incapacitated Patients," *Making Health Care Decisions,* Washington, DC: U.S. Government Printing Office.
  1983a *Screening and Counseling for Genetic Conditions: The Ethical, Social, and Legal Implications of Genetic Screening, Counseling, and Education Programs,* Feb.
  1983b *Implementing Human Regulations: The Adequacy and Uniformity of Federal Rules and Their Implementation,* March.
  1983c *Securing Access to Health Care: The Ethical Implications of Differences in the Availability of Health Services,* March.
  1983d *Deciding to Forego Life-Sustaining Treatment: Ethical, Medical and Legal Issues in Treatment Decisions,* March.
  1983e President's Commission I.R.B. Guidebook. President's Commission on AIDS, *Final Report,* Washington, DC: Department of Health and Human Services, March 4, 1988.

President's Commission on AIDS, *Final Report,* Washington, DC: Department of Health and Human Services, 1988.

Prochaska, J.; Clemente, D.; and Norcross, J. "In Search of How People Change: Application to Addictive Behavior," *American Psychology* 47:4 (1992).

Pro-Life Committee—NCCB Prolife Committee, "Nutrition and Hydration: Moral and Pastoral Reflections," *Origins* April 9, 1992, p. 705.

Prummer, Dominicus M., OP, *Manuale Theologiae Moralis,* 14th ed., 3 vols., Barcelona: Herder, 1958, vol. 1, n. 617–623.

Purviance, Susan. "Kidney transplantation policy: race and distributive justice," *Business and Professional Ethics Journal* 12:2 (Summer 1993): 19–37.

Quaid, Kimberly. "Presymptomatic testing for Huntington's disease in the United States," *American Journal of Human Genetics* 53:3 (September 1993): 785–787.

Quay, Paul, *The Christian Meaning of Sexuality,* San Francisco: Ignatius Press, 1988, 3–10.

Quill, Timothy; Cassell, Christine; and Meier, Diane; "Care of the Hopelessly Ill: Proposed Clinical Criteria for Physician Assisted Suicide." *New England Journal of Medicine,* 327(19), November 5, 1992, 1380–83.

Quill, Timothy; and Suchman, Anthony. "Uncertainty and Control: Learning to Live with Medicine's Limitations," *Human Medicine* (April 9, 1993) p. 109–120.

Rachels, James
    1983 "The Sanctity of Life," in *Biomedical Ethics Review,* James Humber and Robert Almeder, eds., Clifton, NJ: Humana Press, 29–42.
    1986 *The Elements of Moral Philosophy,* New York: Random House.

Rahner, Karl
    1961 "On the question of a formal existential ethics,"
    1963 "The Church and the Sacraments," in *Questiones Disputatae,* no. 9. New York: Herder & Herder.
    1965 *On the Theology of Death,* New York: Herder & Herder.

Ramsey, Paul
    1965 *Deeds and Rules in Christian Ethics,* Edinburgh: Oliver and Boyd, p. 144 ff.
    1970 *The Patient as Person,* New Haven: Yale University Press, 1980 (5th prtg.).
    1973 "Abortion: A Review Article," *Thomist* 37, 174–226.
    1983 *Basic Christian Ethics,* Chicago: University of Chicago Press, reprint of 1950 ed.

Rand, Ayn
    1964 *The Virtue of Selfishness: A New Concept of Egoism,* New York: New American Library, Signet Books.
    1967 *Capitalism: The Uncommon Ideal,* New York: New American Library.

Ratner, Herbert, MD
    1977 "Biology and Biologism," *Child and Family* 16, 194–200.
    1981 "A Physician Speaks on the Right to Life," in *Natural Family Planning: Nature's Way/God's Way,* Anthony Zimmerman, SVD, ed., Collegeville, MN: De Rance, Inc. and Human Life Center, 44–47.

Ratzinger, Cardinal
    1984a "Bishops, Theologians, and Morality," *Origins* 13(40), March 15; 657.
    1984b "Dissent and Proportionalism in Moral Theology," *Origins* 13(40), March 15; 666–670.
    1986 "Letter to Father Charles Curran," *Origins* 16(11), Aug. 23:201–203.
    1987 *Principles of Catholic Theology: Building Stones for a Fundamental Theology,* San Francisco: Ignatius Press.

Rawls, John, *A Theory of Justice,* Cambridge, MA: Harvard University Press, 1971.

Rayport, Stephen, "Cellular and Molecular Biology of the Neuron" in *Textbook of Neuropsychiatry,* American Psychiatric Press, 1992.

RCIA: Rite of Christian Initiation for Adults, Washington, DC: United States Catholic Conference, 1993.

Reardon, David, *Aborted Women: Silent No Longer,* Chicago: Loyola University Press, 1987.

Reed, Sheldon, *Counseling in Medical Genetics,* 3rd ed., New York: Alan R. Liss, Inc., 1980.

Regan, A. "The Human Conceptus and its Personhood," *Studia Moralia* 30 (1992): 97–127.

Reinhardt, Uwe
    1993 "Reorganizing the Financial Flows in U.S. Health Care," *Health Affairs* 12:Supplement:172–194.
    1994 "Demagoguery and Debate over Medicare Reform," *Health Affairs:14:4:101–104.*

Reiser, David; and Rosen, David, *Medicine as a Human Experience,* Baltimore: University Park Press, 1984.

Reiser, Stanley. "The Era of the Patient: Using the Experience of Illness in Shaping the Mission of Health Care," *Journal of the American Medical Association* 269:8 (February 24, 1993), p. 1012–1017.

Rescher, Nicholas, *Unpopular Essays on Technological Progress,* Pittsburgh: University of Pittsburgh Press, 1980.

Restak, Richard M., *Pre-Meditated Man: Bioethics and the Control of Future Human Life,* New York: Viking Press, 1975.

Rice, Nancy; and Doherty, Richard, "Reflections on Prenatal Diagnosis: The Consumer's View," *Social Work on Health Care* 8(1), Fall 1982.

Riddle, John M., *Contraception and Abortion From the Ancient World to the Renaissance* Cambridge, MA: Harvard University Press, 1992.

Rieff, Philip, *The Triumph of the Therapeutic: Uses of Faith After Freud,* New York: Harper & Row Torchbooks, 1968.

Riese, Walther, *The Conception of Disease: Its History, Its Versions, Its Nature,* NY: Philosophical Library, 1953.

Rifkin, Jeremy, *Algeny: A New Word—A New World,* New York: Penguin Books, 1984.

Riskin, Leonard L., "Sexual Relations Between Psychotherapists and Their Patients: Toward Research or Restraint," *California Law Review* 67, 1979, 1000–1027.

Rizzo, Robert; and Yonder, Paul, "Definition and Criteria of Clinical Death," *Linacre Quarterly* 40 (1973): 223–233.

Roach, William et al., *Medical Records and the Law* 2nd edition, Gaithersburg, MD: Aspen, 1994.

Robertson, John A., "What We May Do with Preembryos: A Response to Richard A. McCormick," *Kennedy Institute of Ethics Journal,* 1, 4 (1991): 293–305.

Robinson, James. "The changing boundaries of the American hospital," *Milbank Quarterly* 72:2 (Spring 1994).

Rodd, Rosemary, "Pacifism and Absolute Rights for Animals: A Comparison of Difficulties," *Journal of Applied Philosophy* 2(1), March 1985, 53–61.

Roduin, Marc. *Medicine, Money, and Morals,* NY: Oxford Press, 1993.

Rodwin, MA. "Conflicts in managed care," *NEJM* 332(9) March 2, 1995:604–607.

Roels, L; and Collaborative Group for Transplantation. "Altruism, Self-determination and Organ Procurement Efficiency: The European Experience," *Transplantation Proceedings* 5 Oct 23, 1991, 2514–2515.

Rogers, Carl R., *Client-Centered Therapy,* Boston: Houghton Mifflin, 1951.

Rordorf, Willy. "Sunday: The Fullness of Christian Liturgical Time," Collegeville, MN: Liturgical Press, 1982, 90–96.

Rosenberg, Charles. *The Care of Strangers: The Rise of America's Hospital System,* NY: Basic Books, 1987.

Rosenberg, J.; and Towers, Bernard, "The Practice of Empathy as a Prerequisite for Informed Consent" *Theoretical Medicine* 7(2), June 1986, 181–194.

Rosenfield, Israel
    1987 *The Invention of Memory: A New View of the Brain,* New York: Basic Books.
    1995 *The Strange, Familiar, and Forgotten: An Anatomy of Consciousness,* New York: Vintage.

Rosner, Fred, *Modern Medicine and Jewish Ethics,* New York: Yashiva University Press, 1986.

Rosotti, Sidney, "Ethics of Life Support" (letter) *New England Journal of Medicine* 318(26), June 30, 1988.

Ross, Judith Wilson. "Spirit, emotion, and meaning: the many voices of bioethics—literature, bioethics and the priestly physician," *Hastings Center Report* 24:3 May/June 1994:25–26.

Ross, W. D., *The Right and the Good,* Oxford: Claredon Press, 1930.

Rothman, David J. *Conscience and Convenience: The Asylum and Its Alternatives in Progressive America,* Boston: Little, Brown, 1980.

Rothman, Kenneth; and Michels, Karin. "The continuing use of placebo controls," *NEJM* 331:6 (August 11, 1994):394–398.

Rousseau, Jean Jacques, *Discourse upon Origin and Foundations of Inequality among Mankind in Social Contract and Discourses,* New York: E.P. Dutton, 1976 [1753].

Roy, David, "Created Equal: The Moral Challenge of Prenatal Diagnosis," *Canadian Catholic Health Care Review,* Summer 1984, 13–18.

Rubin, Eva, *Abortion Politics and the Courts,* Westport, CT: Greenwood Press, 1987.

Rubin, Robert, et al., *Critical Condition: America's Health Care in Jeopardy,* Washington, DC: National Committee for Quality Health Care, 1988

Runciman, Steven, *The Medieval Manichee,* Cambridge: Cambridge University Press, 1982 [1947].

Ryder, R., "Natural family planning; effective birth control supported by the Catholic church," *British Medical Journal* (September 18, 1993).

Ryle, A. "Transference and Counter Transference Variations in the Course of Cognitive Analytic Therapy," *British Journal of Medical Psychology* 68:2 (June 1995) p.109–124.

Sacred Penitentiary, 1853/1880, "Responses on Infertile Period, March 2, 1853 and June 16, 1880," in *Natural Family Planning: Nature's Way/God's Way,* Anthony Zimmerman, SVD, ed., Collegeville, MN, DeRance Inc. and Human Life Center, 1981, 44–47.

Sachs, Greg; Rhymes, Jill; and Cassel, Christine. "Biomedical behavioral research in nursing homes: guidelines for ethical investigations," *Journal of the American Geriatric Society* 47:7 (July 1993):771–779.

Sacks, Robert D., *A Commentary on the Book of Genesis,* Ancient Near Eastern Texts and Studies, vol. 6 (Lewiston/Queenston/Lampeter, 1990).

Sadler, Alfred, et al., "The Uniform Anatomical Gift Act," *Journal of the American Medical Association* 206, 1968, 2501–2506.

Sadler, T. W., *Langman's Medical Embryology,* 6th ed., Baltimore: Williams and Wilkins, 1990.

St. John-Stevas, Norman
> 1961   *Life, Death and the Law: Law and Christian Morals in England and the United States,* Bloomington, IN: Indiana University Press.
> 1971   *The Agonizing Choice: Birth Control, Religion and the Law,* Bloomington, IN: Indiana University Press.

Salvendy, J. "Control and Power in Supervision," *British Journal of Psychology* 83:1, February 1992, p.133–145.

Sanders, John H., "Ethical Ingredients in Critical Care," *Bulletin of the American College of Surgeons,* May 1984, 69(5), 14–15.

Sanders, Susan. "Catholic hospitals and community benefit activities," *Health Progress* 1:4 (Jan/Feb 1994):393–400.

Saunders, Cicely, "The Dying Patient" in *Principles of Health Care Ethics,* Raanan Gillon, ed., New York: Wiley, 1994, p. 775–82.

Scherr, L., "AIDS: A Critical Test for Medicine," *American College of Physicians Journal* 7(8), 1987, 2.

Schiff, Robert, et al., "Transfers to a Public Hospital," *New England Journal of Medicine* 314(9), Feb 27, 1986, 552–560.

Schillebeeckx, Edward
> 1981a   *Ministry,* New York: Crossroad Publishing Co.
> 1981b   *Christ: The Experience of Jesus as Lord,* New York: Crossroad Publishing Co.

Schindler, Thomas, "Implications of Prolonging Life," *Health Progress,* Apr. 1988, 12.

Schlitz, Randy, *And the Band Played On,* New York: St. Martin's Press, 1987.

Scott, R. T.; Hoffman, G. E.; Veeck, L. L.; Jones, H. W., Jr.; and Muasher, S. J., "Embryo Quality and Pregnancy Rates in Patients Attempting Pregnancy Through *in Vitro* Fertilization," *Fertility & Sterility,* 55(2), February 1991, 426–8.

Schuller, Bruno. *Die Bergrundung Sittlicher Urteile: Typen Ethiscer Argumentation in der Katholischen Moral Theologie,* Dusseldorf: Patmos Verlag, 1973.

Schwartz, Harold; Applebaum, Paul; and Kaplan, Richard, "Clinical Judgments in the Decision to Commit: Psychiatric Discretion and the Law," *Archives of General Psychiatry* 41(8), Aug. 1984, 811–815.

Schwartz, Lee, "Involuntary Admission: A Century of Experience," *Journals of Clinical Psychiatry* 43(1), Jan. 1982, 28–32.

Schwartz, Mark; Moraczewski, Albert; and Monteleone, James, *Sex and Gender; A Theological and Scientific Inquiry,* St. Louis: Pope John XXIII Center, 1983.

Schwartz, Stephen D. *The Moral Question of Abortion* (forthcoming, against Tooley), Chapter 7.

Scott v. Casey, U.S. District Court, Atlanta Division, Apr. 29, 1983.

Scully, Diana, *Men Who Control Women's Health: The Miseducation of Obstetrician-Gynecologists,* Boston: Houghton Mifflin, 1980.

Seibel, M. M., "In Vitro Fertilization Success Rates: A Fraction of the Truth," *Obstetrics & Gynecology* 72(2), August 1988, 265–6.

Senay, Patrick, "Biblical Teaching on Life and Death," in *Moral Responsibility in Prolonging Life Decisions,* Donald McCarthy and Albert Moraczewski, eds., St. Louis: Pope John XXIII Medical-Moral Research and Education Center, 1981.

Seppälä, Markku; and R. G. Edwards, *In Vitro Fertilization and Embryo Transfer,* ed., New York: Annals of the New York Academy of Science, vol. 442, 1985.

Seppälä, Markku; and Lars Hamberger, eds., *Frontiers in Human Reproduction,* New York: Annals of the New York Academy of Science, vol. 626, 1991.

Seratini, Anthony, "Is Coma Morally Equivalent to Anencephaly?" *Ethics and Behavior* 3(2) 1993, 187–198.

Shaffer, Thomas, *Faith and the Professions,* Albany: State University of New York Press, 1987.

Shalom, Albert, *The Body/Mind Conceptual Framework and the Problem of Personal Identity,* Atlantic Highlands, NJ: Humanities Press International, 1985.

Shannon, M. Jordan, *Decision Making for Incompetent Persons: The Law and Morality of Who Shall Decide,* Springfield, IL: Charles C. Thomas, 1985.

Shannon, Thomas A., *Bioethics: Basic Writings on the Key Ethical Questions that Surround the Major Modern Biological Possibilities and Problems,* 3rd ed., Ramsey, NJ: Paulist Press, 1987.

Shannon, Thomas; and Cahill, Lisa Sowle, *Religion and Artificial Reproduction* (New York: Crossroad, 1988).

Shannon, Thomas; and Wolter, Alan, OFM, "Reflections on the Moral Status of the Pre-Embryo.", *Theological Studies,* 51 (1990):603–626.

Shannon, William H., *The Lively Debate: Response to "Humanae Vitae,"* New York: Sheed & Ward, 1970.

Shapiro, Larry, et al., "New Frontiers in Genetic Medicine," *Annals of Internal Medicine* 104 (4), Apr. 1986, 527–539.

Shapiro, Martin F.; and Charron, Robert, "Scientific Misconduct in Investigational Drug Trials," *New England Journal of Medicine* 312(11), Mar. 14, 1984, 731–736.

Shaw, Margery W., MD, JD; and A. Edward Doudera, J.D., eds. *Defining Human Life: Medical, Legal and Ethical Implications,* Ann Arbor, MI: AUPHA Press, published in cooperation with the American Society of Law and Medicine, 1983.

Shea, M.C.
    1985 "Embryonic Life and Human Life," *Journal of Medical Ethics,* 205–209.
    1987 "Embryonic Life and Human Life," *Journal of Medical Ethics,* 11 (1985):205–209.
    1988 Ensoulment and IVF embryos," *Journal of Medical Ethics,* 13 (1987):95–97.

Shell, Susan Meld, *The Rights of Reason: A Study of Kant's Philosophy and Politics,* Toronto: University of Toronto Press, 1979.

Shirm, M.C., et al., "Contraceptive Failure in the United States: The Impact of Social, Economic, and Demographic Factors," *Family Planning Perspective* 14, 1982, 68.

Showalter, Stuart; and Andrew, Brian, *To Treat or Not to Treat,* St. Louis: Catholic Health Association of the United States, 1984.

Sider, Roger C., "Mental Health Norms and Ethical Practice," *Psychiatric Annals* 13 (4), April 1983, 302–309.

Sider, Roger C.; and Clements, Colleen, "Patients' Ethical Obligation for Their Health," *Journal of Medical Ethics* 10(3), Sept. 1984, 138–142.

Siegel, Eric; and Orr, Robert. "Should religiously oriented HEC name members with opposing views," *HEC Forum* 7:6 (November 1995):364–69.

Sieghart, Paul. "Professions and the Conscience of Society," *Journal of Medical Ethics,* Sept., 1985, 117–122.

Siegl, Karolyn; and Tuchel, Peter, "Rational Suicide and the Terminally Ill Cancer Patient," *Omega* 15(3), 1985, 263–269.

Siegler, Mark, *Medical Innovations and Bad Outcomes: Legal, Social and Ethical Responses,* Ann Arbor: Health Administration Press, 1987.

Siegler, Miriam; and Osmond, Humphrey, *Models of Madness, Models of Medicine,* New York: Macmillan, 1974.

Sigerist, Henry E.
   1951   *History of Medicine,* New York: Oxford University Press.
   1960a   "The Special Position of the Sick," in *Henry E. Sigerist on Medicine,* Milton E. Roemer and James M. MacKintosh, eds., New York: MD Publishers, 9–22.
   1960b   "An Outline of the Development of the Hospital," in *Henry E. Sigerist on Medicine,* Milton E. Roemer and James M. MacKintosh, eds., New York: MD Publishers, 319–326.

Silber, Thomas J., "Amniocentesis and Selective Abortion," *Pediatric Annals* 10 (10), Oct. 1981, 397–400.

Silver, George, "Whom Do We Serve?" *Lancet* (1)8476, Feb. 8, 1986, 315–316.

Silver, Jonathan; and Yudofsky, Stuart, "Pyschopharmocology and Electroconvulsive Therapy," in *Textbook on Psychiatry,* John Talbott, et al., ed., Washington, DC: American Psychiatric Association, 1988, 767–841.

Silvers, E. P. "A Psychotherapeutic Approach to Substance Abuse: Preliminary Observations," *American Journal of Drug & Alcohol Abuse* 19:1 (1993) p. 51–64.

Simmons, H. E. et al, *Comprehensive Health Care Reform and Managed Competition,* NEJM 327, 1992, p. 1525–1528.

Simon, Julian, "The Population Distraction," *New York Times,* op. ed., August 2, 1994.

Simon, Robert, "Forensic Psychiatry and the Perturbation of Psychiatrists," *Bulletin of the American Academy of Psychiatry and the Law,* 22(2) 1993, p. 269–277.

Simon, R. I. "Forensic Psychiatry and the Perturbation of Psychiatrists' Attention and Neutrality During Psychotherapy," *Bulletin of the American Academy of Psychiatry and the Law,* 22:2 (1994) p.269–277.

Simon, Yves. *A General Theory of Authority,* Notre Dame, ID: University of Notre Dame Press, 1962.

Simpson, W. "The Influence of Religion on Sexuality: Implications for Sex Therapy," *Bulletin of the Menniger Clinic* 56:4 (Fall 1992) p. 511–23.

Singer, Peter
   1980   *Practical Ethics,* New York: Cambridge University Press.
   1986   "Animals and the Value of Life," in *Matters of Life and Death,* Tom Regan, ed., New York: Random House.

Skinner, B. F.
   1971   *Beyond Freedom and Dignity,* New York: Alfred A. Knopf.
   1976   *About Behaviorism,* New York: Random House.
   1985   *A Matter of Consequences,* New York: University Press.

Smart, R. G., and Murray, G. F., "Narcotic Drug Abuse in 152 Countries: Social and Economic Factors as Predictors," *International Journal of Addiction* 20, 1985, 737–749.

Smith, Janet E.
   1991   *Humanae Vitae: A Generation Later,* Washington, DC: The Catholic University of America Press.
   1995   "A Tangled Web, Part I: The Moral Terminology of *Veritatis Splendor;* II: Does

Veritatis Splendor Misrepresent Proportionalism?" unpublished essays, University of Dallas.

Smith, Martin, "Futile Medical Treatment and Patient Consent," *Cleveland Clinic Journal of Medicine* 60(2), March 1993, p. 151–4.

Smith, Russell, "Ethical Quandaries: Forming Hospital Partnerships," *The Linacre Quarterly* 63(2), May 1996, 87–97.

Smith, William
1977 "Catholic Hospitals and Sterilization," *Linacre Quarterly* 44, 107–116.
1987 "The Question of Dissent in Moral Theology," *Persona Verita e Morale,* Roma: Citta Nuova Edditrice.

Smith-Bell, M; and Winslade, W. J. "Privacy, Confidentiality and Privilege in Psychotherapeutic Relationships," *American Journal of Orthopsychiatry* 64:2 (April 1994) p. 180–193.

Smythies, John, "The Mind/Brain Problem," in *The Case for Dualism,* Smythies, John; and Beloff, John, eds., Charlottesville, VA: University of Virginia Press, 1989, p. 81–112.

Snaith, R.
1994a "Transsexualism and gender reassignment," *British Journal of Psychiatry* 165:3 (September 1994):418–419.
1994b "Psychosurgery: Controversy and Inquiry," *British Journal of Psychiatry* 165:6 (December 1994) p. 842.

Snyder, Solomon. *Drugs and the Brain,* New York: Scientific Books, 1986.

Speroff, L.; Glass, R. H.; and Kase, N. G., *Clinical Gynecologic Endocrinology and Infertility,* 3rd ed., Baltimore: Williams and Wilkins, 1983, 315ff.

Spiro, Howard, *Doctors, Patients, Placebos,* New Haven: Yale University Press, 1986.

Springer, Robert, "Transsexual Surgery: Some Reflections on the Moral Issues," in *Sexuality and Medicine,* vol. 2, E. Shelp, ed., Boston: D. Riedel, 1987.

St. John-Stevas, Norman
1961 *Life, Death and the Law; Law and Christian Morals in England and the United States,* Bloomington, IN: Indiana University Press.
1971 *The Agonizing Choice: Birth Control, Religion and the Law,* Bloomington, IN: Indiana University Press.

Starr, Paul. "Voluntary Health Risks and Public Policy," *Hastings Center Report* 81, Oct. 18, 26–44.

Steinfels, Peter, "Psychiatrist and Pope Discuss End to Longtime Hostility," *New York Times,* January 3, 1994.

Steel, Knight, et al., "Iatrogenic Illness on a General Medical Service at a University Hospital," *New England Journal of Medicine* 304, 1981, 636–642.

Stenchever, Morton, "Rape, Incest, Abortion," in *Comprehensive Gynecology,* William Droegemueller, ed., St. Louis: C.V. Mosby Co., 1987.

Stephens, Rosemary. *In Sickness and in Health,* NY: Basic Books, 1989.

Stevens, Jay, *Storming Heaven: LSD and the American Dream,* New York: Atlantic Monthly Press, 1987.

Stevens, Richard; Gostin, Lawrence. "Security of Personal Information in a New Health Care System," *JAMA* 27:19, (May 18, 1994) p.1484–1485.

Storch, Janet, *Patient's Rights: Ethical and Legal Issues in Health Care and Nursing,* New York: McGraw-Hill, 1982.

Stover, Eric; and Nightengale, Elena, eds., *The Breaking of Bodies and Minds: Torture, Psychiatric Abuse, and The Health Professions,* New York: W.H. Freeman and Co., 1985

Strasburg-Cohen, T., "The Judicial Aspects of Artificial Insemination," *Medicine and Law* I (1), 1982, 71–80.

Strauss, Anselm, ed., *When Medicine Fails,* San Francisco: University of California, 1984.

Strickler, Ronald C.; Keller, P. W.; and Warren, J. C., "Artificial Insemination with Fresh Donor Semen," *New England Journal of Medicine* 289, 1975, 848–852.

Stroebe, Wolfgang; and Stroebe, Margaret. "Stress and health," in *Social Psychology and Health*, Albany, NY: Brooks Cole Publishing 1995, p.171–1226.

Stumpf, David A., et al., "The Infant with Anencephaly," *The New England Journal of Medicine*, 322 (March 8, 1990):669–674.

Suarez, Antoine, "Hydatidiform Moles and Teratomas Confirm the Human Identity of the Preimplantation Embryo," *The Journal of Medicine and Philosophy*, 15 (1990): 627–635.

Sugar, M. "A clinical approach to childhood gender identity disorder," *American Journal of Psychotherapy*, 49:2 (Spring, 1995):260–281.

Sullivan, Francis
    1983   *Magisterium and Teaching Authority in the Catholic Church*, Dublin: Gill and Macmillan.
    1994   "New Claims for the Pope," *The Tablet* 248, June 18, 767–769.

Sullivan, Joseph V., *The Morality of Mercy Killing*, Westminster, MD: Newman Press, 1952.

Summers, Jim, "Take Patients' Rights Seriously to Improve Patient Care and Lower Cost," *Health Care Management Review* 10(4), Fall 1985, 55–62.

Sumner, L. W., *Abortion and Moral Theory*, Princeton, NJ: Princeton University Press, 1981.

Sumner, William Graham, "A Defense of Cultural Relativism," in *Issues in Moral Philosophy*, Thomas Donaldsen, ed., New York: McGraw-Hill, 1986.

SUPPORT Study Investigators, "A controlled trial to improve care for seriously ill hospitalized patients," *JAMA* 274-20 November 22, 1995:1591–1598.

Swift, Francis W., "An Analysis of the American Theological Reaction to Janssens' Stand on 'The Pill'," *Louvain Studies* 1, Fall 1966, 19–53.

Synod of Bishops, "Message for Christian Families," *Origins* 10(21) November 7, 1980, 321–330.

Szasz, Thomas
    1974   *The Myth of Mental Illness*, rev. ed., New York: Harper & Row (orig. pub. 1961).
    1977   *The Theology of Medicine: The Political-Philosophical Foundations of Medical Ethics*, New York: Harper & Row.
    1987   *Insanity, the Idea and Its Consequences*, New York: John Wiley and Sons.

Szasz, Thomas; and Hollender, Marc H., "The Basic Models of the Doctor-Patient Relationship," *American Medical Association Archives of Internal Medicine* 97, 1956, 585–592.

Talbott, John A.; Hales, Richard E.; Yudolfsky, Stuart C., *Textbook of Psychiatry*, Washington, DC: American Psychiatric Press, 1988.

Taragin, Mark, "The Influence of Standard of Care and Severity of Injury on the Resolution of Medical Malpractice Claims," *Annals of Internal Medicine* 117(9) November 1, 1992:780–784.

Tauer, Carol
    1984   "The Tradition of Probabilism and the Moral Status of the Early Embryo," *Theological Studies*, 45, 3–33.
    1985   "Personhood and Human Embryos and Fetuses," *Journal of Medicine and Philosophy* 10(3), Aug., 253–266.

Taylor, Michael Allyn, *Human Generation in the Thought of Thomas Aquinas: A Case Study on the Role of Biological Fact in Theological Science*, Catholic University of America, (diss.) Ann Arbor, MI: University Microfilms Int'l, 1982.

Taysi, Kutay, "*Genetic Disorders*," *Genetic Medicine and Engineering: Ethical and Social Dimensions*, St. Louis: Catholic Health Association of the United States, 1983.

Temkin, Owsei, "The Scientific Approach to Disease: Specific Entity and Individual Sickness," in *Scientific Change*, A.C. Crombie, ed., London: Heinemann, 1963, 629–660.

Tertullian, (d. 240), *Apolgeticum* IX, 8PL, I, 371–372.

Texas Medical Association, *Second Supplemental Report*, Nov. 20, 1987.

Thayer, Nelson, *Spirituality and Pastoral Care*, Philadelphia: Fortress Press, 1985.

Theological Commission (International), *Thesis on the Relationship between the Ecclesiastical Magisterium and Theology*, Washington, DC: U.S. Catholic Conference, 1976.

Thielicke, Helmut
    1964 *The Ethics of Sex*, New York: Harper & Row.
    1969 "Moral Dilemmas," in *Theological Ethics* 2 vols., Philadelphia: Fortress Press, vol. 1, 609–668.
    1983 *Living with Death*, Grand Rapids: Erdmans.

Thomasma, David, "Telling the Truth to Patients, A Clinical Ethics Exploration," *Cambridge Quarterly of Health Care Ethics*, 3(3), 1994, 375–382.

Thompson, James; and Thompson, Margaret, *Genetics in Medicine*, Philadelphia: W.B. Saunders Co., 1980, rev. ed. 1988, 309.

Thompson, Troy, "Psychosomatic Disorders," in *Textbook of Psychiatry*, edited by Talbott, Washington, DC: American Psychiatric Press, 1988, p.493–532.

Thomson, Judith Jarvis,
    1971 "A Defense of Abortion," *Philosophy and Public Affairs*, Fall, 47–66.
    1983 *Ethics and Public Policy: An Introduction to Ethics*, Tom Beauchamp and Terry Pinkard, eds., Englewood Cliffs, NJ: Prentice-Hall, 268–283.

Thorup, Oscar, et al, "High Tech Cardiology—Issues and Costs: A Panel Discussion," *Pharos* 48(3), Summer 1985, 31–37.

Tillich, Paul, *Systematic Theology 2*, Chicago: University of Chicago Press, 1957.

Tooley, Michael, *Abortion and Infanticide*, Oxford: Clarendon Press, 1983.

Torrens, Paul, "Hospice Care: What Have We Learned?" in *Annual Review of Public Health*, Lester Breslow, et al., eds., 1985, Palo Alto: Annual Reviews.

Tranel, Daniel. "Functional Neuroanatomy: Neuropsychological Correlates of Cortical and Subcortical Damage," in Yudofsky, Stuart; and Hales, Robert, eds., *Textbook of Neuropsychiatry*, 2nd edition, DC: American Psychiatric Press, 1992.

Tresolini, Carol, et al., "An Integrated Conceptual Model for Health Professions Practice and Education," Pew Commission Report, 1993.

Truant, G. S.; and Lohrenz, J. G., "Basic Principles of Psychotherapy, Basic Goals and the Therapeutic Relationship," *American Journal of Psychotherapy*, 47(1), Winter, 1993, 8–18.

Ullmann, Manfred, *Islamic Medicine* (Islamic Surveys II), Edinburgh: Edinburgh University Press, 1978.

Ulmann, André; Georges Teutsch; and Daniel Philibert, "RU 486," *Scientific American*, 262, June, 1990, 42–48.

Underwood, Kenneth, *The Church, the University, and Social Policy*, 2 vols., Middletown, CT: Wesleyan University Press, 1972; vol. 1, 422–436.

United Nations, *Universal Declaration of Human Rights*, New York: United Nations Publications, 1948.

Ursano, Robert; and Silberman, Robert, "Individual Psychotherapies," in *Textbook of Psychiatry*, John Talbott; Robert Hales; and Stuart Yudofsky, eds., Washington, DC: American Psychiatric Press, 1988, 855–891.

USCC: United States Catholic Conference
    1969 Rite of Funerals
    1971a *Ethical and Religious Directives for Catholic Health Facilities*, approved by National Conference of Catholic Bishops and the United States Catholic Conference, Nov., as "the national code, subject to the approval of the bishop for use in the diocese," Washington, DC: United States Catholic Conference; n. 12.
    1971b Rite of Baptism for Children
    1976 *To Live in Christ Jesus*, Washington, DC: USCC.
    1979 *The Deacon, Minister of Word and Sacrament*, Washington, DC: United States Catholic Conference.

1981 *Pastoral Letter on Health and Health Care*, Washington, DC: United States Catholic Conference.

1983 "The Challenge of Peace: God's Promise and Our Response," *Origins* 13(1), May 19.

1986 "Economic Justice for All," *Origins* June 5, p. 33 ff.

1987 "The Many Faces of AIDS: A Gospel Response," *Origins* 7(28), Dec. 24, 481 ff.

1988 "Partners in the Mystery of Redemption: A Pastoral Response to Women's Concerns for Church and Society," *Origins* 17(45), Apr. 21, 97.

1993a "Resolution on Health Care," *Origins* 23(7) July 1, p. 97–102.

1993b "Rite of Christian Initiation for Adults," Washington, DC: USCC.

1994 "Ethical and Religious Directives for Catholic Health Services," *Origins* 24(27) December 15, p. 449–462.

1995 "Remarks on the Christian Coalition's Catholic Alliance," *Origins*, 25(25), Dec. 7, 417–430.

U.S. Congress, Senate Committee on Labor and Human Resources, *Organ Transplantation: Examination of Problems Involved in Obtaining Organs for Transplant Surgery*, Washington, DC: U.S. Government Printing Office, May 25, 1984.

U.S. Congress, Office of Technology Assessment, *Infertility: Medical and Social Choices*, Washington, DC: Government Printing Office, May, 1988.

U.S. Department of Health, Education, and Welfare 1973 Commission on Medical Malpractice.

U.S. Select Committee on Aging, U.S. Congress, *Dying with Dignity: Difficult Times, Difficult Choices*, Washington, DC: U.S. Government Printing Office, 1965.

Vacek, Edward, "Vatican Instruction on Reproductive Technology," *Theological Studies* 49(6), March 1988, 11–130.

Valenstein, Elliot, "Therapeutic Exuberance: A Double Edge Sword," in Harrington, Anne, ed., *So Human a Brain: Knowledge and Value in the Neuro Sciences*, Boston: Birkhauser, 1992, 159–178.

Valliant, P. M.; and Antonowicz, R. A., "Cognitive Behavior Therapy and Social Skills Training," *Psychological Reports*, 68(1), February, 1991, 27–33.

Valsecchi, Ambrogio, *Controversy: The Birth Control Debate, 1958–1968*, Washington, DC: Corpus Books, 1968.

Van Blerkom, Jonathan, "Extragenomic Regulation and Autonomous Expression of a Developmental Program in the Early Mammalian Embryo," Seppälä, Markku; and R. G. Edwards, eds., *In Vitro Fertilization and Embryo Transfer*, New York: Annals of the New York Academy of Science, vol. 442, 1985.

Vande Creek, Leon; and Shopland, Susan. "Sex with Ex-clients: Theoretical Rationales for Prohibition," *Ethics and Behavior* 1919; 1(1):35–44. 1991.

Van Delden, Johannes, et al., "The Remmelink Study: Two Years Later," *Hastings Center Report*, 23(6), November, 1993, 24–27.

Van Kaam, Adrian

1983 *Fundamental Formation*, New York: Crossroad Publishing Co.

1985 *Human Formation*, New York: Crossroad Publishing Co.

1986 *Formation of the Human Heart: Formative Spirituality*, New York: Crossroad Publishing Co.

Varga, Andrew

1984 *The Main Issues in Bioethics*, 2nd ed., Mahwah, NJ: Paulist Press, 42, 81.

Vatican Council II

Documents, quotations and citations are from *Vatican II: The Conciliar and Post Conciliar Documents*, Austin Flannery, OP, ed., Collegeville, MN: Liturgical Press, 1975. See also *The Documents of Vatican II*, Walter M. Abbott, SJ, ed., New York: Association Press, 1966.

1964a *Dogmatic Constitution on the Church* (Lumen Gentium), Nov. 21, 350–426.

1964b *Decree on Ecumenism* (Unitatis Redintegratio), Nov. 21, 452–470.

1965a *Declaration on the Relation of the Church to Non-Christian Religious* (Nostra Aetate), Oct. 28, 738–742.

1965b *Declaration on Religious Liberty* (Dignitatis Humanae) Dec. 7, 799–812.

1965c *Pastoral Constitution on the Church in the Modern World* (Guadium et Spes), Dec. 7, 903–1001.

1965d *Decree on the Training of Priests*, October 28, 707–724.

1984 *The Church*, 15–16.

Vaux, Kenneth L., *This Mortal Coil: The Meaning of Health and Disease,* San Francisco: Harper & Row, 1978.

Veatch, Henry, *For an Ontology of Morals: A Critique of Contemporary Ethical Theory,* Evanston, IL: Northwestern University Press, 1971.

Veatch, Robert

1975 "The Whole-Brain-Oriented Concept of Death: An Outmoded Philosophical Formulation," *Journal of Thanatology* 3(1), 13–30.

1981 *A Theory of Medical Ethics,* New York: Basic Books.

1993 "The impending collapse of the whole-brain definition of death," *Hastings Center Report,* 23(4), July-August, 18–24.

Vitz, Paul, *Psychology as Religion: The Cult of Self-Worship* Grand Rapids: Erdmans, 1977 and 2nd edition, 1994.

Viviano, Benedict, *The Kingdom of God in History,* Wilmington, DE: Michael Glazier, Inc., 1988.

Vogel, Morris J., *The Invention of the Modern Hospital: Boston 1870–1930,* Chicago: University of Chicago Press, 1980.

Von Hildebrand, Dietrich, *Marriage: The Mystery of Faithful Love,* Chicago: Franciscan Press, 1984.

Von Hildebrand, Dietrich; and Von Hildebrand, Alice, *The Art of Living,* Chicago: Franciscan Press, 1965.

Wahlberg, Rachel Conrad

1971 "The Woman and the Fetus: 'One Flesh'?" *Christian Century* 88, 1045–1048.

1973 "Abortion: Decisions to Live With," *Christian Century* 90, 1973, 691–693.

Wallace, William A., "Nature and Human Nature as the Norm in Medical Ethics," in *Catholic Perspectives on Medical Morals,* Edmund D. Pellegrino, eds., Boston, MA: Kluwer Academic Publishers, 1989, 23–53.

Waller, Louis, "Secrets Revealed: The Limits of Medical Confidence," *Journal of Contemporary Health Law and Policy,* Spring, 1993, 183–210.

Warnock Report, *Report of Inquiry into Human Fertilization and Embryology: Medical Research Council Response,* London: The Council, 1985.

Warren, J. W. et al., "Informed Consent by Proxy: An Issue in Research with Elderly Patients," *New England Journal of Medicine* 315(18), Oct. 30 1986, 1124–1128.

Washington Post, "Life is precious, even in the lab," *Washington Post,* December 2, 1994.

Wasserstrom, Richard, "The Status of the Fetus," *Hastings Center Report* 5, 1975, 18–22.

Watson, James D., "Moving Toward the Clonal Man: Is This What We Want?" *The Atlantic,* May 1971, 50–53.

Watson, James D., et al., *Molecular Biology of the Gene: General Principles,* Menlo Park, CA: Benjamin-Cummings, 1987.

Webb, William, "Ethics and psychiatry," in *Textbook of Psychiatry,* Washington, DC: American Psychiatric Press, 1988, 1085–1097.

Webster, Richard, *Why Freud Was Wrong,* New York, NY: Harper Collins, 1995.

Weir, Robert; and Gostin, Larry, "Decisions to Abate Life Sustaining Treatment," *JAMA* 264(14) October 10, 1846–1853.

Weiss, S.J., et al., "Risk of Human Immunodeficiency Virus (HIV-1) Infection Among Laboratory Workers," *Science* 239, 1988, 68–71.

Welch, Gilbert; and Larson, Eric, "Dealing with Limited Resources: The Oregon Decision to Curtail Funding for Organ Transplantation," *New England Journal of Medicine* 319(3) July 21, 1988, 171–173.

Welsby, Phillip, "HIV-III Testing Without Consent," *British Medical Journal* 292(652), Apr. 5, 1986.

Wertheimer, Michael, et al., "Ethics and Communication in the Surgeon-Patient Relationship," *Journal of Medical Education* 60(10), Oct. 1985, 4–6.

Wertz, Dorothy
    1992 "Ethical and Legal Implications of the New Genetics: Issues for Discussion," *Social Science and Medicine* 35(4), 495–505.
    1995 "Reproductive Technologies, II, Sex Selection," in Reich, Warren, ed., *Encyclopedia of Bioethics,* revised edition.

Wertz, Dorothy; and Fletcher, John, "Prenatal Diagnosis and Sex Selection in Nineteen Nations," *Social Science and Medicine* 37(11), December 1993, 1359–1366.

White, Andrew Dickson, *A History of the Warfare of Science with Theology in Christendom* 1896, New York: Dover Publications, 1960, vol. 2, 55–63.

White, Gladys, ed., *Ethical Dilemmas in Contemporary Nursing Practice,* Washington, DC: American Nurses Association, 1992.

White, Michelle, "The value of liability in medical malpractice," *Health Affairs,* Fall, 1994, 75–87.

White, R. J. et al., eds., *Working Group on the Determination of Brain Death and Its Relationship to Human Death,* Vatican City: Pontificia Academia Scientierum, 1992.

Whitehead, Alfred North, *Process and Reality* [1929], New York: Free Press, 1957.

WHO: World Health Organization
    1946 Nuremberg Code, *Encyclopedia of Bioethics,* New York: Free Press, vol. 4:1768.
    1957 "Geneva Declaration on Human Research," *Encyclopedia of Bioethics,* New York: Free Press, vol. 4:1768.
    1958 "Constitution" *The First Ten Years of the World Health Organization,* Geneva, WHO, p. 459.
    1964 "Helsinski Statement on Research on Human Subjects," World Health Association: see *Encyclopedia of Bioethics,* New York: Free Press, vol. 4, 1769.
    1974 World Population Conference, Geneva.
    1981 "A Prospective Multicenter Trial of the Ovulation Method of Natural Family Planning: The Teaching Phase," *Fertility and Sterility* 36, 152.
    1984 "A Prospective Multicenter Study of the Ovulation Method of Natural Family Planning, IV: The Outcome of Pregnancy," *Fertility and Sterility* 41, 573.
    1987 "A Prospective Multicenter Trial of the Ovulation Method of Natural Family Planning, V: Psychosexual Aspects," *Fertility and Sterility* 47, 765.

Wicclair, Mark, *Ethics and the Elderly,* NY: Oxford University. Press, 1993.

Wicks, Robert; Parson, Richard; and Capps, Donald, eds., *Clinical Handbook of Pastoral Counseling,* Mahwah, NJ: Paulist Press, 1985.

Wilcox, Allen, et al., "Incidence of Early Loss of Pregnancy," *New England Journal of Medicine* 319(4), July 28, 1988, 189–194.

Wilcox, Allen; Weinberg, Carlice R.; and Baird, Donna D., "Timing of Sexual Intercourse in Relation to Ovulation," *The New England Journal of Medicine,* 333(23), December 7, 1995, 1517–1522. Corroboration by Joe Leigh Simpson, MD, "Pregnancy and the Timing of Intercourse," *ibid.* issue 1563–1565.

Wiley, James, *Power Recover: 12 Steps for a New Generation,* Mahwah, NJ: Paulist Press, 1995.

Williams, Cornelius, "The Hedonism of Aquinas," *Thomist* 38, 1974, 257–290.

Williams, Janet, "Psychiatric Classification" in Talbott, John; Hales, Robert, Yudofsky, *Textbook of Psychiatry,* Washington, DC: American Psychiatric Association, 1988.

Williams, Oliver; and Houck, John, *The Common Good and U.S. Capitalism,* Lanham, MD: University Press of America, 1987.

Williams, Preston, et al., *Ethical Issues in Biology and Medicine*, Rochester, VT: Schenkman, 1973.

Wilson, Edward O., *On Human Nature*, Cambridge, MA: Harvard University Press, 1978.

Wilson, E. O., *Success and Dominance in Ecosystems: The Case of Social Insects*, Oldendorf, Germany: Ecology Institute, 1990.

Wilson, E. O., *The Diversity of Life*, Cambridge, MA: Belhnap, Harvard University, 1992.

Wilson, James, "On abortion," *Commentary*, 97(1), January, 1994, 29–0000

Winslade, William; and Ross, Judith, *Choosing Life or Death: A Guide for Patients, Families, and Professionals*, New York: Free Press, 1986.

Wolinsky, Howard, "Transplants from the Unborn," *American Health*, Apr. 1988.

Wolf, Naomi, "Our Bodies, Our Souls," *The New Republic*, October 16, 1995, 26–35.

Wolpe, Joseph, "The Comparative Clinical Status of Conditioning Theories and Psychoanalysis," in *The Conditioning Therapies: The Challenge of Psychiatry*, Joseph Wolpe, Andrew Slater, and L.J. Reyna, eds., New York: Holt, Rinehart and Winston, 1966, 3–20.

Woodcock, George. *Anarchism, A History of Libertarian Ideas and Movements*, Cleveland, OH: Meridian Books, 1962.

Yamaguchi, K.; and Kandel, D. B., "Patterns of Drug Use From Adolescence to Young Adulthood," *American Journal of Public Health* 74, 1984, 673–680.

Yankelovich, Daniel, "The debate that wasn't: The public and the Clinton plan," *Health Affairs*, Spring, 1995, 7–24.

Younger, Stuart; and Bartlett, Edward, "Human Death and High Technology: The Failure of the Whole Brain Formulation," *Annals of Internal Medicine* 99(2), Aug. 1983, 252–258.

Zalba, M., "Applicato encyclicae 'Humanae Vitae' apudconferentias episcopales," *Periodica de re Morale, Cononica, et Liturgica* 59, 1970, 371–413.

Zaner, Richard, ed., *Death: Beyond Whole-Brain Criteria*, Norwell, CT: Kluwer Academic Publishers, 1988.

Ziegenfuss, James T., *Patients' Rights and Professional Practice*, New York: Van Nostrand Reinhold, 1983.

Zika, S.; and Chamberlain, K., "On the Relation Between Meaning in Life and Psychological Well-being," *International Journal of Group Psychotherapy*, 43(3), July, 1993, 363–76.

Zimmerman, Anthony, SVD, ed., *Natural Family Planning: Nature's Way/God's Way*, Collegeville, MN: De Rance Inc. and Human Life Center, 1981.

Zuger, Abigail; and Miles, Stephen, "Physicians, AIDS and Occupational Risk," *Journal of the American Medical Association* 258(14), Oct. 8, 1987, 1924–1928.

Name Index

AAMC *see* Association of American Medical Colleges

Adler, Mortimer, 141

Advanced Directive: A Christian Perspective, 432

Age of Reason, 146

AHA *see* American Hospital Association

Alcoholics Anonymous, 386

Allport, Gordon, 20

AMA *see* American Medical Association

American Fertility Society, 233

American Hospital Association, 131

American Medical Association (AMA), 86, 104, 105, 110

American Psychiatric Association (APA), 30, 104, 361, 390

APA *see* American Psychiatric Association

Apostolic Constitution on the Sacrament of Anointing the Sick, 448

Aquinas, Thomas, 20, 167, 207, 228, 284

Aristotelian model of the human person, 357

Aristotle, 20, 78, 144, 151, 156, 207, 228, 229, 236

Asclepius, 77

Association of American Medical Colleges (AAMC) Report, 82

Baby M case, 248

Barber, Bernard, 72

Barnlund, Dean, 95

Becker, Ernst, 71

Belmont Report, The, 349

Benthan, Jeremy, 157, 159

Berger, Peter, 29

Berlant, Jeffery Lionel, 76

Bioethics Line, The, 123

Bloom, Alan, 382

Blum, Henrik, 23

Boisen, Anton, 438

Breggin, Peter, 366

Browning, Don, 35

Buddha, 169

Bultmann, Rudolph, 155

Cassell, Eric, 406

Casti Connubii, 274, 275

Catechism of the Catholic Church, 49, 146, 163, 211, 277, 288, 309, 453, 455

Centesimus Annus, 113

Church in the Modern World, The, 275, 280

Clinical Pastoral Education (CPE), 438

Commission for the Protection of Human Subjects of Biomedical & Behavioral Research (CPHS), 120, 121, 131, 337, 350

Commission of Medical Malpractice, 102, 103

Confucius, 169

Congregation for the Doctrine of the Faith (CDF), 453 (*see* bibliography)

Congressional Biomedical Ethics Board, 121

Connery, John, 192

CPHS *see* Commission for the Protection of Human Subjects of Biomedical & Behavioral Research

Cruzan, Nancy Beth; parents: Lester (Joe); Joyce, 87

Curran, Charles E., 160

Declaration of Independence, 143

Declaration on Certain Problems of Sexual Ethics, 277, 309

Declaration on Euthanasia, 413, 420, 427

Declaration on Procured Abortion, 228, 256, 257

Definition of Death Legislation, 403

Descartes, Rene, 35, 144, 239

Dewey, John, 158, 200

Diamond v. Chakrabarty, 323

Didache, 143, 256

Doe v. Bolton, 266

Doms, Herbert, 208

EAB *see* Ethics Advisory Board

Ecclesial Vocation of the Theologian, The, 185

Ellul, Jacques, 46

Encyclopedia of Bioethics, 123

Engel, Frederick, 45

Engelhardt, Jr., H. Tristam, 5, 9

English, Joseph, 393

Enlightenment, 206, 272

ERD *see Ethical and Religious Directives for Catholic Health Services*

Erikson, Erik, 382

Ethical & Religious Directives for Catholic Health Services, (ERD) 59, 66, 132, 134, 186, 262, 312, 339, 430, 435, 437

Ethical and Judicial Council of the AMA, 337

Ethics Advisory Board (EAB), 121

Ethics and Medics, 123

European Common Market, 118

Fletcher, Joseph, 10, 158, 288, 413

Flexner, Abraham, 82

Ford, Amasa, 84

Ford, Norman, 233

Foucault, Michael, 77

Fra Angelico, 52

Francoeur, Robert, 317

Frankena, William, 154

Freidson, Eliot, 29, 48, 76

Freud, Sigmund, 32, 96, 150, 381, 383, 392, 356, 362, 369, 372

Freudian model, 356

Freymann, John Gordon, 75, 76, 77

Fromm, Erich, 382

Fuchs, SJ, Josef, 160, 164

Galen, 78

Geneva Declaration, The, 418

Gilder, George, 15

Glaser, William, 79

Goffman, Erving, 125

Goode, William, 73

Gospel of Life, The, 66, 249, 256, 259, 268, 310, 352, 419, 422, 425, 427

Greely, Andrew, 413

Grisez, Germain, 167

Gustafson, James, 457

Haring, Bernard, 160

Harvard criteria, 402

Harvey, William, 77, 78

Hastings Center Institute of Society, Ethics, and the Life Sciences, 123

Hastings Center Report, 123

Health Affairs, 109

Health Care Ethics USA, 123

Health Insurance Association of America, 110

Heidegger, Martin, 160

Helsinki Statement of the World Health Organization, 346, 418

Hemlock Society, 413

Hippocrates, 26, 42, 78

Hippocratic Oath, 118, 133, 143, 418

Hitler, Adolph, 54

HMO, (Health Maintenance Organization), 111, 373

Hollender, Marc, 89

Human Genome Project, 323

Humanae Vitae, (HV) 276, 277, 278, 279, 280, 281, 285, 286, 287, 303, 308, 309

Humanist Manifesto, 12

Humanist Manifesto II, 13

Hume, David, 144, 149, 150, 153

Huntington's chorea, 330

Husserl, Edmund, 160

HV, *see Humanae Vitae*

Illich, Ivan, 63, 71

Industrial Revolution, 272

Institute for Public Policy and Ethics, 123

Instruction on Infant Baptism, 453

Instruction on Reconciliation and Penance, 451

Instruction on Respect for Human Life, 237, 229, 244, 245, 246, 248, 277

Instruction on the Good of Marriage, 207

Instruction on the Human Family, 277, 281, 288, 310

James, William, 392

Janssens, Louis, 160, 274

JCAHO *see* Joint Commission for Accreditation of Health Care Organizations

Joint Commission for Accreditation of Health Care Organizations (JCAHO), 131, 336

Jones, Bob, 54

Jung, Carl Gustav, 362, 370

Kant, Immanuel, 146, 153, 154, 157, 218, 239

Kauffmann, Christopher, 124

Kelly, David, 159, 166, 179

Kennedy Institute of Ethics, 123

Kesey, Ken, 361

Kevorkian, Jack, 413, 416

Kingdom of God, 14, 115, 116, 117, 168, 170, 200, 201, 254

Knauer, Peter, 99, 160, 414

Kohlberg, Lawrence, 139

Koresh, David, 54

Krishna, 169

Kubler-Ross, Elizabeth, 407

Lain-Entralgo, R., 26

Lederberg, Joshua, 9

Lejeune, Jerome, 52

Locke, John, 15, 144

London, Peter, 369

Lonergan, Bernard, 166

Luckmann, Thomas, 29

Magna Charta, 16

Marcel, Gabriel, 52

Maritain, Jacques, 52
Martelet, Gustave, 279
Marx, Karl, 45, 115
Maslow, Abraham, 4, 18, 20, 358
Masters and Johnson Foundation, 387, 388
May, Rollo, 382
May, William F., 75
McCormick, Richard, 160, 179, 414
Mcguire, Daniel, 414
Mendel, Gregor, 324
Menninger, Karl, 39
Merton, Thomas, 71
Metz, Johannes, 200
Michelangelo, 52
Mill, John Stuart, 158, 159
Moltmann, Jurgen, 200
Monod, Jacques, 182
Moore, G. E., 157
Moses, 383
Muhammad, 169

Nash, George, 116
National Bioethics Advisory Commission, 121
National Conference of Catholic Bishops (NCCB), 289, 290
National Organ Transplant Act, 411
National Reference Center for Bioethics Literature, 123
Natural Family Planning (NFP), 297, 298, 300, 301
Netherlands, 417
Nietzche, Frederich Wilhelm, 15
Nightingale, Florence, 436
Nozick, Robert, 15
Nuremberg Code, 346, 347

Pannenburg, Wolfhart, 200
Pastoral Care of Homosexual Persons, 277, 309
Patient Self Determination Act, 429
Patient's Bill of Rights, 405, 406
PCEMR *see* President's Commission for the Study of Ethical Problems in Medicine and Biomedical and Behavioral Research
Pew Commission, 82, 83
Piaget, Jean, 139
Planned Parenthood, 298
Plato, 6, 35, 116, 144, 228, 413
Pontifical Commission on Peace and Justice, 16
Pontifical Study Commission on Family, Population, and Birth Problems, 275, 156
Pope John Paul II, 16, 113, 162, 168, 183, 209, 276, 309, 310, 331, 393, 419, 451
Pope John XXIII, 113, 275, 286
Pope John XXIII Medical-Moral Research & Education Center, 123
Pope Leo XIII, 113
Pope Paul VI, 16, 113, 305

Pope Pius XII, 331, 425
President's Commission for the Study of Ethical Problems in Medicine and Biomedical and Behavioral Research (PCEMR), 121, 131
Principles of Medical Ethics of the APA, The, 389
Prometheus, 45
Pythagoreans, 228

Quinlan, Karen Ann, 87, 131
Quinn, Archbishop John, 285

Rahner, SJ, Karl, 160, 164, 165
Ramsey, Paul, 75, 94, 152
Rand, Ayn, 15, 157
Rawls, John, 154
Reproductive Biology Research Foundation, 387
Rieff, Philip, 381
Roe v. Wade, 262, 266, 267, 268
Rogers, Carl, 91
Role of Christian Family, The, 297, 309
Rousseau, Jean Jacques, 150, 152

Sartre, Jean Paul, 155
Scheler, Max, 160
Schuller, SJ, Bruno, 160
Scotus, Duns, 228
Second Vatican Council, 11, 13 46, 51, 113, 114, 116, 131, 146, 160, 166, 178, 256, 257, 264, 275, 280, 297, 298, 438 441
sensus fidei, 285
sensus fidelium, 285
Sigerist, Henry, 41, 124
Skinner, B. F. 372, 374
Smith, Adam, 116
Splendor of Truth, The, 49, 53, 146, 163, 164, 165, 168, 183, 276, 420
St. Augustine, 207
St. Catherine of Siena, 52
St. Teresa of Avila, 52
Stalin, Joseph, 54
SUPPORT Study, 462
Synod of Bishops, 310
Szasz, Thomas, 30, 89, 361

Tarasoff v. Regents of University of California, 100
Teilhard de Chardin, Pierre, 52
Temkin, Owsell, 26
Tertullian, 232

Ulpian, 156
Underwood, Kenneth, 72
Uniform Anatomical Gift Act, 410

United Nations, 297
Universal Declaration of Human Rights, 16, 17, 20, 114
Universal Declaration of Human Rights, 177, 182, 238

Veatch, Henry, 174
Vesalius, Andreas, 77

von Bertalanffy, Ludwig, 24, 29
von Hildebrand, Dietrich, 160, 209
Von Hildebrand, Alice, 209

Warnock Committee, 346
Whitehead, Alfred North, 230
Wilson, E. O., 4
World Health Organization, (WHO) 301, 346

Subject Index

abortion, 50, 227, 252, 312; induced, 253, 255; procured, 253; indirect 253, 254
abortion counselors, 460
abortion in a pluralistic society, 264
abortion, objective morality of, 257
abortion, subjective morality of, 257
abreaction, 357
absolute autonomy of the individual, 416
academic freedom, 52
acceptance of the human condition, 427
Acquired Immunodeficiency Syndrome *see* AIDS
act utilitarianism, 158
action therapy, 369, 370, 371, 379
addiction, 384
addictions and phobias, 204
advance directives, 132, 429
affirmation of life, 40
Age of Darwin, 77
Age of Pasteur, 77
aging, 27
agnostic world view, 12
AID *see* artificial insemination, donor
AIDS, 102, 399
AIDS epidemic, 296
AIDS patients, 102
AIDS patients, ethical & legal responsibilities to care for, 74
AIDS physicians and patients, 73
AIDS testing for, 61
AIH *see* artificial insemination, husband
alcoholism, 36, 360, 376, 386, 398
allocation of organs for transplantation, 334
allocation of resources, 112
amniocentesis, 248, 324, 328
anencephalic infants, 86, 236, 337
angelism, 35
animals, knowledge of, 239
anointing the sick, 448, 455; with oil, 449; meaning of this rite, 449; communal nature of, 449
anovulants, 274
antifertility drugs, 305
apnea, 403
artificial insemination, 241, 242, 244, 321; by husband, 242; by donor, 242

artificial nutrition and hydration, 421
artificial nutrition and hydration for patients in a persistent vegetative state (PVS), 426
artificial reproduction, 227
assisted suicide, 39, 411
autoeroticism, 389
automatization of behavior, 371
autonomous person, 373
autonomy, 105, 153
autopsy, 409

baptism, 452; infant, 452
baptism of desire, 453
basic biological drives, 32
basic health care, 110
basic human needs, 18
basic rights, 143
behavior control, 376, 377, 378
behavior control programs, 379
behaviorism, 374
behavioristic therapy, 374
benefit of earthly life, 426
biological and psychological needs, 19
biological determinism, 4
biological dimension, 18, 19
biological health, 31, 38
biologism, 31, 165, 278
blind submission to God's will, 152
bodily resurrection, 408
brain-death criteria, 337, 402

capitalism, 13
capitalism, criticism of 113
capitation, 111
care for the corpse, 407
casuistry, 164
Catholic health care facilities, identity of 134
Catholic social thought, 118
cerebration, 236
certitude in ethical decision, 56
chaplain, character, 443
chemical dependency, 100, 384, 386
choose the lesser evil, 58

chorionic villi sampling, 324
Christian burial, 409
Christian discernment, 460
Christian ethics, 177
Christian humanism, 144
Christian morality, 459
Christian physician, 79
Christian politics, 14
Christian social teaching, 113
Christian spirituality, 456
Christian understanding of marital sexuality, 210
Church teaching, views of theologians, 461; pastoral experience, 461
circumstances or other intentions, 161
clinical signs for determining human death, 401
Clinical Pastoral Education (CPE), 438, 447
codependency, 380
cognitive therapy, 370, 371, 390
coitus interruptus, 296
commensurate reason, 414
common decency, 150
common good, 113, 114, 218
common good and community, 334
common morality, principles of, 148, 154, 222
Communism, 217
community, 8, 9, 16
community of the Father, Son, and Holy Spirit, 9
computerization of health records, 101
conception, 232, 252
conception, responsible regulation of, 271
confession, 100
confession to a layman, 455
confidentiality, 99
conscience of Christian community, 460
consequentialism, 134, 146, 158, 170, 176
consumer discipline, 105
contemplation, 203
contraception, 203, 271, 272, 287, 312
contraceptives, oral, 295
contrition, 451
conversion, 451, 452
cooperation, formal and material; immediate and mediate; proximate or remote, 195-199
cooperation in creation, 318
corporatism, 117
counseling, 443
counseling contract, 443
counseling relationship, 89
countertransference, 92
covenant, 75, 94
CPE, *see* Clinical Pastoral Education
creative needs, 20
cremation, 409
crisis counseling, 407
criteria for biological health, 37
cultural needs, 19
cultural relativism, 141, 238
custom, 153

D and C *see* dilation and curettage
dangers of a closed social system, 362
death, 397
death is imminent, 422, 423
death with dignity, 417
defining death, 400
definition of Death Legislation, 403
delayed hominization, 228, 238
denying death, 397
deontological, 145
deontological and teleological, difference between, 146
deontological ethics, 145, 147, 156
deontologism, 176
deontologist, 153
depersonalization, 70
determinants of morality, 188
development of doctrine, 184
deviant sexuality, 387, 389
die with dignity, 412
dignity of the human body, 407
dignity of the human person, 136
dilation and curettage (D & C), 304
direct killing, 421
disease, 25, 26
dissent from church teaching, 184, 290
divorce among health care professionals, 398
DNA recombination, 249
DNA splicing, 120
double-blind research, 348
doubts of conscience, 57
drug-induced coma, 402
dualism, 32, 37
dumping, 127
durable power of attorney, 418
duress, 197, 294
duty ethics, 146
dying process, 400
dysfunctions of the central nervous system, 34

ecclesia semper reformanda, (the Church needs constant renewal), 440
ecology, 323
ECT *see* electroencephalogram
ectopic pregnancy, 253
ecumenical method, 457
education, 369
EEG, 403
ego, 356
egoism, 157, 158
electro encephalogram, 493
electroconvulsive therapy (ECT), 364, 365, 377
embodied intelligent freedom, 5, 8, 173, 175
emergency care, 128
emotivism, 144, 150, 151, 154, 176
emotivist reduction of moral statements, 150
Enlightenment, 77, 79, 143, 144
Enlightenment humanism, 124
ensoulment, 228

enzyme immunoassays, 300
equal personal dignity and inequalities in abilities, 216
escalation of health care costs, 109
essentialism, 180
ethical counseling, 456, 457; goal of, 457
ethical counselors, final task, 462
ethical judgments, 47
ethical methodologies, utilitarianism; Kantianism; liberal individualism; communitarianism; ethics of care; casuistry; 148-161
ethical principle, definition, 179
ethical problems in treating mentally ill, 376
ethical standards for professionals, 389
ethics committees, 131
ethics of relationality and responsibility, 147
eucharist, 452, 454
eugenics, negative, 250
European Common Market, 118
euthanasia, 411, 422, 430; passive, 417; active, 417
evolution of the human species, 4
evolution, theory of, 29
evolutionary process of natural selection, 142
exceptionless norms, 147
existentialism, 155
expense, pain, spiritual and social burden, 428
experimental research, 345
experimentation and research on human subjects, 344

faith and reason, harmony between, 140
family limitation, 302
Fascism, 265
fear of death, 397
fee-for-service, 111
fetal testing, 227
fetishism, 389
for-profit corporation, 112
formal cooperation, 198
formalism, 144, 153, 154
forming a prudent conscious, 47
fortitude, 204
four basic needs of human persons, 222
fraternal correction, 106
French Revolution, 79
friendship with God, 168
frontal lobes, 5
frontal lobotomy, 377
functionalism, 116, 117, 118
fundamental human right, 108
fundamental option, 187

gamete intrafallopian tube transfer (GIFT), 244
gender dysphoria syndrome, 342; primary, 343; secondary, 343
gender identity, 342
gender role, 342

general practitioner, 128
generation, aspects of the act of 244
genetic engineering, 45, 120, 316, 317
genetic intervention, 316, 320, 321
genetic manipulation, 319
genetic physiological defects, 359
genetic screening and counseling, 323, 324, 327, 331
genotype, 317, 322
germ-line intervention, 319
GIFT see gamete intrafallopian transfer
good moral decision, 47
group therapy, 375
guidance and reconciliation, 436

healing ministry, 135
health, 22, 23, 24, 25, 36
health and disease, 29, 30
health as optimal functioning, 25
health care counseling, 74
health care ethics, 16
health care ethics and public policy, 120
health care fees, 95
health care ministry, first task of, 439
health care power of attorney statute, 429
health care profession, 69
health care team, 127
health management organization (HMO), 111, 373
heterologous artificial insemination (AID), 242, 245
heteronomy, 153
heterosexuality, 391
heterozygous twins, 234
higher brain centers function, 5
HMO see health management organization
holism, 27
homeostasis, 26, 66
homologous artificial insemination (AIH), 242
homophobia, 390, 391
homosexual orientation, 390
homosexuality, 342
hospital in Western culture, 436
hospitals, 124
human being, 4, 20, 23
human bodily contact as a sign of spiritual presence 448
human brain, 45
human dominion over nature, 317
human health, 3, 7
human life, beginning, 227
human life, goal of, 170
human nature, 4, 140, 180
human nature, common sense understanding, 141
human needs and values, 17
human person, definition of, 4
human person, legal definition, 265
human personhood, 7

human rights of mental patients, 364
human sexuality, 205
human species, 6
human value, 18
humanism, 12, 169, 201, 222, 265, 268, 285, 437
humanist point of view, 436
humanist spiritual care department, 437
humanists, 207
humility, 181
hydatidiform moles, 229
hypothermia, 402

ICSI *see* intracytoplasmic sperm injection
idealism, 239
identical twinning, 235
illness, 26
image and likeness of God, 152
imaginary sickness, 39
immediate material cooperation, 194, 197
implicit consent, 350
implicit formal cooperation, 194
impotency, 387
in vitro fertilization, 121, 185, 321, 244
in vitro fertilization with embryo transfer (IVF-ET), 243
Incarnation, 221
incommensurable moral values, 164
independent physicians' associations (IPA), 110
indicators of humanhood, 10
individualism, 13; and collectivism, 14; and human rights, 15
ineffective medical means, 426
infants who are in danger of death, 452
infants with birth defects, 427
infertility, 240
informed consent, 47, 59, 64, 92, 132, 349, 352
infusion of the spiritual soul, 235
insight therapy, 369, 370, 371, 372, 374, 382
institutional review board (IRB), 347
integral human fulfillment, 169
integrated delivery systems, 112
integrity, anatomical, 333
integrity, functional, 333
intelligent freedom, 16
intention, 190
intention of the object, 166
interface of the ethical and the spiritual, 362
interpersonal communication, 388
intracytoplasmic sperm injection (ICSI), 243
intrastaff problems, 440
intrauterine device, 296
intrauterine diaphragm, 296
intrauterine douche, 305
intrauterine insemination (IUI), 243
intravenous feeding, 220
intrinsically evil, (*malum per se*), 161
intrinsically evil acts, 163
intuitionist ethics, 157

IPA *see* independent physicians' associations
is and the ought, 146

Jesus as model of personalism, 168
Jesus' moral teaching and the Church, 184
joint ventures, 197
just wage, 133
justice, 181

labor unions, 118
laissez faire capitalism, 15, 116
law and ethics, 144
law of Christ, 171
law of gradualness, 310
laws and customs, 153
laxism, 156
lay ministers, 455
legalism, 152, 153
lesser evil, 193
letting die decisions for incompetent persons, 429
liberal welfare state, 217
liberation theologians, 13
libertarianism, 157
lifestyle, 42
limbo, 453
linear salpingostomy, 253
listening, 97
living human embryos, 351
living will, 418
living will statute, 429
logic of bioethical decisions, preconventional phase; conventional phase; postconventional phase, 139
logical link between is and ought, 141
long-term care centers, 124
low tubal ovum transfer (LTOT), 243
LSD *see* lysergic acid diethylamide
LTOT *see* low tubal ovum transfer
lying, 99
lysergic acid diethylamide (LSD), 367

male infertility, 241
malpractice, 103
managed care, 63, 71, 76, 98, 103, 104, 109, 110, 129
managed health care systems, 197
marital therapy, 387
Marxism, 13, 265
masturbation, 389
material cooperation in sterilization, 293
mature personality, 373
mechanistic theory, 28, 37
mediate material cooperation, 194, 195
medical education, 81
medical fees, 97
medical model, 93

medical procedures, 421
medical profession, autonomy, 76; ideals, 77;
    personalistic concept, 77
medical profession in the United States, 82
medical schools; biases, 84
medieval professions, 69
mental health, 34
mental health and mental illness, 355
mental illness, 361
mental illness, genetic basis for some, 363
mental illness, reality of, 363
mercy killing, 417
methotrexate, 253
ministry to the hospital staff, 440
miscarriages, 235
mixed form of ethics, 147
models of therapeutic relationships, 90
modern medical center, 124
modifying the human body, 316
moral agents, 6
moral certitude; two different levels, 58
moral dualism, 164
moral methodologies, evaluation of, 172
moral norms; rational and revealed, 48
moral object, 166
moral object or the purpose of the human
    action, 189
moral objectivity, 47
moral purism, 191
moral relativism, 133, 153
moral sensitivity, 151
moral theology; revision of, 50
morality, 153
morality of suicide, 412
mortal and venial sin, 188
mystery of death, 394

national health care program, 108, 119
natural cycle oocyte retrieval intravaginal fertili-
    zation (NORIF), 243
natural family planning, 284
natural law, 284
natural law ethics, 141, 142, 156
natural law morality, 141
natural law theories, 140
natural methods of delivery and breast-feeding,
    314
natural needs, 20
natural reproduction, 242
nature, 28
nature religions, 12
needs of human persons, 17
negative eugenics, 326
neurotic anxiety, 371
neurotic guilt, 363
neurotic persons, 375
nontherapeutic research, 346
normal or comfort care, 427
normal person, 375

norms of Christian decision making, 177
norms of Christian faith and prudence, 181
norms of Christian hope, 200
norms of Christian love, 213
nurse's proper role, 129
nursing, 76, 83, 125

objective morality, 458
objective sinfulness of an act and the subjective
    guilt, 188
objective truth, 47
ontological concept of disease, 26
open system, 24
operant conditioning, 370, 378
ordinary and extraordinary means to prolong
    life, 420, 425
ordinary and universal magisterium, 184
ordinary teaching of the magisterium, 186
organ donation, 410
orgasmic dysfunction, 387
ought from is, 149
ovulation or Billings method, 299

pain, not of itself a moral evil, 430
paradigms, 86
paraphilias, 389
parental responsibility, 142
partial brain death, 404
passive potentiality, 231
pastoral approach, 307
pastoral care, 130
pastoral care, appointment to the staff, 437
pastoral care, department of, 436
pastoral care, director of team, 437
pastoral care, ethical dimension, 456
pastoral care, history of, 435
pastoral care personnel, 438
pastoral care, responsibility of department in
    medical-moral decisions, 457
pastoral care, spiritual task of, 447
pastoral gradualness, 309
pastoral ministry and the health care team, 435
pastoral ministry in health care, 433
paternalism, 105
patient advocate, 127
patient's representative, 405
patient's rights, 62, 102
peacemaking as a ministerial function, 441
pedophilia, 389, 390
peer relationship and professional discipline,
    102, 103, 105
pelvic inflammatory disease (PID), 296
perplexed conscience, 57
persistent vegatative state; persistent cognitive-
    affective deprivation, 421
person, 5, 20
person and community, 8, 21
person as conscious, intelligent, free adult, 240

personal biography, 6
personal responsibility, 107
personal responsibility for health, 38
personality, 5, 7
personalized sexuality, 240
personhood, 20, 237, 239
pharmacotherapy, 364, 366
phenotype, 317, 322
physical health, 439
physicalism, 33, 165, 278,
physician as charismatic character, 80
physician as priest, 78
physician-assisted suicide, 416
physiological addiction, 384, 385
physiological concept of disease, 26
politics of health care, 14
population control, 298
population explosion, 286, 297
positivism, 152, 153
postcoital douche, 286
pragmatism, 133, 158
prefrontal lobotomy, 365
premature ejaculation, 387
premoral values, ontic, 160
presumed consent, 350
preventive medicine, 42, 119, 324
primary care, 93, 129, 130
primary care gatekeepers, 111
principalism, 180
principle of double effect, 191, 192, 291, 305,
     347, 421, 425
principle of family-oriented sexuality, 201, 212,
     276
principle of free and informed consent, 186, 346
principle of growth through suffering, 201, 212
principle of human dignity in community, 60,
     214, 215, 377, 346
principle of inner freedom, 201, 203, 301
principle of inseparability of the unitive and
     procreative meanings of marriage, 212
principle of legitimate cooperation, 193, 198, 412
principle of love, or charity, 332
principle of moral discernment, 190
principle of moral discrimination, 187
principle of participation, 114, 216, 218, 219,
     264, 297
principle of participation or subsidiarity, 214
principle of personalized sexuality, 204, 273,
     286, 288, 389
principle of professional communication, 199,
     378, 405
principle of proportionate reason, 190
principle of stewardship, 44, 46, 66
principle of stewardship and creativity, 297,
     201, 202, 207, 281, 283, 319, 322, 416
principle of subsidiarity, 117
principle of totality and integrity, 214, 219, 220,
     288, 290, 291, 332, 334, 340, 343, 346, 347
principle of well-formed conscience, 182, 285,
     346

principles of ethics, 380
principles of research on human subjects, 346
pro-choice, 285
pro-choice position, 261
pro-choice views, 150
pro-life, 285
pro-life movement, 267
production of clones, 317
profession; personalistic concept, 71
professional autonomy, 113
professional communication, 97
professional freedom in health care institutions,
     126
professional-patient relationships, 89
professions; depersonalizing trends, 69
profit, 96
progesterone, 274
pronuclear stage tubal transfer (PROST), 243
proportionalism, 133, 159, 160, 172, 188, 276, 278
proportionalism, and magisterium, 162
proportionalists, 414
proportionate and disproportionate, 420
PROST *see* pronuclear stage tubal transfer
protection of rights, 64
proxy consent, 349, 350, 378
prudence, 169, 187
prudence in moral decisions, 58
prudential personalism, 137, 166, 169, 175, 171,
     190
psychoactive drugs, 377, 378
psychoanalytical model, 91
psychological and social activities, 20
psychological coping mechanisms, 384
psychological dependency, 385
psychological experimentation, 345, 352
psychologism, 35
psychopharmacology, 366
psychosexual development, 390
psychosurgery, 364, 365, 377
psychotherapeutic counseling, 359
psychotherapeutic means of therapy, 369
psychotherapeutic methods, 369
psychotherapy, 364, 372, 375, 378
psychotic persons, 375
psychotropic drugs, 367
public policy, 48
punishment, 378
Puritan and Victorian morality, 40
PVS *see* persistent vegetative state

quality of care, 63
quality of life, 422
Quietism, 158

radical healing, 135
radical individualism, 15
randomized clinical trial, 348
rape, prevention of conception, 303

rape victims, 302
ratification of life, 397
rational animal, 7
recombinant DNA, 317, 323, 324
reductionism, 24, 36, 81
relationship of needs, 19
relativism, 134
religion, 362
religious legalism, 151
religious submission of will and intellect, 55, 185
religious versus natural law ethics, 140
removal of life support, 132
Renaissance, 79, 124
reproductive technologies, 240
research, 351
research and human sexuality, 354
research and therapy, 345
research with fetal tissue, 338
rhythm method, 274, 298
right to dissent, 52, 56, 185
rights of patients, 126, 428
rigorism, 156, 191
Rite of Penance, 452
role of the laity, 50
role of the magisterium, 53
role of theologians, 52
rule utilitarianism, 159

Sacrament of Anointing, doubtfully alive, 450
Sacrament of Reconciliation, 451
sadomasochism, 389
sale of organs, 411
scandal, 195, 196, 292, 294
schools of psychiatry, 365
screening for genetic defect, 325
secular humanism, 79, 116, 118, 134, 143, 144
secular humanist system, 415
secularization, 12
secularization of the universities, 52
self-control, 374
self-fulfillment, 16
self-realization, 175
self-righteousness, 152
sensus fidei, 51
sensus fidelium, 51
sentimentalism, 154
Sermon on the Mount, 179
sex therapy, 387, 389
sexual dysfunction, 387, 388, 389
sexual orientation, 390
sexual reassignment, 340
sexual research, 391, 392
sexual revolution and the crisis of the family, 206
sexual therapy, 392
sexuality, 204
shock therapy, 366

sickness, 26
single payer system, 109
situationism, 158, 176
social dimension, 18
social organization of health care, 117
social responsibility for health care, 115
social teaching, 13
socialism, 201, 217
socialism, criticism of 113
socialized medicine, 108
solidarity of a community, 117
somatic cell intervention, 319
spiritual counseling, 456
spiritual counseling differs from psychological counseling, 442
spiritual counseling in health care, 442
spiritual death, 42
spiritual guidance, 456
spiritual health, 37
spiritual or creative activities, 20
spiritual or creative dimension, 18
spiritual purpose of life, 425
spiritual suicide, 42
spirituality, 362
staff relationships, 126
state licensing boards, 104
sterilization, 287, 312
sterilization and hospital policy, 291
sterilization, involuntary, 289
stewardship, 144
stipend for professionals, 97
subjective morality, 458
subsidiarity, 115, 118, 217
substituted judgment or best interest of the patient, 429
suicide, 39, 92, 100, 101, 398, 413
suicide as intrinsically immoral, 415
surgical reconstruction, 316
surrogate motherhood, 247
sympto-thermal method, 299
syngamy, 232, 235
syngamy and implantation, 232

team effectiveness, 131
technological imperative, 317
teleological (means-ends) methodologies, 156
teleological ethics, 145, 156
teleologists, 145
teleology and natural law, 156
temperance, 181
terminal disease, 422
theology of compromise, 57
theonomy, 153
theory of personhood, 9
therapeutic man, 382
therapeutic research, 345
therapy and punishment and rehabilitation, 361
Thomistic revival, 146

to live in Christ Jesus, 168
total brain death, 404
totalitarianism, 220
tradition of Church teaching on sex, 207
transference, 380
transformation of suffering and death, 399
transplantation, financing, 335
transplantation, organ, 331
transplantation, supply of organs, 336
transplants from living donors, 332
transsexual surgery, 341, 342
transsexualism, 341, 342
transvestism, 342, 389
traumatic aspect of being sick, 126
trophoblast, 233
trust, 442, 443
trust between a spiritual guide and the spiri-
    tual pilgrim, 443
trust, professional-patient, 94
trusteeship, 75
truth telling, 97
truth telling to the dying, 405
tubal ligation, 289
twinning, 232, 234
two concepts of disease, 26
types of ethics, 48

ultimate end, 187
unitive and procreative, 244
universal access to health care, 109

unregulated capitalism or free enterprise, 117
utilitarianism, 144, 157, 158, 170, 176

vaginal douche, 305
vaginismus, 387
value system, 144
vasectomy, 288, 289
venereal disease, 101
Viaticum, reception of, 450
vicarious consent, 349, 350
virtues, development of, 146
virtues of temperance, 204
virtuous person, 373
voluntarism, 156
voluntarist legalism, 160
voluntarists, 145
voyeurism, 389

WHO definition of human health, 36
WHO, World Health Organization, 3, 25
will to life and health, 39

xenodochia, 124

zoophilia, 389
zygote, 232
zygote intrafallopian tube transfer (ZIFT), 243